362.196 P974f

Psychiatric aspects of
HIV/AIDS

D1805505

PSYCHIATRIC ASPECTS OF HIV/AIDS

PSYCHIATRIC ASPECTS OF HIV/AIDS

Francisco Fernandez, M.D.
Professor and Chairperson
Department of Psychiatry and Behavioral Medicine
Director, Institute for Research in Psychiatry
University of South Florida College of Medicine
Tampa, Florida

Pedro Ruiz, M.D.
Professor and Vice Chair
Department of Psychiatry and Behavioral Sciences
The University of Texas Medical School
Houston, Texas

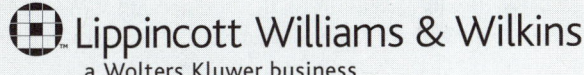

a Wolters Kluwer business
Philadelphia · Baltimore · New York · London
Buenos Aires · Hong Kong · Sydney · Tokyo

Executive Editor: Charles W. Mitchell
Senior Managing Editor: Lisa R. Kairis
Project Manager: Bridgett Dougherty
Manufacturing Manager: Kathleen Brown
Associate Director of Marketing: Adam Glazer
Design Coordinator: Terry Mallon
Production Services: GGS Book Services
Printer: Edwards Brothers, Inc.

© 2006 by LIPPINCOTT WILLIAMS & WILKINS
530 Walnut Street
Philadelphia, PA 19106 USA
LWW.com

All rights reserved. This book is protected by copyright. No part of this book may be reproduced in any form by any means, including photocopying, or utilized by any information storage and retrieval system without written permission from the copyright owner, except for brief quotations embodied in critical articles and reviews. Materials appearing in this book prepared by individuals as part of their official duties as U.S. government employees are not covered by the above-mentioned copyright.
Printed in the USA

Library of Congress Cataloging-in-Publication Data

Psychiatric aspects of HIV/AIDS / [edited by] Francisco Fernandez, Pedro Ruiz.
   p.; cm.
  Includes bibliographical references and index.
  ISBN 1-58255-713-6
  1. AIDS (Disease)—Psychological aspects. 2. HIV infections—Psychological aspects. I. Fernandez, Francisco, 1951- II. Ruiz, Pedro, 1936- III. Title.
  [DNLM: 1. HIV Infections—psychology. 2. HIV Infections—complications. 3. Mental Disorders—complications. WC 503.7 P972 2006]
RA643.83.P759 2006
362.196'9792—dc22

                                                                               2005037604

Care has been taken to confirm the accuracy of the information presented and to describe generally accepted practices. However, the authors, editors, and publisher are not responsible for errors or omissions or for any consequences from application of the information in this book and make no warranty, expressed or implied, with respect to the currency, completeness, or accuracy of the contents of the publication. Application of the information in a particular situation remains the professional responsibility of the practitioner.

    The authors, editors, and publisher have exerted every effort to ensure that drug selection and dosage set forth in this text are in accordance with current recommendations and practice at the time of publication. However, in view of ongoing research, changes in government regulations, and the constant flow of information relating to drug therapy and drug reactions, the reader is urged to check the package insert for each drug for any change in indications and dosage and for added warnings and precautions. This is particularly important when the recommended agent is a new or infrequently employed drug.

    Some drugs and medical devices presented in the publication have Food and Drug Administration (FDA) clearance for limited use in restricted research settings. It is the responsibility of the health care provider to ascertain the FDA status of each drug or device planned for use in their clinical practice.

To purchase additional copies of this book, call our customer service department at (800) 638-3030 or fax orders to (301) 824-7390. International customers should call (301) 714-2324.

Visit Lippincott Williams & Wilkins on the Internet: at LWW.com. Lippincott Williams & Wilkins customer service representatives are available from 8:30 am to 6 pm, EST.

                                                                              10 9 8 7 6 5 4 3 2 1

To our loving wives, Susan P. Fernandez and Angela Ruiz, we thank you for your generous support and understanding always. To our children, Francis Paul and Joseph Richard Fernandez, along with Angela Maria Ruiz Holguin and Pedro Pablo Ruiz whose loving spirits helped us collectively to achieve our goals by more than we had hoped for. Also, to Francisco Antonio Ruiz and Pedro Pablo Ruiz, Jr. as well as Omar Josef Holguin, III, whose smiles were inspiring in this project. Finally, to our patients, who live courageously with HIV and to those who have died from AIDS. We honor the memory of all the beauty that those who live with and die from HIV/AIDS leave in this world for all to enjoy.

Contributors

Jeffrey S. Akman, M.D.
Leon M. Yochelson Professor & Chair
Department of Psychiatry & Behavioral Sciences
George Washington University School of Medicine
Washington, District of Columbia

Margarita Alegría, Ph.D.
Professor of Psychiatry, Department of Psychiatry
Harvard Medical School—Cambridge Health Alliance
Cambridge, Massachusetts
Center for Multicultural Mental Health Research
Cambridge Health Alliance
Somerville, Massachusetts

Kenneth B. Ashley, M.D.
Assistant Professor
Department of Psychiatry & Behavioral Sciences
Albert Einstein College of Medicine
Bronx, New York
Assistant Attending Physician
Department of Psychiatry
Beth Israel Medical Center
New York, New York

Steven L. Batki, M.D.
Professor and Director of Research
Department of Psychiatry
State University of New York Upstate Medical University
Director, VA Center for Integrated Healthcare
VA Medical Center
Syracuse, New York

Janette Beals, Ph.D.
Associate Professor
Department of Psychiatry, School of Medicine
University of Colorado at Denver and Health Sciences Center
Denver, Colorado

Philip A. Bialer, M.D.
Associate Professor of Clinical Psychiatry
Department of Psychiatry
Albert Einstein College of Medicine
Bronx, New York
Chief, Consultation-Liaison Psychiatry and Psychosomatic Medicine
Department of Psychiatry
Beth Israel Medical Center
New York, New York

William Breitbart, M.D.
Professor of Clinical Psychiatry
Department of Psychiatry
Weill Medical College of Cornell University
Chief, Psychiatry Service
Attending Psychiatrist
Department of Psychiatry & Behavioral Sciences
Memorial Sloan-Kettering Cancer Center
New York, New York

Glenn Catalano, M.D.
Professor & Director of Medical Student Education
Department of Psychiatry & Behavioral Medicine
University of South Florida
Medical Director
Department of Psychiatry
Tampa General Hospital
Tampa, Florida

Tiffany Chenneville, Ph.D.
Clinical Assistant Professor
Department of Psychological and Social Foundations
University of South Florida
Tampa, Florida

Mary Ann Cohen, M.D.
Clinical Professor of Psychiatry
Department of Psychiatry
Mount Sinai School of Medicine
Director of AIDS Psychiatry
Department of Psychiatry
Mount Sinai Medical Center
New York, New York

Francine Cournos, M.D.
Professor of Clinical Psychiatry
Department of Psychiatry

Columbia University
Deputy Director
New York State Psychiatric Institute
New York, New York

Karina D'Souza, B.S.
Research Assistant
Division of Infectious Diseases and Internal Medicine
University of South Florida
Tampa, Florida

Nabila El-Bassel, D.S.W.
Professor/Director
Social Intervention Group
Columbia University
School of Social Work
New York, New York

Mark Evans, M.S.W., LCSW
Senior Research Coordinator
Department of Behavioral Science
The University of Texas M.D. Anderson Cancer Center
Houston, Texas

Jacqueline Maus Feldman, M.D.
Patrick H. Linton Professor
Department of Psychiatry and Behavioral Neurobiology
University of Alabama at Birmingham
Birmingham, Alabama

Francisco Fernandez, M.D.
Professor and Chairperson
Department of Psychiatry and Behavioral Medicine
Director, Institute for Research in Psychiatry
University of South Florida College of Medicine
Tampa, Florida

Stephen J. Ferrando, M.D.
Professor of Clinical Psychiatry
Department of Psychiatry
Weill Medical College of Cornell University
Vice Chair for Psychosomatic Medicine
Department of Psychiatry
New York-Presbyterian Hospital
New York, New York

Howard Field, M.D.
Clinical Professor, Department of Psychiatry and Human Behavior
Jefferson Medical College
Attending Physician
Department of Psychiatry
Thomas Jefferson University Hospital
Philadelphia, Pennsylvania

Marshall Forstein, M.D.
Associate Professor
Department of Psychiatry
Harvard Medical School
Boston, Massachusetts
Director of Psychiatry Residency Training
Department of Psychiatry
The Cambridge Health Alliance
Cambridge, Massachusetts

Harold W. Goforth, M.D.
Assistant Professor of Psychiatry
Department of Psychiatry and Behavioral Sciences
Duke University Medical Center
Co-Director, Consultation-Liaison Psychiatry Service
Director, HIV-Psychiatry Liaison Clinic
Durham Veterans Affairs Medical Center
Durham, North Carolina

Michael Golder, M.D.
Assistant Professor
Department of Psychiatry & Behavioral Sciences
The George Washington University Medical Center
Attending Psychiatrist
Department of Psychiatry
The George Washington University Hospital
Washington, District of Columbia

Johanna Goldfarb, M.D.
Professor of Pediatrics
The Cleveland Clinic Lerner College of Medicine at Case Western Reserve University
Head, Section of Pediatric Infectious Diseases in the Division of Pediatrics
The Children's Hospital, The Cleveland Clinic
Cleveland, Ohio

Stephen M. Goldfinger, M.D.
Professor and Chair
Department of Psychiatry
State University of New York/Downstate Medical Center
Chief of Service
Department of Psychiatry
University Hospital of Brooklyn
Brooklyn, New York

María Fernanda Gómez, M.D.
Associate Professor
Department of Psychiatry and Behavioral Sciences
Albert Einstein College of Medicine
Associate Director—Psychosomatic Medicine
Department of Psychiatry and Behavioral Sciences
Montefiore Medical Center
Bronx, New York

Contributors

Karl Goodkin, M.D., Ph.D.
Professor, Departments of Psychiatry and
    Behavioral Sciences, Neurology, and
    Psychology
University of Miami Miller School of Medicine
Miami, Florida

Cheryl Gore-Felton, Ph.D.
Associate Professor
Department of Psychiatry and Behavioral
    Sciences
Stanford University School of Medicine
Medical Staff
Department of Psychiatry
Stanford University Medical Center, Stanford
    Hospital & Clinics
Stanford, Connecticut

James L. Griffith, M.D.
Professor of Psychiatry and Neurology
Department of Psychiatry and Behavioral
    Sciences
The George Washington University Medical
    Center
Director, Psychiatric Consultation-Liaison Service
Department of Psychiatry
The George Washington University Hospital
Washington, District of Columbia

Daniel W. Hicks, M.D., DFAPA, FAPM
Associate Professor
Director, Psychosomatic Medicine
Department of Psychiatry
Georgetown University Medical Center
Washington, District of Columbia

Vicenzio Holder-Perkins, M.D.
Assistant Clinical Professor, Department of
    Psychiatry & Behavioral Sciences
George Washington University, School of
    Medicine
Washington, District of Columbia
Staff Psychiatrist
Department of Psychiatry
Northern Virginia Mental Health Institute
Falls Church, Virginia

Ewald Horwath, M.D., M.S.
Clinical Professor, Department of Psychiatry
Columbia University
Medical Director
Columbia University Mental Health Training
    Project
New York State Psychiatric Institute
New York, New York

Cynthia L. Hoyler, M.D.
Assistant Professor
Department of Psychiatry
University of Texas Health Science
    Center at San Antonio
Private Practice of Psychiatry
San Antonio, Texas

Janice G. Hutchinson, M.D., M.P.H.
Assistant Professor of Pediatrics
    and Psychiatry
Program Director
Department of Psychiatry
Howard University
Washington, District of Columbia

Alison R. Jones, M.D.
Clinical Assistant Professor
Department of Psychiatry
University of Texas Health Science Center at
    San Antonio
Staff Psychiatrist
Department of Veterans Affairs South Texas
    Veterans Health Care System
Audie L. Murphy Hospital
San Antonio, Texas

Sara Jumping Eagle, M.D.
Instructor, Department of Psychiatry and
    Pediatrics, School of Medicine
University of Colorado at Denver and Health
    Sciences Center
Aurora, Colorado
Physician
Department of Adolescent Medicine
Denver Children's Hospital
Denver, Colorado

Kyle S. Kato, M.D.
Assistant Professor of Psychiatry and
    Behavioral Sciences
Albert Einstein College of Medicine
Bronx, New York
Attending Physician
Department of Psychiatry
Beth Israel Medical Center
New York, New York

Carol E. Kaufman, Ph.D.
Assistant Professor
Department of Psychiatry, School
    of Medicine
University of Colorado at Denver and Health
    Sciences Center
Denver, Colorado

Michael D. Knox, Ph.D.
Distinguished University Professor
Mental Health Law & Policy, Medicine, and
    Global Health
University of South Florida
Director
USF Center for HIV Education and Research
Louis de la Parte Florida Mental Health
    Institute
Tampa, Florida

CONTRIBUTORS

Janet Konefal, Ph.D., M.P.H., L.Ac.
Director
Center for Integrative and Complementary/Alternative Medicine
University of Miami Miller School of Medicine
Miami, Florida

Lukasz M. Konopka, AM, Ph.D.
Associate Professor
Department of Psychiatry and Pharmacology
Loyola Medical Center
Maywood, Illinois
Director of Clinical Neuroscience
Hines Veterans Affairs Hospital
Hines, Illinios

Cheryl Koopman, Ph.D.
Associate Professor (Research)
Department of Psychiatry & Behavioral Sciences
Stanford University
Stanford, California

Elisabeth J. S. Kunkel, M.D.
Professor, Department of Psychiatry & Human Behavior
Jefferson Medical College
Vice Chair for Clinical Affairs, Department of Psychiatry & Human Behavior
Thomas Jefferson University
Philadelphia, Pennsylvania

Isabel T. Lagomasino, M.D., M.S.H.S.
Assistant Professor
Department of Psychiatry & Behavioral Sciences
Keck School of Medicine of USC
Los Angeles, California

Vassilios Latoussakis, M.D.
Fellow in C/L Psychiatry
Department of Psychiatry
Beth Israel Medical Center
New York, New York

William B. Lawson, M.D., Ph.D., DFAPA
Professor
Department of Psychiatry
Howard University
Chairman
Department of Psychiatry
Howard University Hospital
Washington, District of Columbia

Jon A. Levenson, M.D.
Associate Clinical Professor of Psychiatry
Columbia University
College of Physicians and Surgeons
Attending Psychiatrist
New York Presbyterian Hospital
New York, New York

Joel K. Levy, Ph.D.
Neuropsychologist
Department of Internal Medicine, Section of Geriatrics
Baylor College of Medicine
Houston, Texas

Jessica Lillisand, M.D.

Maria D. Llorente, M.D.
Professor of Psychiatry
Division of Geriatric Psychiatry
University of Miami Miller School of Medicine
Chief of Psychiatry
Miami VA Healthcare System
Miami, Florida

Francis G. Lu, M.D.
Professor of Clinical Psychiatry
Department of Psychiatry
University of California, San Francisco
Attending Psychiatrist
Department of Psychiatry
San Francisco General Hospital
San Francisco, California

Constantine G. Lyketsos, M.D., M.H.S., DFAPA, FAPM
Professor of Psychiatry
Department of Psychiatry/Gero-NeuroPsychiatry
Johns Hopkins Medicine
Baltimore, Maryland

Julie E. Malphurs, Ph.D.
Assistant Professor
Department of Psychiatry & Behavioral Sciences
University of Miami Miller School of Medicine
Health Science Specialist
Mental Health and Behavioral Science Service
Miami VA Healthcare System
Miami, Florida

Dimitri D. Markov, M.D.
Instructor, Department of Psychiatry & Human Behavior
Jefferson Medical College
Attending Psychiatrist, Department of Psychiatry & Human Behavior
Thomas Jefferson University Hospital
Philadelphia, Pennsylvania

Annette M. Matthews, M.D.
Assistant Professor
Department of Psychiatry
Oregon Health & Science University
General Psychiatrist
Department of Behavioral Health & Neurosciences

Portland VA Medical Center
Portland, Oregon

Angela M. McBride, Ph.D.
Director
Neuropsychology Services
Center for Integrated Counseling and
   Neuropsychology
Tampa, Florida

Katherine A. McQueen, M.D.
Assistant Professor
Department of Internal Medicine
Baylor College of Medicine
Medical Director
InSight
Harris County Hospital District
Houston, Texas

Lynette J. Menezes, Ph.D.
Director of International Programs
Division of Infectious Diseases and
   International Medicine
University of South Florida
Tampa, Florida

Christina M. Mitchell, Ph.D.
Associate Professor
Department of Psychiatry, School
   of Medicine
University of Colorado at Denver and Health
   Sciences Center
Denver, Colorado

Ellen A. B. Morrison, M.D., M.P.H.
Assistant Professor of Clinical Medicine and
   Clinical Epidemiology
Department of Medicine and Mailman School
   of Public Health
Columbia University
Assistant Attending Physician
Department of Medicine
New York-Presbyterian Hospital
New York, New York

Wade C. Myers, M.D.
Professor of Psychiatry
Chief, Division of Child and Adolescent
   Psychiatry
University of South Florida
Tampa, Florida

Herbert Ochitill, M.D.
Clinical Professor
Department of Psychiatry
University of California at San Francisco School
   of Medicine
Chief, Psychiatric Consultation Service
Department of Psychiatry, San Francisco
   General Hospital
San Francisco, California

Mary Alice O'Dowd, M.D.
Professor of Clinical Psychiatry
Department of Psychiatry
Albert Einstein College of Medicine
Director, Psychosomatic Medicine
Department of Psychiatry
Montefiore Medical Center
Bronx, New York

Andres J. Pumariega, M.D.
Chair
Department of Psychiatry
The Reading Hospital and Medical Center
Reading, Pennsylvania
Clinical Professor of Psychiatry
Temple University School of Medicine
Philadelphia, Pennsylvania

JoAnne B. Pumariega, M.A.
Adjunct Faculty, Department of Mathematics
East Tennessee State University
Johnson City, Tennessee

Dianne L. Reynolds, M.D.
Assistant Professor of Psychiatry and
   Neurology
Department of Psychiatry
Howard University
Washington, District of Columbia

Gustavo Rodriguez, B.A.
Research Assistant
Department of Psychiatry
USC Keck School of Medicine
Los Angeles, California

Meghan M. Ross, M.D.
Resident Physician
Department of Psychiatry and Behavioral
   Medicine
University of South Florida
Tampa, Florida

Pedro Ruiz, M.D.
Professor and Vice Chair
Department of Psychiatry and Behavioral
   Sciences
The University of Texas Medical School
Houston, Texas

Deborah L. Sanchez, M.D., M.P.H.
Resident Physician
Department of Psychiatry and Behavioral
   Medicine
University of South Florida
Tampa, Florida

Carlos A. Santana, M.D.
Associate Professor
Chief of Outpatient Services

Department of Psychiatry and Behavioral Medicine
University of South Florida College of Medicine
Tampa, Florida

James Satriano, Ph.D.
Assistant Professor, Department of Psychiatry
Columbia University
New York, New York

Shelly L. Sayre, M.P.H.
Research Associate, Department of Psychiatry
University of Texas-Houston Medical School
Houston, Texas

Margaret A. Shugart, M.D., M.S.
Associate Professor, Department of Psychiatry & Behavioral Sciences
James H. Quillen College of Medicine
East Tennessee State University
Johnson City, Tennessee

Khenu Singh, M.D.
Assistant Clinical Professor
Department of Psychiatry
University of California, San Francisco
Staff Psychiatrist
Department of Psychiatry
San Francisco General Hospital
San Francisco, California

David Spiegel, M.D.
Willson Professor and Associate Chair
Department of Psychiatry and Behavioral Sciences
Stanford University, Stanford School of Medicine
Medical Director
Stanford Center for Integrative Medicine
Stanford Hospital and Clinics
Stanford, California

Andrea Stolar, M.D.
Assistant Professor, Department of Psychiatry
Case Western Reserve University School of Medicine
Associate Residency Program Director
Department of Psychiatry
University Hospitals of Cleveland
Cleveland, Ohio

Angela L. Stotts, Ph.D.
Assistant Professor, Psychiatry & Behavioral Sciences
The University of Texas Medical School at Houston
Houston, Texas

Sarah Train, B.A.
Research Assistant
Center for Muticultural Mental Health Research
Cambridge Health Alliance
Somerville, Massachusetts

Manuel Trujillo, M.D.
Professor of Psychiatry
Department of Psychiatry
New York University School of Medicine
Director of Psychiatry
Bellevue Hospital Center
New York, New York

Doryliz Vila, M.S.
Adjunct Professor
Department of Biochemistry
University of Puerto Rico, Medical Sciences Campus
San Juan, Puerto Rico

Milton L. Wainberg, M.D.
Associate Clinical Professor
Department of Psychiatry
Columbia College of Physicians and Surgeons
Attending Physician
Department of Psychiatry
New York State Psychiatric Institute
New York, New York

Sandra Williams, B.A.
Center for Multicultural Mental Health Research
Cambridge Health Alliance
Somerville, Massachusetts

Todd Wills, M.D.
Assistant Professor
Department of Internal Medicine
Division of Infectious Diseases and International Medicine
University of South Florida College of Medicine

Claire Zilber, M.D.
Clinical Assistant Professor
Department of Psychiatry and Medicine
University of Colorado School of Medicine
Director, Mental Health Program
Infectious Disease Group Practice
University Hospital
Denver, Colorado

Preface

We are in the third decade of the human immunodeficiency virus (HIV) pandemic. Following its identification in 1983, the spread of HIV/AIDS (acquired immunodeficiency syndrome) intensified quickly due to a lack of concerted efforts to target treatment interventions in the environment of scarce global resources. With the cooperation of the world community, a plan was developed to improve the skills and intervention ability of the medical workforce, and information on the needs of the medical community to cope with the growth of HIV/AIDS worldwide.

Medical research on HIV infection and AIDS continues to improve our understanding of the infection throughout all stages of HIV disease. Just as with cancer before, as disease-modifying treatments evolve and new, more-effective treatments are investigated, it is vitally important that we move beyond the systemic aspects of this disease and focus on the psychological, social, cultural, spiritual, psychiatric, and neurobehavioral aspects of HIV infection and AIDS. Much knowledge has been acquired and joint efforts between medicine and psychiatry have been developed and successfully implemented. We must be sure that knowledge about the psychiatric aspects of HIV/AIDS will become quickly on par with the biologic and clinical knowledge base of this disease.

This is how the idea for this book was born. After more than 20 years of close collaboration in HIV/AIDS from clinical, educational, research, prevention, and public policy viewpoints, we have decided to accept the challenge and produce a groundbreaking book focusing on the "psychiatric aspects" of HIV/AIDS. We wanted to bridge existing gaps in knowledge and communication among clinicians working in HIV/AIDS and others who are concerned with the psychological, social, cultural, spiritual, psychiatric, and neurobehavioral complications of HIV infection and AIDS.

With our team of expert contributors, we worked to highlight the salient topics and discuss the relevant issues in the field from multiple perspectives. This collaboration has produced comprehensive and up-to-date coverage of all psychiatric aspects of HIV/AIDS within a single text, accessible to clinicians, researchers, and allied professional groups.

This book is composed of seven sections. Each focuses on a set of relevant topics pertaining to HIV/AIDS and all offer the most pertinent and up-to-date description of all significant psychological, behavioral, social, cultural, spiritual, psychiatric, and neurobiological aspects of HIV infection and AIDS. Section I presents background information and reviews the relevant scientific and clinical aspects of the HIV/AIDS epidemic. Chapter 1 offers a comprehensive review of the current epidemiologic trends of HIV infection and AIDS, the co-occurrence aspects of psychiatric comorbidities, the factors leading to an increase in psychiatric morbidity, the social and psychological challenges of living with HIV/AIDS, and the epidemiologic implications in the delivery of mental health and psychiatric care to persons suffering from HIV/AIDS. Chapter 2 presents an in-depth review of the understanding of the human immunodeficiency virus, the process of initial infection, and its systemic and neuropathogenesis. This chapter also addresses the modes of transmission of HIV and the progression of HIV disease. Chapter 3 introduces an overview of the initial medical evaluation, treatment of medical complications, principles of antiretroviral therapy, and risk of exposure in health care settings as well as its prophylaxis.

Section II reviews the most appropriate assessment strategies to psychiatrically evaluate persons suffering with HIV/AIDS. Collectively, the chapters become a practical discussion that will assist clinicians in identifying the psychiatric manifestations and complications of HIV/AIDS. Chapter 4 focuses on methods of psychiatric assessment. Chapter 5 depicts the methods of psychological and neuropsychological assessment of HIV infection and/or AIDS. Chapter 6 reviews electrophysiological diagnostic testing that could play a substantial role in the diagnosis of HIV-related neurobehavioral conditions and their progression. They all represent a solid, up-to-date approach to the diagnosis and assessment of comorbid psychiatric conditions in persons living with HIV infection and/or AIDS.

Section III focuses on the psychological, psychosocial, and psychiatric complications from varying theoretical frameworks and presumed etiologies. Each chapter presents a thorough review and description of the most relevant issues pertaining to each of these conditions. They are: Chapter 7, Psychological Reactions; Chapter 8, Stress-Distress Spectrum and Adjustment Disorders; Chapter 9, Anxiety Disorders; Chapter 10, Mood Disorders; Chapter 11, Personality Disorders; Chapter 12, Cognitive Disorders; Chapter 13, Psychotic Disorders; Chapter 14, Substance Use Disorders; and Chapter 15, Sleep Disorders. Chapter 12 also introduces the reader to the use of neuroimaging in the differential diagnostic process.

Section IV presents the major medical issues that exacerbate comorbidity. Chapter 16 discusses psychotropic drug interactions with antiretroviral medications. Chapter 17 represents an overview of pain syndromes and their treatment. Chapter 18 describes all relevant sexually transmitted infections as they relate to HIV/AIDS. Finally, Chapter 19 focuses on the management of medically hospitalized psychiatric patients with HIV/AIDS. Together, these chapters offer an excellent review of the most significant aspects of medical comorbidities and therapeutic considerations in HIV/AIDS.

Chapters 20–32 comprise Section V and they focus on the unique and specific characteristic pertaining to HIV/AIDS among special populations. It encompasses four ethnic minorities, sexual minorities, neonates and infants, children and adolescents, and older adults; and unique groups such as the homeless and prisoners. Special issues concerning the patient in the context of family and support systems is also reviewed. As a group, our experts examine the specific characteristics and issues pertaining to each of these special populations. The objective is to offer culturally competent care and psychosocially relevant services to all patients. We also offer the most relevant and current clinical, investigational, and preventive knowledge related to these special populations.

Section VI focuses on clinically relevant aspects of patient care. Chapter 33 discusses the most important ethical, forensic, and legal considerations of persons who are HIV-infected or suffering from AIDS. Chapter 34 reviews all-important religious and spiritual considerations among persons with HIV/AIDS. Chapter 35 focuses on psychotherapy while Chapter 36 discusses complementary and alternative medicine. Chapter 37 alludes to the most relevant psychosocial aspects of living with HIV/AIDS. Finally, Chapter 38 explores issues pertaining to suicide and end-of-life care among persons suffering from HIV/AIDS. On the whole, these chapters present and examine very significant issues pertaining to persons who suffer from HIV/AIDS.

Section VII consists of two chapters. These chapters address very important key policy issues in the field of HIV/AIDS care. Chapter 39 relates to prevention and education strategies. Chapter 40 discusses physician-assisted suicide—a controversial but richly stimulating topic.

We wish to take this opportunity to deeply thank the tireless efforts of our contributing authors. Because of their hard work, the book is an exemplary compilation and synthesis of significant and up-to-date scientific information concerning the psychiatric aspects of HIV/AIDS. They too shared our vision of educating clinicians and their students in a truly multidisciplinary endeavor. Likewise, we wish to recognize two very caring professionals at Lippincott Williams & Wilkins: Charles W. Mitchell, Executive Editor, and Lisa Kairis, Senior Managing Editor. Without their generous and intelligent efforts on our behalf, this text would not have been produced. We are much indebted to them for their guidance and encouragement throughout the process. In addition, we wish to thank our support staff, Shawn Hood and Marie O. Gonzales-Arms, who worked hard on our behalf to complete this book on time. Finally, we remain indebted to our patients who, we hope, will be the true beneficiaries of this collaborative effort.

Francisco Fernandez, M.D.
Tampa, Florida

Pedro Ruiz, M.D.
Houston, Texas

Contents

Contributors   vii
Preface   xiii

SECTION I
Background   1

1   Epidemiology   3
Margarita Alegría, Doryliz Vila, Sarah Train, Sandra Williams, Nabila El-Bassel

2   Virology, Immunology, Transmission, and Disease Stage   11
Karl Goodkin

3   Medical Treatment and Occupational Exposure   23
Ellen A. B. Morrison, Jon A. Levenson

SECTION II
Diagnostic Tools   37

4   Psychiatric Assessment   39
María Fernanda Gómez, Mary Alice O'Dowd

5   Psychological and Neuropsychological Testing   48
Joel K. Levy

6   Electrophysiology and Brain Mapping   63
Harold W. Goforth, Lukasz M. Konopka

SECTION III
Psychiatric Comorbidity   69

7   Psychological Reactions   71
Vicenzio Holder-Perkins, Jeffrey S. Akman

8   Stress-Distress Spectrum and Adjustment Disorders   79
Dimitri D. Markov, Elisabeth J. S. Kunkel, Howard Field

9   Anxiety Disorders   86
Annette M. Matthews, Manuel Trujillo

10   Mood Disorders   93
Pedro Ruiz

11	Personality Disorders Khenu Singh, Herbert Ochitill	101
12	Cognitive Disorders Angela M. McBride, Francisco Fernandez	111
13	Psychotic Disorders Ewald Horwath, Francine Cournos	119
14	Substance Use Disorders Stephen J. Ferrando, Steven L. Batki	127
15	Sleep Disorders Carlos A. Santana, Francisco Fernandez	137

SECTION IV
Medical Comorbidity — 147

16	Psychotropic Drug Interactions with Antiretroviral Medications Philip A. Bialer, Kyle S. Kato, Vassilios Latoussakis	149
17	Pain Syndromes William Breitbart	161
18	Sexually Transmitted Infections Angela L. Stotts, Mark Evans, Shelly L. Sayre, Katherine A. McQueen	188
19	Psychiatric Comorbidities in Medically Ill Patients with HIV/AIDS Stephen J. Ferrando, Constantine G. Lyketsos	198

SECTION V
Special Populations — 213

20	HIV/AIDS Among Hispanic Americans Pedro Ruiz, Francisco Fernandez	215
21	HIV/AIDS Among African Americans William B. Lawson, Janice G. Hutchinson, Dianne L. Reynolds	223
22	HIV/AIDS Among Asian and Pacific Islander Americans Lynette J. Menezes, Todd Wills, Karina D'Souza	232
23	HIV/AIDS Among American Indians and Alaska Natives Carol E. Kaufman, Janette Beals, Sara Jumping Eagle, Christina M. Mitchell	241
24	HIV/AIDS Among Neonates and Infants Andrea Stolar, Johanna Goldfarb	250
25	HIV/AIDS Among Children and Adolescents Andres J. Pumariega, Margaret A. Shugart, JoAnne B. Pumariega	259
26	HIV/AIDS Among Older Adults Maria D. Llorente, Julie E. Malphurs	267
27	HIV/AIDS Among Women Isabel T. Lagomasino, Gustavo Rodriguez	277
28	HIV/AIDS Among Men Who Have Sex with Men Milton L. Wainberg, Kenneth B. Ashley	288
29	HIV/AIDS Among Women Who Have Sex with Women Alison R. Jones, Cynthia L. Hoyler	299

30	HIV/AIDS Among the Homeless Jacqueline Maus Feldman, Stephen M. Goldfinger	308
31	HIV/AIDS Among Prisoners Wade C. Myers, Glenn Catalano, Deborah L. Sanchez, Meghan M. Ross	316
32	HIV/AIDS and the Patient's Family James L. Griffith, Michael Golder	328

SECTION VI
Special Issues — 339

33	Ethical, Forensic, and Legal Considerations James Satriano	341
34	Religious and Spiritual Considerations Daniel W. Hicks, Francis G. Lu	347
35	Psychotherapeutic Strategies Claire Zilber	355
36	Complementary and Holistic Medicine Janet Konefal, Jessica Lillisand	365
37	Biopsychosocial Aspects Cheryl Gore-Felton, Cheryl Koopman, David Spiegel	378
38	Suicide and End-of-Life Care Mary Ann Cohen	383

SECTION VII
Policy Issues — 393

39	Prevention and Education Strategies Michael D. Knox, Tiffany Chenneville	395
40	Physician Assisted Suicide and Voluntary Euthanasia Marshall Forstein	404

Index — 415

SECTION 1

Background

CHAPTER 1

Epidemiology

Margarita Alegría, Doryliz Vila, Sarah Train,
Sandra Williams, Nabila El-Bassel

This chapter provides an overview of the epidemiology of the human immunodeficiency virus and acquired immunodeficiency syndrome (HIV/AIDS) and its co-occurrence with psychiatric morbidity. It is organized into six general topics: (a) the epidemiology of HIV; (b) the psychiatric epidemiology and types of co-occurring psychiatric disorders of patients with HIV; (c) psychiatric morbidity and HIV disease progression and mortality; (d) factors associated with increased psychiatric morbidity or psychological distress in persons living with HIV/AIDS; (e) the social, psychological, and contextual challenges of living with HIV; and (f) epidemiologic implications for the delivery of mental health and substance abuse services. It is critical to identify and treat comorbid mental illness among people living with HIV/AIDS, for such identification will improve their quality of life, increase their health outcomes, and augment their survival. The elevated risk for psychiatric conditions may be directly caused by HIV/AIDS, be exacerbated by the illness, or be a precursor to the HIV disease. Understanding the manifestations and challenges of the co-occurrence of psychiatric disorders and HIV/AIDS will help practitioners provide strategies to persons with these co-occurring disorders so they can adapt well to the challenges, avoid disease progression, and receive appropriate care.

EPIDEMIOLOGY AND RISKS

According to the Centers for Disease Control and Prevention (CDC) HIV/AIDS surveillance report through 2003, approximately 850,000 to 950,000 persons in the United States are living with HIV and an estimated 929,985 (749,887 cases in males and 170,679 cases in females) have a diagnosis of AIDS.[1] Worldwide, 38 million people are living with HIV. U.S. surveillance reports from 2000 to 2003 indicate that the overall annual rate of diagnosis of HIV/AIDS has remained stable over this period, with an increase of 3% in the annual rate in males and a decrease of 3.7% in the annual rate in females.[2]

The ranking of transmission using age-adjusted rates demonstrates that men who have sex with men (MSM), injection drug users (IDUs), those who are both MSM and IDU, and people exposed to high-risk heterosexual contact had the higher annual rates of diagnosis in

2000 to 2003. The transmission categories with the largest proportion of males with HIV were MSM (61.2%), high-risk heterosexuals (17.3%), and IDUs (14.6%); the transmission categories for the largest proportion of women were high-risk heterosexuals (77.7%) and IDUs (19.4%).[2]

There is a disproportionate incidence of HIV by race and ethnicity. Incidence of HIV is greater in minority men compared with that in White men, independent of the route of transmission.[3] The disparity in the HIV rate of non-Latino Black women is 19 times higher than White women.[2] A change in annual age-adjusted rates from 2000 to 2003 shows that the rates among non-Latino White males (6.2% change) and Asian Pacific Islander males (39.7% change) are increasing while the rate for non-Latino Black females is decreasing (6.0%), with no statistically significant change in the other racial or ethnic groups.[2] However, it should be noted that non-Latino Black women accounted for 13% of the population included for surveillance purposes but represented 51.3% of the HIV/AIDS diagnoses during 2000 to 2003. Women also account for an increasing percentage of all AIDS cases (6.7% in 1986 to 18% in 1999),[4] with a disproportionate increase for Black women living in the South. Also of importance is the finding—using trends of AIDS surveillance data to estimate the past incidence of HIV infection—that 66% of HIV-infected young people who had acquired the infection heterosexually were minorities, although they represented only 27% of the total U.S. population born during 1988 and 1993.[3]

Homosexual contact appeared as the major means of transmission among young men, whereas heterosexual contact was the key mode of infection for young women.[3] In White, Black, and Latino male teenagers and young adults, risk of HIV transmission through homosexual contact was considerably higher during the adolescent years but decreased as they became young adults. HIV incidence ascribed to heterosexual contact was found to be rising or constant in the successive birth cohorts, particularly among women. While HIV prevalence dropped approximately 50% for White young men aged 20 to 25, HIV prevalence increased 36% to 45% for women in that same age cohort.

There is a growing recognition of the necessity to identify social and structural factors that have an impact on HIV risk. Isolating the risk environments (i.e., those risk factors that are exogenous to the individual but place the individual at risk for the disease)[5] is critical because these environments appear linked to variation in population behavior in response to divergent social, cultural, economic, and political forces.[6] For example, residence in neighborhoods where there is a preponderance of sex work and crack cocaine is a predictor of increased HIV risk.[7] However, this finding may be a surrogate for "risk that an individual's sex partner is HIV positive" rather than represent an environmental risk.

There are many independent predictors of HIV infection in community samples: having a history of sexually transmitted diseases (STDs), Latino having multiple sexual partners, and exchanging money or drugs for sex.[7] The main risk factors may differ among groups. A recent case-control study of older adults found that in this population a history of STDs, positive hepatitis B status, and certain medical history parameters (including the albumin to globulin ratio) were more likely in HIV-positive adults than in controls.[8] A study of 1,800 IDUs found that risk factors for HIV differed by gender. For males, drug-related risk factors (such as needle sharing) and homosexual activity were the most important predictors, but for females, factors related to high-risk sexual activity were the most important predictors.[9]

PSYCHIATRIC EPIDEMIOLOGY AND TYPES OF CO-OCCURRING PSYCHIATRIC DISORDERS

Psychiatric morbidity in persons with HIV was detected early in the epidemic.[10] A 1996 epidemiological study of a nationally representative sample of adults (aged ≥ 18 years) receiving care for HIV in the United States showed that 47.9% demonstrated positive status for at least one psychiatric disorder on screening in the previous 12 months.[11] More people receiving care for HIV demonstrated positive status for major depression (36.0%) and dysthymia (26.5%) than for generalized anxiety disorders (15.8%) and panic attacks on screening in the previous 12 months (10.5%).[11] The positive screen rates for current psychiatric disorder in HIV-infected persons receiving medical care compared to rates in the general population were eight times greater for generalized anxiety disorder, five times greater for major depression, and four times greater for panic attacks.[11]

Estimates of the lifetime and past year prevalence of psychiatric disorders in persons living with HIV/AIDS may differ substantially depending on the sample and comparison groups. Data on HIV-infected women at the South Texas AIDS Center for Children and Their Families demonstrated that over 60% met criteria for at least one current Axis I psychiatric disorder, with major depressive disorder and substance disorders being the most prevalent.[12] However, studies of gay men have established few differences in current psychiatric disorders between infected and uninfected gay men.[13] A study of inmates diagnosed with HIV infection revealed that psychiatric disorders were significantly more common among the HIV-infected inmate population (89% men) than their noninfected counterparts, even after age, gender, and race adjustments: current major depression (6.05% versus 2.21%), dysthymia (3.24% versus 0.72%), bipolar disorder (1.51% versus 0.98%), and schizoaffective disorders (1.12% versus 0.53%).[14]

A wide spectrum of psychiatric disorders have been directly or indirectly associated with HIV/AIDS: delirium, HIV-associated dementia, HIV-associated mania, minor cognitive motor disorder, adjustment disorders, anxiety disorders, mood disorders, personality disorders, psychotic disorders, sexual disorders, sleep disorders, and substance disorders. Some investigators argue that the high prevalence of psychiatric disorders among persons with HIV may reflect high rates of preexisting affective and substance abuse disorders or increased risk for HIV infection among those with mental disorders and drug abuse. Others posit that anxiety, depression, and emotional distress may be, for some, a response to learning that they are seropositive or to subsequent symptoms and disability associated with HIV.[15]

Major depression and substance disorders appear as frequent co-occurring psychiatric disorders in persons living with HIV/AIDS. In a longitudinal cohort study of HIV infection in women, a diagnosis of current major depressive disorder was four times greater in HIV-seropositive compared to HIV-seronegative women (19.4% versus 4.8%).[16]

There is evidence of increased risk of suicidal ideation and attempts in people with HIV/AIDS, particularly among HIV-positive women.[17] Data from Project WAVE (Women, AIDS, and Violence Epidemic) revealed that HIV-positive women were five times more likely than HIV-negative women to have ever attempted suicide.[18]

Cognitive disorders such as dementia, delirium, neurobehavioral impairments, and myelopathy from the neuropathic effects of HIV disease also occur frequently. AIDS dementia complex (ADC), or HIV-associated dementia (HAD), has an unpredictable course, with some HIV-infected persons reporting subtle cognitive dysfunction and others deteriorating rapidly, with signs of profound dementia.[19] Psychomotor retardation (e.g., slow speech or response time), impaired concentration and attention, lack of visuospatial memory (e.g., misplacing things), reduced speed in information processing, impaired verbal memory (e.g., word-finding abilities), loss of balance, lack of visuomotor coordination (e.g., eye movement abnormalities), decreased executive functioning, and decreased learning efficiency are some usual symptoms of persons living with HIV/AIDS.[20]

PSYCHIATRIC MORBIDITY, DISEASE PROGRESSION, AND MORTALITY

Major depression and substance disorders are frequent co-occurring psychiatric disorders in persons living with HIV/AIDS, but there is inconsistent evidence of their effect on HIV progression and mortality.[16] Some studies have demonstrated a significant association between depression and increased HIV disease progression. For example, previous research has identified associations among depression, immune system suppression, and disability.[21] Ickovics et al.[22] found that, controlling for clinical characteristics, substance use, and sociodemographic characteristics, depressive symptoms among women with HIV are associated with disease progression.

FACTORS ASSOCIATED WITH INCREASED PSYCHIATRIC MORBIDITY OR PSYCHOLOGICAL DISTRESS IN PERSONS LIVING WITH HIV/AIDS

Several factors have been identified as being linked with HIV-related psychiatric morbidity and psychological adjustment. For example, a prior history of psychiatric or substance abuse disorder has been positively associated with augmented risk for subsequent psychiatric disorders in women and men with HIV/AIDS.[15,16] Unemployment and work-related disability in persons with HIV/AIDS was also related to increased odds of positive status on screening for a comorbid psychiatric disorder among people receiving care for HIV disease.[11]

Coping style and levels of stress also appear to play a significant role in the likelihood of developing a comorbid psychiatric disorder or reduced psychological adjustment for those with HIV/AIDS.[15] There is evidence that coping styles that involve planned problem-solving, searching for information, and seeking support are related to improved adaptation and reduced emotional distress.

The occurrence of negative life events has been found to predict increased psychological distress in people living with HIV.[23] At the same time, abusive relationships can increase the risk for psychiatric morbidity in women with HIV. For example, HIV-positive women who were consistently abused compared to HIV-negative nonabused women were seven times more likely to indicate the presence of depression, 4.9 times more likely to experience anxiety problems, and 12.5 times more likely to have attempted suicide.[18] Although the highest rates of these indicators were found in HIV-positive abused women, women with only one of these risk factors (abuse or positive HIV status) were also more likely than HIV-negative non-abused women to indicate the presence of these mental health indicators. Depression symptoms have also been correlated with domestic abuse in both HIV-positive and HIV-negative women.[24]

Certain personality characteristics have also been associated with comorbid psychiatric disorders or higher psychological distress in persons with HIV/AIDS. Dispositional optimism among men at risk for HIV/AIDS[25] and personality hardiness[26] are described as resilience factors in people at risk for or living with HIV/AIDS. There is some suggestion that a positive personal meaning ascribed to HIV/AIDS may benefit adaptation to the disease and reduced risk for psychiatric morbidity.

Availability of social networks, sense of integration, and quality of social supports have additionally been associated with better psychological adjustment and reduced distress in persons with HIV infection. Conversely, social isolation and rejection resulting from negative labeling of people with HIV/AIDS is another negative consequence of the disease. Living alone or with someone other than a partner or spouse has been correlated with positive status on screening for a current psychiatric disorder among people receiving care for HIV disease.[11]

SOCIAL, PSYCHOLOGICAL, AND CONTEXTUAL CHALLENGES OF LIVING WITH HIV

Individuals with HIV must confront a number of adverse psychological and social consequences common to those suffering from a chronic illness. Some of the psychological challenges evolve from having a life-threatening disease and the coping process related to receiving an initial diagnosis, the onset of opportunistic infections, and the abrupt changes in physical and neurocognitive functioning.[20] Other psychosocial challenges may develop in the adaptation to having HIV, such as social stigma, changes in social roles, decisions linked to disclosure of illness status, changes in sexual practices, and uncertainty of financial and material resources.[20]

In addition, women living with HIV are vulnerable to many stressors, including higher rates of loss events such as losing family members, jobs, and health. Some of these stressors include worries about meeting caregiving responsibilities, issues of stigma and shame, rejection, and lack of social support. Physical symptoms and decreased functioning among HIV-infected mothers also appear to have an impact on parental monitoring, parental self-efficacy, and the quality of parent–child relationships. At the same time, single mothers with late-stage HIV/AIDS displayed extremely elevated distress rates in the Psychiatric Symptom Index (mean in mothers with HIV = 36.3 versus 10.5 in community samples), associated with restrictions in their abilities to perform usual daily activities such as housework, shopping, and childcare.[27] Losing one's usual social roles may negatively affect the well-being of HIV-positive individuals.

There is also some indication that HIV-infection may have adverse sexual consequences for both men and women. Delayed ejaculation has been reported in seropositive gay men,[15] possibly associated with fears of infecting sexual partners. Psychosexual dysfunction subsequent to a diagnosis of HIV/AIDS has also been more commonly described by HIV-seropositive women compared to HIV-seronegative women. Loss of interest in sex has been typically mentioned by women living with HIV infection, with half or more reporting abstinence or reduced frequency of intercourse.[28]

Dealing with the power differentials of intimate relationships in which one partner exerts substantial power over the other might additionally be necessary to initiate safer sex practices that reduce the sexual transmission of HIV. This reduction is critical because 40% of female HIV cases can be attributed to heterosexual transmission.[29]

HIV may also affect socioeconomic circumstances because of the high cost of medical care and intermittent job interruptions, as well as increased arrangements for child care. However, HIV/AIDS is also evidenced in populations that previous to the illness had inadequate economic and social resources. Zierler et al.[30] studied the relationship between incidence of AIDS and economic deprivation in Massachusetts, finding that economically depressed areas where 40% or more of the population was below the poverty line had a cumulative incidence of AIDS nearly seven times higher than those in areas where less than 2% of the population was below the poverty line. The magnitude of the relationship between AIDS incidence and poverty varied by race/ethnicity and sex; the highest rates were among non-Hispanic Black men living in the most densely populated areas, followed by non-Hispanic Black men and Hispanic men living in the poorest areas; the lowest rates were among White women living in the least impoverished areas. Additionally, Strathdee et al.[9] found that among male IDUs, both lower income and homelessness were associated with HIV seroconversion, although this relationship was not found for women.

Communicating with family, children, friends, and co-workers may be particularly stressful, especially in response to disruption of social roles or as an outcome of hospitalizations. Qualitative work on this topic has found that people with HIV and AIDS may avoid disclosing their status, even to sexual partners. Relationship quality is particularly important in selecting to whom to disclose one's status, and a complex set of factors may be considered when deciding whether to disclose.

EPIDEMIOLOGIC IMPLICATIONS FOR THE DELIVERY OF MENTAL HEALTH AND SUBSTANCE ABUSE SERVICES

There are many obstacles to the recognition and treatment of psychiatric disorders or symptoms in persons with HIV/AIDS. For example, psychiatric symptoms or syndromes may be regarded as merely a manifestation of HIV/AIDS, not as pathology leading to the need of professional mental health care. Furthermore, mental health services for persons with HIV are typically provided in primary or secondary health care. Primary care providers who self-perceive lack of competence in the management of mental health problems may be discouraged from assessing mental health problems in their HIV-positive patients. The fear of being stigmatized by the medical profession may also keep persons with comorbid psychiatric conditions and HIV from seeking mental health care. For women, the criminalization of substance abuse during pregnancy in some states, fear of losing children to the foster care system, and treatment programs designed without adequate child care mechanisms may also prevent mental health service utilization.

At present, little information is available on mental health service use among people living with HIV/AIDS.[12] Most literature regarding this topic has limited generalizability because of reliance on convenience samples of individuals with HIV. Some studies have examined mental health service utilization among persons living with HIV receiving care in the United States using one nationally representative probability survey of HIV-infected adults, the HIV Cost and Services Utilization Study.

Burnam et al.[12] estimated 6-month rates of use of services for mental health and substance abuse problems among adults with HIV using a national probability survey of 2,864 HIV-infected adults receiving medical care in the United States in 1996. Half of the population demonstrated positive status for at least one mental or drug dependence disorder within the previous year on screening, and approximately 61% of individuals infected with HIV used mental health or substance abuse services, mostly those with positive status on screening for psychiatric disorders. These investigators found that of the approximately 141,154 adults under care for HIV who used mental health or substance services, 1.8% of HIV-infected adults were admitted to psychiatric inpatient units, 3% received residential substance abuse treatments, 6% used outpatient treatments, 12% used substance abuse self-help groups, 15% used group mental health services, nearly 30% used psychiatric medication, and 40% discussed mental health issues with medical providers. The disabled and those individuals living in the Northeast and West regions of the country or in large metropolitan areas were more likely to receive outpatient mental health treatment. Homosexuals, those with more HIV symptoms, and those with greater HIV symptom burdens were more likely to access mental health treatment through the general health sector. Predictors of type of treatment received included employment status, region of residence, sexual orientation, severity of HIV symptoms and burdens, age, insurance status, and race/ethnicity. Those unemployed because of disability, persons residing in the Northeast, heterosexuals, individuals with more severe HIV symptoms and burdens, older individuals, persons with public health insurance, and Whites were more likely to receive specialty treatments such as outpatient therapy or psychiatric medication than were members of more disenfranchised groups. Members of disenfranchised groups were likely to receive treatment in group therapy situations, substance abuse treatment programs, or residential treatment programs.

Unmet needs for mental health services among adults with significant mood disturbances and substance abuse problems with HIV/AIDS have been linked to negative health behaviors such as poor adherence to HIV therapy and difficulty in accessing HIV medication once it is prescribed. Although antiretroviral therapy has proven to be effective in HIV survival, women may be less likely than men to use these therapies. In addition, drug use, high-risk sexual behaviors, depression, and unmet social needs may disrupt or limit women's HIV prevention and treatment resources.[4]

In a longitudinal study of 1,716 HIV-seropositive women, Cook et al.[31] found that AIDS-related deaths were more likely to occur among women with chronic depressive symptoms and that mental health service utilization was significantly associated with reduced mortality in people living with HIV. These findings have implications for the importance of monitoring and improving access to mental health services for individuals with comorbid psychiatric disorders and HIV. Increasing access to services may augment the quality of life of individuals with HIV/AIDS and the opportunities for survival.

SUMMARY

Surveillance data indicate that the distribution of HIV and the primary means through which it is transmitted have continuously shifted (although the overall annual rate of diagnosis of HIV/AIDS has remained stable), with various populations carrying the heaviest incidence of disease burden at any given time. Minorities represent a disproportionate percentage of HIV cases, suggesting the need to target efforts to minority populations, as well as those living in risk environments. HIV incidence attributed to heterosexual contact is found to be increasing, particularly among women, indicating the necessity to provide them HIV counseling, facilitate partner empowerment, and build improved couple communication and safe-sex negotiation.

Our review demonstrates that lifetime and past-year prevalence of psychiatric disorders and suicidality in persons living with HIV/AIDS diverges considerably (19% to 89%) as a function of the sample and contrast groups employed. Psychiatric morbidity has been detected in a substantial proportion of persons living with HIV infection (47.9%) in a national sample of adults (aged ≥18 years) receiving care for HIV in the United States.[11]

The current model used in understanding health behavior and health outcomes for individuals faced with chronic illnesses integrates biological, social, contextual, and psychosocial factors, acknowledging that these elements contribute to the well-being and quality of life of HIV-infected individuals. On the one hand, it is necessary to assess specific neuropathic effects of HIV, opportunistic infections, metabolic dysfunction, drug-drug interactions, and medication side effects for differential diagnosis.[20] On the other hand, it is essential to establish the patient's perceptions of physical symptoms, physical limitations, and pain-related discomfort to realize potential factors increasing the risk for psychiatric morbidity. Also relevant are screening for cognitive impairment and identification of substance use patterns. A comprehensive evaluation of sexual functioning, risk behavior practices, social networks, living situation, and socioeconomic circumstances can facilitate provider awareness of the daily challenges or constraints of those living with HIV.

Because premorbid psychiatric disorders, including depression and substance disorders, are predictive of higher psychological distress and negative overall adjustment in individuals with HIV disease, psychiatric assessments must be a requisite for appropriate care. In keeping with this understanding, it has been proposed by some that treating the medical aspects of HIV alone without addressing mental health, social, and interpersonal concerns do not meet best practice standards of care for the HIV population. Global management of HIV disease requires considering psychiatric assessments and treatments as a vital component of HIV treatment. This chapter is intended to facilitate a better grasp of the multidimensional forces that impinge on psychiatric morbidity and adaptation of persons living with HIV.

REFERENCES

1. Centers for Disease Control and Prevention. *HIV/AIDS Surveillance Report: HIV Infection and AIDS in the United States*. Atlanta: Centers for Disease Control and Prevention; 2003.
2. Centers for Disease Control and Prevention. Diagnoses of HIV/AIDS-32 States, 2000–2003. *MMWR Morb Mortal Wkly Rep*. 2004;53:1106–1110.
3. Rosenberg PS, Biggar RJ. Trends in HIV incidence among young adults in the United States. *JAMA*. 1998;279:1894–1899.
4. Hader SL, Smith DK, Moore JS, Holmberg SD. HIV infection in women in the United States. *JAMA*. 2001;285:1186–1192.
5. Rhodes T. The 'risk environment': a framework for understanding and reducing drug-related harm. *Int J Drug Policy*. 2002;13:85–94.
6. Singer M. Toward a biocultural and political economic integration of alcohol, tobacco and drug studies in the coming century. *Soc Sci Med*. 2001;53:199–213.
7. Ellerbrock TV, Chamblee S, Bush TJ, et al. Human immunodeficiency virus infection in a rural community in the United States. *Am J Epidemiol*. 2004;160:582–588.
8. Szerlip MA, Desalvo KB, Szerlip HM. Predictors of HIV-infection in older adults. *J Aging Health*. 2005;17:293–305.

9. Strathdee SA, Galai N, Safaiean M, et al. Sex differences in risk factors for HIV seroconversion among injection drug users: a 10-year perspective. *Arch Intern Med.* 2001;161:1281–1288.
10. Hoffman RS. Neuropsychiatric complications of AIDS. *Psychosomatics.* 1984;25:393–395.
11. Bing EG, Burnam MA, Longshore D, et al. Psychiatric disorders and drug use among human immunodeficiency virus-infected adults in the United States. *Arch Gen Psychiatry.* 2001;58:721–728.
12. Burnam MA, Bing EG, Morton SC, et al. Use of mental health and substance abuse treatment services among adults with HIV in the United States. *Arch Gen Psychiatry.* 2001;58:729–736.
13. Kemeny ME, Dean L. Effects of AIDS-related bereavement on HIV progression among New York City gay men. *AIDS Educ Prev.* 1995;7:36–47.
14. Baillargeon J, Ducate S, Pulvino J, Bradshaw P, Murray O, Olvera R. The association of psychiatric disorders and HIV infection in the correctional setting. *Ann Epidemiol.* 2003;13:606–612.
15. Catalan J, Klimes I, Day A, Garrod A, Bond A, Gallwey J. The psychosocial impact of HIV infection in gay men: a controlled investigation and factors associated with psychiatric morbidity. *Br J Psychiatry.* 1992;161:774–778.
16. Morrison MF, Petitto JM, Ten Have T, et al. Depressive and anxiety disorders in women with HIV infection. *Am J Psychiatry.* 2002;159:789–796.
17. Komiti A, Judd F, Grech P, et al. Suicidal behavior in people with HIV/AIDS: a review. *Austr N Z J Psychiatry.* 2001;35:747–757.
18. Gielen AC, McDonnell KA, O'Campo PJ, Burke JG. Suicide risk and mental health indicators: do they differ by abuse and HIV status? *Womens Health Issues.* 2005;15:89–95.
19. AIDS Institute. *Mental Health Care for People with HIV Infection: HIV Clinical Guidelines for the Primary Care Practitioner.* New York: New York State Department of Health; 2004.
20. Farber EW, McDaniel SJ. Clinical management of psychiatric disorders in patients with HIV disease. *Psychiatr Q.* 2002;73:5–16.
21. Reichlin S. Mechanisms of disease: neuroendocrine-immune interactions. *N Engl J Med.* 1993;329:1246–1253.
22. Ickovics JR, Hamburger ME, Vlahov D, et al. Mortality, CD4 cell count decline, and depressive symptoms among HIV-seropositive women: longitudinal analysis from the HIV Epidemiology Research Study. *JAMA.* 2001;285:1466–1474.
23. Blaney NT, Goodkin K, Morgan RO, et al. A stress-moderator model of distress in early HIV-1 infection: concurrent analysis of life events, hardiness and social support. *J Psychosom Res.* 1991;35:297–305.
24. Richardson J, Barkan S, Cohen M, Back S, Fitzergald G, Feldman J. Experience and covariates of depressive symptoms among a cohort of HIV infected women. *Soc Work Health Care.* 2001;32:93–111.
25. Taylor SE, Kemeny ME, Aspinwall LG, et al. Optimism, coping, psychological distress, and high-risk sexual behavior among men at risk for acquired immune deficiency syndrome (AIDS). *J Pers Soc Psychol.* 1992;63:460–473.
26. Farber EW, Schwartz JAJ, Schaper PE, et al. Resilience factors associated with adaptation to HIV disease. *Psychosomatics.* 2000;41:140–146.
27. Silver EJ, Bauman LJ, Camacho S, Hudis J. Factors associated with psychological distress in urban mothers with late-stage HIV/AIDS. *AIDS Behav.* 2003;7:421–431.
28. Brown GR, Rundell JR. Prospective study of psychiatric morbidity in HIV-seropositive women without AIDS. *Gen Hosp Psychiatry.* 1990;12:30–35.
29. Centers for Disease Control and Prevention. *HIV/AIDS Surveillance Report.* Atlanta: Centers for Disease Control and Prevention; 1999.
30. Zierler S, Krieger N, Tang Y, et al. Economic deprivation and AIDS incidence in Massachusetts. *Am J Public Health.* 2000;90:1064–1073.
31. Cook JA, Grey D, Burke J, et al. Depressive symptoms and AIDS-related mortality among a multisite cohort of HIV-positive women. *Am J Public Health.* 2004;94:1133–1140.

CHAPTER 2

Virology, Immunology, Transmission, and Disease Stage

Karl Goodkin

THE VIRUS

Human immunodeficiency virus (HIV) is a retrovirus. Retroviruses have a ribonucleic acid (RNA) core. The term *retrovirus* refers to the fact that these viruses reverse transcribe their RNA to deoxyribonucleic acid (DNA) during the replication process. To accomplish this, HIV uses the enzyme reverse transcriptase (RT). Not coincidentally, this enzyme is a major target for anti-HIV (or antiretroviral) therapy. The predominant type of HIV worldwide is type 1 (HIV-1). HIV-1 has 9,749 nucleotides and is about the same size as other retroviruses. HIV-1 is further subdivided into subtypes (also known as clades), designated A through K (collectively referred to as group M), N, and O. More than 98% of HIV-1 infections in the United States are due to subtype B. Human immunodeficiency virus type 2 (HIV-2) has also been identified and likewise causes AIDS, though HIV-2 is not endemic in the United States. Originally, retroviruses were not thought to cause human disease. The HIV/AIDS epidemic has permanently changed that perception.

The HIV-1 genome has nine open reading frames, although 15 proteins are produced. The structural genes are *gag, pol,* and *env*. The *gag* gene and the *gag-pol* complex are translated into large polyproteins. These polyproteins are cleaved by a protease that is part of the Pol polyprotein. Gag polyprotein is cleaved into four proteins that are found in mature virions: matrix (MA), capsid (CA), nucleocapsid (NC), and p6 (a core protein). Pol polyprotein is cleaved into protease (PR) (a target for antiretroviral therapy), RT, and integrase (IN). The *env* gene codes for the envelope glycoprotein, gp160 (which comprises gp120 and gp41). The regulatory genes include *tat, rev, nef, vpr, vif,* and *vpu*. The gene *tat* (*t*rans-*a*ctivator of *t*ranscription) is a positive regulator of viral protein synthesis and produces the protein Tat, which is known to have direct neurotoxic effects.[1] The gene *vpr* (*v*iral *p*rotein *R*) produces a protein that can bind glucocorticoid receptors, enhancing glucocorticoid resistance and increasing stimulation of the limbic-hypothalamic-pituitary-adrenal axis. *vif* (*v*irion *i*nfectivity *f*actor) is known to control viral infectivity; the protein Vif is needed for production of infectious virus because it inhibits an antiviral pathway in the cells that involves a host enzyme called APOBEC3G. The Rev (*r*egulator of *v*irion protein *e*xpression) and Nef (*n*egative *r*egulatory *f*actor) proteins are involved in viral replication. Vpu (*v*iral *p*rotein *u*), among other functions, enhances viral particle release from the host cell.

The glycoprotein coat of HIV-1, referred to as gp160 (molecular weight 160 kilodaltons [kD]) comprises two major proteins, the globular portion gp120 and the transmembrane portion gp41. gp120 is of great importance because it interacts with the primary target of HIV-1, the CD4+ T "helper" lymphocyte, a critical cell for immune system function. gp120 contributes to HIV-1 infection of the CD4 cell by binding to the CD4 receptor, which is followed by a conformational change and then by binding to a coreceptor on the surface of the cell (Figure 2.1). These coreceptors include cysteine-cysteine chemokine receptor 5 (CCR5) (on monocytes and macrophages) and cysteine-X-cysteine receptor 4 (CXCR4) (on lymphocytes). gp41 then changes its conformation, allowing membrane fusion to occur between the CD4 cell's surface membrane and the viral glycoprotein envelope. It is through this mechanism that the viral core enters the cell. Once the core of HIV-1 has gained entry into the host cell, it is translocated to the nucleus. There, two outcomes may occur. The cell may begin a process of productive infection, or the cell may integrate HIV-1 into its genome (through the DNA complementary to the genomic RNA of HIV-1). In the latter case, the virus enters a latent (inactive) state (as a "provirus").

Various factors may cause viral replication to be reactivated from the latent state. Latency is abrogated when the CD4 cell is stimulated during the normal immune response. One stimulant to reactivation of replication from the latent state is nuclear factor NF kappa B (NFκB), a host transcription factor. The latent state is known to be established in a number of cells and tissues (including CD4+ T helper lymphocytes in the peripheral blood and in macrophages in brain tissue). On reactivation from the latent state, viral messenger RNAs (mRNAs) are transcribed, viral proteins are translated, and whole virions are packaged. In the case of the CD4 cell, these virions bud off of the cell surface, resulting in a lytic form of cell death.

In addition to the glycoprotein envelope proteins described above, the virus also has core proteins, including p24, p17, p7, and p6. Of these, p24 (molecular weight 24 kD) is the best known; in an earlier stage of the epidemic this protein was quantified in serum to assess the probability of HIV-1 disease progression. The level of production of the core antigen

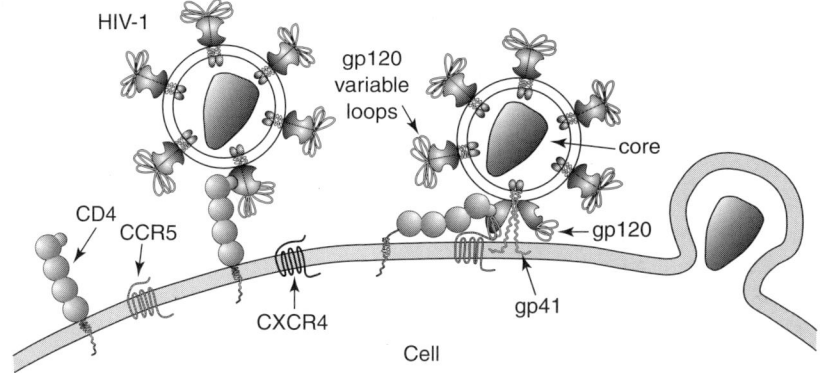

FIGURE 2.1 The hypervariable loop of gp120 (the globular portion of the envelope glycoprotein of HIV-1) binds to CD4 receptor (see interaction with HIV-1 at left). gp120 then changes its conformation and binds to one of the chemokine coreceptors for HIV-1 (e.g., CCR5 or CXCR4) (the latter in the interaction with HIV-1 at right). gp41 (the transmembrane portion of the envelope glycoprotein of HIV-1) then changes conformation, allowing fusion with the host cell membrane, culminating in viral entry (pictured at the far right). (Courtesy of HIV InSite, a project of the UCSF Center for HIV, hivinsite@ucsf.edu.)

correlated well with the level of production of whole virions. Thus, it was used as a surrogate measure of viral replication, which is directly related to the likelihood of clinical disease progression.[2] In fact, before the routine quantification of HIV-1 RNA copy number in plasma ("viral load"), the quantification of the p24 core antigen—enhanced by acid dissociation of antigen–antibody complexes ("complexed antigen") before measurement—was felt to hold great promise as a measure of viral replication and proxy for clinical disease progression. This measure has remained useful and is currently recommended as a surrogate marker for plasma viral load for resource-limited settings internationally.

PROCESS OF INITIAL INFECTION

It was discovered early that HIV-1 infects cells expressing CD4 receptor on their surfaces, particularly T helper lymphocytes and monocytes in the blood. Monocytes differentiate into macrophages that express CD4 receptor on migration into the tissues. More recently, coreceptors required for the entry of HIV-1 into the cell were discovered. Of great importance are CCR5 and CXCR4. CCR5-using strains predominate in the early phase and infect monocytes, which are known to carry HIV-1 into the brain past an intact blood–brain barrier (mediating the subsequent infectious process in brain). CXCR4 is the coreceptor on the CD4+ T lymphocyte. CXCR4-using strains are associated with disease progression and predominate in later stages of HIV-1 disease.

When HIV-1 replicates in CD4 cells, the progeny virions produced bud off the cell, causing a lytic form of cell death. In macrophages, the cell is not killed; instead, it becomes a warehouse for a large number of virions. The presence of these virions affects the macrophage's function in such a way that a chronic activated state is maintained. This activated state is associated with the secretion of several cytokines (soluble proteins released by immune cells that communicate with other cells). One of these cytokines, tumor necrosis factor-alpha (TNF-α) is associated with both demyelination and upregulation of HIV-1 replication. Another such cytokine, interleukin-1 (IL-1), is also associated with the upregulation of HIV-1 replication.

SYSTEMIC VIRAL PATHOGENESIS

HIV-1 depends on the CD4 cell for its replication and survival. As HIV-1 infection becomes established, antibodies are generated to its glycoprotein envelope. These antibodies are detected by the HIV antibody test, which is a combination of an enzyme-linked immunosorbent assay (ELISA) and a confirmatory, more specific test, the Western immunoblot assay. The HIV antibody test generally becomes positive an average of 6 weeks after exposure, although it can require as long as 6 months for this change to occur. Although longer periods for this process (termed seroconversion) have been described, this is now thought to be very rare.

When seroconversion has occurred and HIV-1 infection is initially established (versus an exposure after which no seroconversion occurs), the count of CD4 cells at this early point is generally maintained at a high level. However, this does not indicate a quiescent or latent stage, as was originally thought. Rather, the viral dynamics are very active at this stage, with 10^8 to 10^9 virions produced per day. The impact of this high level of viral replication is balanced by the capacity of the bone marrow to produce more CD4+ T lymphocytes at a daily rate of $2(10)^9$/day (5% of the body's total). Although the CD4 cell count does not change significantly in the peripheral blood during this period, there is a loss of lymph node architecture due to a similarly high level of activity of HIV-1 infection in the lymph nodes. As the infectious process progresses, the ability of the virus to replicate itself eventually overcomes the ability of the bone marrow to replace the killed lymphocytes. Thereafter the CD4 cell count in the peripheral blood declines and immunologic disease progression is the result.

SYSTEMIC IMMUNOPATHOGENESIS

Early in the process of HIV-1 infection, the CD4 cell count remains in the normal range and there is no clinical manifestation of the infection. However, as viral replication with CD4+ T lymphocyte death overcomes the replacement of CD4+ T lymphocytes by the bone marrow, the CD4 cell count begins to decline in the peripheral blood. When the CD4 cell count falls below 500 cells/mm^3, a clinically significant decrement has occurred. At this level of immune progression, the initiation of antiretroviral therapy has formally begun. However, more recently, the antiretroviral treatment guidelines have been modified to begin consideration of treatment at a CD4 cell count between 200 and 350 cells/mm^3, depending on the level of plasma viral load.[3] As the decline of CD4 cell number continues, the CD4 cell count eventually decreases below 200 cells/mm^3, a landmark value. At this point, AIDS is defined on a laboratory basis, regardless of whether there has been any evidence of clinical disease progression.[4] The risk for clinical disease is heightened at this severe immunologic stage of progression. Specifically, at this level, AIDS-indicator conditions commonly occur. Finally, at a CD4 cell count below 50 cells/mm^3, a very severe level of immunoprogression has occurred in which the risk for mortality within 6 months increases.

The immunopathogenesis of HIV-1 infection is not solely related to the decline of the CD4 cell count over time. For example, the CD8+ T lymphocyte cell subset generally expands and becomes activated, as measured by coexpression of CD38 and HLA-DR.[5] In addition, there is a shift in the pattern of cytokines produced by the CD4+ T lymphocytes over time. The level of cytokines produced by the subset known as Th1 cells decreases, while the level of those produced by the Th2 subset increases. As the Th1 cytokines (e.g., interferon-γ [IFN-γ], IL-2, and IL-12) stimulate cellular immune functions, their decrement is associated with decreased immunologic monitoring of HIV-1 infection by cytotoxic T lymphocytes (CTLs) and systemic disease progression. The Th2 cytokines, in contrast, increase and are associated with stimulation of the humoral immune system and with abnormal, chronic, polyclonal B lymphocyte stimulation in HIV-1 infection. These changes are likewise associated with systemic disease progression.

PATHOPHYSIOLOGY OF CENTRAL NERVOUS SYSTEM DISEASE

Before the introduction of today's highly active antiretroviral therapy (HAART) regimens (now referred to as combination antiretroviral therapy [CART]), the cumulative prevalence of HIV-1–associated dementia (HAD) over the course of AIDS could be expected to be 21%, with an incidence rate during AIDS of about 7% a year.[6] After the implementation of CART, the incidence rate of HAD has been documented to have decreased by 40% to 50% in the United States. The HAD prevalence rate has been suggested to have decreased to a lesser extent than the incidence rate because HAD patients are now living longer.

Minor cognitive motor disorder (MCMD) is a diagnosis that can properly be associated with the early symptomatic disease stage or with AIDS. It formerly was expected to be prevalent in as many as 25% of early symptomatic patients and as many as 50% of late symptomatic patients. However, recent data suggest that the incidence of MCMD, like that of HAD, has been reduced by CART. Currently, the cumulative prevalence rate of MCMD has been estimated at 14% in the early symptomatic stage and at 24.4% in AIDS.

HAD has been noted to be associated with ventricular enlargement and with cortical atrophy (as well as with brain atrophy generally). However, brain atrophy is not necessarily associated with the development of cognitive-motor disorder and is a nonspecific measure of risk for it. HIV-1 infection of brain has been widely described as a subcortical disease. In the basal ganglia, atrophy of the caudate nucleus has been noted to occur with HAD and has been specifically associated with decreased performance on neuropsychological (NP) tests requiring psychomotor speed, manual dexterity, sustained attention, and flexibility of set shifting and sequencing. Likewise, white matter lesions are seen in HIV-1 infection of the brain. Although white matter hyperintensities on T2-weighted structural magnetic resonance imaging (MRI) imaging have been challenged regarding their clinical import, leukoariosis has been associated with decreased information processing speed. In contrast, cortical dysfunction has been thought to be restricted to late-stage HIV-1 disease in the brain.

HIV-1 penetrates into brain tissue as early as 2 weeks after infection, but rarely, if ever, directly infects neurons. Of seven brain regions examined in one important study, the hippocampus (Ammon's horn) and the basal ganglia demonstrated the highest genomic HIV-1 RNA loads, with cerebellar and midfrontal cortices showing lower loads.[7] An excess of multispliced RNAs over single-spliced RNAs suggests a contribution by abortive HIV-1 infection.[8] Abortive infection in brain is related to the transient and restricted infection of astrocytes. Although abortive, this form of infection nevertheless expands the total viral burden in brain beyond the combination of genomic RNA (representing recent replication) and proviral DNA (representing the archive of virus infecting brain tissue).

Of note regarding a measure described earlier, significant correlations of free p24 antigen level in cerebrospinal fluid (CSF) have been reported with HIV-1 associated neurologic disease, especially in HAD patients. One study found a significant negative correlation ($r = -0.31$, $p = .03$) between a global NP z-score from a 23-score NP test battery and the total p24 antigen level in serum in a sample of 214 HIV-1–seropositive individuals with cognitive-motor impairment.[9] In contrast, the correlation of this z-score with the free p24 antigen level was not significant. Hence, empirical data exist to support that the total p24 antigen level may prove advantageous over free p24 antigen levels for monitoring NP impairment in HIV-1–infected individuals, as is true for the prediction of systemic disease progression. The p24 core antigen is a viral product for which no direct toxicity has been described, though it may reflect the overall discrepancy between replication of whole virions and the elaboration of viral products (some of which have established toxicity for brain tissue). With the inefficiency of HIV-1 replication over time, as well as the use of protease inhibitors in CART regimens, specific viral proteins are produced that are not packaged into whole virions but are nevertheless toxic in and of themselves.

The sequence of gp120 comprises five hypervariable domains (V1 to V5), interspersed among relatively conserved regions. The "third" hypervariable domain (the V3 loop) contains an epitope localized at its tip (the crown tetrapeptide), which acts as the major binding site for type-specific neutralizing antibodies and as an epitope for CTL activity against virus-infected cells. Variation in sequence analysis of gp120 has been related to the regional clustering of HIV-1 across brain regions.[10] The functional relevance of this viral diversity for increased neurovirulence or CTL immunologic escape may account for a possible association of specific HIV-1 variants with the cognitive-motor disorders.

Tat protein, like gp120, carries its own neurotoxicity. Tat increases intracellular free calcium levels in a dose-dependent fashion. It also increases glutamate-induced excitotoxicity, a favored mechanism associated with neuronal cell death in HIV-1 infection and, in turn, with the therapeutic rationale for memantine. Moreover, Tat has been demonstrated to increase monocyte chemoattractant protein (MCP)-1, drawing monocytes to the site of infection. Tat (and gp120 as well) may induce neuronal apoptosis (or programmed cell death). Thus Tat antagonists are being developed therapeutically.

Regardless of viral load (measured by genomic RNA or by proviral DNA) and the additional burden of viral proteins in the brain, the inflammatory response to HIV-1 is a largely independent pathophysiologic focus for the cognitive-motor disorders that has continued to be a principal research focus. Macrophages infected by HIV-1 become chronically activated and produce proinflammatory cytokines. As mentioned earlier, TNF-α is one of the most frequently cited cytokines regarding potential destructive effects in the brain. TNF-α induces a nuclear factor 6B (NF6B), the host transcriptional factor that stimulates viral reactivation from the latent state. NF6B is a cytoplasmic factor that dissociates from an inhibitory protein (I6B) and translocates to the cell nucleus, binding to the enhancer sequence of the long terminal repeat (LTR) and activating HIV-1 replication. Neurotoxic effects may also be seen with chronic overexpression of interleukin (IL)-1 (produced by activated macrophages as well). Such effects may also be seen with the β isoform of S100, a small (10 kD), soluble calcium-binding protein synthesized and released by astroglia that is associated with increased nitric oxide concentrations. Increased nitric oxide concentrations are, in turn, associated with neuronal cell loss. Like TNF-α and IL-1, IL-6 is a proinflammatory cytokine produced on macrophage activation. This cytokine has been associated with an increased production of autoantibodies, including brain-reactive antibodies. One such brain-reactive antibody is the antisulfatide antibody; however, this type of antibody could also be produced as an epiphenomenon of myelin destruction. IFN-γ is a cytokine that is salutary for CTL function in the periphery but may be damaging in the central nervous system (CNS), because macrophages stimulated with IFN-γ in vitro produce large amounts of quinolinic acid, a neurotoxin and convulsant.[11] IFN-α, another type of interferon, may cause specific CNS neuronal damage associated with Parkinsonism, which occurs in early CNS HIV-1 infection. In contrast to the previously discussed cytokines, IL-4 is known to suppress macrophage activation and is salutary in the CNS, although it is a Th2 cytokine known to be associated with systemic disease progression in the periphery.

Much less research has been conducted on the specific association of the chemokines with HIV-1–associated cognitive-motor disorder than has been conducted with the larger group of cytokines. Chemokines are a subgroup of cytokines that are specifically involved in regulation of the process of inflammation through the mobilization and activation of white blood cells. They are protective against HIV-1 infection of the cell by occupying their own receptors, which are the coreceptors for HIV-1. However, in the CNS, their endogenous effects of enhancing the inflammatory process may prove deleterious. For example, CSF levels of MCP-1 are correlated with CSF viral load and with the severity of HAD. Macrophage inflammatory protein (MIP)-1α, MIP-1β, and "regulated on activation, normal T-cell expressed and secreted" (RANTES) have been shown to upregulate the secretion of matrix metalloproteinases (MMPs). MMPs disrupt the basal lamina underlying brain capillary endothelium and damage the blood–brain barrier. Thus, repeated bursts of macrophage activation over time may be associated with cycles of MMP secretion that impair the integrity of the blood–brain barrier. This would promote HIV-1–infected monocyte infiltration, microglial activation, and the enhancement of an inflammatory focus in the brain through recruitment of additional activated macrophages to the site.

TRANSMISSION

Transmission of HIV-1 infection may be accomplished by high-risk sexual behaviors, injection substance use, giving birth ("vertical" transmission), breast feeding, and other means of blood or mucocutaneous tissue exposure to HIV-1–infected body fluids (including inadequate HIV preventive techniques during blood transfusion and other medical procedures, as well as occupational exposures). HIV-1 does not survive well in the environment, rendering the probability of environmental transmission remote.[12] Although HIV-1 has been transmitted in a household setting, this type of transmission is very rare and is thought to result from exposure of skin or mucous membrane to infected blood. There is no risk identified for HIV-1 transmission to co-workers, clients, or consumers from industries such as food-service establishments or personal service industries (such as hairdressers, barbers, cosmetologists, and massage therapists). There is also no risk identified for HIV-1 transmission through contact with saliva, tears, or perspiration. Insect bites, likewise, are not associated with HIV-1 transmission risk. Closed-mouth ("social") kissing does not present an HIV transmission risk; however, open-mouth ("French") kissing is thought to represent a very low risk. Similarly, a human bite represents a very low HIV transmission risk. When consistently and correctly used, latex and polyurethane condoms prevent pregnancy in 98% of cases, conferring a high degree of protection against sexually transmitted disease, including HIV-1, as well.

Regarding sexual activity, in "pattern I" countries, men who have sex with men (MSM) have been the initial group most widely infected in the epidemic. In "pattern II" countries, heterosexual transmission was the major route of HIV-1 transmission from the beginning of the epidemic. The increased HIV-1 transmission risk associated with rectal intercourse in both epidemiologic patterns relates to the fact that the rectal mucosa is more friable than the vaginal mucosa. This issue is equally relevant for heterosexuals and MSM during rectal intercourse, although rectal intercourse had been a previously underestimated sexual behavior amongst heterosexuals. With rectal intercourse, increased exposure to blood occurs and, with such an exposure, an increased risk of HIV-1 transmission occurs as well. It has been found that there is greater risk of exposure to HIV-1 for the receptive partner than for the insertive partner during rectal intercourse. Regarding heterosexual transmission, it has been found that there is a greater risk for male-to-female transmission than for female-to-male transmission in European and U.S. populations. The transmission risk per coital act (i.e., infectivity) for vaginal intercourse has been estimated to vary from 1/10,000 to 14/10,000. Higher transmission rates of 56/1,000 to 1 in 10 have been reported among men who have had sexual contacts with commercial sex workers in Thailand and Kenya.[13] Other factors that increase transmission risk include a high plasma viral load and a low CD4 cell count.

Injection substance use is another major source of HIV-1 transmission risk. This route yields an increased risk for transmission due to direct exposure of the virus to the blood. Injection use in "shooting galleries" may be related to a particularly high risk, because virus may be transmitted not only by direct needle sharing but also by sharing of the equipment used to prepare psychoactive substances for injection over time.[14] Programs teaching injection substance users how to clean needles with bleach and programs distributing free needles and syringes have been associated with decreased HIV-1 transmission in this population, although the introduction of such programs has created controversy surrounding the attendant ethical issues. It should be noted that injection substance users also may be exposed to HIV-1 through sexual activity with HIV-1–infected partners. In addition, use of substances by noninjection routes (drinking alcohol and inhaling cocaine) are also associated with increased HIV-1 transmission risk, indirectly, by increasing the likelihood that risk reduction practices will not be observed.

Originally, vertical transmission was estimated to be a route with a transmission rate of 30% to 45% with breast feeding (18 to 24 months) and of 15% to 25% without breast feeding.[15] Studies suggest that transmission risk during passage through the vaginal canal may be more important than fetal exposure to HIV-1. Thus Cesarean section is recommended for pregnant HIV-1–seropositive women. Breast feeding itself has been difficult to link with a clearly determined level of HIV-1 transmission risk; however, it has been determined that colostrum (the milk first expressed) is no different from later breast milk in HIV-1 transmission risk. Vertical transmission risk, overall, can be relatively easily addressed by the combination of effective HIV-1 antibody test screening of pregnant women, antiretroviral therapy at the time of birth, and the avoidance of breast feeding. International studies have shown that a single dose of nevirapine before birth is effective in averting vertical transmission, expanding the availability of this prevention technique to resource-limited settings worldwide. It is recommended that the avoidance of breast feeding in HIV-1–seropositive women should be uniform, because mixing breast feeding with use of infant milk formulas has been associated with a higher transmission risk than that occurring with breast feeding alone. After zidovudine (formerly "AZT" [azidothymidine]) was FDA approved in 1987, the target of elimination of vertical transmission was viewed as eventually attainable. In the landmark national AIDS Clinical Trials Group 076 study, zidovudine treatment (given to the mother [prenatally and intrapartum] and to the baby [postpartum]) decreased vertical transmission from 25.5% to 8.3%. If plasma viral load is suppressed below 1,000 HIV-1 RNA copies/ml, vertical transmission can be further decreased to 1% to 2%. Progress toward the international goal of minimizing vertical transmission will continue to improve with expanded access to antiretroviral medications.

HIV-1 exposure through inadequate medical care can occur in numerous situations. Before the routine screening of blood banks in the United States for HIV by the HIV-1 antibody test in 1985, blood transfusion was associated with a significant transmission rate. In fact, transfusion recipients currently remain relatively numerous among the subgroup of older HIV-1–seropositive persons (defined by the Centers for Disease Control and Prevention [CDC] as ≤50 years old). The most frequent form of exposure through medical care worldwide involves the reuse of needles because of insufficient resources for obtaining new needles or for cleaning needles after each use (in resource-limited settings). Another type of exposure associated with medical care is accidental exposure by needle stick, estimated to be associated with a transmission risk of 1/250 without intervention. This form of exposure can be essentially reduced to nil with proper use of CART prophylaxis postexposure, per current CDC guidelines.[16] It should also be pointed out here that nonoccupational postexposure prophylaxis has been shown to be effective as well and that the CDC has recently disseminated guidelines for the use of this prevention technique.[17]

Though great strides have been made in stemming the tide of the HIV epidemic in the United States, an estimated 40,000 new cases continue to be reported annually. The CDC has now set a goal of preventing half of these cases.[18] In 2004, the CDC provided $415.5 million to state and local health departments to achieve this goal, of the $668 million total budgeted domestically for HIV-1 prevention. It may be concluded that it is now time for a cost-effectiveness approach to HIV-1 prevention, which can and should be both empirically derived and quantitative.

PROGRESSION OF THE DISEASE PROCESS

The clinical progression of HIV-1 infection comprises several well-defined stages. After initial exposure, the acute phase of HIV-1 infection occurs and symptoms occur in 40% to 90% of patients. This phase is incorporated within the asymptomatic clinical stage of disease, which is typically accompanied by a normal or minimally decreased CD4 cell count (seen in CDC immunologic Stage 1).[4] The asymptomatic stage can continue for over a decade without antiretroviral therapy. This stage is eventually followed by the first symptoms referable to HIV-1, which are typically those seen in the early symptomatic stage (with a moderate decline in the CD4 cell count). The early symptomatic stage comprises non–AIDS-defining conditions such as CDC-defined "constitutional" symptoms (weight loss of at least 10% and diarrhea) and non–AIDS-defining infections such as "thrush" (oral candidiasis) and oral hairy leukoplakia. Finally, with a severe CD4 cell count decline, the late symptomatic stage (AIDS) is defined. The late symptomatic stage is documented by the occurrence of clinical AIDS-defining conditions (e.g., *Pneumocystis jeroveci* [previously named *carinii*] pneumonia [PCP] and Kaposi's sarcoma) or by a CD4 cell count less than 200 cells/mm^3.[4] With CART today, there is significant immune reconstitution and increases in the CD4 cell count post-treatment. Thus the parallel predictive clinical utility of the CD4 cell count pre-CART can be provided now only by a historical review for the CD4 nadir (the lowest documented CD4 cell count) rather than by a recent CD4 cell count with the patient on treatment.

ACUTE HIV INFECTION

The diagnosis of acute infection is missed in the majority of cases, because other viral illnesses (e.g., the flu) are often assumed to be the cause of the symptoms. Thus the diagnosis therefore requires a high degree of clinical suspicion. Following HIV transmission, approximately 40% to 90% of individuals will develop a flulike illness with most or all of the following: swollen lymph nodes, oral ulcers, rash, myalgia, sore throat, headache, diarrhea, and nausea or vomiting. A small number will develop hepatosplenomegaly. In 12% of patients the symptoms may be neurologic or neuropsychiatric. The onset of symptomatic acute HIV-1 infection occurs 1 to 6 weeks after exposure and may continue for 1 to 3 weeks. It should be noted that the HIV antibody test may be negative at this time, although quantitative HIV-1 RNA polymerase chain reaction testing or a complementary HIV-1 DNA test may be positive.

Extremely high levels of HIV-1 RNA copy number are seen in the peripheral blood during the acute stage. Within 2 weeks, HIV-1 reaches sanctuary sites (lymph nodes, brain, skin, the reticuloendothelial system, gastrointestinal cells, and bone marrow) (Figure 2.2). Safer sex practices must be emphasized at this stage to decrease the likelihood of transmission to others. A very high plasma viral load persists until 4 months post-transmission, when a viral set point is generally reached. The set point reached is known to be predictive of the subsequent clinical course of disease. A higher than average set point is consistent with rapid disease progression, whereas a lower than average set point is consistent with delayed disease progression.

ASYMPTOMATIC STAGE

After the acute phase of HIV-1 infection, asymptomatic infection is observed. During this period there are no clinical symptoms of the infectious process or signs on physical examination. Some patients without symptoms may demonstrate enlarged lymph nodes (persistent generalized lymphadenopathy [PGL]). For the purposes of the CDC, acute HIV-1–infected patients, patients with PGL, and postacute, asymptomatic patients without PGL are all categorized as CDC clinical disease stage A. Destruction of CD4 cells is actively ongoing during this stage, although it is first confined to the lymph nodes. Later, this process starts to deplete the

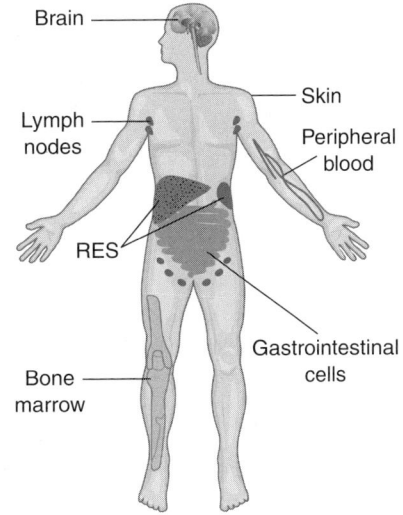

FIGURE 2.2 Shortly after initial infection, HIV-1 reaches sanctuary sites where it may become latent and is protected from the immune response and the effects of treatment (lymph nodes, brain, skin, the reticuloendothelial system, gastrointestinal cells, and bone marrow). The brain has been documented to be a large reservoir for HIV-1 provirus. (Courtesy Anthony Fauci, MD, Formulating a Comprehensive HIV/AIDS Research Agenda in Developing Countries symposium, First International AIDS Society Conference on HIV Pathogenesis and Treatment, Buenos Aires, Argentina, July 7, 2001.

CD4 cell count in the peripheral blood, becoming abnormal slowly and without clinical evidence of immunodeficiency until the CD4 cell count decreases below 500 cells/mm^3. This is consonant with a change from the mild immunologic stage ($\leq$500 cells/mm^3, Stage 1) of HIV-1 disease to the moderate stage (200 to 499 cells/mm^3, Stage 2).[4] Concomitantly, plasma viral load steadily increases over this stage in the absence of effective antiretroviral treatment. Individuals may remain at this apparently inactive clinical stage (formerly inaccurately referred to as the "latent" stage) for 12 to 15 years without treatment. The actual length of this stage in a particular patient is affected by how high the viral load set point is and by the starting point of antiretroviral therapy.

EARLY SYMPTOMATIC STAGE

In the early symptomatic CDC clinical disease Stage B, the first symptom referable to HIV-1 infection occurs (unless that symptom is a symptom of an AIDS-defining condition). Many patients experience nonspecific, constitutional symptoms at this stage; thus this transition can frequently occur without the suspicion of the patient or primary health care provider. This may also be true with the occurrence of non–AIDS-defining infections as well, such as oral hairy leukoplakia. However, some symptoms experienced at this stage cause clear-cut discomfort and bring the individual to seek medical attention, such as oral candidiasis, peripheral neuropathy, MCMD, and recurrent multidermatomal herpes zoster.[4] Other diseases that typically occur during this stage are cervical dysplasia, listeriosis, and pelvic inflammatory disease. Although it is no longer common to initiate CART with a treatment-naïve, asymptomatic patient having a CD4 cell count of 500 cells/mm^3 or higher, CART is recommended for all treatment-naïve, symptomatic patients. It is also recommended for treatment-naïve, asymptomatic patients with a CD4 cell count of 350 cells/mm^3 or less; provisions are also made in the current recommendations for initiation of treatment for those asymptomatic patients with a CD4 cell count greater than 350 cells/mm^3, if the plasma viral load is 100,000 HIV-1 RNA copies/ml or greater.[3]

LATE SYMPTOMATIC STAGE

When the CD4 cell count declines below 200 cells/mm^3, the severe level of immunologic progression is defined (CDC immunologic Stage 3). This CD4 cell count also defines a case of AIDS, regardless of prior clinical symptomatology.[4] However, it is uncommon for individuals to reach this stage of immunologic decline without any prior clinical symptoms. Independently of the CD4 cell count, the late symptomatic clinical stage may be clinically defined by the list of AIDS-indicator conditions (or AIDS-defining illnesses). These conditions include: PCP, candidal esophagitis, *Mycobacterium avium* complex (MAC) infection, CNS toxoplasmosis, progressive multifocal leukoencephalopathy, extrapulmonary tuberculosis, invasive squamous cell carcinoma of the cervix, Kaposi's sarcoma, and cytomegalovirus (CMV) disease (e.g., retinitis, hepatitis). Another of these conditions is HAD, which occurs as the AIDS-defining illness in 5% to 10% of persons with AIDS.

Changes in antiretroviral therapy frequently may be called for during this stage, including the use of "salvage regimens." These regimens may offer limited immune reconstitution potential but nevertheless are preferable to alternative regimens shown to be liable to antiretroviral medication resistance demonstrated by genotypic or phenotypic viral resistance monitoring techniques. In genotypic monitoring, the RNA sequence of the virus determines the potential for resistance to antiretroviral medications in the major classes of the nucleoside reverse transcriptase inhibitors, non-nucleoside reverse transcriptase inhibitors, protease inhibitors, and fusion/entry inhibitors. With phenotypic resistance monitoring, the process of viral replication is monitored in response to specific antiretroviral agents. The late symptomatic clinical disease stage is also characterized by the use of primary and secondary prophylactic therapies. These include the prevention of PCP using trimethoprim/sulfamethoxazole, dapsone, or atovaquone when the CD4 cell count decreases below 200 cells/mm^3. When the CD4 cell count drops further, to fewer than 50 cells/mm^3, primary MAC prophylaxis is indicated with azithromycin or clarithromycin.

A decrease to this level is also consistent with an increased risk of mortality within the following 6 months. Nevertheless, in the CART era, a significant improvement has been made in the longevity of this group. In addition to the decreased incidence of AIDS diagnoses and HIV-related deaths (50% or more), the causes of death have changed since the introduction of CART. Deaths resulting from non-AIDS illnesses and suicide have increased. Deaths due to cardiovascular disease, renal disease, and viral coinfections (such as hepatitis C virus), as well as bacterial infections and systemic lymphoma, have also risen. Although the overall mortality rate has clearly decreased in the CART era, HIV-1–seropositive persons still have an abnormally high death rate—about 7.8 times higher than that of the general population. Further, there has been a slowing in the rate of decline in the mortality rate since 1997. This suggests that a concern for the future will be how to avert an increased rate of failure of current antiretroviral therapy regimens due to medication resistance, toxicities, and other causes.

SUMMARY

In this chapter we have reviewed the HIV-1 infectious process from the points of view of virology, immunology, the process of initial infection, systemic viral pathogenesis, systemic immunopathogenesis, CNS pathogenesis, viral transmission, and clinical disease progression (across the acute, asymptomatic, early symptomatic, and late symptomatic disease presentations). HIV-1 is a retrovirus with a high capacity for response to its microenvironment and to the pressure to mutate in the setting of CART. The process of initial infection at the cellular level involves the interactions of viral components, predominantly the glycoprotein coat (gp120 and gp41) of HIV-1, with host cells bearing the CD4 receptor and chemokine coreceptors (such as CXCR4 and CCR5). Transmission may occur by sexual activity, injection substance use, birth, breast feeding, as well as inadequate protections and accidental exposures in the medical care environment. Immunopathogenesis is associated not only with decreases in the function and (subsequently) the number of CD4+ T lymphocytes but also with abnormal increases in immunologic activation that occur with HIV-1 infection over time. In the CNS, some effects may be opposite to those occurring in the periphery. CNS HIV-1 disease is thought to be mediated primarily by indirect effects of the virus manifested by the extent of the inflammatory process. The clinical disease presentations of acute HIV-1 infection, the asymptomatic stage, the early symptomatic stage, and the late symptomatic stage/AIDS were explicitly reviewed. Following acute HIV-1 infection (during which plasma viral load is very high), with subsequent disease progression, the CD4 cell count in the peripheral blood tends to decline in parallel with an increase in plasma viral load (without treatment). This progression may be significantly deterred by current-day CART regimens; however, regardless of optimal control of viral replication indicated by nondetectable levels of HIV-1 RNA copy number in the plasma, active viral replication is not eliminated and HIV-1 nevertheless finds sanctuary in selected areas of the body, including the brain. Over time, in the face of CART, the infectious process may still continue to the point that severe immunodeficiency or treatment toxicities are reached, resulting in an increased likelihood of mortality.

ACKNOWLEDGMENTS

I acknowledge NIMH grants MH58532 and MH/AG61629 and NIDA grant DA018085.

REFERENCES

1. Bansal AK, Mactutus CF, Nath A, et al. Neurotoxicity of HIV-1 proteins gp120 and Tat in the rat striatum. *Brain Res.* 2000;879:42–49.
2. Fiscus SA, Wallmark EB, Folds JD, et al. Detection of infectious immune complexes in human immunodeficiency virus type 1 (HIV-1) infections: correlation with plasma viremia and CD4 cell counts. *J Infect Dis.* 1991;164:765–769.
3. U.S. Department of Health and Human Services. *Guidelines for the Use of Antiretroviral Agents in HIV-1 Infected Adults and Adolescents.* Washington, DC: U.S. Department of Health and Human Services; April 7, 2005.
4. Centers for Disease Control and Prevention. 1993 revised classification system for HIV infection and expanded surveillance case definition for AIDS among adolescents and adults. *MMWR Morb Mort Wkly Rep.* 1992;41:1–19.
5. Ho HN, Hultin LE, Mitsuyasu RT, et al. Circulating HIV-specific CD8+ cytotoxic T cells express CD38 and HLA-DR antigens. *J Immunol.* 1993;150:3070–3079.
6. McArthur JC, Hoover DR, Bacellar H, et al. Dementia in AIDS patients: incidence and risk factors. *Neurology.* 1993;43:2245–2252.
7. Wiley CA, Soontornniyomkij V, Radhakrishnan L, et al. Distribution of brain HIV load in AIDS. *Brain Pathol.* 1998;8:277–284.
8. Fujimura RK, Khamis I, Shapshak P, Goodkin K. Regional quantitative comparison of multispliced to unspliced ratios of HIV-1 RNA copy number in infected human brain. *J Neuro AIDS.* 2004;2:45–60.
9. Goodkin K, Wilkie F, Vitiello B, et al. HIV-1 induced cognitive impairment and p24 antigen levels. In: *The 150th Meeting of the American Psychiatric Association: New Research Abstracts.* Washington, DC: American Psychiatric Association; 1997:153.
10. Shapshak P, Segal SM, Crandall KA, et al. Independent evolution of HIV type 1 in different brain regions. *AIDS Res Hum Retrovir.* 1999;15:811–820.
11. Shapshak P, Duncan R, Minagar A, et al. Elevated expression of IFN-gamma in the HIV-1 infected brain. *Front Biosci.* 2004;9:1073–1081.
12. Centers for Disease Control and Prevention. *HIV and its transmission* (fact sheet). Available at: http://www.cdc.gov/hiv/pubs/facts/transmission.htm. Accessed 2006.
13. Gray RH, Wawer MJ, Brookmeyer R, et al. Probability of HIV-1 transmission per coital act in monogamous, heterosexual, HIV-1-discordant couples in Rakai, Uganda. *Lancet.* 2001;357:1149–1153.
14. Shah SM, Shapshak P, Rivers JE, et al. Detection of HIV-1 DNA in needle/syringes, paraphernalia, and washes from shooting galleries in Miami: a preliminary report. *J Acquir Immun Defic Syndr.* 1996;11:301–306.
15. World Health Organization. *HIV Transmission Through Breastfeeding: A Review of Available Evidence.* Geneva: World Health Organization; 2004:1–25.
16. Centers for Disease Control and Prevention. *Updated U.S. Public Health Service Guidelines for the Management of Occupational Exposures to HIV and Recommendations for Postexposure Prophylaxis.* Atlanta: Centers for Disease Control and Prevention; September 30, 2005.
17. Centers for Disease Control and Prevention. *Management of Possible Sexual, Injecting-Drug-Use, or Other Nonoccupational Exposure to HIV, Including Considerations Related to Antiretroviral Therapy.* Atlanta: Centers for Disease Control and Prevention; January 21, 2005.
18. Cohen D, Wu S-Y, Farley TA. Cost-effective allocation of government funds to prevent HIV infection. *Health Aff.* 2005;24:915–926.

CHAPTER 3

Medical Treatment and Occupational Exposure

Ellen A. B. Morrison, Jon A. Levenson

In the early years of the acquired immunodeficiency syndrome (AIDS) epidemic, AIDS was a rapidly fatal disease. Patients died of infections caused by opportunistic pathogens, microbes that do not usually cause disease in people who are immunologically normal or from wasting, malignancies, and a variety of other complications. The survival of individuals with AIDS improved over time because of advances in diagnosing and treating the complications that result from advanced immunosuppression. Beginning in the mid-1990s, the development of effective antiretroviral combination therapies made it possible to actually suppress the human immunodeficiency virus (HIV). Antiretroviral treatment strategies have led to dramatically reduced risk of opportunistic infections, improved functional status, and astounding improvements in patient survival.[1] Although the opportunistic infections, malignancies, and neurologic problems characteristic of advanced AIDS are now theoretically avoidable, these complications remain commonplace.[2] Failure to diagnosis HIV infection before advanced immunosuppression, nonadherence to medications, complex psychosocial- and mental health–related issues, and problems with the long-term efficacy and tolerability of current HIV treatment regimens are all contributing factors.

HIV DIAGNOSIS AND INITIAL MEDICAL EVALUATION

The diagnosis of HIV infection is made by the detection of antibodies against HIV in blood or oral secretions. Rapid HIV antibody tests, which are easy to use and provide results in as little as 10 minutes, have been developed in recent years. These tests are quite accurate; sensitivities and specificities are comparable to those of the standard serum enzyme-linked immunosorbent assay tests that have been used for many years. Because false positive results may occur with any methodology, a second test (usually a Western blot) is required to confirm the diagnosis.

The initial medical evaluation of a newly diagnosed HIV-infected patient focuses on determining the current extent of immunologic damage, as reflected in the CD4 count, and the rate of disease progression, as determined by a quantitative assay of HIV-1 ribonucleic acid (RNA). Recommendations for the initial medical evaluation, including laboratory testing, and immunizations are summarized in Table 3.1.

TABLE 3.1	Initial Medical Evaluation of the Newly Diagnosed HIV-Infected Patient
History and examination	History should address sexual behaviors, substance use (including tobacco), the importance of notifying exposed partners, knowledge about HIV, mental health and coping, diagnosis disclosure, and other psychosocial needs
	Examination should be complete and comprehensive, including funduscopic, genitourinary, and cognitive/neurologic examinations
HIV staging and assessment	Quantitative plasma HIV-1 RNA (viral load)
	CD4 cell count
	HIV genotype* (if patient recently infected or in geographic areas where resistant strains are prevalent)
Other laboratory tests	Complete blood count, glucose-6-phosphate dehydrogenase,* electrolytes, blood urea nitrogen, creatinine, fasting blood glucose, liver function tests, amylase, lipid panel, serologic testing for *Toxoplasma* spp., syphilis, cytomegalovirus, hepatitis B, C, and A,* screening for other sexually transmitted diseases (especially gonorrhea chlamydia)
Cervical Papanicolaou smear (females)	
Tuberculin skin test	
Chest radiograph*	
Vaccinations	*Streptococcus pneumoniae*, influenzae, hepatitis B, hepatitis A*
Infection prophylaxis	Based on CD4 count (refer to text)
Routine health maintenance	

*Applicable to some patients or advised by some authorities.
Adapted from Hammer S. Management of newly diagnosed HIV infection. *N Engl J Med*. 2005;353:1702–1710; Aberg JA, Gallant JE, Anderson J, et al. Primary care guidelines for the management of persons infected with human immunodeficiency virus: recommendations of the HIV Medicine Association of the Infectious Diseases Society of America. *Clin Infect Dis*. 2004;39:609–629.

TREATMENT OF THE MEDICAL COMPLICATIONS OF HIV

Increased susceptibility to medical problems begins early in HIV infection. Early manifestations of HIV may include community-acquired bacterial pneumonia, outbreaks of oral or genital herpes, zoster (shingles), pulmonary tuberculosis, or cervical dysplasia (abnormalities that may progress to cervical cancer). Malignancies, including cervical or vulvar cancer, anal cancer, Kaposi's sarcoma, and B cell lymphomas may occur in early HIV infection, even when the CD4 count suggests that immunosuppression is mild. Because these illnesses are common in the general population, the possibility of underlying HIV infection is often overlooked.

The likelihood of complications increases further as HIV-related immunosuppression advances. Although current knowledge does not predict exactly when a given patient will begin to suffer from opportunistic infections or other medical complications of HIV infection, there is reasonable correlation between the patient's CD4 count and the development of complicating illnesses. The CD4 count at which patients become susceptible to infection has been defined for most common opportunistic pathogens. As the CD4 count drops further, the risk of infection continues to increase.

Although there is some geographic variability in opportunistic infections, primarily reflecting geographic variability in exposure to microorganisms, the infections reviewed here represent the most common opportunistic infections of HIV in the developed world. This represents a brief overview, but more extensive reviews are readily available.[2]

PNEUMOCYSTIS PNEUMONIA

Pneumocystis jiroveci (previously named *P. carinii*) is a fungus that causes pneumonia in patients with advanced HIV infection (CD4 count <200) or other severe immune impairment, such as immunosuppression from organ transplantation or cancer chemotherapy. Early in the AIDS epidemic, *Pneumocystis* pneumonia (PCP) was the AIDS-defining illness for more than 60% of HIV-infected patients and was a leading cause of death. PCP continues to be a common presenting illness for patients who have undiagnosed HIV infection.

Improved techniques for diagnosing PCP using bronchoscopy or sputum induction, use of monoclonal antibodies for the detection of *P. jiroveci* in sputum or bronchoscopy specimens, availability of effective antibiotics, and use of adjuvant steroids for patients with severe pneumonia have significantly decreased the morbidity and mortality from this infection. Treatment of PCP requires a prolonged course (3 weeks) of antibiotics. Effective antibiotics include combinations of trimethoprim and sulfamethoxazole, clindamycin and primaquine, or dapsone and trimethoprim or single-agent therapy with pentamidine, trimetrexate, or atovaquone. Steroids may be added to prevent the worsening of oxygenation that is otherwise common early in treatment. Guidelines for adding steroids are based on abnormalities in the patient's oxygenation.

More importantly, PCP can be prevented by the ongoing administration of low doses of trimethoprim and sulfamethoxazole, dapsone, or atovaquone. It is standard practice to prescribe these antibiotics to symptomatic HIV-infected individuals or those who have CD4 counts under 200. This practice, termed primary prophylaxis, has dramatically decreased morbidity and mortality from PCP.

TOXOPLASMA GONDII

Toxoplasma gondii is a parasite that causes focal encephalitis in patients who have advanced HIV infection. The initial infection is acquired by eating infected, undercooked lamb, pork, or beef or by the ingestion of oocysts shed into the environment in the feces of infected cats. After ingestion, the parasite migrates and encysts in tissues throughout the body. Although this may cause fever and lymphadenopathy, it is usually a mild, self-limited illness that does not come to clinical attention. Subsequently, toxoplasmosis remains as asymptomatic, quiescent cysts in a variety of body sites.

HIV-infected patients with advanced immunosuppression (usually those who have CD4 counts <100) may experience a reactivation of infection, most commonly in the central nervous system (CNS). Patients present with focal neurologic abnormalities such as hemiplegia, tremor, diplopia, or more generalized CNS symptoms such as headache, personality change, confusion, lethargy, disorientation, coma, myoclonus, or seizures. Neurologic abnormalities can be quite profound, making it difficult to imagine that the patient will ever recover functional status. Nevertheless, antibiotic treatment (using combinations of sulfa drugs, pyrimethamine, clindamycin, and/or atovaquone) often leads to complete or nearly complete recovery. Trimethoprim with sulfamethoxazole or dapsone with pyrimethamine are used as prophylaxis to prevent reactivation of infection in patients who have very low CD4 counts (CD4 <100).

CYTOMEGALOVIRUS

The cytomegalovirus (CMV) herpes virus is transmitted perinatally (from mother to baby at or near the time of birth) or through close interpersonal contact, causing a mild viral syndrome in healthy individuals. The virus then establishes a latent, clinically silent infection. Individuals who become severely immunosuppressed (including patients with AIDS who have CD4 counts <50) can experience viral reactivation with devastating consequences.

In patients with AIDS, the most common sites of reactivation include the eyes and the gastrointestinal (GI) tract. Ocular CMV infection, a focal chorioretinitis, leads to retinal necrosis, with loss of vision in the affected areas of the retina. Patients often report curtain-like areas of darkness in their vision, floaters, or more generalized blurring. Because the infection can progress quickly and irreversibly, new or changing visual complaints in a patient with advanced HIV disease should prompt an urgent ophthalmologic assessment.

CMV infection in the GI tract occurs most commonly in the esophagus or colon. The spectrum of disease ranges from minor inflammation to very large, deeply penetrating ulcers. Symptoms include pain, diarrhea, weight loss, anorexia, and fever.

CMV infection may involve the nervous system, presenting as a rapidly progressive peripheral neuropathy that causes burning or shooting pains in the arms or hands or involving the brain itself (ventriculitis or encephalitis). Hepatitis, biliary tract disease, and pneumonitis may also occur.

Treatment of CMV infection is difficult because available medications prevent CMV from replicating, but do not kill the virus. All have significant side effects. Ganciclovir is available intravenously, in a device that can be surgically implanted into the eye, or as a formulation (valganciclovir) that can be taken orally. Foscarnet and cidofovir must be given intravenously. Although medical treatments for CMV infection are suboptimal, treatment of HIV infection with antiretroviral medications often leads to significant immunologic recovery and eventual immunologic control of CMV infection.

MYCOBACTERIUM AVIUM COMPLEX

Mycobacterium avium is a distant relative of the bacterium that causes tuberculosis. Although *M. avium* complex (MAC) is common in the environment and humans are exposed through both ingestion and inhalation, it rarely causes disease in healthy people. Patients with far-advanced HIV disease (usually those with a CD4 count of less than 50) may develop disseminated infection that involves the bloodstream, lymph nodes, liver, other sites in the GI tract, or bone marrow. The patient experiences progressive weakness, fever, chills, sweats, weight loss, enlarged lymph nodes, abnormal liver function tests (increased alkaline phosphatase and gamma-glutamyl transferase (GGT)), abdominal pain, pulmonary infiltrates, and bone marrow suppression. Patients usually do not die of MAC per se, but MAC contributes to wasting, catabolism, and susceptibility to other problems; systemic MAC infection is associated with a high short-term mortality rate.

Treatment of MAC with antibiotics is marginally successful. Furthermore, two or more drugs must be used in combination to prevent the rapid development of drug resistance. Azithromycin or clarithromycin, ethambutol, and rifabutin are the drugs of choice. Given the marginal efficacy of these antibiotics, treatment is continued indefinitely unless the patient's immunologic status improves. Prophylactic antibiotics are moderately effective in preventing MAC; prophylaxis is usually prescribed to HIV-infected patients who have very low CD4 counts (<100).

CRYPTOCOCCUS NEOFORMANS

Cryptococcus is a ubiquitous environmental fungus. It typically enters the body through inhalation, causes a mild pneumonitis, and then disseminates via the blood stream to the CNS. In patients with AIDS, it is a frequent cause of subacute or chronic meningitis. Patients with cryptococcal meningitis experience vague symptoms such as fever, headache, nausea, vomiting, malaise, and cognitive dysfunction that worsen gradually over days to weeks. Patients sometimes present with altered mentation, personality changes, or behavioral disturbances as the predominant symptoms. A test for cryptococcal antigen can be performed using serum or cerebrospinal fluid (CSF). This test is relatively simple and widely available.

Although ultimately fatal if untreated, this infection usually responds to a prolonged course of antifungal agents (amphotericin or fluconazole with or without flucytosine). Recent attention has focused on the importance of addressing increased intracranial pressure in the setting of cryptococcal meningitis. Repeated lumbar puncture or CSF shunts are helpful when patients have persistently elevated intracranial pressure.

There are numerous other infectious complications of HIV, including some infections that are seen only in limited geographic areas. A full discussion is beyond the scope of this text, but excellent references are available.[2]

TREATMENT OF THE HIV INFECTION (ANTIRETROVIRAL TREATMENT)

HISTORICAL CONTEXT

Zidovudine was the first antiviral agent available to treat HIV infection. Clinical trials testing zidovudine against placebo in patients who had AIDS demonstrated significantly improved survival among those who received the drug. These results were met with great enthusiasm. A number of antiviral agents with similar mechanisms of action were developed over the next few years. Unfortunately, these agents were able to only partially suppress the virus. After a few weeks or months of treatment, replication and mutation of the HIV virus facilitated the development of drug resistance and resulted in progression of the infection.

In the mid-1990s, new classes of antiretroviral medications (protease inhibitors and non-nucleoside reverse transcriptase inhibitors) became available. Clinical trials verified dramatically improved efficacy when these medications were used in combinations of three or more agents. Initial skepticism about HIV treatment yielded to overly enthusiastic claims that AIDS would soon be cured.

Although it is now clear that currently available therapies do not cure HIV, antiretroviral combination treatment reduces viral replication dramatically. Such combinations have been referred to as highly active antiretroviral therapy (HAART). Effective antiretroviral therapy stops the progression of immunologic damage, leading to significant recovery of the immune system and a rebound in CD4 counts. Even debilitated patients with advanced AIDS may experience dramatic improvement with restoration of functional status and control or resolution of infections. The development of effective therapies was followed by a precipitous drop in hospitalizations for AIDS and dramatic decreases in AIDS mortality.[1]

PRINCIPLES OF ANTIRETROVIRAL THERAPY

HIV infection is not curable with currently available therapies. However, HIV infections can be controlled such that HIV infection has become a chronic disease. The initial enthusiasm for antiretroviral medications has been tempered by realization that antiretroviral medications have significant long-term toxicity and that patients have great difficulty with adherence to complicated medical regimens over long periods of time. These realities mean that decisions about initiating HAART should be carefully considered, weighing the risks and benefits for the individual patient. Current guidelines advise antiretroviral treatment for all patients who have experienced opportunistic infections or severe HIV-related illnesses and for patients who have significant immunosuppression, as measured by CD4 counts <200.[3,4] Conversely, most experts suggest careful clinical monitoring without HAART for patients who have a CD4 count greater than 350. There is continued controversy about management of patients who have CD4 counts between 200 and 350. Some authorities favor treatment, whereas others favor close clinical monitoring, deferring medications for as long as possible. Given the medical uncertainty, patient preference, motivation, and readiness for treatment should weigh heavily in the decision process.

An additional possible indication for HIV treatment is pregnancy.[5] The first trial of zidovudine for perinatal transmission of HIV revealed a 70% reduction in perinatal infection. A number of trials using a variety of treatment regimens have subsequently been conducted. Perinatal transmission rates of less than 2% have been documented using current combination antiretroviral therapies.

TREATMENT REGIMENS

To avoid the rapid development of resistance, effective antiretroviral regimens include at least three drugs.[3,5] Initial regimens usually include one protease inhibitor (PI) and two drugs from the nucleoside analog reverse transcriptase inhibitors (NRTI) group or a non-nucleoside reverse transcriptase inhibitor (NNRTI) with two NRTIs. Table 3.2 lists currently available

TABLE 3.2　Antiretroviral Medications

Nucleoside Reverse Transcriptase Inhibitors

Generic Name	Trade Names	Common Side Effects	Significant Drug–Drug Interactions*
Abacavir	Ziagen, Trizivir†, Epzicom†	Hypersensitivity reactions (including fever, rash, nausea, fatigue, abdominal discomfort, lactic acidosis with hepatic steatosis)	
Didanosine	Videx, Videx EC	Pancreatitis, peripheral neuropathy, lactic acidosis with hepatic steatosis	
Emtricitabine	Emtriva, Truvada†	Lactic acidosis with hepatic steatosis (rarely)	
Lamivudine	Epivir, Combivir†, Epzicom†, Trizivir†	Lactic acidosis with hepatic steatosis (rarely)	
Stavudine	Zerit	Lactic acidosis with hepatic steatosis, lipodystrophy, hyperlipidemia, peripheral neuropathy	
Tenofovir‡	Viread, Truvada†	Headache, asthenia, GI upset, lactic acidosis with hepatic steatosis (rarely)	
Zalcitabine	Hivid	Peripheral neuropathy, oral ulcers, pancreatitis, lactic acidosis	
Zidovudine	Retrovir, Combivir†, Trizivir†	Anemia, neutropenia, headache, fatigue, GI upset, lactic acidosis	

Non-Nucleotide Reverse Transcriptase Inhibitors (NNRTIs)

Delavirdine	Rescriptor	Rash, hepatitis, headache	Alprazolam, + midazolam, + triazolam, + St. John's wort, + methadone

Efavirenz	Sustiva	Rash, CNS symptoms (refer to text), false positive cannabinoid test, hepatitis	Midazolam, + triazolam, + alprazolam, St. John's wort, + methadone, sertraline
Nevirapine	Viramune	Rash (may be life-threatening), hepatitis (may be fatal)	St. John's wort, + methadone

Protease Inhibitors (PIs)

Atazanavir	Reyataz	GI upset, rash, hyperbilirubinemia, first-degree heart block, hyperglycemia, lipodystrophy	Pimozide, + midazolam, + triazolam, + St. John's wort, + sildenafil, vardenafil, tadalafil, tricyclic antidepressants
Fosamprenavir	Lexiva	Rash, GI upset, headache, hyperlipidemia, lipodystrophy	Pimozide, + midazolam, + triazolam, + St. John's wort, + methadone, sildenafil, vardenafil, tadalafil, tricyclic antidepressants
Indinavir	Crixivan	Kidney stones, GI upset, hyperbilirubinemia, hyperglycemia, lipodystrophy	Pimozide, + midazolam, + triazolam, + alprazolam, + St. John's wort, + venlafaxine, methadone, sildenafil, vardenafil, tadalafil
Lopinavir	Kaletra†	GI upset, hyperglycemia, lipodystrophy, hepatitis	Pimozide, + midazolam, + triazolam, + St. John's wort, + methadone, sildenafil, vardenafil, tadalafil, disulfiram+
Nelfinavir	Viracept	Diarrhea	Pimozide, + midazolam, + triazolam, + St. John's wort, + methadone, sildenafil, vardenafil, tadalafil
Ritonavir	Norvir Kaletra* Aptivus*	GI upset, hyperlipidemia, hyperglycemia, lipodystrophy, hepatitis, oral numbness, taste changes	Pimozide, + midazolam, + triazolam, + other sedative/hypnotics, St. John's wort, + methadone, sildenafil, vardenafil, tadalafil, disulfiram, + SSRIs, tricyclics, bupropion, nefazodone, neuropeptics, meperidine
Saquinavir	Invirase Fortovase	GI upset, hyperlipidemia, hyperglycemia, lipodystrophy, hepatitis	Pimozide, + midazolam, + triazolam, + St. John's wort, + methadone, sildenafil, vardenafil, tadalafil, tricyclic antidepressants
Tipranavir	Aptivus†	GI upset, hyperlipidemia, hyperglycemia, hepatitis	fentanyl, flecainide, amiodarone, bepridil, flecainide, propafenone, quinidine, ergotamine, pimozide, midazolam, triazolam, St. John's wort

Fusion Inhibitors

Enfuvirtide	Fuzeon	Local injection site reactions (must be given by subcutaneous injection), hypersensitivity	

GI, Gastrointestinal; CNS, central nervous system; SSRIs, selective serotonin reuptake inhibitors.
*This list is not complete but focuses on medications commonly used in psychiatric care. Many listed medications may be used with caution or dose adjustment. Those with + are contraindicated.
†The listed medication is one component of a combination pill.
‡Tenofovir is technically a nucleotide.

medications, along with common side effects and drug interactions that are particularly relevant to mental health providers.

Nucleoside Analog Reverse Transcriptase Inhibitors
Zidovudine, the first available antiretroviral agent, is the prototype NRTI. This group includes abacavir, didanosine, emtricitabine, lamivudine, stavudine, zalcitabine, and tenofovir. This last agent is technically a nucleotide because it has already been phosphorylated. Drugs in this class are structurally similar to the endogenous cellular nucleotides adenosine, guanosine, thymidine, and cytidine, the basic building blocks of deoxyribonucleic acid (DNA). HIV reverse transcriptase, the enzyme that copies viral RNA into DNA, cannot distinguish between the phosphorylated nucleoside analogs and their natural counterparts. Incorporation of NRTIs into the viral DNA blocks the addition of further nucleotides, aborting HIV replication.

Non-Nucleoside Reverse Transcriptase Inhibitors
Non-nucleoside reverse transcriptase inhibitors (NNRTIs) inhibit the reverse transcriptase of HIV by binding to the enzyme. These agents, efavirenz, nevirapine, and delavirdine, are very active and have long half-lives. Unfortunately, HIV can easily develop resistance to these medications; viral strains that are resistant to one drug in this class are almost always resistant to all NNRTIs.

The unique neuropsychiatric side effects of efavirenz should be noted.[6] About 40% of patients who begin treatment with efavirenz experience dizziness, sedation or excitability, loss of motor coordination (similar to that experienced with alcohol intoxication), peculiarly vivid dreams, and/or anxiety. Reports of more extreme reactions include precipitation of mania, panic attacks, psychotic episodes, and severe depression. Because neuropsychiatric effects are most pronounced in the hours immediately after taking the medication, efavirenz is usually prescribed for administration at bedtime. Neuropsychiatric side effects usually decrease over the first 10 to 14 days of treatment, often resolving entirely. Nevertheless, in cases of more extreme reactions, discontinuation of the medication is sometimes necessary.

Protease Inhibitors
The HIV protease is a viral enzyme that is essential for HIV replication. It acts at a late step of HIV replication, cleaving both structural and functional proteins from precursor viral polyprotein strands. Without appropriate cleavage by HIV protease, HIV replication produces only immature noninfectious virions. When combined with reverse transcriptase inhibitors, protease inhibitors (PIs) are quite potent in suppressing viral replication. Available PIs include atazanavir, fosamprenavir, indinavir, lopinavir, nelfinavir, ritonavir, and saquinavir.

Although PIs have revolutionized the treatment of HIV infection and are largely responsible for the decrease in HIV mortality, they have some significant limitations. All protease inhibitors are metabolized in the liver, and all have some potential for hepatotoxicity. They are poorly orally bioavailable, often requiring the patient to take large pills or large numbers of pills. They both induce and inhibit the hepatic metabolism of many other medications, leading to long lists of potentially dangerous drug–drug interactions. Ritonavir, one of the oldest drugs in this class, has the greatest potential for drug–drug interaction. Although ritonavir is not well tolerated at therapeutic doses, small doses of ritonavir block the hepatic metabolism of many other PIs, greatly increasing the blood level of the coadministered PI. Such combinations decrease the number of pills or frequency of dosing while increasing the effectiveness of the regimen.

Fusion Inhibitors
This new class of antiretroviral medications work by blocking HIV's entry into the cell. Thus fusion inhibitors are the only medications that truly prevent HIV infection. Although only one fusion inhibitor, enfuvirtide, is marketed in the United States, other agents are in development.

Although enfuvirtide is effective against HIV strains that are resistant to other classes of antiviral medications, it is very expensive and must be given by twice daily subcutaneous injections.

VIRAL RESISTANCE

Suboptimal antiretroviral therapy can result from the use of insufficiently potent medication combinations, use of regimens to which the virus has already become partially resistant, factors such as poor absorption or unusually rapid metabolism of medications or patient nonadherence to the prescribed regimen. HIV mutates frequently during replication. Suboptimal therapy favors the selection for drug-resistant mutants, in effect creating treatment-resistant "superviruses." Such viruses may be poorly responsive to currently available treatments and can be transmitted to other individuals.

Laboratory tests are frequently used to detect resistance to HIV medications. Although these tests are complicated, time consuming, and expensive, they are very useful in designing optimal treatment regimens. Several types of resistance tests are commercially available. Genotypic tests look for mutations in the HIV virus that are known to be associated with resistance. Phenotypic tests look at the ability of a virus cloned from the patient to replicate in the presence of medication.

Viral mutations that confer resistance to one medication often confer resistance to other medications. This cross resistance can greatly limit treatment options. Treatment of patients who have highly resistant strains of HIV not uncommonly requires regimens of four of more antiretroviral medications.

ADHERENCE

Studies of adherence to medications suggest that most people take fewer than half of prescribed doses.[7] Studies of adherence to antiretroviral medications suggest that a much higher level of adherence is required for long-term successful antiretroviral treatment.[8] Unlike the situation faced in treating hypertension, where cardiovascular injury may occur as a result of poor blood pressure control when patients miss medication doses, but blood pressure responds appropriately when the patient takes the medication, nonadherence to antiretroviral medication can lead to viral resistance. Patients who continue to take medication, but frequently miss doses, seem to be at higher risk of resistance than untreated patients or those who seldom take their medications. Once resistance has developed, resumption of the medication is ineffective. Furthermore, cross resistance between antiretroviral agents may permanently limit other treatment options.

Given the fact that many patients with HIV infection have significant psychosocial and medical problems, the challenge of long-term, high-level adherence is great. Factors that may adversely affect adherence must be assessed before initiating treatment and at regular intervals thereafter. Several such variables have been identified.[9,10] Regimens that include many pills, pills that are too large, frequent dosing, food restrictions, or unpleasant side effects may contribute to poor adherence. Substance and alcohol abuse, issues in the patient–provider relationship, and issues related to the system of care may be problematic. Sociodemographic characteristics, quality of life issues, CD4 count, patient belief systems, patient satisfaction with health care, and untreated depression[11] may contribute. Addressing these issues may require assistance from outside resources.

It is also critical that patients understand the goals of treatment and necessity of taking every dose of prescribed medication. Given that available data suggest that suppression of viral replication is directly correlated to adherence,[8] a goal of 95% of prescribed doses taken is optimal.

Formal interventions to improve patient adherence are often labor intensive and difficult to implement outside of a research setting. Further work in this area is sorely needed.[7,12] Although data on efficacy are limited, there are a number of simple tools that may assist in maintenance of adherence. These include the incorporation of medication into the patient's usual daily routine (e.g., learning to take your pills when you brush your teeth), use of programmable watches or beepers as medication reminders, and use of pillboxes. Pillboxes with separate compartments for each dose facilitate patient self-monitoring of adherence. By providing visible evidence (whether or not the pills are still in the box) of adherence, pillboxes eliminate the confusion that can lead to double dosing or missed doses. Furthermore, patients frequently discover that their actual adherence is considerably less than their perceived adherence. This knowledge can be a vital first step toward improvements in adherence.

Even patients who have been adherent to their medications for long periods may have periods of nonadherence. Depression, drug use, or psychosocial stressors may contribute. In addition, patients often complain of being tired of following complicated medication regimens. This phenomenon has been referred to as "pill fatigue." During periods of suboptimal adherence, it may be most prudent to stop medications entirely. Such "medication holidays" can be used to address the issues that led to nonadherence and to provide psychological respite. Although immunologic damage resumes during these periods, the immunologic damage of HIV is usually slowly progressive and moderately reversible. On the other hand, the development of resistance to antiretroviral medications is often irreversible.

TRANSMISSION OF HIV IN THE HEALTH CARE SETTING

Sexual activity, perinatal transmission, and exposure to blood via injection or blood transfusion are the major ways that HIV is transmitted from person to person. Although many individuals think of HIV infection as a disease of men who have sex with men, heterosexual sex is the major risk for HIV transmission worldwide. In addition, rare instances of HIV transmission have been documented involving nonsexual mucous membrane exposure (such as eyes or mouth), transmission of HIV through abraded or injured skin, or transmission by human bite.

Although exposure to HIV in the health care setting is not infrequent, occupationally acquired HIV infection is extremely uncommon. Data from 1997 and 1998 suggested that there were 384,325 percutaneous injuries to health care workers annually in the United States.[13] However, the Centers for Disease Control and Prevention (CDC) recorded only 57 definite and 139 possible cases of occupationally acquired HIV during the first two decades (1981 to 2002) of the epidemic.[14] Nevertheless, the medical care and follow-up of health care providers exposed to HIV requires significant resources.[15] In addition, health care providers who have been exposed to HIV in the workplace report significant associated anxiety.[16]

RISKS FOR HIV TRANSMISSION IN THE MENTAL HEALTH CARE SETTING

In health care settings, the major risk of HIV transmission comes from accidental percutaneous injuries.[14] Needles previously used to draw blood or give intramuscular injections are often the source of such injuries. Care involving violent or psychotic patients may pose particular challenges; dealing with such patients requires caution and planning to avoid injury. For example, staff members should have assigned and coordinated tasks when restraining or medicating an agitated patient. Occupational exposure to HIV may also occur when infectious materials, including blood, bloody body fluids, semen, or vaginal fluids are splashed onto mucous membranes or skin that has been chapped or abraded.[15] Although no documented cases of occupational HIV transmission have been attributed to assault, sexual assault or traumatic assault in which the blood of an HIV-infected perpetrator has contact with the mucous membranes (eye, nose, or mouth) or abraded or injured skin of another individual carries risk of transmitting HIV.

Many health care workers present with concerns about workplace exposures that do not pose a risk of HIV transmission. Intact skin (skin without chapping, abrasions, rash, or injury) is an effective protective barrier against HIV. A splash of HIV-infected blood onto intact skin should be washed away with soap and water. This exposure does not constitute a risk for HIV transmission. Urine, feces, sweat, tears, saliva, and vomitus do not contain significant HIV unless they are contaminated with blood. Contact with these substances does not transmit HIV.

When a human bite has occurred, it is important to consider that both the individual who was bitten and the individual who inflicted the bite may have been exposed to bloodborne pathogens. Although no documented cases of occupationally acquired HIV due to human bite have been reported, case reports have documented transmission of HIV by bite in other settings. In these cases, exposure to HIV was most likely due to blood in the individual's mouth at the time the bite was inflicted.

ASSESSING THE MAGNITUDE OF THE RISK

The risk of HIV transmission by mucous membrane splash in the occupational setting has been estimated at 0.09%. The risk for transmitting HIV by percutaneous injury with an HIV-contaminated sharp instrument has been estimated to be 0.3% per exposure, but the circumstances of the individual accident can greatly increase or decrease the risk of a specific exposure. Increased risk has been associated with an injury caused by a needle that was previously in the patient's vein or artery (as opposed to needles used for subcutaneous or intramuscular injection), injury from a hollow needle (rather than a lancet or suture needle), a particularly deep or serious injury, or an injury caused by an overtly bloody device. Factors related to the source patient also modify risk. Source patients who have advanced HIV infection, likely a surrogate for high HIV viral load, are more likely to transmit HIV.[17] Although definitive data are not available, it is reasonable to assume that patients on effective antiretroviral therapy may pose less risk than untreated patients.

MEDICAL EVALUATION

Antiretroviral medications are commonly prescribed to health care workers who have been exposed to HIV in an attempt to prevent infection,[15] a practice termed postexposure prophylaxis (PEP). Although PEP has not been studied in randomized clinical trials, data from experiments in animals, observational data of babies born to HIV-infected mothers, and follow-up of occupationally exposed health care workers suggest that antiretroviral therapy after HIV exposure greatly decreases the likelihood that the exposed individual will become HIV infected.

In addition to occupational PEP, some authorities advocate the use of PEP for survivors of sexual assault. Recent guidelines endorse the selective use of PEP for a variety of nonoccupational exposures to HIV.[18] These may include sex between HIV-discordant individuals, sex with condom breakage or failure, sexual assault, traumatic assault, or exposures related to drug use. PEP should never substitute for behavioral interventions to reduce HIV exposure. Nevertheless, it is appropriate to consider the use of PEP in a variety of situations relevant to mental health care.

Animal data suggest that the efficacy of PEP declines significantly as the time since HIV exposure increases. PEP is most likely to confer benefit if given in the first hours after an exposure. Treatment should not be delayed during attempts to ascertain the HIV status of the source patient.

ASSESSMENT OF THE HIV STATUS OF THE SOURCE OF AN EXPOSURE

Because an HIV-uninfected patient cannot transmit HIV to another individual, a determination that the patient who was the source of the exposure is not HIV infected can relieve anxiety and permit PEP to be discontinued. Legal regulations concerning HIV testing and access to medical records regarding prior HIV testing vary by jurisdiction. In some states, HIV testing a source patient in a case of occupational exposure does not require the patient's consent. In other areas, it is not legally permissible to test source patients unless they consent to the test. Every health care site should have a protocol for dealing with potential exposure to bloodborne pathogens and be aware of applicable federal, state, and local laws.

In making final decisions about PEP and medical follow-up, it is critical that the limitations of HIV antibody testing be considered. Patients who have been very recently infected by HIV may have high titers of bloodborne HIV for several weeks before the development of antibodies. Such patients may be hyperinfectious, yet have a negative HIV test result. Issues relevant to other infectious pathogens such as hepatitis B or C are beyond the scope of this chapter, but must also be considered after occupational exposure.[19]

MEDICAL TREATMENT: POST EXPOSURE PROPHYLAXIS

Various PEP regimens have been advocated. The strategy endorsed by the CDC advocates the use of two medications for low-risk exposures and three or more medications for high-risk exposures.[15] It is reasonable to alter the drug regimen if the source patient is known to be infected with an HIV strain that is resistant to medications or if the individual receiving PEP has side effects or difficulties tolerating the medications. Expert advice should be sought when such problems or issues arise. Telephone consultation regarding PEP can be obtained via the National Clinicians' Post-Exposure Prophylaxis Hotline (888-448-4911).

PEP should be continued for 4 weeks. The individual receiving PEP should be counseled to use condoms for sexual activity until a final HIV test is conducted 6 months after the exposure. Support, reassurance, and attention to medication side effects are important throughout.

SUMMARY

Although treatment of opportunistic infections, wasting, and malignancies remain major focuses in HIV care, advances in antiretroviral treatment have dramatically improved the health and life expectancy of patients with advanced HIV. Achievement of strict adherence to complex drug regimens over long periods of time presents numerous challenges, but remains critically linked to treatment success. In addition, antiretroviral medications are widely used to decrease the risk of acquiring HIV infection after exposure to HIV due to occupational or other types of exposures.

REFERENCES

1. Palella FJJ, Delaney KM, Moorman AC, et al. Declining morbidity and mortality among patients with advanced human immunodeficiency virus infection. *N Engl J Med*. 1998;338:853–860.
2. Benson CA, Kaplan JE, Masur H, et al. Treating opportunistic infections among HIV infected adults and adolescents. *MMWR Recomm Rep*. 2004;53:1–112.
3. Yeni PG, Hammer SM, Hirsch MS, et al. Treatment of adult HIV infection: 2004 recommendations of the International AIDS Society-USA Panel. *JAMA*. 2004;292:251–265.
4. Panel on Clinical Practices for Treatment of HIV Infection Convened by the Department of Health and Human Services. *Guidelines for the Use of Antiretroviral Agents in HIV-1-Infected Adults and Adolescents: April 7, 2005*. Bethesda, Md: National Institutes of Health; 2005.
5. Perinatal HIV Guidelines Working Group. *Public Health Service Task Force Recommendations for Use of Antiretroviral Drugs in Pregnant HIV-1-Infected Women for Maternal Health and Interventions to Reduce Perinatal HIV-1 Transmission in the U.S.* Bethesda, Md: National Institutes of Health; 2005.

6. Wichers M, van der Ven A, Maes M. Central nervous system symptoms related to the use of efavirenz in HIV-seropositive patients. *Curr Opin Psychiatry*. 2002;15:643–647.
7. Haynes RB, McDonald H, Garg AX, Montague P. Interventions for helping patients to follow prescriptions for medications. *Cochrane Database Syst Rev*. 2002;2:CD000011.
8. Low-Beer S, Yip B, O'Shaughnessy MV, Hogg RS, Montaner JS. Adherence to triple therapy and viral load response. *J Acquir Immune Defic Syndr*. 2000;23:360–361.
9. Ammassari A, Trotta MP, Murri R, et al. Correlates and predictors of adherence to highly active antiretroviral therapy: overview of published literature. *J Acquir Immune Defic Syndr*. 2002;31(suppl):123–127.
10. Chesney MA. Factors affecting adherence to antiretroviral therapy. *Clin Infect Dis*. 2000;30(suppl 2):171–176.
11. Starace F, Ammassari A, Trotta MP, et al. Depression is a risk factor for suboptimal adherence to highly active antiretroviral therapy. *J Acquir Immune Defic Syndr*. 2002;31(suppl 3):136–139.
12. Tuldra A, Wu AW. Interventions to improve adherence to antiretrovirals. *J Acquir Immune Defic Syndr*. 2002;31(suppl):154–157.
13. Panlilio AL, Orelien JG, Srivastava PU, et al. Estimate of the annual number of percutaneous injuries among hospital-based healthcare workers in the United States, 1997-1998. *Infect Control Hosp Epidemiol*. 2004;25:532–535.
14. Do AN, Ciesielski CA, Metler RP, et al. Occupationally acquired human immunodeficiency virus (HIV) infection: national case surveillance data during 20 years of the HIV epidemic in the United States. *Infect Control Hosp Epidemiol*. 2003;24:86–96.
15. Panlilio AL, Cardo DM, Grohskopf LA, Heneine W, Ross CS. Updated U.S. Public Health Service guidelines for the management of occupational exposures to HIV and recommendations for postexposure prophylaxis. *MMWR Recomm Rep*. 2005;54:1–17.
16. Meienberg F, Bucher HC, Sponagel L, Zinkernagel C, Gyr N, Battegay M. Anxiety in health care workers after exposure to potentially HIV-contaminated blood or body fluids. *Swiss Med Wkly*. 2002;132:321–324.
17. Cardo DM, Culver DH, Ciesielski CA, et al. A case-control study of HIV seroconversion in health care workers after percutaneous exposure. *N Engl J Med*. 1997;337:1485–1490.
18. Smith DK, Grohskopf LA, Black RJ, et al. Antiretroviral postexposure prophylaxis after sexual or injection-drug, or other nonoccupational exposure to HIV in the United States: recommendations from the U.S. Department of Health and Human Services. *MMWR Recomm Rep*. 2005;54:1–20.
19. Centers for Disease Control and Prevention. Updated U.S. Public Health Service guidelines for the management of occupational exposures to HBV, HCV, and HIV and recommendations for postexposure prophylaxis. *MMWR Recomm Rep*. 2001;50:1–42.

SECTION II

Diagnostic Tools

… CHAPTER 4

Psychiatric Assessment

María Fernanda Gómez, Mary Alice O'Dowd

A thorough psychiatric evaluation is the cornerstone of diagnosis and treatment. Despite the popularity of "check list" evaluations that meet the requirements of third party payers, there is still much to be learned through an assessment based on both open- and closed-ended questions that enhance understanding of a patient and develop a life narrative. This is certainly true in the assessment of the patient with human immunodeficiency virus infection (HIV) or acquired immunodeficiency syndrome (AIDS), given the complex interaction of biopsychosocial factors at every stage of infection, including the risk behaviors underlying transmission, barriers to adherence, the stigma of diagnosis, cultural issues, and the impact of progressive illness and its treatment in an impaired population, more than 50% of whom may have psychiatric disorders antedating HIV infection.[1]

The form and completeness of the psychiatric assessment in a population with physical illness may be dictated in part by the stage of illness. The debilitated patient may be unable to participate in an extensive interview or may be unable to recall details of past history, giving collateral informants a more central role. Issues of discomfort, whether physical due to illness or its treatment, or emotional, due to the lack of privacy in a hospital or clinic setting may limit the assessment possible or may require changes in strategy. In such situations the assessment may need to be completed in a series of brief interviews or to be more problem focused, leaving more complete assessment for a time when the patient is better able to participate. In a multidisciplinary clinic setting, the interviewer may have the advantage of the data available in the medical chart, which can be mined for clues as to the patient's past and present history and behaviors. Useful information can be found in the notes from social workers and other care providers, as well as in the medical progress notes, laboratory values, neuroimaging reports, and medication lists. This chapter reviews the wider range of topics that could be covered in the complete psychiatric assessment of an HIV-infected patient, but the actual assessment of a particular patient will be dictated by the circumstances.

INITIAL ASSESSMENT

The first step to the achievement of a successful psychiatric assessment is the formation of an alliance in which the patient experiences a level of trust and comfort with the interviewer that permits sharing of intimate information and feelings. Different interview settings may have an impact on the development of such an alliance. The individual who presents voluntarily to the psychiatrist's office may have at least some level of insight into the need for mental health services and thus may be more open to participation in the assessment. A different situation may unfold when a patient in a multidisciplinary clinic is referred for psychiatric assessment. Here, the patient may not understand the reasons for referral and may even see the psychiatric assessment as an assault, as evidence that caregivers think him or her "crazy." In addition to reluctance in being identified as a psychiatric patient, patients may be hesitant to participate in an in-depth interview due to experiences of stigmatization when HIV infection or risk behaviors have been divulged in other settings. It is also not unusual for a patient to feel uncomfortable initially discussing personal details with an interviewer perceived to differ in age, race, gender, sexual orientation, or socioeconomic status. The most effective way to build an alliance in this situation is by initially focusing not on psychiatric issues but on the patient's experience of his or her illness. Discussing the patient's illness, a story that patients usually never tire of telling, most often sets the patient at ease and offers an assurance of the examiner's interest and understanding. While reviewing the patient's experience with his or her illness, it is possible at the same time to gain considerable information about memory, insight, and judgment. At this point, it is almost always possible to move toward an examination of psychiatric issues, even in patients who are initially resistant or even hostile.

The psychiatric interviewer must be an acute observer on many levels. The interviewer must listen to what the patient is saying, as well as retain awareness of what is not being said. The patient's behavior, appearance, and dress should be observed for appropriateness to the situation. Observed interactions with the examiner, clinic staff, and even other patients can provide insight into social skills. Motor skills and coordination can be examined directly or inferred from the ability to sign an insurance form or button a coat before leaving the office. The following sections do not include every topic that could be covered in the psychiatric assessment of a patient with HIV infection but do attempt to cover the topics of most concern.

CLINICAL APPROACH TO THE PSYCHIATRIC ASSESSMENT

The following guidelines detail areas that should be covered in the patient psychiatric assessment.

1. Determine from the patient or referring clinician the reason why the patient has been referred for assessment. Knowing what problem areas have been identified will help focus the assessment.
2. Gather a history from the patient or collateral sources, including the history of the psychiatric complaint; the past psychiatric history; the family psychiatric history; social history, including school and work history; history of trauma or abuse; and legal history. Identify social supports available to the patient, and explore the patient's strengths in coping with this and prior stressors.
3. Pay special attention to a careful history of past and present substance abuse, including the age at which use of each substance began, quantities used, and the impact of substance use on all aspects of the patient's life. It is important for the examiner to be familiar with evolving patterns of substance use in the community and direct the examination accordingly. In eliciting an accurate history of substance abuse, it may be useful to remember that users may underestimate use, deceiving both themselves and examiners. Questions assuming use and phrased in terms of quantities and even exaggerated quantities may elicit a more

honest response. Thus, rather than asking, "Do you drink beer?" the questioner might ask, "How many quarts of beer do you drink daily?" and so on.
4. Take a careful medical history, including medications used to treat HIV-related disorders and other illnesses. Understanding of and adherence to treatment regimens should be reviewed. Height, weight, body mass index, and vital signs should be recorded. Further elements of the physical and neurologic examination should be included when suggested by the history.
5. Take a sexual history, emphasizing behaviors that may put the patient or others at risk. Here, again, questions phrased so as to assume that behaviors are part of a patient's expression of sexuality may lead to a more honest dialog than questions that encourage a simple "yes" or "no" response.
6. Perform a mental status examination, through a combination of questioning and observation. The spheres to be examined include the following:

Behavior and appearance: Does the patient sit quietly or move restlessly in the chair or about the room. Is his or her behavior appropriate for the interview? Are hygiene, clothing, grooming, and makeup appropriate? Are there abnormal movements?

Mood and affect: Does the patient acknowledge any disturbance in mood, whether sadness or elation? Is the affect displayed by the patient appropriate to the self-described mood? Does the patient exhibit lability or irritability during the examination? Does the patient endorse any symptoms of depression when asked specifically about anhedonia, helplessness, hopelessness, or worthlessness? Does the patient endorse any current or past symptoms of mania, including decreased need for sleep, overspending, or unusual sense of creativity? What was the duration of these episodes and how did they resolve? Was treatment ever sought and what was the outcome?

Speech and thoughts: Does the patient speak at a normal rate and rhythm or is speech slowed, rapid, or pressured? Is there any evidence of dysarthria or aphasia? Are the patient's thoughts organized and logical or are the thinking processes concrete, vague, disjointed, loose, or disorganized? Does the patient ever think life is not worth living? Does the patient acknowledge any past or present suicidal, homicidal, or paranoid ideation? If suicidal or homicidal ideations are present, does the patient feel able to control these ideas?

Perceptions: Is there any evidence of acute or chronic perceptual disturbance, such as auditory, visual, gustatory, tactile, or olfactory hallucinations? If present, are these experiences culturally syntonic? Is the patient able to ignore or de-emphasize these experiences or are they central to or interfering with daily activity?

Insight, judgment, and impulse control: Does the patient demonstrate a good understanding of his or her illness and its treatment? Do the choices that the patient makes in this and other areas reflect his or her best long-term interests? What is the patient's life-long pattern of decision making and do current decisions conform to that pattern?

Cognitive testing: Formal orientation to person, place, and time should be tested. Orientation to person seems the most obvious, but should include awareness of age, relationship to significant others, and other indicators of "personhood," beyond the simple recognition of or response to a name.

Recent and remote memory: Memory is tested in the course of gathering a history, but should also be tested by giving specific memory tasks. Working memory can be tested by giving the patient a task (remembering three words) and then asking for the material to be recalled.

Attention: The ability to sustain attention is tested by nonautomatic, moderately demanding tests, such as spelling backward or serial subtraction. In assigning such tasks, information on a patient's level of education is helpful, because this is not a test of knowledge. More simple tasks (serial 3s or even serial 1s) should be substituted if these are more reflective of the patient's abilities.

Executive function: Executive function is the ability to plan, organize, and perform actions within a reasonable time frame, skills necessary for normal professional or social functioning. Dysfunctional behavior is marked by impulsivity, disorganization, or amotivation. Evidence of dysfunction can be elicited by examining a patient's ability to function in real-life situations. More formal testing can include naming items in a category (animals, things that begin with letter D, etc.) within a minute or completion of a complex task. One such task is the "Marie Three Paper test," in which the patient is given three pieces of paper and the instructions to return the largest to the examiner, throw the smallest on the ground, and place the middle one in his or her pocket or elsewhere. Abstractions also test executive function.

- *Instruments to aid in testing:* Because deterioration can be expected in patients with HIV-associated dementia complex (HAD) and early signs of dysfunction can be subtle, it is useful to establish a baseline for each patient at the initial visit with more formal testing. The Internet offers literally millions of references to instruments that can be used as adjuncts to the psychiatric examination.*

The ideal instrument for neurocognitive testing in the clinical setting should be simple and within the purview of any examiner. Repeating such testing over time provides an invaluable monitor of cognitive change. An instrument that has proved useful in this population, although not specific to it, is clock drawing, which assesses planning and executive function. Advantages of this test are its simplicity, its lack of correlation with formal education, and the ease both of administration and of comparing repeated drawings over time. Difficulty in performing this test is linked to nonspecific cognitive dysfunction and slowing on electroencephalogram.[2] Various strategies for scoring have been suggested.†

The Folstein-McHugh Mini-Mental Status Examination, which is commonly used in the assessment of mental state in medically ill patients, is insufficiently sensitive to HIV-related cognitive change. The HIV Dementia Scale was developed to focus specifically on the domains affected by HIV, including timed tasks that are more sensitive to executive dysfunction and cognitive slowing.[3] However, one item, the antisaccadic eye movement task, which assesses attention, proved cumbersome to use and the test has been recalibrated without this item, with a score of 7.5 or less suggesting impairment.[4] Trail Making A and B,‡ which are timed and structured versions of the "follow the dots" drawing enjoyed by children, have been used extensively with an HIV-infected population to quantify and track cognitive impairment. They are sensitive to the slowing and decline in executive function seen in the HIV-infected patient.

Numerous instruments to assist in other diagnostic parameters have been developed, both those that can be filled out by the patient and those that require questioning by the examiner. Although originally designed for primary care,[5] the General Health Questionnaire has stood the test of time, comes in versions ranging from 12 to 60 items, and examines the domains of somatization, anxiety, depression, and social function. It can be administered at baseline and repeated at intervals to monitor change in these domains. The Beck and Hamilton rating scales are well-known adjuncts to both diagnosis and follow-up. Instruments that have been developed to look more specifically at HIV-related distress and quality of life can be accessed through the previously cited websites.

---

*Samples of such sites include http://www.popcouncil.org/horizons/aidsquest/appendix_d-part_1.html and http://www.mentalhealthaids.samhsa.gov/Fall2004/fall2004_assess.asp.
†One such method can be accessed at http://www.seniorpsychiatry.com/pages/articles/10ptclocktest.html.
‡Trail Making A and B can be accessed at http://www.angelfire.com/retro/michaelpoon168/trail_making_test.htm.

DIFFERENTIAL DIAGNOSTIC CONSIDERATIONS

The general format of the psychiatric assessment of patients with HIV infection or AIDS does not vary from the assessment of any patient with medical and psychiatric illness, but a different emphasis is given to certain areas of the examination. The course of HIV infection suggests some of the areas to which special attention should be paid: barriers to risk reduction, adherence to treatment, substance abuse, the presence of Axis I or Axis II psychiatric disorders, and cognitive impairment. Obviously these factors do not exist in a vacuum but interact in the production of both symptoms and behaviors of concern.

BARRIERS TO RISK REDUCTION

Changes in behavior have contributed to the decline in the incidence of AIDS in the last decade. However, multiple studies have found that knowledge of HIV and its modes of transmission may not be sufficient to change behavior. Although some groups at risk have been able to adopt safer behaviors, other subgroups have continued at-risk behaviors or may have changed their perception of risk as the treatment of HIV infection has improved. Younger men who see HIV as a problem that has been solved or those using methamphetamines may abandon safer practices, and the Internet has expanded the options for seeking partners willing to engage in high-risk activities. Use of other drugs or alcohol, including "club drugs," such as Ecstasy, may lower inhibitions and lead to unsafe sexual activities. Men engaging in sexual activities with both men and women may consider women "safer" partners and may not use condoms; women in coercive or abusive relationships may feel less able to require partners to practice safer sex. The examiner should be familiar with evolving patterns of risk behavior and be comfortable discussing them in a nonpejorative fashion. Strategies for prevention and education are reviewed in Chapter 39.

BARRIERS TO TREATMENT AND ADHERENCE

Studies have shown multiple barriers to adherence to medications and medical treatment in general, but the particular demands of HIV treatment make adherence essential and the most important factor affecting outcome of treatment. Patients should be asked about adherence to all aspects of treatment, including the keeping of appointments and taking of medications for other medical conditions as well as antiretrovirals. Barriers to adherence should be explored. The causes for nonadherence are multiple[6] and can include denial, fear of side effects, and fear of being identified as an AIDS patient by friends or family. The Internet can serve as a source of disinformation, encouraging the use of unproven "natural" remedies that are perceived as benign over regimens seen as medical and thus "unnatural" and dangerous; herbal remedies may be favored by patients from different cultural backgrounds. Financial constraints may play a role for some patients. Those who continue drug use or have cognitive impairment may find it difficult to adhere to the routines required for successful antiretroviral treatment. Poor language and literacy skills, which a patient may be ashamed to discuss with care providers, can also be a barrier to adherence. Patients may be reluctant to acknowledge nonadherence for fear of angering or disappointing care providers. Addressing issues of nonadherence and developing an understanding of specific barriers to adherence are essential in the assessment of the patient with HIV infection or AIDS.

SUBSTANCE ABUSE

Ongoing substance abuse clearly can have an impact on all aspects of a patient's ability to care for himself or herself. Drugs or alcohol may affect liver function already compromised by HIV infection or by the commonly comorbid hepatitis B and C, making adherence to highly active antiretroviral therapy (HAART) more difficult. Patients are often reluctant to acknowledge the extent of past and current substance abuse. It may be appropriate to include urine toxicology examinations as a standard part of the initial psychiatric assessment because patients cannot be helped if the problem is not identified. Unexpected positive status may be the result of such screening, and patients may continue to deny drug use or blame the results on laboratory error. However, the value of such information outweighs the risk of the patient's hurt feelings. Repeat testing and further discussion may help elucidate the nature of the patient's substance abuse, with movement toward and achievement of recovery—the ultimate goal. The comorbidity of substance use disorders and HIV infection is discussed in Chapter 14.

AXIS I DIAGNOSES

PSYCHOTIC DISORDERS

Studies over two and a half decades suggest a complex relationship between HIV infection and psychiatric illness. The presence of a major psychiatric illness may make it more difficult for a patient to take care of his or her HIV infection. At the same time, studies have also found that having a psychotic disorder may put a patient at higher risk of contracting HIV infection.[7] This may be due to the extensive comorbidity between substance abuse and psychosis, as well as to poor decision making or victimization during periods of illness. The age of highest incidence for the development of schizophrenic disorders is also a period of high risk for HIV infection. The risk that HIV infection presents to the seriously mentally ill may be underestimated by these patients and by their care providers. It is thus important both to discuss HIV risk factors and suggest HIV testing if the history suggests the presence of risk behaviors in a patient with a psychotic disorder and to rule out the presence or history of a psychotic disorder in patients who have HIV disease. Once a patient with psychiatric illness has been diagnosed as HIV-positive, the most important factor in promoting wellness with this patient, as with any other, is promoting adherence to care. This is a multilayered challenge for the mentally ill patient because adherence to psychotropic medication may be essential before adherence to HAART can be established and periods of relapse from psychotropic medication may lead to nonadherence to HAART or an increase in risk behaviors. When such multiproblemed individuals are identified, careful assessment and close coordination between medical and psychiatric caretakers are essential to maintain patients in treatment and to maximize wellness. One recent study found that rates of adherence to treatment were actually higher in patients with schizophrenia, perhaps because of the closer scrutiny they receive.[8] The appearance of new psychotic symptoms in the later stages of HIV infection suggest an organic cause, and a neurologic workup may be appropriate before ascribing the symptoms to another Axis I disorder. The interrelationship between psychosis and HIV infection is further explored in Chapter 13.

DEPRESSIVE DISORDERS

Comorbidity with depression is common in HIV infection, with a meta-analysis of 10 published studies finding a frequency of major depression almost two times higher in HIV-positive than HIV-negative subjects.[9] The presence of depressive symptoms has been linked to nonadherence and may be a more important factor in nonadherence than neurocognitive impairment.[10] Depression may be primary and contribute to risk behaviors or may be a response to HIV infection, with both biologic and psychological factors playing a role. Patients who are not psychologically minded may not identify themselves as depressed, but may complain of fatigue, insomnia,[11] or even memory loss. Medication side effects and disease state should be taken into consideration when patients complain of decreased mood or lack of energy. When physically ill patients are assessed, the diagnosis of depression should be made by the examiner based on the totality of the symptoms presented by the patient, including vegetative signs, rather than on the patient's self-identification as depressed or not depressed. Bereavement is a particular feature of HIV infection because most HIV-positive individuals have lost friends or family to the infection. They may have sadness associated with "survivor's guilt," feeling they are less worthy of pleasure and even of life itself than those who died before them. Reviewing symptoms of sadness, grief, and depression, both past and present, as well as family history of affective disorder, should figure prominently in the psychiatric assessment of an HIV-positive patient.

BIPOLAR DISORDERS

The presence of manic disorders has been noted in conjunction with HIV infection since the earliest days of the epidemic. Again, mania can be primary or secondary, with HIV infection itself, AIDS-related central nervous system (CNS) infections or neoplasms, and medications all implicated. Comorbid substance abuse can also play a role. It has been suggested that patients with onset of manic symptoms later in the course of infection are less likely to have personal or family history of mood disorder and are more likely to have evidence of neurocognitive compromise, suggesting a secondary mania.[12] These patients also present with irritability more prominent than euphoria and may have more frequent relapses. Thus, with any patient it is important to inquire about family history as well as the individual's history of mania or hypomania to put present or future episodes into context. Chapter 10 discusses mood disorders in HIV-positive individuals.

ANXIETY DISORDERS

Anxiety, a common corollary of HIV infection, may present at different stages of the infection, including testing, initial diagnosis, changes in CD4 or viral load, beginning medications, weight loss, or other markers of illness progression. In addition, anxiety about identification as being HIV-positive, stigmatization, and rejection persist. Medications can give rise to subjective sensations of anxiety, as can withdrawal from drugs or alcohol, precipitated by hospitalization or changes in drug metabolism due to other prescribed medications. It is important to take a good history of a patient's experience with anxiety over his or her lifetime and of how such experiences have been dealt with. Anxiety may be part of another psychiatric disorder, including adjustment disorders or major affective disorder. In addition, patients with post-traumatic stress disorder due to traumatic experiences earlier in life may be more likely to engage in high-risk behaviors, while those behaviors themselves may put individuals at risk for further traumatic experiences.[13] Finally, having HIV itself can be a traumatic event.[14] Chapter 9 reviews the anxiety disorders commonly seen in this population, and Chapter 8 discusses adjustment and stress-related disorders.

PAIN

Pain is frequent in the course of HIV infection. The complete psychiatric assessment should inquire about the presence of pain and the patient's past experience with pain and its treatment. Chapter 17 presents a more detailed review.

SEXUAL DYSFUNCTION

Sexual dysfunction is a common result of HIV infection. It can be due to hypogonadism; it can also be a marker of possible depression, substance abuse, or medication side effects. Patients should be asked about changes in libido and sexual dysfunction.

SUICIDAL BEHAVIORS

Concern has been raised since the early days of the epidemic about increased risk of suicide in this population. Earlier in the epidemic, it appeared that there was a higher risk, perhaps not an unexpected finding at a time when treatment options were extremely limited and supportive resources unavailable. As knowledge and treatment options have grown, the risk of suicide in this population appears to have decreased and seems to be related to factors well known to increase risk of suicide in other populations—family history, the availability of support, the presence of affective disorder, history of past suicidality, or substance abuse.

Chronic illness, particularly when painful or involving neurologic symptoms, has been noted to be associated with increased risk of suicide in other patient populations. Losses due to HIV infection, including financial or personal losses, as well as the loss of health, may increase risk. Exploration of suicidal ideation, as well as past suicidal behaviors and specific risk factors, should be part of any psychiatric assessment. Current suicidal ideation and intent is a psychiatric emergency, requiring immediate assessment and even hospitalization if the patient feels unable to control his or her behaviors. Chapter 38 reviews suicidal behaviors in HIV infection, and physician-assisted suicide is discussed in Chapter 40.

PERSONALITY DISORDERS

Some studies have suggested that the prevalence of personality disorders is higher in patients with HIV infection than in control populations.[15] This is not unexpected given the high prevalence of substance abuse in patients with certain personality disorders and the link between impulsivity and risk behaviors for HIV infection. Personality disorders in Cluster B, which are marked by impulsivity and interpersonal difficulty, are the most common in the HIV-positive population and may portend difficulty in complying with the demands of treatment. Such individuals may have difficulty with the concept of delayed gratification and thoughtful decision making that underlie adherence. Studies have found such personality disorders in HIV-positive individuals are associated with a higher rate of depression, maladaptive coping, and a higher rater of injection drug use.[16] Careful review of the patient's history should focus on assessment of pervasive patterns of behavior that suggest impulsivity, instability in interpersonal relationships, difficulty in conforming to social norms, and other markers of personality disorder as reviewed in the *Diagnostic and Statistical Manual (DSM-IV-TR)*.

COGNITIVE DISORDERS

Ambrosino et al.[17] suggest a hierarchical approach to differential diagnosis in the HIV-positive patient, especially in assessment of the patient with more advanced disease, always examining first for symptoms of delirium, then ruling out HADc, then assessing for medical diagnoses, and only then considering other psychiatric diagnoses. The rationale behind this hierarchical approach is the high prevalence of neurocognitive disorders in this population and the need for a high index of suspicion to avoid underdiagnosis. Delirium is a medical emergency and can be confused with psychiatric disorders such as psychosis or depression. Patients with a history of prior psychiatric disorder may be at higher risk for misdiagnosis, and a missed diagnosis of delirium, as confusion, paranoia, hallucinatory experiences, and misperceptions, may be wrongly attributed to psychosis. A sudden change in level of alertness or sudden or subacute presentation of psychiatric symptoms in an HIV-positive patient should always lead to a complete evaluation, including physical and neurologic examination, Serum MultipleAnalysism-6 (SMA 6), complete blood count, liver function texts, electroencephalogram, lumbar puncture, and neuroimaging, to rule out a potentially treatable opportunistic infection, neoplasm, or metabolic derangement. HADc is a multifaceted syndrome, with cognitive, affective, motoric, and behavioral symptoms. Common symptoms include mental and motoric slowing, apathy, loss of fine motor coordination, and difficulty with the manipulation of knowledge (executive functions). The prevalence and severity of the symptoms increase as patients develop other sequelae of progressive HIV infection. Assessment of attention, concentration, memory, and executive function, which can be done in the course of eliciting a history, as well as through formal testing, will help determine the presence and severity of delirium or dementia. AIDS-related cognitive disorders are discussed in Chapter 12.

SUMMARY

A substantial proportion of those living with HIV may still be unaware of being infected. Thus any psychiatric assessment may be the assessment of an HIV-positive individual, and it is up to the clinician to consider the possibility of HIV infection in the evaluation of any new patient, as well as using the opportunity each clinical encounter provides to educate patients about risk reduction and prevention. Once a patient has been identified as HIV-positive and referred for evaluation, a psychiatric assessment presents the opportunity to diagnose and treat the psychiatric syndromes commonly seen in HIV infection, lessening the burden of distress for these individuals with the triple diagnoses of medical illness, psychiatric illness, and substance use disorders. The information gleaned from a thorough psychiatric assessment can assist an interdisciplinary HIV care team to help a patient make the best use of the services available and guide the team in determining the most useful means of providing services to a given patient. It all starts with a thorough assessment, sensitive to the special needs of this special population.

REFERENCES

1. McDaniel JS, Fowlie E, Summerville MB, et al. An assessment of rates of psychiatric morbidity and functioning in HIV disease. *Gen Hosp Psychiatry*. 1995;17:346–352.
2. Manos P, Wu R. The ten point clock test: a quick screen and grading method for cognitive impairment in medical and surgical patients. *Intl J Psychiatry Med*. 1998;24:229–244.
3. Power C, Selnes OA, Grim JA, et al. HIV Dementia Scale: a rapid screen test. *J Acquir Immune Defic Syndr Human Retrovirol*. 1995;8:273–278.
4. Davis HF, Skolasky RL, Selnes OA, et al. Assessing HIV-associated dementia: Modified HIV Dementia Scale versus the grooved pegboard. *AIDS Read*. 2002;12:29–38.
5. Goldberg DP, Hillier VF. A scaled version of the General Health Questionnaire. *Psychol Med*. 1979;9:139–145.
6. Mehta A, Moore RD, Graham NMH: Potential factors affecting adherence with HIV therapy. *AIDS*. 1997;11:1665–1670.
7. Kalichman SC, Kelly JA, Johnson JR, et al. Factors associated with risk for HIV infection among chronically mentally ill adults. *Am J Psychiatry*. 1994;151:221–227.
8. Walkup J, Sambamoorthi U, Crystal S. Incidence and consistency of antiretroviral use among HIV-infected Medicaid beneficiaries with schizophrenia. *J Clin Psychiatry*. 2001;62:174–178.
9. Ciesla J, Roberts J. Meta-analysis of the relationship between HIV infection and risk for depressive disorders. *Am J Psychiatry*. 2001;158:725–730.
10. Ammassari A, Antinori A, Aloisi MS, et al. Depressive symptoms, neurocognitive impairment, and adherence to highly active antiretroviral therapy among HIV-infected persons. *Psychosomatics*. 2004;45:394–402.
11. Perkins DO, Leserman J, Stern RA, et al. Somatic symptoms of HIV infection: relationship to depressive symptoms and indicators of HIV disease. *Am J Psychiatry*. 1995;152:1776–1781.
12. Lyketsos CG, Schwartz J, Fishman M, et al. AIDS mania. *J Neuropsychiatry Clin Neurosci*. 1997;9:277–279.
13. Stiffman AR, Dore P, Earls F, et al. The influence of mental health problems on AIDS related risk behaviors in young adults. *J Nerv Ment Dis*. 2000;180:314–320.
14. Kelly B, Raphael B, Judd F, et al. Post traumatic stress disorder in response to HIV infection. *Gen Hosp Psychiatry*. 1998;20:345–352.
15. Della Penna ND, Triesman GJ. HIV/AIDS. In: Levenson JL, ed. *Textbook of Psychosomatic Medicine*, Washington, DC: American Psychiatric Press; 2005.
16. Perkins DO, Davidson EJ: Personality disorder in patients affected with HIV: a controlled study with implications for clinical care. *Am J Psychiatry*. 1993;150:309–313.
17. Ambrosino Wyszynski A, Bruno B, Ying P, et al. The HIV infected patient. In: Ambrosino Wyszynski A, Wyszynski B, eds. *Manual of Psychiatric Care for the Medically Ill*. Washington, DC: American Psychiatric Press; 2005.

CHAPTER 5

Psychological and Neuropsychological Testing

Joel K. Levy

One of the common complications of human immunodeficiency virus (HIV)-1 infection is neurocognitive impairment. This alteration of brain-behavior functioning may range from a subjective sense that one has slowing of thinking and difficulty with memory retrieval to a severe dementia with confusion, mutism, and gross neurologic signs. Numerous studies indicate the percentage of HIV-1–infected patients having any cognitive impairment during the course of their illness to be 38.8% to 54.4% overall[1–3] and meeting the full criteria for dementia to be 10.4% to 25.2%,[1–3] despite more and more effective antiretroviral therapy.[3] With this percentage of people with potential cognitive loss, it follows that clinicians working with HIV-1–infected patients must be sensitive to any signs that cognition is declining, be prepared to refer for a formal neurocognitive evaluation to fully delineate the problems, and, if results show that there are deficits, have a regimen ready for their relief.[4,5]

Since 1987, neurocognitive dysfunction in the form of HIV-associated dementia complex has been one of the case-defining criteria conditions for the diagnosis of fully developed acquired immunodeficiency syndrome (AIDS).[6] Indeed, the presence of severe neurocognitive impairment has been associated with a shortened life expectancy,[7–9] although now lengthened since the introduction of highly active antiretroviral therapy (HAART).[10] At the beginning of the epidemic, when opportunistic infections were less controllable, the causes of cognitive impairment and dementia were multifactorial, in that those infections and central nervous system (CNS) neoplasia could result in cognitive decline.[11–13] This was in addition to the diffuse effects of HIV infection in the brain. Opportunistic infections and tumors could also be reflected as focal neuropsychological deficits, such as strokes. There may also be complications from substance-induced psychiatric disorders (by illicit or prescribed drugs, or chemotherapy.[14–16] All of the cognitive, behavioral, and emotional conditions just discussed may be characterized, differentiated, and followed by quantitative behavioral methods such as psychological and neuropsychological assessments.

Later in the epidemic, in 1991, as more research confirmed that HIV infection alone could result in significant dementia or subdementia syndromes, a committee of the American Academy of Neurology (AAN) convened to standardize the nomenclature of HIV-associated neurocognitive impairment.[17] This nomenclature remains in force to date and is irrespective of viral load, CD4 count, or physical symptoms. These diagnostic categories depend on cognitive performance and its impact on daily functioning.

Table 5.1 lists the diagnostic criteria for the HIV-1–associated minor cognitive motor disorder (MCMD) that manifest early in the course of the HIV-1 infection. Complaints such as forgetfulness, inattention, difficulty concentrating, mental slowing, and loss of interest or pleasure in everyday activities have often been misinterpreted as a psychological reaction to having contracted this serious illness. Indeed, a number of studies indicate that often the self-report of subjective cognitive disturbance is correlated more with mood disorder rather than with cognitive dysfunction.[18–20] However, many patients do recognize and report their own mental, physical, and mood changes early in the course of the illness, and, whether a sign of cognitive or mood dysfunction, all reports should be taken seriously and thoroughly investigated. This is because it is also known that HIV-1–related cognitive impairment, whether subjectively reported or not, can occur at any time during the course of the systemic infection.[21] Several investigators have reported that asymptomatic HIV-1–positive patients have measurable cognitive dysfunction compared with HIV-1–negative controls.[22–24] These findings are unrelated to the level of immunosuppression or to depression. Persons with certain risk factors, which lower their "cognitive reserve,"[25–27] are even more prone to early cognitive decline. Moreover, now into the third decade of the epidemic, there are individuals who are surviving into their 50s and 60s with the infection and elderly who are acquiring the infection at a later age.[28] Thus, one now has to consider the possibility of the interaction of the CNS effects of the virus with age-related cognitive changes,[29] or, because of its high overall base rate, an incipient dementia of the Alzheimer's type.

Table 5.2 lists the diagnostic criteria for HIV-1–associated dementia complex. Moderate to severe cognitive deficits, confusion, psychomotor slowing, and seizures may develop as the course of the dementia advances. Patients may appear mute and catatonic. Socially inappropriate behavior, psychosis, mania, and marked motor abnormalities, including ataxia, spasticity, hyperreflexia, hypertonia, and incontinence of bladder and bowel can occur.

TABLE 5.1 Criteria for Clinical Diagnosis of HIV-1–Associated Minor Cognitive Motor Disorder

1. Cognitive/motor/behavioral abnormalities (each of the following):
    a. At least two of the following present for at least 1 month:
        (1) Impaired attention or concentration
        (2) Mental slowing
        (3) Impaired memory
        (4) Slowed movements
        (5) Incoordination
        (6) Personality change, irritability or emotional lability
    b. Acquired cognitive/motor abnormality verified by clinical neurologic examination or neuropsychological testing (e.g., fine motor speed, manual dexterity, perceptual motor skills, attention/concentration, speed of processing information, abstraction/reasoning, visuospatial skills, memory/learning, or speech/language)
2. Disturbance from No. 1 causes mild impairment of work or activities of daily living
3. Does not meet criteria for HIV-1–associated dementia complex or HIV-1–associated myelopathy
4. No evidence of another etiology, including active CNS opportunistic infection or malignancy, severe systemic illness, active alcohol or substance use, acute or chronic substance withdrawal, adjustment disorder, or other psychiatric disorders
5. HIV seropositivity (enzyme-linked immunoabsorbent assay [ELISA] test confirmed by Western blot, polymerase chain reaction, or culture)

Adapted from Janssen RS, Saykin AJ, Cannon L, et al.; American Academy of Neurology AIDS Task Force. Nomenclature and research case definitions for neurologic manifestations of human immunodeficiency virus-type-1 (HIV-1) infection. *Neurology*. 1991;41:778–785.

TABLE 5.2 Criteria for Clinical Diagnosis of HIV-1–Associated Dementia Complex

Must have each of the following:
1. Acquired abnormality in at least two of the following cognitive abilities for at least 1 month: Attention/concentration, speed of processing information, abstraction/reasoning, visuospatial skills, memory/learning, and speech/language. Cognitive dysfunction causing impairment of work or activities of daily living should not be attributable solely to severe systemic illness.
2. At least 1 of the following:
   (a) Acquired abnormality in motor function or performance verified by clinical examination, neuropsychological testing, or both.
   (b) Decline in motivation or emotional control, or change in social behavior.
3. Absence of clouding of consciousness during a period long enough to establish the presence of No. 1.
4. No evidence of another etiology, including active CNS opportunistic infection or malignancy, other psychiatric disorders (e.g., depression), active alcohol or substance use, or acute or chronic substance withdrawal.
5. HIV seropositivity (enzyme-linked immunoabsorbent assay [ELISA] test confirmed by Western blot, polymerase chain reaction, or culture).

Adapted from Janssen RS, Saykin AJ, Cannon L, et al.; American Academy of Neurology AIDS Task Force. Nomenclature and research case definitions for neurologic manifestations of human immunodeficiency virus-type-1 (HIV-1) infection. *Neurology*. 1991;41:778–785.

Similar to the operationalized diagnostic categorization for Dementia of the Alzheimer Type,[30] this classification system requires demonstration of impairment in one or more cognitive domains. The criteria for impairment have been established as a consensus of performance levels on standardized neuropsychometric tests. These tests most reliably and reproduceably express performance in quantitative terms and can do so with considerable precision. The metric often used is a statistical value in terms of units and fractions of the standard deviation from the test's normative mean.[31] The patient's performance at two standard deviations below the published normative mean is usually taken to indicate severe impairment on that test, and thus in the cognitive domain for which that test taps representative abilities. This level corresponds to a ranking at or below the first percentile. Lesser impairment, but at a level considered lower than the low end of the normal range, is operationalized as one and one-half standard deviations (fifth percentile) below the test's normative mean, and this level has been used to indicate sub–dementia syndromal states such as HIV-related MCMD.

The complete assessment of any patient with neurocognitive impairment should include several areas: the patient's background and details of current illness; a neuropsychological assessment of the various cognitive domains, an assessment of the impairments' impact on daily functioning, and measures of any psychological distress. The most basic of assessments are the history and mental status examination.

NEUROBEHAVIORAL EVALUATION IN HIV-1 INFECTION

THE STRUCTURED PSYCHOLOGICAL AND NEUROPSYCHOLOGICAL HISTORY

A comprehensive cognitive history is essential for initiating the assessment and designating which tests may be used in the evaluation battery. In combination with the pattern of neuropsychological test results, the history can be key in the differential diagnosis of etiologies of cognitive dysfunction in HIV-1–infected patients with cognitive complaints. Sometimes, the interview identifies the basis of the problem when neuropsychological testing is not possible or available. Table 5.3 lists the essentials of the interview for formulating this history.[32] Answers to these questions can help associate patient complaints with the AAN criterion system for defining HIV-1–associated cognitive disorders.

TABLE 5.3　HIV Cognitive History

Name
Age and birthday
Handedness
First language at home
Educational background
 Best subjects, grades
 Worst subjects
Occupational background
 How long
Medical history
 Childhood diseases or injuries
 Head injuries with loss of consciousness
 Strokes
 High fevers
 Toxin exposure
 Major illness, injuries, or surgeries
 Medicines: prescription, nonprescription
Duration of diagnosis of HIV infection; AIDS
 Current problem
  Change in thinking functions: how long or over what period of time
Change in ability to concentrate
Periods of confusion or mental "fuzziness"
 When talking with people, or on the phone, watching TV or a movie, reading
Problem with following a train of thought
Difficulties with handwriting
Word-finding problems; difficulties with slurring or stammering
Slowing of thinking or understanding, trouble with mental arithmetic such as making change or balancing checkbook
Wear glasses
Blurring vision, double vision, or flashing lights in eyes
Change in understanding what is seen; do things look right in their relation to each other?
Overlook things when right in front of you
Hear unusual sounds, see unusual things, have strange feelings
Changes in any other senses
 Decreased hearing; ringing or buzzing sounds
 Change in smell or taste
 Numbness, "pins or needles," loss of feeling, tingling, or burning feelings
 Severe pain
Memory
 Areas of memory that are better or worse
 Memory for recent information

(continued)

TABLE 5.3	HIV Cognitive History (Continued)

Information from a long way back in life
Difference in memory for situations versus rote facts and figures
Kinds of things most easily forgotten: names, addresses, directions, reading
How long things can be remembered; more notes written than previously
Lapses
Getting lost or forgetting where you are
New difficulties with thinking through problems or solving them, making decisions, staying organized—on job, at home
Sleep: trouble getting to sleep; night versus daytime; awakenings from which you cannot immediately return to sleep
Inability to move parts of the body
    Muscle weakness, twitching, spasms, trouble walking, coordination problems, tremors or shakiness, problems with dropping things, feeling like moving more slowly; difficulty using tools or household utensils, getting dressed, telling right from left
Headaches or dizziness, instances thought to be seizures (staring off into space for a long time, uncontrollable movements, periods where you seemed "lose" time, incontinence)
Changes in mood, feelings, ideas
    Mood swings, loss of patience or change in temper, increase in irritability, change in amount of worry, sense of panic
(Continue with Hamilton Depression and Anxiety Scales)

Adapted from Levy JK, Fernandez F. HIV infection of the CNS: implications for neuropsychiatry. In: Yudofsky SC, Hales RE, eds. *The American Psychiatric Press Textbook of Neuropsychiatry*. 3rd ed. Washington, DC: American Psychiatric Press; 1996.

THE MENTAL STATUS EXAMINATION

The introductory cognitive history should include an appropriate mental status examination. A standard examination, such as the Mini-Mental State Examination (MMSE),[33,34] is frequently performed because it is well known and many practitioners have developed a sense of what its score means in terms of overall cognitive functioning. This test was developed to help identify the cortical type of dementia associated with Alzheimer's disease. It has a concentration of items associated with language and orientation and a visuospatial task. However, it may miss the types of memory, speed of information processing, and attention/concentration problems often associated with HIV-1 CNS infection. The HIV Dementia Scale is better suited for the subcortical type of cognitive involvement associated with HIV-1 CNS infection.[35–37] It contains a learning and memory section, two speed of processing tasks (one involving language and one involving visuospatial analysis and construction), and a saccadic control task that can double as a behavioral inhibition test. Studies have validated this brief task as an indicator of HIV-related impairment.[38,39] Another screening task, the High Sensitivity Cognitive Screen (HSCS), may be useful in screening for simple presence or absence of cognitive dysfunction.[40,41] The creators of this measure report high correlations between this test and the overall result of neuropsychological testing. They note that the HSCS is also correlated with electroencephalographic results in medical psychiatric inpatients and with functional status in HIV-infected community-dwelling subjects. Results on this measure may then establish the eligibility of the patient for more in-depth neuropsychological assessment.

NEUROPSYCHOLOGICAL ASSESSMENT

The most prevalent components of cognitive impairment related to HIV-1 infection include, by stages, early, mild problems with abstraction, attention and concentration, learning and memory, and psychomotor speed that progress to more serious difficulties with these functions, as well as impaired cognitive flexibility, nonverbal problem solving, and visuospatial integration and construction.[42,43]

As with the language-heavy MMSE, neuropsychological tests for assessment of other forms of dementia include tasks that gauge such cortical functions as complex language-associated functions (such as aphasia and apraxia), higher level cognitive functions of verbal and nonverbal abstract reasoning and problem solving, and perceptual functioning. These tasks are still necessary when one suspects or has information that the patient is experiencing dysfunction related to focal disturbances in the CNS. These can be caused by such conditions as an abscess created by an HIV-1–related opportunistic infection or tumor; a stroke caused by illicit use of drugs that have vasoconstricting properties, such as cocaine; or an HIV-related process such as varicella-zoster vasculitis. Other tasks often used in comprehensive batteries for evaluation of memory, attention and concentration, and psychomotor speed are more useful for detecting the often-subtle impairments of the early stages of HIV-1's effects on the CNS. Table 5.4 shows

TABLE 5.4 | National Institute of Mental Health Neuropsychological Battery

A. Indication of premorbid intelligence
   1. Vocabulary (Weschler Adult Intelligent Scale–Revised[WAIS-R])
   2. National Adult Reading Test (NART)
B. Attention
   1. Digit Span (Weschler Memory Scale–Revised [WMS-R])
   2. Visual Span (WMS-R)
C. Speed of processing
   1. Sternberg search task
   2. Simple and choice reaction time
   3. Paced Auditory Serial Addition Test (PASAT)
D. Memory
   1. California Verbal Learning Test (CVLT)
   2. Memory working test
   3. Modified Visual Reproduction test
E. Abstraction
   1. Category Test
   2. Trail Making Test, parts A and B
F. Language
   1. Boston Naming Test
   2. Letter and category fluency tests
G. Visuospatial
   1. Embedded figures test
   2. Money's standardized road-map test of direction sense
   3. Digit Symbol substitution
H. Construction abilities
   1. Block Design Test
   2. Tactual Performance Test
I. Motor abilities
   1. Grooved pegboard

(continued)

TABLE 5.4	National Institute of Mental Health Neuropsychological Battery (Continued)

  2. Finger-tapping test
  3. Grip strength
J. Psychiatric assessment
  1. Diagnostic Interview Schedule (DIS)
  2. Hamilton Depression Scale
  3. State-Trait Anxiety Scale
  4. Mini-Mental State Examination

Adapted from Butters N, Grant I, Haxby J, et al. Assessment of AIDS-related cognitive changes: recommendations of the NIMH Workgroup on Neuropsychological Assessment Approaches. *J Clin Exp Neuropsychol.* 1990;12:963–978.

an early neuropsychological battery recommended by the National Institute of Mental Health (NIMH) for HIV patients.[44] This battery was comprehensive, but lengthy, and could tax the sometimes-limited stamina of the patient. Moreover, some of the instruments in this battery were not easily available from commercial suppliers and had to be obtained from the developing investigators. Some of the items in the battery had only one form, and repeated testings that are necessary for follow-up of treatments could be problematic because of carry-over effects.

A brief form of this battery was developed, but, when this short form was used longitudinally for measurement of intervention effects, unsatisfactory practice or carry-over effects were discovered.[45] More recent efforts at developing a briefer, more available battery have produced one that more economically answers the questions about the patient's neurocognitive stage.[46,47] Table 5.5 lists the tests that make up this battery. The tests included have previously and individually been validated in applications in HIV cases. Examples of these are the Hopkins Verbal Learning Test-Revised,[48] the Trail Making Test,[49–52] verbal fluency measures,[53,54] digit-symbol or symbol-digit substitution tasks,[55–57] and the Grooved Pegboard psychomotor speed test.[58,59] The psychomotor and neuromotor tasks especially may reveal early detection of HIV-1–related cognitive impairment.[60]

These tests, as well as the NIMH battery, taken together, yield an appreciable number of scores that individually may be difficult to interpret in isolation. Neuropsychologists have often tried to summarize or digest multiple scores into indices that correspond to diagnostic levels (e.g., the Halstead-Reitan Impairment Index[61,62]). Associated with the HNRC battery, those co-workers have advanced a rating system that ranks test scores and then summarizes the ranks to fit within the AAN framework for HIV cognitive diagnostic categories.[63,64] This system has been found reliable and has been validated for HIV neurocognitive impairment.[65]

At rare times, in neuropsychological testing, situational factors such as potential monetary compensation or increase in benefits, or a number of psychological issues, suggest that persons may wish to portray themselves in less than the most favorable light and not expend their best effort in performing the tests. This is also an issue often alleged in litigation, regardless of HIV status. Neuropsychologists often employ instruments that can indicate effort or symptom validity as a control to the other tests. Lezak[31] details some of these procedures and describes how validity indices may be derived from the most commonly used neuropsychological instruments. However, in employing these measures, one must know their limitations, especially with regard to generation of false positive results. As a health care provider, one may be hesitant to believe that patients are trying to mislead, yet one wants to help them in the most appropriate way. Additionally, in doing research with these populations, it is essential to enter subjects who validly carry the diagnoses under investigation. With regard to one of the most generally used instruments, the Rey 15-Item Test,[66,67] several investigators have

TABLE 5.5	HNRC Neuropsychological Battery

A. Indication of Premorbid Intelligence
 1. Vocabulary (Wide Range Achievement Test–III Reading Subtest)
B. Attention/Working Memory
 1. Digit Span Subtest (Weschler Memory Scale–Revised [WMS-R])
 2. Wechsler Adult Intelligence Scale–III Letter-Number Sequencing Subtest
C. Speed of Information Processing
 1. Trail Making Test–Part A
 2. Wechsler Adult Intelligence Scale–III Digit Symbol Subtest
 3. Paced Auditory Serial Addition Test (PASAT)–First Trial
D. Memory
 1. Hopkins Verbal Learning Test–Revised (HVLT-R)
 2. Brief Visual Memory Test–Revised (BVMT-R)
E. Abstraction/Executive Function
 1. Wisconsin Card Sort Test–Computer Version
 2. Trail Making Test–Part B
F. Language
 1. Letter (FAS) and Category (Animals) Fluency Tests
G. Visuospatial
 1. Wechsler Adult Intelligence Scale–III Digit Symbol Subtest
 2. Brief Visual Memory Test–Revised (BVMT-R)–Copy Trial
H. Motor Abilities
 1. Grooved Pegboard
I. Psychological Assessment
 1. Beck Depression Inventory

Adapted from Woods SP, Childers M, Ellis RJ, et al.; HIV Neurobehavioral Research Center (HNRC) Group. A battery approach for measuring neuropsychological change. *Arch Clin Neuropsychol.* 2006;21:83–89.

shown that genuine conditions may yield false positive results, and clinical judgment must ultimately determine validity of this task's performance. A more recently developed method, the forced two-choice selection task,[68] in which correct selections below the 50% level (actually, from the research, a much higher cutoff score[69]) may imply an attempt to deceptively manipulate the task, appears to be less problematic. This task has even been validated in the HIV-infected population,[70] and, unless the patient is obviously severely demented or delirious, there can be high confidence that results reflect the patient's actual effort.

PSYCHOLOGICAL FUNCTIONING

Psychiatric conditions have received much attention because they arise often in HIV neurobehavioral spectrum disorders. The position of opportunistic infection foci or tumors in the brain, the emotional distress caused by HIV infection and all the influences it has on a person, and preexisting psychiatric disorders and/or neurologic syndromes caused by other medical circumstances may necessitate a psychiatric consultation. A number of screening and more comprehensive measures have been used or validated in HIV disease.

In addition to severe and persistent illnesses, which by their epidemiology and base rates probably occurred before or were unrelated to HIV infection (e.g., schizophrenia and bipolar disorder), depression and anxiety have been extensively researched in HIV-infected patients.[71–74] The screening instruments Beck Depression Inventory[75–77] and Symptom Checklist-90[78] (or its brief form, the Brief Symptom Inventory[79,80]) have appeared frequently in the AIDS literature[81–83] and are simple to administer and score. These instruments and the more comprehensive Minnesota Multiphasic Personality Inventory-2 (MMPI-2[84]) have been used to assess psychological difficulties in HIV-infected patients.[85,86] A common problem and point of debate is the overlap[87] of somatic or vegetative symptoms (e.g., fatigue[88]) of depression and the systemic effects of HIV and/or its treatments. A newer, multifactor screening instrument, the Hospital Anxiety and Depression Scale (HADS[89]), attempts to avoid this problem by focusing on the psychological distress elements. For psychological evaluations beyond the screening level, the MMPI-2 and a structured interview would provide information required for a full psychological diagnosis.

Additional specialized areas of psychological measurement of importance to HIV-infected patients, for both research and clinical care, include: (a) surveys of AIDS risk knowledge[90,91] to direct educational efforts for the prevention of further transmission and morbidity; (b) surveys of potential for adherence to AIDS pharmacotherapeutic regimens,[92] to attempt to avoid lapses in treatment that may foster the development of viral resistance to successful medications; (c) measures of patients' impressions of and satisfaction with the care provided,[93] so that they may maintain an alliance with their providers; (d) patients' self-report of comfort with their body image,[94] especially in this era of lipodystrophy syndromes associated with some HIV pharmacotherapies, so that their self-esteem may be optimized; (e) and indicators of patients' quality of life,[95-99] so that care can be adjusted to provide the best possible levels for their comfort and survival.

FUNCTIONAL INDICATORS

Because AAN classification of the fully developed HIV-related cognitive syndrome requires evidence of a significantly adverse impact on daily functioning, both at home and in one's occupation, the battery of these neuropsychometric tests must include a measure of these abilities, too. These types of instruments tend to be based on the observations of the clinician or a collateral informant and psychometrically are, at best, ordinal in their scaling. They may be constructed on a Lickert-type scale in which various abilities are ranked numerically from one extreme to the other—normal for the individual and unchanged from premorbid levels to severely impaired or the inability occurring as a continual problem.

Brew and colleagues characterized functional disabilities and established a scale for the clinical staging of fully developed HIV-1–associated dementia (HAD).[100,101] Table 5.6 shows this staging system, somewhat similar in structure to the Zubrod Performance Scale[102] in cancer or the Clinical Dementia Rating[103] in Alzheimer's disease. It is specific for HAD, and

TABLE 5.6 Clinical Staging System for HIV-1–Associated Dementia Complex

Stage 0 (normal)
+ Normal mental and motor function. Neurologic signs are within the normal age-appropriate spectrum.

Stage 0.5 (subclinical)
+ Minimal or equivocal symptoms without impairment of work or capacity to perform activities of daily living (ADL). Mildly abnormal signs may include reflex changes (e.g., generalized increase in deep tendon reflexes with active jaw jerk, snout, or glabellar sign) or mildly slowed ocular/limb movements, but without clear loss of strength (must be differentiated from fatigue).

Stage 1 (mild)
+ Able to perform all but the more demanding aspects of work or ADL but with unequivocal evidence (symptoms or signs including performance on neuropsychological testing) of intellectual or motor impairment. The abnormal clinical motor signs usually include slow or clumsy movements of extremities, but the patient can walk without assistance.

(continued)

TABLE 5.6 Clinical Staging System for HIV-1–Associated Dementia Complex (Continued)

Stage 2 (moderate)
+ Able to perform basic activities of self-care at home but cannot work or maintain more demanding aspects of daily life (e.g., maintain finances, read text more complex than newspaper). Ambulatory but may require single prop (e.g., cane).

Stage 3 (severe)
+ Major incapacity in intellectual capacity (cannot follow news or personal events, cannot sustain conversation of any complexity, considerable slowing of all output) and motor ability (cannot walk unassisted, requiring walker or personal support, usually with slowing and clumsiness of arms as well).

Stage 4 (end stage)
+ Nearly vegetative. Intellectual and social comprehension and output limited to rudimentary understanding. Nearly or absolutely mute. Paraparetic or plegic with double incontinence.

Adapted from Brew BJ, Sidtis JJ, Petito CK, et al. The neurologic complications of AIDS and human immunodeficiency virus infection. In: Plum F, ed. *Advances in Contemporary Neurology*. Philadelphia: FA Davis; 1994:1–49.

it ranks cognitive, behavioral, and neurologic/motoric functioning commensurate with the stages of progression within the AIDS diagnosis.

However, because of the possibility of early cognitive impairment before the diagnosis of HAD, a means of ranking cognitive functioning needed to be developed to define cognitive disabilities at earlier stages of involvement. The Global Deterioration Scale of Reisberg et al.[104] was adapted from Alzheimer's disease use and is helpful in this respect because of its capability to characterize cognitive functioning in daily activities (Table 5.7).

TABLE 5.7 Global Deterioration Scale (GDS) for Age-Associated Cognitive Decline

GDS stage
1. No cognitive decline
   + Normal
   + No subjective complaints of memory deficit. No memory deficit evident on clinical interview.
2. Very mild cognitive decline
   + Forgetfulness
   + Subjective complaints of mild memory deficit, most frequently in following cognitive areas: (a) forgetting where one has placed familiar objects; (b) forgetting names one formerly knew well. No objective evidence of memory deficit on clinical interview. No objective deficits in employment or social situations. Appropriate concern with respect to symptomatology.
3. Mild cognitive decline
   + Early confusional
   + Earliest clear-cut deficits. Manifestations in more than one of the following areas: (a) patient may have gotten lost when traveling to an unfamiliar location; (b) co-workers become aware of patient's relatively poor performance; (c) word- and name-finding deficits become evident to intimates; (d) patient may read a passage or a book and retain relatively little material; (e) patient may demonstrate decreased facility in remembering names on introduction to new people; (f) patient may have lost or misplaced an object of value; (g) concentration deficit may be evident on clinical testing.

(continued)

TABLE 5.7 Global Deterioration Scale (GDS) for Age-Associated Cognitive Decline (Continued)

4. Moderate cognitive decline
   + Late confusional
   + Clear-cut deficit on careful clinical interview. Deficit manifested in following areas: (a) decreased knowledge of current and recent events; (b) possibly some deficit in memory of one's personal history; (c) concentration deficit elicited on serial substractions; (d) decreased ability to travel, handle finances, etc.
   + + Frequently, no deficit in following areas: (a) orientation to time and person; (b) recognition of familiar persons and faces; (c) ability to travel to familiar locations.
   + + Inability to perform complex tasks. Denial is dominant defense mechanism. Flattening of affect and withdrawal from challenging situations occur.

5. Moderately severe cognitive decline
   + Early dementia
   + Patients can no longer survive without some assistance. Patients are unable during interview to recall a major relevant aspect of their current lives: e.g., their address or telephone number of many years, the names of close members of their family, the name of the high school or college from which they graduated.
   + + Frequently some disorientation to time (date, day of week, season, etc.) or to place. An educated person may have difficulty counting back from 40 by 4s or from 20 by 2s.
   + + Persons at this stage retain knowledge of many major facts regarding themselves and others. They invariably know the name of their significant others. They require no assistance with toileting or eating, but may have some difficulty choosing the proper clothing to wear.

6. Severe cognitive decline
   + Middle dementia
   + May occasionally forget the name of significant others upon whom they are entirely dependent for survival. Will be largely unaware of recent events and experiences in their lives. Retain some knowledge of their past lives, but this is very sketchy. Generally aware of their surrounding, the year, the season, etc. May have difficulty counting backward from 10, and sometimes forward. Will require some assistance with activities of daily living, e.g., may become incontinent, will require travel assistance but occasionally will display ability to travel to familiar locations. Diurnal rhythm frequently disturbed. Almost always recall their own name. Frequently continue to be able to distinguish familiar from unfamiliar persons in their environment.
   + + Personality and emotional changes occur. These are quite variable and include: (a) delusional behavior, e.g., patients may accuse their significant others of being an impostor, may talk to imaginary figures in the environment or to their own reflection in the mirror; (b) obsessive symptoms, e.g., person may continually repeat simple cleaning activities; (c) anxiety symptoms, agitation, and even previously nonexistent violent behavior may occur; (d) cognitive abulia, i.e., loss of will power because an individual cannot carry a thought long enough to determine a purposeful course of action.

7. Very severe cognitive decline
   + Late dementia
   + All verbal abilities are lost. Frequently, there is no speech at all, only grunting. Incontinent of urine; requires assistance toileting and feeding. Loses basic psychomotor skills, e.g., ability to walk. The brain appears no longer to be able to tell the body what to do.
   + + Generalized and cortical neurologic signs and symptoms.

Adapted from Reisberg B, Ferris SH, de Leon MJ, et al. The global deterioration scale (GDS): an instrument for the assessment of primary degenerative dementia (PDD). *Am J Psychiatry*. 1982;139:1136–1139.

Application of the Global Deterioration Scale to a sample of HIV-1–infected patients determined that 21% of the patients at an early stage of symptomatic infection, such as progressive generalized lymphadenopathy (PGL), had Global Deterioration Scale stage 1 (meaning normal), but 42% of the sample had cognitive impairment ranging from forgetfulness to early dementia.[105] As HIV-1 disease progressed, 27% of these patients were shown to have forgetfulness and almost 30% qualified for classification of early, middle, or late dementia.[105] Thus the Global Deterioration Scale can provide a summary quantification of the decline of cognitive function clinically as it relates to an HIV-1–infected person's performance of daily activities, even before the patient fulfills the diagnostic criteria for the HIV-1–associated cognitive/motor complex. The Global Deterioration Scale is also of benefit to research and planning investigations because it is capable of comparing the cognitive impairment associated with HIV-1 infection with the cognitive impairment found in non–HIV-1–related dementias.

SUMMARY

HIV-1 infection, in its 20th year of the epidemic (as of this writing), continues to defy efforts to conquer it, although extensive and untiring efforts have been mounted. It continues to spread around the world, changing its genetic signature as it goes. In countries where the latest advances in antiretroviral therapies are available, it has changed in its course from a relatively rapidly fatal disease to a more controlled, chronic one.[106] The infection continues to invade the brain and cause psychological, behavioral, and cognitive disturbances. The new antiretroviral therapies have been shown to help cognitive functioning, but as yet there is no specific agent to target the virus in the CNS. Thus there is still a need for quantification of the disease's effects on neurobehavioral status, to determine the breadth and depth of the problems, and to measure changes in the various components of functioning in the course of pharmacotherapy. Newer and more sensitive neurocognitive tests are being utilized in these assessments. Efforts are being made to standardize the ways that neuropsychometric results are combined to form a diagnosis of these disorders. Signs of neuropsychiatric disorders may now be detected earlier, allowing prompt and aggressive management of these potentially devastating complications of the HIV-1 infection.

REFERENCES

1. Cysique LA, Maruff P, Brew BJ. Prevalence and pattern of neuropsychological impairment in human immunodeficiency virus-infected/acquired immunodeficiency syndrome (HIV/AIDS) patients across pre- and post-highly active antiretroviral therapy eras: a combined study of two cohorts. *J Neurovirol*. 2004;10:350–357.
2. Valcour V, Shikuma C, Shiramizu B, et al. Higher frequency of dementia in older HIV-1 individuals: the Hawaii Aging with HIV-1 Cohort. *Neurology*. 2004;63:822–827.
3. Neuenburg JK, Brodt HR, Herndier BG, et al. HIV-related neuropathology, 1985 to 1999: rising prevalence of HIV encephalopathy in the era of highly active antiretroviral therapy. *J Acquir Immune Defic Syndr*. 2002;31: 171–177.
4. Fernandez F. Neuropsychiatric aspects of human immunodeficiency virus (HIV) infection. *Curr Psychiatry Rep*. 2002;4:228–231.
5. Hinkin CH, Castellon SA, Hardy DJ, Farinpour R, Newton T, Singer E. Methylphenidate improves HIV-1-associated cognitive slowing. *J Neuropsychiatry Clin Neurosci*. 2001;13:248–254.
6. Centers for Disease Control and Prevention (CDC). Revision of the CDC surveillance case definition for acquired immunodeficiency syndrome. *MMWR Morb Mortal Wkly Rep*. 1987;36(suppl 1):1S–15S.
7. Farinpour R, Miller EN, Satz P, et al. Visscher Psychosocial risk factors of HIV morbidity and mortality: findings from the Multicenter AIDS Cohort Study (MACS). *Br J Clin Exp Neuropsychol*. 2003;25:654–670.
8. Tozzi V, Balestra P, Serraino D, et al. Neurocognitive impairment and survival in a cohort of HIV-infected patients treated with HAART. *Res Hum Retroviruses*. 2005;21:706–713.
9. Wilkie FL, Goodkin K, Eisdorfer C, et al. Mild cognitive impairment and risk of mortality in HIV-1 infection. *J Neuropsychiatry Clin Neurosci*. 1998;10:125–132.
10. Dore GJ, McDonald A, Li Y, Kaldor JM, Brew BJ. National HIV Surveillance Committee: marked improvement in survival following AIDS dementia complex in the era of highly active antiretroviral therapy. *AIDS*. 2003;17:1539–1545.

11. Price RW, Brew BJ. The AIDS dementia complex. *J Infect Dis.* 1988;158:1079–1083.
12. Bredesen DE, Levy RM, Rosenblum ML. The neurology of human immunodeficiency virus infection. *Q J Med.* 1988;68:665–677.
13. Del Valle L, Pina-Oviedo S. HIV disorders of the brain: pathology and pathogenesis. *Front Biosci.* 2006;11:718–732.
14. Hestad K, Aukrust P, Ellertsen B, Klove H, Wilberg K. Neuropsychological deficits in HIV-1 seropositive and seronegative intravenous drug users. *J Clin Exp Neuropsychol.* 1993;15:732–742.
15. Langford D, Adame A, Grigorian A, et al.; HIV Neurobehavioral Research Center Group. Patterns of selective neuronal damage in methamphetamine-user AIDS patients. *J Acquir Immune Defic Syndr.* 2003;34:467–474.
16. Clifford DB, Evans S, Yang Y, et al. Impact of efavirenz on neuropsychological performance and symptoms in HIV-infected individuals. *Ann Intern Med.* 2005;143:714–721.
17. Janssen RS, Saykin AJ, Cannon L, et al.; American Academy of Neurology AIDS Task Force. Nomenclature and research case definitions for neurologic manifestations of human immunodeficiency virus-type 1 (HIV-1) infection. *Neurology.* 1991;41:778–785.
18. Carter SL, Rourke SB, Murji S, Shore D, Rourke BP. Cognitive complaints, depression, medical symptoms, and their association with neuropsychological functioning in HIV infection: a structural equation model analysis. *Neuropsychology.* 2003;17:410–419.
19. van Gorp WG, Satz P, Hinkin C, et al. Metacognition in HIV-1 seropositive asymptomatic individuals: self-ratings versus objective neuropsychological performance: Multicenter AIDS Cohort Study (MACS). *J Clin Exp Neuropsychol.* 1991;13:812–819.
20. Claypoole KH, Elliott AJ, Uldall KK, et al. Cognitive functions and complaints in HIV-1 individuals treated for depression. *Appl Neuropsychol.* 1998;5:74–84.
21. Villa G, Solida A, Moro E, et al. Cognitive impairment in asymptomatic stages of HIV infection: a longitudinal study. *Eur Neurol.* 1996;36:125–133.
22. Pereda M, Ayuso-Mateos JL, Gomez Del Barrio A, et al. Factors associated with neuropsychological performance in HIV-seropositive subjects without AIDS. *Psychol Med.* 2000;30:205–217.
23. Bornstein RA, Nasrallah HA, Para MF, Whitacre CC, Rosenberger P, Fass RJ. Neuropsychological performance in symptomatic and asymptomatic HIV infection. *AIDS.* 1993;7:519–524.
24. Stern Y. The impact of human immunodeficiency virus on cognitive function. *N Y Acad Sci.* 1991;640:219–223.
25. Stern RA, Silva SG, Chaisson N, et al. Influence of cognitive reserve on neuropsychological functioning in asymptomatic human immunodeficiency virus-1 infection. *Arch Neurol.* 1996;53:148–153.
26. Green JE, Saveanu RV, Bornstein RA. The effect of previous alcohol abuse on cognitive function in HIV infection. *J Int Neuropsychol Soc.* 2004;10:298–300.
27. Basso MR, Bornstein RA. Estimated premorbid intelligence mediates neurobehavioral change in individuals infected with HIV across 12 months. *J Clin Exp Neuropsychol.* 2000;22:208–218.
28. Cherner M, Ellis RJ, Lazzaretto D, et al.; HIV Neurobehavioral Research Center Group. Effects of HIV-1 infection and aging on neurobehavioral functioning: preliminary findings. *AIDS.* 2004;18(suppl 1):S27–S34.
29. Valcour VG, Shikuma CM, Watters MR, Sacktor NC. Cognitive impairment in older HIV-1-seropositive individuals: prevalence and potential mechanisms. *AIDS.* 2004;18(suppl 1):S79–S86.
30. McKhann G, Drachman D, Folstein M, Katzman R, Price D, Stadlan EM. Clinical diagnosis of Alzheimer's disease: report of the NINCDS-ADRDA Work Group under the auspices of Department of Health and Human Services Task Force on Alzheimer's disease. *Neurology.* 1984;34:939–944.
31. Lezak MD, Howieson DB, Loring DW. *Neuropsychological Assessment.* 4th ed. New York: Oxford University Press; 2004.
32. Levy JK, Fernandez F. HIV infection of the CNS: implications for neuropsychiatry. In: Yudofsky SC, Hales RE, eds. *Textbook of Neuropsychiatry.* 3rd ed. Arlington, Va: American Psychiatric Press; 1996.
33. Folstein MF, Folstein SE, McHugh PR. "Mini-mental state": a practical method for grading the cognitive state of patients for the clinician. *J Psychiatr Res.* 1975;12:189–198.
34. Anthony JC, LeResche L, Niaz U, von Korff MR, Folstein MF. Limits of the "Mini-Mental State" as a screening test for dementia and delirium among hospital patients. *Psychol Med.* 1982;12:397–408.
35. Power C, Selnes OA, Grim JA, McArthur JC. HIV Dementia Scale: a rapid screening test. *J Acquir Immune Defic Syndr Hum Retrovirol.* 1995;8:273–278.
36. Dougherty RH, Skolasky RL Jr, McArthur JC. Progression of HIV-associated dementia treated with HAART. *AIDS Read.* 2002;12:69–74.
37. Berghuis JP, Uldall KK, Lalonde B. Validity of two scales in identifying HIV-associated dementia. *J Acquir Immune Defic Syndr.* 1999;21:134–140.
38. Richardson MA, Morgan EE, Vielhauer MJ, Cuevas CA, Buondonno LM, Keane TM. Utility of the HIV Dementia Scale in assessing risk for significant HIV-related cognitive-motor deficits in a high-risk urban adult sample. *AIDS Care.* 2005;17:1013–1021.
39. von Giesen HJ, Haslinger BA, Rohe S, Koller H, Arendt G. HIV Dementia Scale and psychomotor slowing: the best methods in screening for neuro-AIDS. *J Neuropsychiatry Clin Neurosci.* 2005;17:185–191.
40. Fogel BS. The high sensitivity cognitive screen. *Int Psychogeriatr.* 1991;3:273–288.
41. Faust D, Fogel BS. The development and initial validation of a sensitive bedside cognitive screening test. *J Nerv Ment Dis.* 1989;177:25–31.
42. Bornstein RA, Nasrallah HA, Para MF, et al. Neuropsychological performance in symptomatic and asymptomatic HIV infection. *J Acquir Immune Defic Syndr.* 1993;7:519–524.
43. Van Gorp WG, Miller E, Satz P, et al. Neuropsychological performance in HIV-1 immunocompromised patients. *J Clin Exp Neuropsychol.* 1989;11:35.

44. Butters N, Grant I, Haxby J, et al. Assessment of AIDS-related cognitive changes: recommendations of the NIMH Workgroup on Neuropsychological Assessment Approaches. *J Clin Exp Neuropsychol.* 1990;12:963–978.
45. McCaffrey RJ, Cousins JP, Westervelt HJ, et al. Practice effects with the NIMH AIDS abbreviated neuropsychological battery. *Arch Clin Neuropsychol.* 1995;10:241–250.
46. Woods SP, Childers M, Ellis RJ, Guaman S, Grant I, Heaton RK; The HIV Neurobehavioral Research Center (HNRC) Group. A battery approach for measuring neuropsychological change. *Arch Clin Neuropsychol.* 2006;21:83–89.
47. Carey CL, Woods SP, Rippeth JD, et al.; HNRC Group. Initial validation of a screening battery for the detection of HIV-associated cognitive impairment. *Clin Neuropsychol.* 2004;18:234–248.
48. Woods SP, Scott JC, Dawson MS, et al; The HIV Neurobehavioral Research Center (HNRC) Group. Construct validity of Hopkins Verbal Learning Test-Revised component process measures in an HIV-1 sample. *Arch Clin Neuropsychol.* 2005;20:1061–1071.
49. Basso MR, Bornstein RA. Effects of past noninjection drug abuse upon executive function and working memory in HIV infection. *J Clin Exp Neuropsychol.* 2003;25:893–903.
50. Sacktor NC, Lyles RH, Skolasky RL, et al. Combination antiretroviral therapy improves psychomotor speed performance in HIV-seropositive homosexual men: Multicenter AIDS Cohort Study (MACS). *Neurology.* 1999;52:1640–1647.
51. Jones BN, Teng EL, Folstein MF, Harrison KS. A new bedside test of cognition for patients with HIV infection. *Ann Intern Med.* 1993;119:1001–1004.
52. Hestad K, McArthur JH, Dal Pan GJ, et al. Regional brain atrophy in HIV-1 infection: association with specific neuropsychological test performance. *Acta Neurol Scand.* 1993;88:112–118.
53. Millikin CP, Trepanier LL, Rourke SB. Verbal fluency component analysis in adults with HIV/AIDS. *J Clin Exp Neuropsychol.* 2004;26:933–942.
54. Woods SP, Conover E, Rippeth JD, et al.; HIV Neurobehavioral Research Center (HNRC) Group. Qualitative aspects of verbal fluency in HIV-associated dementia: a deficit in rule-guided lexical-semantic search processes? *Neuropsychologia.* 2004;42:801–809.
55. Grassi MP, Perin C, Borella M, Mangoni A. Assessment of cognitive function in asymptomatic HIV-positive subjects. *Eur Neurol.* 1999;42:225–229.
56. Becker JT, Salthouse TA. Neuropsychological test performance in the acquired immunodeficiency syndrome: independent effects of diagnostic group on functioning. *J Int Neuropsychol Soc.* 1999;5:41–47.
57. Llorente AM, van Gorp WG, Stern MJ, et al. Long-term effects of high-dose zidovudine treatment on neuropsychological performance in mildly symptomatic HIV-positive patients: results of a randomized, double-blind, placebo-controlled investigation. *J Int Neuropsychol Soc.* 2001;7:27–32.
58. Chang L, Ernst T, Witt MD, Ames N, Gaiefsky M, Miller E. Relationships among brain metabolites, cognitive function, and viral loads in antiretroviral-naive HIV patients. *Neuroimage.* 2002;17:1638–1648.
59. Sacktor NC, Skolasky RL, Lyles RH, Esposito D, Selnes OA, McArthur JC. Improvement in HIV-associated motor slowing after antiretroviral therapy including protease inhibitors. *J Neurovirol.* 2000;6:84–88.
60. Davis HF, Skolasky RL Jr, Selnes OA, Burgess DM, McArthur JC. Assessing HIV-associated dementia: modified HIV dementia scale versus the Grooved Pegboard. *AIDS Read.* 2002;12:29–31, 38.
61. Hestad K, Aukrust P, Ellertsen B, Klove H, Wilberg K. Neuropsychological deficits in HIV-1 seropositive and seronegative intravenous drug users. *J Clin Exp Neuropsychol.* 1993;15:732–742.
62. Elias MF, Podraza AM, Pierce TW, Robbins MA. Determining neuropsychological cut scores for older, healthy adults. *Exp Aging Res.* 1990;16:209–220.
63. Heaton R, Kirson D, Velin RA, et al. The utility of clinical ratings for detecting cognitive change in HIV infection. In: Grant I, Martin A, eds. *Neuropsychology of HIV Infection.* New York: Oxford University Press; 1994:188–206.
64. Carey CL, Woods SP, Gonzalez R, et al.; HNRC Group. Predictive validity of global deficit scores in detecting neuropsychological impairment in HIV infection. *J Clin Exp Neuropsychol.* 2004;26:307–319.
65. Woods SP, Rippeth JD, Frol AB, et al. Interrater reliability of clinical ratings and neurocognitive diagnoses in HIV. *J Clin Exp Neuropsychol.* 2004;26:759–778.
66. Hays JR, Emmons J, Stallings G. Dementia and mental retardation markers on the Rey 15-item Visual Memory Test. *Psychol Rep.* 2000;86:179–182.
67. Frederick RI. Mixed group validation: a method to address the limitations of criterion group validation in research on malingering detection. *Behav Sci Law.* 2000;18:693–718.
68. Hiscock M, Hiscock CK. Refining the forced-choice method for the detection of malingering. *J Clin Exp Neuropsychol.* 1989;11:967–974.
69. Guilmette TJ, Whelihan W, Sparadeo FR, Buongiorno G. Validity of neuropsychological test results in disability evaluations. *Percept Mot Skills.* 1994;78(3 Pt 2):1179–1186.
70. Woods SP, Conover E, Weinborn M, et al.; HIV Neurobehavioral Research Center (HNRC) Group. Base rate of Hiscock Digit Memory Test failure in HIV-associated neurocognitive disorders. *Clin Neuropsychol.* 2003;17:383–389.
71. Tsao JC, Dobalian A, Moreau C, Dobalian K. Stability of anxiety and depression in a national sample of adults with human immunodeficiency virus. *J Nerv Ment Dis.* 2004;192:111–118.
72. Carter SL, Rourke SB, Murji S, Shore D, Rourke BP. Cognitive complaints, depression, medical symptoms, and their association with neuropsychological functioning in HIV infection: a structural equation model analysis. *Neuropsychology.* 2003;17:410–419.
73. Rabkin JG, Goetz RR, Remien RH, Williams JB, Todak G, Gorman JM. Stability of mood despite HIV illness progression in a group of homosexual men. *Am J Psychiatry.* 1997;154:1632–1633.

74. Joyce GF, Chan KS, Orlando M, Burnam MA. Mental health status and use of general medical services for persons with human immunodeficiency virus. *Med Care.* 2005;43:834–839.
75. Beck AT, Ward CH, Mendelson M, Mock J, Erbaugh J. An inventory for measuring depression. *Arch Gen Psychiatry.* 1961;4:561–571.
76. Judd FK, Mijch AM. Depressive symptoms in patients with HIV infection. *Aust N Z J Psychiatry.* 1996;30:104–109.
77. Rabkin JG, Ferrando SJ, Lin SH, Sewell M, McElhiney M. Psychological effects of HAART: a 2-year study. *Psychosom Med.* 2000;62:413–422.
78. Derogatis LR. *Symptom Checklist-90-Revised.* Minneapolis: Pearson Assessments; 1975.
79. Derogatis LR. *Brief Symptom Inventory.* Minneapolis: Pearson Assessments; 1993.
80. Rabkin JG, Rabkin R, Wagner G. Effects of fluoxetine on mood and immune status in depressed patients with HIV illness. *J Clin Psychiatry.* 1994;55:92–97.
81. Skoraszewski MJ, Ball JD, Mikulka P. Neuropsychological functioning of HIV-infected males. *J Clin Exp Neuropsychol.* 1991;13:278–290.
82. Abbott PJ, Moore BA, Weller SB, Delaney HD. AIDS risk behavior in opioid dependent patients treated with community reinforcement approach and relationships with psychiatric disorders. *J Addict Dis.* 1998;17:33–48.
83. Nnadi CU, Better W, Tate K, Herning RI, Cadet JL. Contribution of substance abuse and HIV infection to psychiatric distress in an inner-city African-American population. *J Natl Med Assoc.* 2002;94:336–343.
84. *Minnesota Multiphasic Personality Inventory-2.* Minneapolis: The University of Minnesota Press; 1989.
85. Inman TH, Esther JK, Robertson WT, Hall CD, Robertson KR. The Minnesota Multiphasic Personality Inventory-2 across the human immunodeficiency virus spectrum. *Assessment.* 2002;9:24–30.
86. McMahon RC, Mallow RM, Penedo FJ. Psychiatric symptoms and HIV risk in MMPI-2 cluster subgroups of polysubstance abusers in treatment. *J Addict Dis.* 2001;20:27–40.
87. Kalichman SC, Rompa D, Cage M. Distinguishing between overlapping somatic symptoms of depression and HIV disease in people living with HIV-AIDS. *J Nerv Ment Dis.* 2000;188:662–670.
88. Millikin CP, Rourke SB, Halman MH, Power C. Fatigue in HIV/AIDS is associated with depression and subjective neurocognitive complaints but not neuropsychological functioning. *J Clin Exp Neuropsychol.* 2003;25:201–215.
89. Savard J, Laberge B, Gauthier JG, Ivers H, Bergeron MG. Evaluating anxiety and depression in HIV-infected patients. *J Pers Assess.* 1998;71:349–367.
90. Kelly JA, St Lawrence JS, Hood HV, Brasfield TL. An objective test of AIDS risk behavior knowledge: scale development, validation, and norms. *J Behav Ther Exp Psychiatry.* 1989;20:227–234.
91. Leake B, Nyamathi A, Gelberg L. Reliability, validity, and composition of a subset of the Centers for Disease Control and Prevention acquired immunodeficiency syndrome knowledge questionnaire in a sample of homeless and impoverished adults. *Med Care.* 1997;35:747–755.
92. Martin J, Escobar I, Rubio R, Sabugal G, Cascon J, Pulido F. Study of the validity of a questionnaire to assess the adherence to therapy in patients infected by HIV. *HIV Clin Trials.* 2001;2:31–37.
93. Hekkink CF, Sixma HJ, Wigersma L, et al. QUOTE-HIV: an instrument for assessing quality of HIV care from the patients' perspective. *Qual Saf Health Care.* 2003;12:188–193.
94. Martinez SM, Kemper CA, Diamond C, Wagner G; California Collaborative Treatment Group. Body image in patients with HIV/AIDS: assessment of a new psychometric measure and its medical correlates. *AIDS Patient Care STDS.* 2005;19:150–156.
95. Jacobson DL, Wu AW, Feinberg J; Outcomes Committee of the Adult AIDS Clinical Trials Group. Health-related quality of life predicts survival, cytomegalovirus disease, and study retention in clinical trial participants with advanced HIV disease. *J Clin Epidemiol.* 2003;56:874–879.
96. WHOQOL HIV Group. WHOQOL-HIV for quality of life assessment among people living with HIV and AIDS: results from the field test. *AIDS Care.* 2004;16:882–889.
97. Fang CT, Hsiung PC, Yu CF, Chen MY, Wang JD. Validation of the World Health Organization quality of life instrument in patients with HIV infection. *Qual Life Res.* 2002;11:753–762.
98. Cohen SR, Hassan SA, Lapointe BJ, Mount BM. Quality of life in HIV disease as measured by the McGill quality of life questionnaire. *AIDS.* 1996;10:1421–1427.
99. Jacobson DL, Wu AW, Feinberg J; Outcomes Committee of the Adult AIDS Clinical Trials Group. Health-related quality of life predicts survival, cytomegalovirus disease, and study retention in clinical trial participants with advanced HIV disease. *J Clin Epidemiol.* 2003;56:874–879.
100. Price RW, Brew BJ. The AIDS dementia complex: I. Clinical features. *Ann Neurol.* 1986;19:517–524.
101. Navia BA, Cho E-S, Petito CK, et al. The AIDS dementia complex. *J Infect Dis.* 1988;158:1079–1083.
102. Marder K, Albert SM, McDermott MP, et al. Inter-rater reliability of a clinical staging of HIV-associated cognitive impairment. *Neurology.* 2003;60:1467–1473.
103. Burke WJ, Miller JP, Rubin EH, et al. Reliability of the Washington University Clinical Dementia Rating. *Arch Neurol.* 1988;45:31–32.
104. Reisberg B, Ferris SH, de Leon MJ, et al. The global deterioration scale (GDS): an instrument for the assessment of primary degenerative dementia (PDD). *Am J Psychiatry.* 1982;139:1136–1139.
105. Fernandez F, Levy JK. Adjuvant treatment of HIV dementia with psychostimulants. In: Ostrow D, ed. *Behavioral Aspects of AIDS and Other Sexually Transmitted Diseases.* New York: Plenum Publishing; 1990:279–286.
106. Selwyn PA, Goulet JL, Molde S, et al. HIV as a chronic disease: implications for long-term care at an AIDS-dedicated skilled nursing facility. *J Urban Health.* 2000;77:187–203.

CHAPTER 6

Electrophysiology and Brain Mapping

Harold W. Goforth, Lukasz M. Konopka

Electrophysiologic diagnostic testing can play a substantial role in the diagnosis of human immunodeficiency virus (HIV)-related neurobehavioral disorders and can assist in narrowing what is often a substantial differential diagnosis associated with a highly complex and evolving disease. The purpose of this chapter is to review the current state of electrophysiologic data associated with HIV disease as measured by traditional and quantitative electroencephalography, evoked potentials, and polysomnographic techniques.

ELECTROENCEPHALOGRAPHY

Seizures can occur at any stage of HIV infection and were the presenting symptom in 18% of patients as described by Holtzman, Kaku, and So.[1] Seizures as the presenting symptom may reflect advanced HIV disease, and thus may be associated with poor outcome, as noted by Aronow, Brew, and Price,[2] who reported that 7 of 7 patients with status epilepticus died within 1 month of the presenting episode. Initial data regarding HIV-associated seizures suggested that approximately 50% of new-onset seizures were related directly to HIV and the remainder were secondary to HIV-associated complications. However, current thought reflects the more dynamic view that multiple processes may occur simultaneously and overlap significantly.[3]

New-onset seizures in HIV-positive patients are most commonly generalized tonic-clonic and not infrequently (13%) involve status epilepticus upon presentation.[4] A retrospective review of all patients with new-onset generalized seizures presenting to St. Vincent's Hospital in New York identified 26 patients who were known to be HIV-positive. Of this cohort, 31% (8 patients) were determined to have idiopathic seizures; in another 31% (8 patients), the seizure etiology was judged to be HIV encephalopathy. The remaining etiologies were determined to be central nervous system (CNS) toxoplasmosis (5 patients, 18%), alcohol withdrawal (2 patients, 8%), progressive multifocal leukoencephalopathy (2 patients, 8%), and CNS lymphoma (1 patient, 5%). A comparison group of 120 patients without HIV infection was judged to have idiopathic causes (43 patients) or alcohol-related seizures (29 patients) as the two most common diagnoses. Of interest, of the 6 HIV-positive patients with mass-occupying lesions requiring admission to the hospital, only 2 presented with focal signs on admission that would have suggested the need for hospital admission under then-existing seizure guidelines written for patients without HIV infection, which highlights the need for a thorough evaluation for new-onset seizures in patients with known or suspected HIV disease.[5]

Electroencephalograms (EEGs) in patients with HIV infection and acquired immunodeficiency syndrome (AIDS) frequently demonstrate epileptiform features, including sharp waves, spikes, and focal slowing associated with epileptic foci. AIDS dementia complex (ADC) frequently demonstrates low-amplitude, slow, monotonous EEG patterns that are quite indistinct from patterns identified with other types of dementing illness.[6,7] Gabuzda, Levy, and Chiappa[7] demonstrated the presence of frequent EEG abnormalities identified in a series of patients with AIDS, with the most common pattern being generalized slowing (38%), compared to unremarkable patterns (37%), focal slowing (19%), and epileptiform activity (6%). Among those patients with a clinical diagnosis of seizure disorder, half demonstrated sharp wave patterns and another 17% demonstrated focal slowing.[7] The presence of focal slowing on an EEG in these patients is especially important, because such patterns can be derived from an underlying seizure disorder as well as the presence of focal abnormalities, including tumor and infection. Accompanying neuroimaging is almost always advisable in such instances and remains a mandatory part of the initial evaluation of most new-onset seizures.[8]

In contrast to patients with active HIV infection and AIDS, there is conflicting evidence to indicate that asymptomatic HIV infection may or may not lead to EEG abnormalities. Nuwer et al.[9] conducted visual and quantitative EEG testing in 200 asymptomatic homosexual men, half of whom were HIV-positive, and found abnormalities or borderline slowing in 32%. However, EEG changes did not appear related to HIV serostatus, but rather to underlying impaired neuropsychological test performance. The authors used this evidence to highlight the importance of further evaluation in patients with HIV infection and an abnormal EEG, rather than cursorily attributing the EEG changes to an effect of the serostatus of the individual.[9] This finding was replicated by Tinuper et al.,[10] who noted that EEGs correlated with CNS involvement and that neurologically asymptomatic individuals demonstrated no abnormal tracings. These data clearly strengthen the approach that borderline or abnormal EEGs should be further investigated before assigning seropositivity as the primary determinant of the abnormal rhythm.

QUANTITATIVE ELECTROENCEPHALOGRAPHY

Quantitative EEG (qEEG) results in patients with HIV disease have more consistently demonstrated the evolution of electrophysiologic abnormalities across the HIV disease spectrum; however, caution should be appropriately used when examining qEEG studies, because qEEG is an investigative technique for research purposes and has not demonstrated a routine clinical role in the evaluation or management of HIV-infected patients or patients with neurologic disease. Nevertheless, the results provide interesting data and demonstrate the promise of an increasing role for these techniques in the foreseeable future.

Quantitative techniques across multiple studies appear to confirm the essential absence of clinical EEG abnormalities in asymptomatic HIV-positive patients compared to healthy controls, and they have confirmed this pattern using methods suitable for statistical analysis, which strengthens the data further.[11] Quantitative EEG measures have also served to strengthen the concept of HIV disease as having a disproportionate impact on subcortical processes and eventually producing a subcortical-type dementia. At least one study examined the relationship between cerebral metabolism and brain electrical activity in patients with AIDS by the use of positron emission tomography and qEEG and found that data were suggestive that coherence abnormalities may reflect the presence of subcortical AIDS-related disease, but perhaps more importantly supported the validity of coherence measures in studies of AIDS-associated neuropsychiatric dysfunction.[12]

There is preliminary evidence that qEEG may be used potentially to monitor antiviral effectiveness in the CNS. Baldeweg et al.[13] demonstrated that in a group of asymptomatic HIV-1–positive patients administered zidovudine versus placebo, patients receiving zidovudine did not experience the progressive increase in delta and theta slow-frequency qEEG activity over the study period that was identified in the placebo group. Long-term studies examining the role of other pharmacologic agents involved in highly active antiretroviral therapy (HAART) and their potential CNS protective effects are needed, and data correlating measured qEEG abnormalities to clinical or neuropsychological deficits are required for optimal interpretation of available qEEG data.[13]

qEEG changes in patients who have already progressed to AIDS or AIDS-related complex (ARC) have high rates of clinical abnormalities, and abnormal rates have been reported to be as great as 67%. Two of the most common etiologies of abnormal EEGs include AIDS-related dementia and opportunistic infections, with AIDS dementia associated with intermittent or continuous slowing, whereas focal slowing or sharp activity was more reflective of underlying neuronal irritability associated with focal CNS processes such as toxoplasmosis and lymphoma. These data demonstrate that EEG may be especially helpful in the differential diagnosis of dementia versus other mental status changes.[14] A careful investigation of all observed clinical EEG abnormalities is required to adequately detect and diagnose the myriad of complications of this disease.

EVOKED AND EVENT-RELATED POTENTIALS

The roles of evoked and event-related potentials in the routine diagnosis and management of HIV disease are even less uncertain than the role of qEEG and primarily relate to the diagnosis of polyneuropathy and myopathy states, which are found as a result of both direct HIV toxicity and iatrogenically induced by HAART. AIDS-associated vacuolar myelopathy has been reported in greater than 50% of autopsy cases, but is underdiagnosed in clinical situations. Clinical assessment is difficult, and the high comorbidity of peripheral neuropathy makes the diagnosis challenging under optimal circumstances. Somatosensory evoked potentials (SEPs) have enjoyed widespread utility in the evaluation of central conduction velocities, but have not enjoyed as widespread use in the differential diagnosis of vacuolar myelopathy, in spite of evidence that the combined use of median, posterior tibial, and peroneal SEPs with a derived spinal conduction time appeared valuable in differentiating these abnormalities.[15]

Other evoked potential evidence exists suggestive of a relationship between immune impairment and neurophysiologic function, with an inverse relationship being identified between brainstem auditory evoked potential (BAEP) interpeak latencies and CD4 count. This finding was strongly suggestive of a direct immunomodulatory effect of HIV on central neuronal processes.[16] Similar findings were reported by the HIV Neurobehavioral Research Center (HNRC) Group,[17] which concluded that asymptomatic seropositive individuals may have evidence of subclinical central somatosensory dysfunction and that the degree of neurologic involvement increases with disease progression.

The sensitivity of event-related potential (ERP) abnormalities in early, asymptomatic HIV infection also suggests that ERPs may play a role in the evaluation of antiviral therapy and its potential ability to stabilize or prevent further cognitive deterioration. This hypothesis was best tested in Husstedt et al.'s study[18] from Muenster, Germany in 2002, in which ERPs were obtained on 214 seropositive patients without secondary neurologic signs in a cross-sectional manner, and antiviral treatment status was recorded (no treatment; zidovudine monotherapy; zidovudine in combination with didanosine, zalcitabine, or lamivudine; or HAART). Fifty-four of these subjects then enrolled in a prospective, longitudinal design study in which ERPs were evaluated over the course of 1 year. A significant negative correlation between CD4 count and P300 latency was identified in all patients in the cross-sectional study, and patients enrolled in HAART therapy demonstrated significantly lower P300 latencies compared to patients with no treatment. Furthermore, patients enrolled in HAART therapy experienced significantly decreased P300 latencies over 1 year as opposed to patients receiving no antiretroviral therapy, who experienced significantly increased latencies over the same time period.[18] The results of this well-designed study strongly support the role of HAART in the treatment of HIV disease, as well as provide ample evidence that HAART therapy may have a direct impact on the progression of HIV-mediated CNS disease.

Other investigations have supported a similar, potentially valuable role for P300 in evaluation and treatment studies.[19,20] Data have shown that P300 latencies remain stable in zidovudine-treated patients compared to untreated patients over 2 years of follow-up; this finding was observed across different stages of HIV infection and provided ERP-based evidence that zidovudine was beneficial across the entire spectrum of HIV disease.[19,20]

Additional longitudinal studies are required to determine whether ERP results are a significant predictor in the development of encephalopathy or progression to dementia. Given the uncertainty that exists regarding the presence of neurophysiologic abnormalities in early, asymptomatic HIV-infected patients, it appears certain that any such noted abnormalities on testing require appropriate clinical evaluation and treatment.

POLYSOMNOGRAPHY AND SLEEP STUDIES

The existence of a sleep disturbance specific to HIV disease is a controversial proposition, but HIV-positive patients do manifest a high rate of sleep disturbances relative to the general population, which may be secondary to the disease itself or potentially iatrogenically induced from certain antiviral agents.[21] HIV-infected patients also are subject to unusual complications, such as HIV-induced adenotonsillar hypertrophy, which may serve as a risk factor for obstructive sleep apnea.[22] In addition, patients with HIV disease enjoy a similar incidence of unrelated sleep abnormalities as found in the general population, which necessitates a thorough evaluation of sleep-related complaints in this population.[21]

A preliminary study of sleep architecture of 14 patients with HIV infection was characterized by longer onset latencies, reduced total sleep time, reduced sleep efficiency, and significantly reduced stage 2 sleep compared to healthy controls.[23] Other studies have found that wakefulness, slow-wave sleep (SWS), and rapid eye movement (REM) sleep were more evenly dispersed throughout the night than in controls and SWS was associated especially with the second half of the night in contrast to controls.[24,25] This reversal of SWS/REM sleep patterns may reflect underlying immune dysfunction,[26] but the existence of a specific sleep abnormality associated with HIV disease remains a controversial position, as illustrated by a review of 29 available studies that proved inconclusive in providing evidence for the existence of such a disorder. The review identified treatment with efavirenz and the presence of cognitive impairment as significant risk factors for sleep disturbance, but the strongest risk factor was the presence of psychological comorbidities such as depression and anxiety, which reinforces the necessity of screening for psychiatric comorbidities in the evaluation of HIV-infected individuals.[21]

HIV-associated sleep disturbance can be easily underdiagnosed and undertreated due to the many psychosocial factors experienced by the HIV-positive population. Distinguishing between sleep disturbance and HIV-associated fatigue is critical to the effective diagnosis and treatment of the appropriate disorder and often can be best achieved initially with a thorough history and physical examination, including mental status examination. No specific treatment exists for HIV-associated sleep disorder, and clinicians should employ behavioral techniques initially either alone or in combination with pharmacotherapy for effective management.[27] Knowledge of the metabolism, pharmacokinetics, and protein binding features of sleep agents is essential to the correct and safe initiation of any pharmacotherapeutic strategy in this complicated population.

Poor sleep, daytime fatigue, and a reduction of cognitive ability coexist during all stages of HIV infection, and these features have been demonstrated to contribute to both a poor quality of life and eventual disability.[28] Somnogenic inflammatory process peptides have been shown to be increased in HIV disease, and physiologic couplings have been demonstrated between tumor necrosis factor-α (TNF-α) and TNF-δ amplitude during sleep. A lessened likelihood of TNF-α and TFN-δ amplitude coupling may partially explain HIV-associated fatigue and sleep-related disturbances.[29] Growth hormone dysregulation may also contribute to sleep pathology early in the course of HIV disease.[28]

Efavirenz antiviral therapy has been associated with a variety of sleep disturbances, including vivid dreams, increased sleep latency, and an increased number of sleep awakenings throughout the night. It has also been associated with impaired sleep architecture compared to that in healthy controls, and efavirenz-treated patients suffered from increased sleep latency and reduced SWS (stages 3 and 4), regardless of insomnia complaints. Sleep efficiencies below 90% were approximately twice as common in efavirenz-treated patients with serum concentrations above 4 mg/ml than among patients with lower blood concentrations, which supports insomnia as a dose-related effect. The role of efavirenz in producing these sleep disturbances is unknown, but it has been speculated to result from a direct inhibition of serotonergic hypothalamic pathways.[30] Zidovudine was not demonstrated to have a significant influence on reported sleep quality in one study, but sleep quality was significantly linked to the stage of HIV infection, with patients with AIDS reporting increased sleep difficulties.[31]

As a final note, sleep disturbances have been noted to mediate potentially the association between psychological distress and immune status in HIV-positive patients on antiretroviral therapy. High levels of subjective psychological distress were predictive of reduced numbers of T cytotoxic/suppressor (CD3,CD8) cells, and this relationship was demonstrated through a path analysis to be mediated by poor subjective sleep quality, which illustrates the growing importance of sleep physiology in understanding immune function.[32] No studies to date have examined whether interventions designed to improve sleep quality have an effect on improved immune function status, reduced viral load, or improved survivability.

SUMMARY

Routine use of EEG and evoked potentials and ERPs can provide the clinician with meaningful clinical information in collaboration with a history and physical examination. Neurologic comorbidities in HIV infection are common, and EEG can provide valuable diagnostic information in new-onset seizures and when discrete lesions are considered, including tumors, lymphomas, and foci of toxoplasmosis. Evoked potentials and ERPs are helpful in assisting with the differential diagnosis of peripheral versus central neurologic lesions and may serve as potential indicators of early CNS dysfunction, although the data are too limited to support a routine clinical role in assessing cognitive changes. Polysomnographic changes elicited by HIV are controversial, but appear to link sleep disturbances with both psychological distress and immune dysfunction, as well as direct adverse events from specific antiviral agents.

REFERENCES

1. Holtzman DM, Kaku DA, So YT. New-onset seizures associated with human immunodeficiency virus infection: causation and clinical features in 100 cases. *Am J Med.* 1989;87:173–177.
2. Aronow HA, Brew BJ, Price RW. The management of the neurological complications of HIV infection and AIDS. *AIDS.* 1988;2(suppl 1):S151–S159.

3. Britton CB. Acquired immunodeficiency syndrome. In: Rowland LP, ed. *Merritt's Textbook of Neurology.* Baltimore: Williams & Wilkins; 1995:179–193.
4. Berger JR, Simpson DM. Neurologic complications of AIDS. In: Scheld WM, Whitley RJ, Durack DT, eds. *Infections of the Central Nervous System.* Philadelphia: Lippincott-Raven; 1997:255–271.
5. Pesola GR, Westfal RE. New-onset generalized seizures in patients with AIDS presenting to an emergency department. *Acad Emerg Med.* 1998;5:905–911.
6. Harden CL, Daras M, Tuchman AJ, Koppel BS. Low amplitude EEGs in demented AIDS patients. *Electroencephalogr Clin Neurophysiol.* 1993;87:54–56.
7. Gabuzda DH, Levy SR, Chiappa KH. Electroencephalography in AIDS and AIDS-related complex. *Clin Electroencephalogr.* 1988;19:1–6.
8. King MA, Newton MR, Jackson GD, et al. Epileptology of the first-seizure presentation: a clinical, electroencephalographic, and magnetic resonance imaging study of 300 consecutive patients. *Lancet.* 1998;352:1007–1011.
9. Nuwer MR, Miller EN, Visscher BR, et al. Asymptomatic HIV infection does not cause EEG abnormalities: results from the Multicenter AIDS Cohort Study (MACS). *J Neurol Neurosurg Psychiatry.* 1998;65:301–307.
10. Tinuper P, de Carolis P, Galeotti M, Baldrati A, Gritti FM, Sacquegna T. Electroencephalogram and HIV infection: a prospective study in 100 patients. *Clin Electroencephalogr.* 1990;21:145–150.
11. Newton TF, Leuchter AF, Miller EN, Weiner H. Quantitative EEG in patients with AIDS and asymptomatic HIV infection. *Clin Electroencephalogr.* 1994;25:18–25.
12. Newton TF, Leuchter AF, Walter DO, et al. EEG coherence in men with AIDS: association with subcortical metabolic activity. *J Neuropsychiatry Clin Neurosci.* 1993;5:316–321.
13. Baldeweg T, Riccio M, Gruzelier J, et al. Neurophysiological evaluation of zidovudine in asymptomatic HIV-1 infection: a longitudinal placebo-controlled study. *J Neurol Sci.* 1995;132:162–169.
14. Comi G, Leocani L. Electrophysiological correlates of dementia. *Suppl Clin Neurophysiol.* 2000;53:331–336.
15. Tagliati M, Di Rocco A, Danisi F, Simpson DM. The role of somatosensory evoked potentials in the diagnosis of AIDS-associated myelopathy. *Neurology.* 2000;54:1477–1482.
16. Pierelli F, Garrubba C, Tilia G, et al. Multimodal evoked potentials in HIV-1-seropositive patients: relationship between the immune impairment and the neurophysiological function. *Acta Neurol Scand.* 1996;93:266–271.
17. Iragui VJ, Kalmijn J, Thal LJ, Grant I. Neurological dysfunction in asymptomatic HIV-1 infected men: evidence from evoked potentials. HNRC Group. *Electroencephalogr Clin Neurophysiol.* 1994;92:1–10.
18. Husstedt IW, Frohne L, Bockenholt S, et al. Impact of highly active antiretroviral therapy on cognitive processing in HIV infection: cross-sectional and longitudinal studies of event-related potentials. *AIDS Res Hum Retroviruses.* 2002;18:485–490.
19. Polich J, Basho S. P3a and P3b auditory ERPs in HIV patients receiving anti-viral medication. *Clin Electroencephalogr.* 2002;33:97–101.
20. Evers S, Grotemeyer KH, Reichelt D, Luttmann S, Husstedt IW. Impact of antiretroviral treatment on AIDS dementia: a longitudinal prospective event-related potential study. *J Acquir Immune Defic Syndr Hum Retrovirol.* 1998;17:143–148.
21. Reid S, Dwyer J. Insomnia in HIV infection: a systematic review of prevalence, correlates, and management. *Psychosom Med.* 2005;67:260–269.
22. Epstein LJ, Strollo PJ Jr, Donegan RB, Delmar J, Hendrix C, Westbrook PR. Obstructive sleep apnea in patients with human immunodeficiency virus (HIV) disease. *Sleep.* 1995;18:368–376.
23. Wiegand M, Moller AA, Schreiber W, Krieg JC, Holsboer F. Alterations of nocturnal sleep in patients with HIV infection. *Acta Neurol Scand.* 1991;83:141–142.
24. Norman SE, Chediak AD, Kiel M, Cohn MA. Sleep disturbances in HIV-infected homosexual men. *AIDS.* 1990;4:775–781.
25. Wiegand M, Moller AA, Schreiber W, et al. Nocturnal sleep EEG in patients with HIV infection. *Eur Arch Psychiatry Clin Neurosci.* 1991;240:153–158.
26. Norman SE, Chediak AD, Freeman C, et al. Sleep disturbances in men with asymptomatic human immunodeficiency (HIV) infection. *Sleep.* 1992;15:150–155.
27. Sciolla A. Sleep disturbance and HIV disease. *Focus.* 1995;10:1–4.
28. Darko DF, Mitler MM, Miller JC. Growth hormone, fatigue, poor sleep, and disability in HIV infection. *Neuroendocrinology.* 1998;67:317–324.
29. Darko DF, Miller JC, Gallen C, et al. Sleep electroencephalogram delta-frequency amplitude, night plasma levels of tumor necrosis factor alpha, and human immunodeficiency virus infection. *Proc Natl Acad Sci USA.* 1995;92:12080–12084.
30. Gallego L, Barreiro P, del Rio R, et al. Analyzing sleep abnormalities in HIV-infected patients treated with efavirenz. *Clin Infect Dis.* 2004;38:430–432.
31. Moeller AA, Oechsner M, Backmund HC, Popescu M, Emminger C, Holsboer F. Self-reported sleep quality in HIV infection: correlation to the stage of infection and zidovudine therapy. *J Acquir Immune Defic Syndr.* 1991;4:1000–1003.
32. Cruess DG, Antoni MH, Gonzalez J, et al. Sleep disturbance mediates the association between psychological distress and immune status among HIV-positive men and women on combination antiretroviral therapy. *J Psychosom Res.* 2003;54:185–189.

SECTION III

Psychiatric Comorbidity

CHAPTER 7

Psychological Reactions

Vicenzio Holder-Perkins, Jeffrey S. Akman

Over the past two decades, the medical and psychosocial needs of people with human immunodeficiency virus (HIV) infection have changed considerably. The introduction of highly active antiretroviral therapy (HAART) has had a profound effect on the epidemic and the prognosis of people affected by HIV. Numerous studies have shown that HAART extends life expectancy, reduces significantly the progression of HIV-related illness, decreases HIV viral loads, and increases CD4 counts. However, the verdict is still out on whether the experience of living longer with HIV disease and its related illnesses is significantly less stressful today than before the introduction of HAART. It is the extension of life for many individuals treated with HAART that has defined HIV infection as a chronic illness. Even though many may feel healthier and are living longer, HAART is not without its problems. Furthermore, these very complex antiretroviral regimens are a constant reminder of one's HIV status. Thus, inherent in living with HIV infection as a chronic illness is the coexistence of emotional and psychological reactions.

Psychological stress, demoralization, and distress are ubiquitous with chronic illness. The uncertainty regarding one's future state of health, potential shortening of one's life trajectory, unpredictability of physical discomfort or ailments, and the impact on the individual's partner, spouse, and family are common sources of psychological stress in individuals with chronic illness. Studies of individuals facing grave illness have identified the key themes for maintaining emotional equilibrium to be a search for meaning, attempts to gain mastery or control over illness, and attempts to enhance self-worth. For many, the meaning and experience of having HIV disease remains difficult and challenging.

The passage of time and modern advances of medicine have not diminished the complexity of social and psychological issues that confront those living with HIV disease. The immediate psychological impact of learning one's HIV seropositivity is frequently one of acute distress expressed as depressed mood, anxiety, shock, and anger. Sexual avoidance is not an uncommon phenomenon, because patients may perceive sex as an activity that is associated with illness and death. These symptoms often take the form of transient and situational adjustment disorders. Seropositive individuals wonder if they can continue with their activities of daily living and responsibilities, including jobs and social relationships. Persons with HIV can become preoccupied with becoming ill and dying, as do persons with any life-threatening disease. Some confront the failure of antiretroviral or protease inhibitors, whereas others live apprehensively, wondering how long they will escape an opportunistic infection. In these situations, hopelessness is a prominent theme. The social impact of HIV infection can also be distressing. People living with HIV-related illness have been stigmatized since the epidemic began. Fear of stigma has interfered with disclosure of seropositive status to sexual partners, family, and friends. The shame imposed by societal beliefs ("they deserve their illness") may adversely affect care-seeking behaviors and adherence to HAART. Furthermore, HAART may be a double-edge sword. On the one hand, it decreases mortality and morbidity, and on the other it produces disturbing physical side effects, including neuropathy, chronic diarrhea, fatigue, and lipodystrophy syndrome. This new treatment adds to the "stressor chest" of HIV infection. The additional impact of physical anguish on mental health can be significant.

The psychological distress linked with the social and physical pressures of HIV infection manifest in the form of depressive symptomatology, including heightened anxiety, worries, tension, perceived stress, and avoidant, intrusive, and overwhelming thoughts. The prevalence of these reactive symptoms has not been determined. Although these symptoms are usually mild and self-limiting, they can be severe and disabling to the extent that they may meet criteria for an adjustment disorder or another *Diagnostic and Statistical Manual of Mental Disorders (DSM-IV)* Axis I diagnoses. HIV infection is also experiential because it is expressed emotionally as shame, guilt, grief, and numbness. An "emotional roller coaster" is often the core of one's experience of living with HIV disease. These emotional responses may elicit maladaptive defense mechanisms, such as denial, regression, or isolation of affect.

Persons with HIV-related illness experience significant psychological and emotional vulnerabilities at each of the key milestones of its clinical course (HIV testing, notification of HIV seropositivity, development of HIV disease, diagnosis of acquired immunodeficiency syndrome [AIDS], development of cognitive dysfunction, progressive disability, and terminal deterioration). Even with the clear advantages of HAART treatment, current research does not, as of yet, support the notion that individuals transverse these clinical milestones with less psychological distress during the era of HAART.

PSYCHOLOGICAL IMPACT AT DIFFERENT STAGES OF HIV/AIDS

PSYCHOLOGICAL REACTIONS TO ANTIBODY STATUS NOTIFICATION

HIV testing is a crucial step in the continuum of HIV disease care. Yet people undergo or avoid HIV antibody testing for many reasons. The decision to test for the presence of HIV antibody can be associated with considerable psychological distress. Fear and denial are the most common obstacles to HIV testing among those acknowledging that they have been at risk.[1] Other reasons for avoiding testing include worries about confidentiality, and wishing to avoid anxiety while waiting for the results. The psychological consequences of choosing to know or not to know one's HIV serostatus were examined in a group of 224 men who had been tested for HIV.[2] Results indicate that men who avoided testing had AIDS-related preoccupations significantly higher than those who were aware of their serostatus, whether seronegative or seropositive. This led to the suggestion that learning what might appear as threatening information may be more psychologically beneficial than avoiding it.

Although it may seem intuitive that a positive HIV antibody test result is an extremely emotional distressing experience, the research findings however, are reflecting a changing picture. Kelly and Murphy[3] observed that studies conducted before 1988 generally report high and pervasive levels of distress following positive HIV serostatus notification, whereas later studies generally indicate relatively lower levels of distress. This observable change may be explained by different conceptual and methodological approaches utilized by the investigator(s) in studying the psychological impact of notification of HIV serostatus over time. Other possible explanations may be related to the level of satisfaction with the communication of test results by the provider or an awareness of the widespread combined use of viral load monitoring and combination therapy (HAART) that has led to a dramatic decrease in morbidity and mortality.

Most studies examining the psychological impact of notification of HIV serostatus before 1988 were restricted to cohorts of gay/bisexual men, hemophiliacs, and intravenous drug users, regardless of gender. Several of these studies found that notification of a positive HIV serostatus was associated with persistent psychological distress manifested in the form of depression, anxiety, suicidal ideations, suicide attempts, and other somatic and psychological symptoms of distress.[4,5] Cleary et al.[5] studied the psychological effects of HIV antibody testing of 173 seropositive individuals (135 men and 38 women) at the completion of a notification session in which antibody test results were provided. They reported higher depression scores on the Center for Epidemiologic Studies Depression Scale (CES-D) in seropositive individuals than in community samples postnotification.[5]

In contrast to these earlier studies, others did not find strong associations between initial positive HIV serostatus notification and persistent psychological distress. Perry et al.[6] found that those most distressed after notification of HIV seropositivity were also most distressed before it. This observation reflects a limitation in retrospective studies of whether certain HIV seropositive individuals are particularly vulnerable for psychiatric symptoms, and whether their psychiatric risk factor profile differs from that found in HIV-seronegative samples. This methodological limitation was not present in some prospective studies performed in later years of the epidemic, such as seen in the Perry et al.[6] investigational study. They were interested in studying the psychological reactions of HIV testing in adults. They followed 328 homosexual and heterosexual men at perceived risk for HIV infection but without AIDS. Over a 1-year period, they found a decline in severity of symptoms on both clinician and self-rated scales, but no difference between HIV-positive and HI- negative participants on any occasion. These investigators concluded that regardless of serostatus, a notable percentage of at-risk adults had sustained levels of psychiatric symptoms.[7] A similar conclusion was echoed by Dew et al.[8] in a multivariate analyses of 113 HIV-positive and 57 HIV-negative men. They reported that persons at risk for HIV infection (regardless of serostatus) had higher rates of some psychiatric disorders than the general population.

Early in the epidemic, relatively few women were included in clinical trials and psychological research. As a result, there is a relative lack of information on the psychological well-being related to HIV testing in women. A literature review by Nakajima and Rubin[9] showed 31 studies examining the psychosocial aspects of HIV infection in 2,438 patients.

THE PSYCHOLOGICAL REACTIONS TO ANTIBODY TESTING IN WOMEN

The work that has been done regardless of where in the clinical spectrum of HIV/AIDS disease suggests that HIV-positive women may experience even higher levels of psychological distress than HIV-positive men.[10,11] In studying the gender differences in HIV-related psychological distress in heterosexual couples, Kennedy et al.[11] reported that women (regardless of serostatus) in couples affected by HIV disease had more distress than men. The explanation of this perceived reality lies within the context of their socioeconomic status. Many women who are seropositive for HIV live in poverty and were already poor when they learned their serostatus. Women at highest risk for HIV infection may already be highly stigmatized. Further, stigma has been associated with lower self-concept, poorer emotional outcomes, and greater psychological distress in mothers with HIV disease.[12] Their role as primary caretakers leads to a different set of challenges not often experienced by men. Life with HIV-related illness is qualitatively different from that of men. Additionally, HIV-infected women are at risk for psychological, physical, and sexual violence.[13] These life stressors pose a more imminent threat to their mental and physical well-being than does HIV/AIDS disease.

PSYCHOLOGICAL REACTION TO DISCLOSURE OF ANTIBODY STATUS

The decision to disclose or notify others of a seropositive antibody test is also fraught with emotional and psychological distress. Disclosure of serostatus ranked second in degree of stressfulness behind testing and receiving a positive diagnosis.[14] Self-blame, loneliness, rejection, abandonment, and isolation have been shown to be negative emotional expressions of disclosure. However, the disclosure of HIV infection reduces stress with resultant positive health consequences. That is, disclosure facilitates the initiation and adherence to medical treatment (e.g., HAART) that may restore health and extend survival.

We live in a dynamic social and interpersonal network of relationships. People living with HIV/AIDS disease have an effect on and are affected by this network of relationships in ways that are not experienced by HIV-seronegative individuals. They may experience disruptions on various levels of personal and interpersonal functioning. "To tell or not to tell" is a weighted decision measured by one's psychological adjustment of being HIV-positive and by the anticipated responses or reactions of the recipient within the individual's network of personal and social relationships. If the anticipated response is a negative one, it is likely that disclosure will not occur, which may result in increasing stress because of social isolation and conflictual social interactions. In contrast, if the anticipated reaction is supportive, the person will likely disclose. Moreover, the woven relationship between social support and disclosure may influence psychological adjustment to living with HIV disease.

Stigma is also viewed as a weighted measure in whether or not to disclose HIV-seropositive status. Social stigma and its accompanying negative consequences are sources of stress that can very easily intensify the anxiety and feelings of helplessness and hopelessness that frequently accompany the course of HIV-related illnesses. Many infected individuals may internalize the societal stigmatization of HIV to the extent that they may feel ashamed and embarrassed, ultimately loathing and blaming themselves. Others may react to the stigma and ostracism of being HIV-positive with silence and denial. Research has shown that HIV stigma can have a negative effect on the willingness to disclose one's status and on receiving and requesting social support. The inter-relationship among stigma, disclosure, and psychological functioning has been studied. Clark et al.[15] collected data at four points across a 6-year period of 244 African-American women (98 HIV-positive and 146 HIV-negative) and found that among HIV-infected African-American women, as the level of perceived stigma increased, the level of disclosure and psychological functioning decreased. The perception of stigma did not significantly change over time for the entire sample. It can be said that there is a linear correlation between psychological distress and the persistence of stigma, whether perceived or enacted. Stigma can be both demoralizing and a life-altering experience for many living with HIV disease.

Emotional and psychological disturbances can remain relatively absent during the asymptomatic phase of HIV disease. Progression from HIV-seropositive status to AIDS can result in a reemergence of significant distress. AIDS-related complex (ARC) is the term used to signal the transition from HIV infection to HIV disease in the pre-HAART era. Today, this stage where symptoms have begun to manifest but before the development of AIDS is known as "early symptomatic HIV infection." There were no distinct comparative or empiric studies examining psychological reactions during the early symptomatic HIV phase but is likely that the reactions reported in the pre-HAART era still prevail.

Comparative studies on the progression from HIV-seropositive status to ARC performed in the pre-HAART era identified this stage as a period of significant psychological and emotional distress. Persons with ARC are at great risk for emotional distress, likely as a result of their persistent uncertainty about developing AIDS. During this symptomatic phase of HIV illness the result of closely monitoring their viral load and CD4 count is a vacillation between fear and relief and despair. Tross et al.[16] reported that men with ARC scored at least as high as and sometime higher than those with AIDS on several parameters, including somatization, anxiety, and intrusive worries with the topic of AIDS.

The development of AIDS is another well-defined time of vulnerability for an acute psychological reaction during the course of HIV disease. The notification of having AIDS is a major event at which a decision must be made to take preventive measures (e.g., antibiotic prophylaxis) and, if HAART has not been initiated, to begin antiretroviral medications. The psychological reaction to the news of having AIDS may include dysphoric mood, hopelessness, helplessness, anhedonia, and heightened rejection sensitivity. The intensity of these reactions may well be influenced by one's perceived vulnerability to the development and onset of opportunistic infections, as well as the development of cognitive difficulties, to the extent that it may have a negative impact on one's social and occupational functioning. Suicidal ideations are common, but actual plans or attempts are rare phenomena. Anxiety may also be experienced in the form of heightened sensitivity to physical symptoms, preoccupations with body image, and verbalized fears of the fatality of HIV disease.

PSYCHOLOGICAL ATTRIBUTIONS TO HIGHLY ACTIVE ANTIRETROVIRAL THERAPY

In the early years of the HIV epidemic it was said that when someone became infected with HIV, there was little to offer. A seropositive status then was "a death sentence." Hope and optimism were measured in weeks and months. Persons with HIV disease or AIDS, regardless of where they were in the continuum of disease progression in those early years, undoubtedly experienced significant levels of psychological distress (not syndrome disorders), especially as the immune system collapsed and opportunistic infections and neoplasms developed. Today there is a widely held belief that HAART has reintroduced hope and optimism for a restored psychological and emotional state for persons seropositive for HIV. But empirical findings indicate that those whose medical markers (CD4 and HIV RNA viral load) reflect successful treatment are no more likely than others to be relieved of distress and hopelessness.[17]

The improvements in the clinical spectrum of HIV/AIDS since the introduction of HAART have not come without a cost; antiretroviral combination regimens are complicated and add to the stress associated with HIV infection. New worries have emerged while old ones persist. The combination of antiretroviral therapies is often toxic and linked with substantial adverse reactions that may influence tolerability and effectiveness. These regimens are also extremely difficult to follow, and yet once started they require strict adherence for an unprecedented length of time. The daunting task of adhering to numerous dosing times, meticulous timing of doses, alterations of eating patterns, and the knowledge of possible virus resistance, if not perfectly adhered to, may be worrisome to many HIV-seropositive persons. Meystre-Agustoni et al.[18] described many of the worries linked to antiretroviral therapy and adherence, including the worry about adverse side effects, a preoccupation with the relatively small choice of available antiretrovirals, and the fear that by taking the drugs individuals might signal to others that they were HIV-positive. Another anxiety-provoking reality for many is that antiretroviral therapies are not equally effective for all. Moreover, pointed clinical arguments in the literature of when to start treatment do not allay the uncertainties associated with HAART.

Self-blame, guilt, and a feeling of personal failure of not adhering to antiretroviral therapies are not uncommon psychological responses. The current stress on adherence may mean that when antiretroviral therapies are unsuccessful, patients are more likely to reproach themselves for having missed doses of medication that would have "saved" them, even when adherence is achieved and some are still not "saved." The absence of health gains despite adherence may lead to feelings of anger, hopelessness, anxiety, and fear.[19] The distress of treatment failure may be magnified by the knowledge of the triumphant experiences of others in treatment. Achieving health gain from treatment does not necessarily translate to an appropriate psychological reaction. "Survivors' guilt" and the uncertainty about the probable magnitude and length of improvement are likely reactions by those who have adhered to treatment and received "the miracle of a second life." Some patients may find having this second chance of life to be worrisome as they face the daunting question of what to do with the rest of their lives.

The physical changes and side effects caused by HAART and, in particular, the protease inhibitors, can lead to significant stress for the individual. The typical changes in one's facial appearance and the redistribution of truncal fat may communicate that the individual has HIV/AIDS. It may affect one's body image and self-esteem. Furthermore, elevations of cholesterol and blood glucose, along with the potential additional complications of pancreatitis, diabetes, or heart disease add an additional level of concern for someone already struggling with living with HIV/AIDS.

HIV/AIDS AS A CHRONIC MEDICAL ILLNESS

The efficacy of HAART and the increased life expectancy of individuals with HIV/AIDS require the clinician to consider HIV/AIDS as a chronic medical illness with many of the same psychological features of other medical illnesses. For many, medical illness frequently leads to various degrees of helplessness and hopelessness. And as part of this response the individual may develop a sense of demoralization, which has been considered a "universal human experience" to be differentiated from a depressive disorder. Griffith and Gaby[20] state that although demoralization shares symptoms seen in depression (e.g., sleep, appetite, energy disturbances, and even suicidal ideation), responsivity of mood is usually preserved in that the cessation of adversity rapidly restores a capacity to feel enjoyment and hope. To that end, these authors deconstructed demoralization into its existential components to address psychotherapeutic interventions.

Griffith and Gaby[20] identified seven existential "postures" of vulnerability and resilience to illness that provide potential avenues for psychotherapeutic intervention in medically ill patients. The seven postures include confusion versus coherence, isolation versus communion, despair versus hope, helplessness versus agency, meaninglessness versus purpose, cowardice versus courage, and resentment versus gratitude. Psychotherapeutic interventions that specifically address these polarities can assist in helping individuals with medical illness sustain the existential postures of resilience.

DISTINGUISHING BETWEEN NORMAL AND PATHOLOGIC PSYCHOLOGICAL REACTIONS

Psychological reactions such as anger, fear, and sadness are human responses to illness. It is the intensity, frequency, and duration of these reactions; the ability or lack thereof to develop adaptive ways to cope with them; and the degree of disability that exists from them that determine if the reaction to the illness is pathologic. One of the most important considerations, regarding adjustment and coping with having HIV disease is the patient's perception of HIV disease. The patient's beliefs about HIV infection and previous experience with illness ought to be understood in order to determine psychiatric problems if and when they occur.

TREATMENT CONSIDERATIONS

Although some individuals adjust well with the challenges posed by HIV-related illness, others experience psychological distress. And given the variability of psychological and emotional reactions and the heterogeneity of HIV-infected individuals, it is likely that there is no single treatment strategy that would be universally successful. However, the existence of a strong, respectful, therapeutic alliance is unquestionably a strong determinant in the success of any treatment option being considered.

Individuals seeking HIV testing should be counseled at the time of HIV testing and again when results are given. Psychoeducation should be provided about HIV and its course, treatment, and effects. The HIV antibody testing process is also a unique opportunity for clinicians to provide and reinforce HIV prevention messages.

After notification of a seropositive result, many individuals cannot take in much information, so the post-test experience should be mainly supportive and provide assistance in obtaining appropriate services. Well thought out counseling efforts may effectively reduce the psychological distress associated with HIV-seropositive results. A suicide risk assessment is indicated if suicidal thoughts or feelings of hopelessness are expressed.

There are no exclusive psychotherapeutic or counseling interventions for people living with HIV/AIDS. Therefore treatment must be tailored to the person's needs and capacity. There are various psychotherapies (cognitive-behavior, interpersonal, supportive, psychodynamic, and psychoanalytical) that may be used. Other effective therapeutic modalities in the management of psychological distress include biofeedback, stress-reduction/relaxation exercises, complementary therapies (e.g., acupuncture), and group therapy. The management of HIV-related psychological issues is detailed in Chapter 35. Pharmacological therapies such as antidepressants and anxiolytics may be useful in the management of reactive symptoms such as anxiety and depression.

SUMMARY

Although life expectancy has dramatically increased for people living with HIV disease and AIDS, the psychological and emotionally picture of living with these is still fraught with stress, adjustment issues, and potentially significant psychiatric symptoms. The key issues of a potentially shortened life expectancy, stigma and shame, living with a chronic medical illness, and taking complicated medication regimens that can cause multiple side effects, including changes in one's physical appearance, require health care professionals to pay close attention to an individual's psychological adjustment and to intervene with psychoeducation, counseling, psychotherapy, and psychopharmacology when appropriate.

REFERENCES

1. Seigel K, Ravies VH, Gorey E. Barriers and pathways to testing among HIV infected women. *AIDS Educ Prev*. 1998;10:114–127.
2. Conley TD, Taylor SE, Kemeny ME, et al. Psychological sequelae of avoiding HIV-serostatus information. *Basic Appl Soc Psychol*. 1991;21:81–90.
3. Kelly JA, Murphy DA. Psychological interventions with AIDS and HIV: prevention and treatment. *J Consult Clin Psychol*. 1992;60:576–585.
4. Jacobsen PB, Perry SW, Hirsch DA, Scavuzzo D, Roberts RB. Psychological reactions of individuals at risk for AIDS during an experimental drug trial. *Psychosomatics*. 1988;29:182–187.

5. Cleary PD, Singer E, Rogers TF, et al. Sociodemographic and behavioral characteristics of HIV antibody-positive blood donors. *Am J Public Health.* 1988;78:953–957.
6. Perry SW, Jacobsberg LB, Fishman B. Suicidal ideation and HIV testing. *J Am Med Assoc.* 1990;263:679–682.
7. Perry SW, Jacobsberg LB, Card CAL, Ashman T, Frances A, Fishman B. Severity of psychiatric symptoms after HIV testing. *Am J Psychiatry.* 1993;150:775–779.
8. Dew MA, Becker JT, Sanchez R, et al. Prevalence and predictors of depressive, anxiety and substance use disorders in HIV infected and uninfected men: a longitudinal evaluation. *Psychol Med.* 1997;27:395–409.
9. Nakajima C, Rubin H. Lack of racial, gender and behavior-risk diversity in psychiatric research on HIV/AIDS in the United States. *Proc 7th Int Conf AIDS.* 1991;1:193, Florence, Italy.
10. Rabkin JG, Johnson J, Lin S, Lipsitz JD. Psychopathology in male and female HIV-positive and negative injecting drug users: longitudinal course over 3 years. *AIDS.* 1997;11:507–515.
11. Kennedy CA, Skurnick JH, Foley M, Louria DB. Gender differences in HIV-related psychological distress in heterosexual couples. *AIDS Care.* 1995;7(suppl 1):S33–S38.
12. Miles MS, Burchinal P, Holdtich-Davis D, Wasilewski Y, Christian B. Personal, family and health-related correlates of depressive symptoms in mothers with HIV. *J Fam Psych.* 1997;11:23–34.
13. Zierler S, Cunningham WE, Andersen R. Violence victimization after HIV infection in a US probability sample of adult patients in primary care. *Am J Public Health.* 2000;90:208–215.
14. Duffy VJ. Crisis points in HIV disease. *AIDS Patient Care.* 1994;8:28–32.
15. Clark HJ, Lindner G, Armistead L, et al. Stigma, disclosure and psychological functioning among HIV infected and non-infected African-American women. *Women Health.* 2003;38:57–71.
16. Tross S, Holland J, Hirsch DA, Schiffman M, Gold J, Safai B. Psychological and social impact of AIDS spectrum disorders. *Proc Second Int Conf Acquir Immunodef Syndr.* p. 157, June 23–26, 1986, Paris, France.
17. Rabkin JG, Fernando SJ, Lin SH, Sewell M, McElhiney M. Psychological effects of HAART: a 2-year study. *Psychosom Med.* 2000;62:413–422.
18. Meystre-Agustoni G, Dubois-Arber F, Cochand P, Telenti A. Antiretroviral therapies from the patient's perspective. *AIDS.* 2000;12:717–721.
19. Kalichman SC, Ramachandran B, Ostrow D. Protease inhibitors and the new AIDS combination therapies: implications for psychological services. *Prof Psychol.* 1998;29:349–356.
20. Griffith J, Gaby L. Brief psychotherapy at the bedside: countering demoralization from medical illness. *Psychosomatics.* 2005;46:109–116.

CHAPTER 8

Stress-Distress Spectrum and Adjustment Disorders

Dimitri D. Markov, Elisabeth J. S. Kunkel, Howard Field

To the confusion of readers, the term *stress* has been used to describe environmental stressors as well as the individual's reaction to those stressors. More specifically, *distress* refers to the person's emotional reaction to various inner or external events. Stressors are the agents, events, or circumstances that may evoke the stress response. They may vary in severity and can be acute or chronic. Distress may originate in inner biologic or psychic factors as in mood or anxiety disorders or as a response to external events. Although it is generally believed that all types of stress affect disease, individual responses to similar stressors vary widely. Furthermore, not all stress can be shown to affect immune parameters and disease outcome. The relationships between stress, distress, immunity, and disease outcomes is complex and not well understood.[1]

Patients living with acquired immunodeficiency syndrome (AIDS) face many stressors: declining health; unpredictability of disease progression; the need for constant monitoring of viral load and CD4+ cell counts; insomnia; opportunistic infections; chronic pain; cognitive decline; physical wasting; chronic diarrhea; medication side effects; loss of significant others; and disclosure of HIV status, resulting in financial losses and health; and social discrimination. The cognitive impairments seen in patients with AIDS impose additional limitations on an individual's ability to function and add to stress. All of these stressors impair the patient's quality of life and interfere with the ability to adhere to a complicated medication regimen. When the patient's emotional resources are overwhelmed by stress, he or she may have difficulty participating in social, occupational, and interpersonal activities.

Until the introduction of highly active antiretroviral therapy (HAART) in the 1990s, patients infected with HIV faced near-certain death. The patients for whom HAART is available now find themselves confronting the stress of living with a chronic illness. Studies of psychiatric symptoms in patients now receiving HAART have yet to be published. Even before contracting the virus, populations at risk for HIV infection have more stressors in their daily lives and fewer resources for coping than the population at large. The fear of being diagnosed as HIV-positive plays a significant part in the decision by many of those at risk to postpone or avoid being tested. The discovery that one is infected may precipitate an acute emotional crisis, overwhelming a person's ability to cope and disrupting the person's life.

ADJUSTMENT DISORDERS

According to the *Diagnostic and Statistical Manual of Mental Disorders (DSM IV-TR)*, adjustment disorders are characterized by the development of emotional or behavioral symptoms in response to an identifiable stressor(s).[2] The symptoms or behaviors are considered clinically significant when they cause impairment in social or occupational function that is in excess of what would be expected from exposure to the stressor. Patients experience anxiety, depression, or a mixture of emotional and behavioral symptoms. Patients positive for HIV infection are at higher risk for developing adjustment disorders for several reasons. The initial fear of becoming HIV-positive is followed by emotional responses to the diagnosis, treatment, and ongoing disease-related stressors. Such stressors often overwhelm the patient's capacity to cope emotionally with HIV and AIDS. In advanced stages of AIDS, many patients are increasingly physically and emotionally dependent on their caretakers. An increased need for dependency is particularly conducive to developing symptoms of adjustment disorder. Finally, people most vulnerable to HIV infection, such as intravenous drug users and persons with multiple sex partners, are also at risk of having a history of exposure to chronic stress throughout their lives. Individuals with a history of exposure to chronic stress may have more symptoms of distress when exposed to minor adverse events.[3] Most patients with adjustment disorder return to normal functioning or to a new emotional equilibrium once the stress abates; patients with HIV, however, are faced with repetitive, multiple, concurrent stressors, making resolution of the adjustment disorder much less likely.

The stress connected with the onset of the HIV epidemic, once experienced by the entire nation, now affects mostly patients, their lovers, caretakers, and families. Caretakers of persons living with HIV disease and AIDS must deal with the stigma of HIV infection, uncertainty about the future, and increasing demands of caretaking as the disease progresses. Couples, especially HIV-discordant couples, face the risk of sexual transmission of the virus, the challenges of maintaining a safe and satisfying intimate relationship, and prospect of the loss of a lover. Not only do both HIV-positive and HIV-negative members of HIV-discordant male couples experience elevated levels of distress compared to the general population, but also there is concordance noted in the level of distress reported by each partner of the HIV-discordant couple.[4]

When a mother or father learns that she or he is HIV-positive, the entire family is confronted with multiple stressors. The unaffected parent may fear sexual transmission, and both parents may worry about disease transmission to their children. Parents must continue caring for children while coping with the unpredictable course of the illness, declining health, and complicated medication regimens. Additionally, parents must decide how to tell children about their HIV status. Children who are coping with the anticipatory loss of a parent may need to assume the responsibility of caring for younger siblings, doing housework, or providing emotional support to the ailing parent. Role functions within the family often are renegotiated, abandoned, or reorganized. Thus the emotional distress of the HIV-positive parent is experienced by the entire family.[5] In a cohort of perinatally HIV-infected children, Mellins et al.[6] reported that higher caregiver distress, worse parent–child communication, and lower caregiver quality of life predicted nonadherence of infected children to antiretroviral therapy. Managing such problems becomes critical because successful viral suppression requires 90% or better adherence to HAART medication regimens, and thus nonadherence becomes a life-threatening issue.

The following case illustrates the impact of stress in a family with an HIV-infected father:

Theresa, an Italian-American woman, mother of three young children, had been caring for her husband, who was dying of AIDS. He had acquired HIV infection through multiple extramarital affairs. Theresa felt ashamed of her husband's illness and his affairs and worried that if her church, friends, or family found out, she would be ostracized because of their fears of contracting HIV infection. The patient isolated herself and, as a result, had no support system while caring for three children and a dying husband. Her oldest child began to miss school as a result of worrying about his mother and father. Theresa was concerned about her son's progress in school, but felt unable to approach his teacher for fear that either she or her son would be ostracized. As a result, she felt even more helpless and isolated. After her husband died, things grew worse. Although Theresa no longer had to provide care for her dying husband, she was left with grief and unresolved anger. She was unable to express or process any of these emotions, and the distraction of caring for her husband, which previously had provided her only method of coping, was gone. Her psychiatric treatment is described in the discussion of treatment considerations.

COPING WITH STRESS

The response to stressors is affected by the individual's appraisal and coping. Effective coping may have a restorative effect on the immune system and slow HIV progression.[7] Gray and Cason[8] defined effective coping as a process in which the individual accurately appraises the stressor and the available supports and mobilizes resources to master a particular stressor. In HIV-discordant male couples, Remien et al.[4] reported higher levels of distress in each partner when self-blame and avoidance coping strategies were employed and HIV-related issues were not discussed.

In a study of women living with HIV/AIDS, mastery over stress was positively correlated with social support and a spiritual perspective. Interpersonal conflict correlated with decreased mastery over stress, possibly by reducing the available social support.[8]

Leserman et al.[9] noted that use of active coping strategies and less use of denial were associated with a decreased likelihood of developing HIV-related symptoms. In men living with HIV who reported greater satisfaction with social support, Leserman et al.[9] found a decreased disease progression. According to O'Cleirigh et al.,[10] in patients with rheumatoid arthritis and asthma, the frequency of expressing either positive or negative emotions about one's medical condition was linked to better clinical outcomes. In 2003, the same authors reported that compared to an HIV-seropositive comparison group, a cohort of long-term HIV survivors reported higher levels of emotional expression and depth processing of traumatic events (depth processing is a measure of the extent to which an individual worked through or attempted to resolve the stressor). Both emotional expression and depth processing were related to long-term survival; depth processing mediated the relationship between emotional expression and long-term survival. Depth processing of traumatic experiences by HIV-infected persons was related to perceived stress and antiretroviral medication adherence. In women, depth processing was positively related to CD4+ lymphocyte count, and emotional expression was both positively related to CD4+ lymphocyte count and negatively related to viral load.[10] Recently bereaved men who reported finding meaning in bereavement had a slower decline in CD4+ cells and lower rates of mortality due to AIDS at a 2- to 3-year follow-up.[10]

The stress of AIDS extends through the life span. The number of older adults living with HIV disease or AIDS has been growing rapidly in the United States. According to Chesney et al.,[11] older people living with HIV disease have a higher rate of progression to AIDS, experience more HIV-related losses, have fewer resources available for support, and have greater levels of psychological distress than their younger counterparts.

STRESS, IMMUNE PARAMETERS, AND DISEASE PROGRESSION

In view of the high burden of stressors faced by HIV-seropositive individuals and the known relationship of stress to the progression of many illnesses, it is important to review the relationship between stress and immune parameters in HIV infection. This is explored in more detail in Chapters 2 and 37. In HIV infection, disease progression parallels the impairment of the immune system, which results in the development of opportunistic infections and AIDS-defining malignancies. Leserman et al.,[12] in five consecutive studies, reported an association between severe life stressors and progression of asymptomatic HIV-positive gay men to AIDS. Severe life stressors were reported to have an association with lower levels of natural killer (NK) cells and subsets of cytotoxic T lymphocytes, both lymphocytes involved in defense against viral illness and those capable of lysing HIV-infected host cells. Higher levels of stress were associated with greater reduction in CD4+ lymphocytes in children and in adults. HIV-seropositive women are at increased risk for reactivation of latent viruses, such as human papilloma viruses (HPVs), and progression of other viral diseases due to immune suppression. HPV types 16 and 18 are associated with development, progression, or persistence of cervical intraepithelial neoplasia (CIN). Higher levels of life stress in HIV-seropositive women who also had a history of at least one abnormal Pap smear, increased the odds of developing progressive CIN 7-fold.[13] Greater numbers of stressful life events have a cumulative effect on decreasing the lymphocytes involved in host defense. Decreased reported satisfaction with social support and more passive coping strategies, such as coping by means of denial, correlated with worse immune parameters and a greater likelihood of HIV disease progression.[9,14-16] The physiologic mechanisms connecting life stressors to changes in the immune system and progression of disease in people living with HIV are not well understood. We know that neurons interact with the immune system via complex and bi-directional networks of hormones and neurotransmitters. Cortisol and norepinephrine are believed to be the most likely hormonal mediators of the stress response. Because synthetic corticosteroids are known to inhibit the immune function, it is hypothesized that elevated levels of endogenous steroids (e.g., cortisol), released in response to life stress, are associated with inhibition of the immune response.[1,13,15,16] Studies attempting to link stressful events to levels of endogenous steroids, immune parameters, and HIV progression have yielded mixed results. As an example of a link between stress and cortisol, Goodkin et al.[17] reported increased plasma cortisol levels in bereaved HIV-seropositive men. After participation in a bereavement support group, the authors measured a reduction in plasma cortisol levels.

Bereavement is a frequent and significant stressor among people at risk for HIV infection and their partners. Following the loss of a friend, partner, or a lover, psychological distress may persist for a long time. Bereavement has been found to be associated with declines in immune measures. Goodkin et al.[17] reported decrements in NK cell cytotoxicity and absolute CD4+ T lymphocyte counts in bereaved, HIV-seropositive homosexual men at 6 months after the loss of a friend or a lover. At 12 months after the loss, a decrement in the proliferative response of lymphocytes to phytohemagglutinin was noted and NK cell cytotoxicity was still significantly suppressed. Although not all studies support the association between stress and immunity, the weight of evidence favors the view that psychological factors and stress influence immunity and immune-based diseases such as AIDS. Some factors that may contribute to discrepancies in research findings are differing study designs, outcome measures, follow-up periods, and criteria for defining and measuring stress.

Sleep disturbances are common among persons living with HIV disease. For detailed discussion about sleep in persons living with HIV disease, see Chapter 15. It is worth mentioning here that numerous life stressors encountered by persons living with HIV disease may contribute to decreased sleep quality. In a recent study, Cruess et al.[18] reported a relationship between greater psychological distress and greater subjective sleep disturbance in HIV-seropositive individuals receiving antiretroviral therapy. Additionally, higher levels of reported distress and higher reported sleep disturbance were significantly associated with lower levels of CD3+ and CD8+ cell counts. The authors concluded that psychological distress may affect the immune system in part through a sleep disturbance mechanism.[18]

TREATMENT CONSIDERATIONS

Early on in the AIDS epidemic, homosexuals living with HIV organized peer support groups as a means of helping them cope. Subsequently, mental health providers have developed clinical and educational interventions to help HIV-infected patients and their partners cope with stress associated with HIV infection and AIDS. Such interventions include individual, couple, family, and group therapies. A variety of standardized individual and group interventions have now been studied and are effective in treating distress in HIV-affected individuals.

The case presented previously and continued here exemplifies the multimodal clinical interventions typically used in patients with HIV and their loved ones.

> Theresa came for treatment complaining of difficulty sleeping, feeling tired, and being unable to make decisions about the care of her children. Theresa was diagnosed with adjustment disorder with anxiety. Supportive therapy was initiated to help Theresa cope with anger and grief. Trazodone was prescribed to restore sleep. Over 3 months, Theresa began to re-engage her support system in her family and the church. She had sufficient energy and focus to start a part-time job, which helped her to feel productive. She started to resume her role as a caretaker for her children, who were able in turn to return to their usual roles. Her oldest son resumed regular attendance in school.

There are only a few studies examining the effectiveness of individual psychotherapy in patients with adjustment disorders. When treating individuals with adjustment disorders, it is important to understand the meaning of stressors to the patient, the reasons behind the patient's maladaptive response, and the patient's capacity to cope with stressors effectively. The goals of psychotherapy should include decreasing the impact of stressors on the patient's daily functioning and facilitating the patient's ability to cope with stress. Various treatment modalities may be useful, such as cognitive-behavioral, supportive, psychodynamic, and crisis intervention therapies.[3] Parents with HIV infection or AIDS may need specific guidance on how to tell their children what disease they have. Disclosure to children must be age appropriate. It may be sufficient to tell a younger child that, "Mommy is sick." An older child may need more detailed information.

Coping Effectiveness Training, a group intervention based on the framework of the stress and coping theory, was designed to help HIV-infected homosexual men cope with stressors in their lives. This experimental intervention incorporates stress management techniques with a cognitive framework aimed at choosing a coping strategy that will best address a given stressor. The authors concluded that coping effectiveness training can be effective for managing psychological distress, based on a significant decrease in perceived stress and burnout.[11,19] Rotheram-Borus et al.[5] designed a coping skills intervention for HIV-positive parents and their adolescent children that involved group therapy based on the framework of cognitive behavioral and social learning theories. At 6-year follow-up, the intervention cohort had significantly reduced rates of reliance on public welfare, had fewer psychosomatic symptoms, were more likely to be employed, and were more likely to have better problem-solving skills in intimate relationships.[5]

Cognitive behavioral stress management, a group intervention based on the cognitive-behavioral framework, was designed to teach HIV-infected persons how to build social support, improve coping skills, and modify cognitive distortions about HIV-related issues. The sessions included a relaxation component, and participants were also instructed to practice relaxation techniques at home. Lutgendorf et al.[20] reported that the intervention improved cognitive coping strategies and the ability to improve social support.

Bereavement support group intervention was designed to help bereaved homosexual men cope with the loss of a close friend or a lover. This brief group intervention was created by integrating support group and bereavement group models. The protocol consists of grief work followed by stress management over a total of 20 sessions. The stress management training focuses on three tasks: assessment of stressor burden, utilization of social support, and selecting functional coping strategies. The authors reported that the intervention significantly reduced overall distress, accelerated the resolution of bereavement-specific distress, and had beneficial effects on immune system parameters.[1,17]

In addition to the patient's personal support network, much reassurance and emotional support for the individual with HIV may come from the primary care or HIV-specialist physician. In select cases, patients who have major psychiatric disorders (major depression, bipolar disorder, schizophrenia, etc.) will need referral for more extensive psychiatric evaluation. Those individuals with cognitive impairment should have both psychiatric and neurologic assessments. Certainly, any patients expressing suicidal, homicidal, or psychotic ideation should get urgent psychiatric evaluation and management.

In regard to pharmacologic treatment, there are only a few published studies examining medication management of adjustment disorders. Few data are available on treatment of any subsyndromal psychopathologic conditions. Traditionally, adjustment disorders have been treated primarily with psychotherapy; pharmacologic treatment has been reserved for major mood and anxiety disorders. With the advent of safer, better tolerated medications that target mood, anxiety, and insomnia symptoms, clinicians may initiate psychopharmacologic treatment in patients with adjustment disorder. Medications may be useful in patients experiencing more severe symptoms and more functional impairment. Pharmacologic interventions include the use of benzodiazepines to target symptoms of anxiety; selective serotonin reuptake inhibitors (SSRIs) to target symptoms of anxiety and depression; and γ-aminobutyric acid (GABA) receptor agonists (e.g., zolpidem and zaleplon) or trazodone for the treatment of insomnia. The role of pharmacotherapy in the treatment of adjustment disorders should be limited to augmentation of psychotherapeutic interventions and symptomatic relief, rather than as a primary treatment modality.[3]

SUMMARY

People living with HIV disease and their loved ones face multiple stressors in their lives. In response to external stressors, individuals may experience emotional distress. Severe life stressors may influence the progression of HIV infection to AIDS. The physiologic mechanisms connecting life stressors to disease progression are complex and not well understood. Mental health interventions aimed at helping individuals living with HIV disease to cope with stress are effective in reducing distress and may improve disease outcomes. Most studies of the effects of stress on people living with HIV disease were performed before the introduction of HAART; less is known about the effects of chronic external stressors on emotional distress since the advent of HAART. Future areas of research should investigate the physiology of stress and disease and the effects of stress on various subgroups of people living with HIV disease. It should also define the mental health needs of the population. Specific mental health interventions for helping women, children, and elderly HIV-seropositive patients may improve the quality of life in such populations.

REFERENCES

1. Goodkin K, Visser AP, eds. *Psychoneuroimmunology*. Washington, DC: American Psychiatric Press; 2000:1–41, 317–395.
2. American Psychiatric Association. *Diagnostic and Statistical Manual of Mental Disorders*. 4th ed, Text Rev. Washington, DC: American Psychiatric Association; 2000:679–685.
3. Sadock BJ, Sadock VA, eds. *Kaplan and Sadock's Comprehensive Textbook of Psychiatry*. Philadelphia: Lippincott Williams & Wilkins; 2000:1714–1722.
4. Remien RH, Wagner G, Dolezal C, et al. Levels and correlates of psychological distress in male couples of mixed HIV status. *AIDS Care*. 2003;15:525–538.

5. Rotheram-Borus MJ, Lee M, Lin YY, et al. Six-year intervention outcomes for adolescent children of parents with the human immunodeficiency virus. *Arch Pediatr Adolesc Med.* 2004;158:742–748.
6. Mellins CA, Brackis-Cott E, Dolezal C, et al. The role of psychosocial and family factors in adherence to antiretroviral treatment in human immunodeficiency virus-infected children. *Pediatr Infect Dis J.* 2004;23:1035–1041.
7. Antoni MH, Cruess DG, Klimas N, et al. Stress management and immune system reconstitution in symptomatic HIV-infected gay men over time: effects on transitional naive T cells (CD4(+)CD45RA(+) CD29(+)). *Am J Psychiatry.* 2002;159:143–145.
8. Gray J, Cason CL. Mastery over stress among women with HIV/AIDS. *J Assoc Nurses AIDS Care.* 2002;13:43–51.
9. Leserman J, Petitto JM, Golden RN, et al. Impact of stressful life events, depression, social support, coping, and cortisol on progression to AIDS. *Am J Psychiatry.* 2000;157:1221–1228.
10. O'Cleirigh C, Ironson G, Antoni M, et al. Emotional expression and depth processing of trauma and their relation to long-term survival in patients with HIV/AIDS. *J Psychosom Res.* 2003;54:225–235.
11. Chesney MA, Chambers DB, Taylor JM, et al. Social support, distress, and well–being in older men living with HIV infection. *J Acquir Immune Defic Syndr.* 2003;33(suppl 2):S185–S193.
12. Leserman J, Petitto JM, Gu H, et al. Progression to AIDS, a clinical AIDS condition and mortality: psychosocial and physiological predictors. *Psychol Med.* 2002;32:1059–1073.
13. Pereira DB, Antoni MH, Danielson A, et al. Life stress and cervical squamous intraepithelial lesions in women with human papillomavirus and human immunodeficiency virus. *Psychosom Med.* 2003;65:427–434.
14. Kopnisky KL, Stoff DM, Rausch DM. Workshop report: the effects of psychological variables on the progression of HIV-1 disease. *Brain Behav Immun.* 2004;18:246–261.
15. Howland LC, Gortmaker SL, Mofenson LM, et al. Effects of negative life events on immune suppression in children and youth infected with human immunodeficiency virus type 1. *Pediatrics.* 2000;106:540–546.
16. Petitto JM, Leserman J, Perkins DO, et al. High versus low basal cortisol secretion in asymptomatic, medication-free HIV-infected men: differential effects of severe life stress on parameters of immune status. *Behav Med.* 2000;25:143–151.
17. Goodkin K, Feaster DJ, Tuttle R, et al. Bereavement is associated with time-dependent decrements in cellular immune function in asymptomatic human immunodeficiency virus type 1-seropositive homosexual men. *Clin Diagn Lab Immunol.* 1996;3:109–118.
18. Cruess DG, Antoni MH, Gonzalez J, et al. Sleep disturbance mediates the association between psychological distress and immune status among HIV-positive men and women on combination antiretroviral therapy. *J Psychosom Res.* 2003;54:185–189.
19. Chesney MA, Chambers DB, Taylor JM, et al. Coping effectiveness training for men living with HIV: results from a randomized clinical trial testing a group-based intervention. *Psychosom Med* 2003;65:1038–1046.
20. Lutgendorf SK, Antoni MH, Ironson G, et al. Changes in cognitive coping skills and social support during cognitive behavioral stress management intervention and distress outcomes in symptomatic human immunodeficiency virus (HIV)-seropositive gay men. *Psychosom Med.* 1998;60:204–214.

CHAPTER 9

Anxiety Disorders

Annette M. Matthews, Manuel Trujillo

Estimated rates of lifetime and current anxiety disorder and specific types of anxiety disorders in the human immunodeficiency virus (HIV)-positive population are highly variable. The prevalence of anxiety disorders over the lifetime in the HIV-positive population is estimated to be 4% to 19% compared with those in the general population, in which the estimates are 15% to 25%. The prevalence of current anxiety disorders in the HIV-positive population is estimated to be 5% to 15% compared with those in the general population, in which the estimates are 13% to 17%. The distribution of the types of anxiety disorders is thought to be different in the HIV-positive population than in the general population. In the general population the most common anxiety disorders are simple and social phobias, whereas in the HIV-positive population there is a much greater rate of social phobia and generalized anxiety disorder, although some authors have found that there is a greater incidence of panic disorder in the HIV-positive population.[1,2]

It is important to recognize and treat anxiety disorders in the HIV-positive population. Increased rates of anxiety disorders have been associated with flight from treatment; poor treatment compliance; increased rates of high-risk behaviors, including high-risk sexual behaviors; increased rate of disease progression; and increased use of health care services.[3] Suicide in the HIV-positive patient is associated with both positive and negative changes in treatment status.[4] Quality of life is also adversely affected by the stress of having to cope with both an HIV diagnosis and an anxiety disorder.[3,5]

There is a spectrum of anxiety-related issues related to the diagnosis and treatment of HIV infection. These include preexisting and new-onset primary anxiety disorders, adjustment disorders or acute stress reactions related to phases of illness, and chronic subsyndromal problems with anxious mood. As patients become more ill, they may develop problems related to their medical condition, including minor cognitive motor disorder (MCMD) and subcortical HIV-associated dementia, which may present as anxiety disorders. It is important for mental health providers to entertain this broad differential when an HIV-positive patient presents with symptoms of anxiety.

PSYCHOLOGICAL STRESSORS

Throughout the course of HIV exposure, infection, diagnosis, and treatment, there are several stressful milestones that can produce normal anxiety responses. It is important to be aware of the anxiety-provoking nature of these events not only because of their treatment implications, including the increased risk of suicide, but also because they may present opportunities to make meaningful mental health interventions.

Getting tested for HIV is one of the first milestones in HIV disease. Patients with high-risk behaviors should be encouraged to get HIV tested and to follow up on the results of testing. New, rapid methods of testing decrease the time from test to result, prevent patients from being lost to follow-up, and decrease the period of anxiety associated with waiting for results. This allows for earlier education about the disease, transmission, and treatment. As stressful as HIV testing is for the general population, HIV-exposed health care providers face unique choices in having to weigh the risks and benefits of taking postexposure prophylaxis for HIV (see Chapter 3).

After the diagnosis of HIV is confirmed, patients commonly experience a series of milestones as they adapt to and cope with their diagnosis and disease progression. These events can be classified into early, middle, and late phases of HIV disease; however, anxiety disorders can and do occur at any phase of illness, and providers should be ready to address them when they arise. When working with patients whose disease is progressing, providers should initiate discussions of the more difficult topics, such as loss of physical and mental health, lack of treatment response, and planning for death, if they do not naturally arise in the course of treatment[6] (Table 9.1).

TABLE 9.1 Milestones in HIV Care

Phase	Treatment Approaches
Early Phase	
Adjusting to new diagnosis of HIV seroconversion	Provide opportunity for patient to address questions and worries as they arise.
Disclosing to others	Help patient determine to whom, when, and how to disclose. Offer to provide additional information or be present during disclosure.
Adapting safer sexual and drug-using behaviors	Provide harm reduction education.
Accessing appropriate HIV medical and psychiatric care	Provide information on treatment options, which may include both allopathic and alternative care.
Assessing substance use	Determine need for detoxification, treatment, methadone maintenance.
Accommodating to medical evaluation and assessment of level of illness (e.g., laboratory results)	Educate patient in coping skills used to accommodate to being in the medical system.
Middle Phase	
Accommodating work and family needs to physical and emotional impact of illness	Refer to social work, vocational rehabilitation, family, couples, or group or individual psychotherapy.
Dealing with learning about the nature of the illness and the potential treatments	Provide patient education and information on local and national peer-support groups.
Adherence issues	Use motivational interviewing techniques.
Decisions about working, going on disability, back-to-work issues, feeling productive	Refer to family, couple, group, or individual psychotherapy.
Maintaining relationships and managing normal developmental issues in the context of the uncertainty of the progression of illness	Refer to family, couple, group, or individual psychotherapy.

(continued)

TABLE 9.1	Milestones in HIV Care (Continued)
Dealing with untoward effects of illness and treatment	Consider medications that are used to improve quality of life, including testosterone, psychostimulants, or other psychotropic agents.
Late Phase	
Advance directives	Discuss early in the course of treatment.
Existential issues	Consider psychodynamic psychotherapy.
Preparations for death	Consider supportive and psychodynamic psychotherapy.

Modified from Forstein M. Psychosocial issues in antiretroviral treatment. In: Cournos F, Forstein M, eds. *What Mental Health Practitioners Need to Know About HIV and AIDS.* San Francisco: Jossey-Bass; 2000:17–24.

In the early phase of HIV diagnosis, stresses include adjusting to the diagnosis of HIV seroconversion, disclosing to others, adopting safer sexual and drug-using behaviors, and accommodating to medical treatment. Patients may experience fear of imminent death, guilt of infecting others or the risk thereof, and resentment at having to adapt their behaviors to their illness. Providers can help through this phase of illness by educating patients on the disease and making referral to education classes, peer-support groups, or other psychotherapies as appropriate (see also Chapters 7 and 8).

In the middle phase of HIV diagnosis, stresses include accommodating work and family needs to the physical and emotional impact of illness, learning about the illness and potential treatments, and adherence issues. Patients can face difficult decisions related to the uncertainty of the progression of illness and for some this can manifest as premature grief or traumatic death anxiety.[3] Cognitive behavioral therapy, coping skills training, and individual psychotherapy can be particularly helpful to address these feelings. When patients begin antiretroviral treatment, they are faced with the challenges of medication side effects, they must adapt to living "by the numbers" of CD4 cells and viral load, and they adapt to the side effects of the medications, including fatigue and depression. Patients may have body-image problems related to lipodystrophy and wasting that may serve as constant reminders, to themselves and others, of their disease and add to their fear and anxiety. Treatments for HIV infection may physiologically induce anxiety and can cause a relapse to premorbid anxiety disorders, such as post-traumatic stress disorder (PTSD) or panic disorder, that had been considered to be in remission.[7]

In the late phase of HIV diagnosis, stresses include planning for death, making provisions for partners and children, and choosing advance directives. Patients also face existential and spiritual issues about the meaning of one's life and one's death. Throughout the course of the illness, patients may be confronted with the repeated need to grieve the death of their HIV-positive peers.

Partners of HIV-positive patients go through their own phases of education, adaptation, planning, anxiety, fear, grief, and loss. They may be forced to undertake different roles in the relationship, home, or financial responsibilities. They may need to decide on the level of caregiving they are able and willing to provide. Some studies of those who provide care have shown that positive coping methods tend to predict better mental health outcomes for the caregivers. Some of these positive ways of coping include positive reframing of situations; goal-directed, problem-focused coping; incorporating spiritual beliefs and practices; and the infusion of ordinary events with positive meaning[8] (see also Chapter 32).

The stress of the illness progression may trigger mood, anxiety, or substance-abuse disorders in the partner or unveil unhealthy relationship patterns, including physical or mental abuse. Providers can help the partner of the HIV-infected patient by discussing caregiver stress, encouraging development and maintenance of a support network, and referring to individual, family, or couples counseling, short-term psychotherapies, and respite services where appropriate.[9,10]

ANXIETY DISORDERS IN HIV-POSITIVE PATIENTS

Rates of the individual Axis I anxiety disorders in HIV-positive patients are difficult to ascertain because the studies are generally not large enough to break out rates for the individual disorders, do not use sufficiently detailed diagnostic criteria, or are limited to a specific cohort or stage of HIV disease. Generally it is thought that HIV-positive patients have rates of anxiety disorders similar to those in the general population, with the exception of relatively increased rates of generalized anxiety disorder.[1] This increased rate may be due to sensitization by repeated stressful disease phases as described above or to substance abuse comorbidity, particularly intravenous drug use, in the HIV-positive individual.[11]

The HIV-positive population is at particular risk for PTSD. Certain subpopulations of the HIV-positive population, including sex workers and gay, lesbian, transgender, or bisexual patients, may be at higher risk than is the general population for complex PTSD from multiple traumatic experiences (see Chapters 28 and 29). For the HIV-positive patient, having a PTSD diagnosis predicts having increased pain intensity and morbidity, more health-related complaints, and more HIV-related illness.[12,13] Treatment of PTSD through cognitive behavioral and other therapies with or without adjunctive pharmacotherapy may not only decrease PTSD symptoms but may also decrease pain response and improve health outcomes.

Some studies have suggested that those with HIV may have a higher rate of panic disorder than the general population. Some patients will have the onset of panic-like symptoms after the start of particular antiretroviral agents, including efavirenz and lamivudine. Patients with new-onset panic disorder should have their antiretroviral regimen reviewed. One study has shown that those with HIV and unresolved grief or multiple traumas are more likely to have panic attacks, suggesting that HIV-positive patients with panic attacks should be screened for grief reactions.[14]

There are several case reports of AIDS-related obsessive compulsive disorder, and these were successfully treated with exposure and response prevention and selective serotonin reuptake inhibitors (SSRIs).[15] People with HIV infection or AIDS may develop specific illness-related obsessions. They may obsess about numerous details of the illness or its management, such as viral loads, CD4 counts, adequate completion of medication schedules, the presence and significance of relatively minor physical symptoms, and many other items. There are also several cases of non–HIV-infected patients developing delusional beliefs about having or possibly contracting HIV infection. Like other forms of delusional parasitosis, delusional beliefs about being infected can sometimes respond to treatment with SSRIs or low-dose antipsychotics.

CONDITIONS THAT MAY MIMIC ANXIETY DISORDERS

Frequently, anxiety and depression run hand in hand. Mood disorders are the most common mental health problem in the HIV-positive patient. An undiagnosed, untreated mood disorder or bereavement may result in significant agitation and psychomotor activation, masquerading as generalized anxiety disorder or panic attacks. Treatment of the underlying mood disorder may result in the decrease or disappearance of anxiety symptoms (see Chapter 10).

Some subpopulations of HIV-positive patients have high rates of comorbid substance dependence. Various substances of abuse can masquerade as anxiety disorders: depressant drugs such as alcohol and heroin have withdrawal symptoms that are anxiety provoking, and stimulants such as methamphetamine or cocaine can result in anxiety when one is intoxicated. Patients with anxiety disorders are also at increased risk for substance abuse, particularly alcohol abuse, and should be screened for this.

As patients become sicker, they may develop mental status changes, including MCMD, HIV dementia, and delirium. Subtle changes in their personality associated with MCMD and decline in emotional control associated with HIV dementia may appear like new-onset generalized anxiety disorder. Delirium can present in an agitated, anxious form. Patients with acute mental status changes should be screened with tests such as the Delirium Assessment Scale or the Confusion Assessment Method to rule out delirium as a cause of anxiety-like symptoms. Somatic symptoms, including fatigue, pain, and loss of appetite can be anxiety-provoking for HIV-positive patients, and sometimes their treatment can help reduce anxiety (see also Chapter 12).

Some of the common medications that are used to improve quality of life and health in those with HIV disease may also provoke anxiety-like conditions. Testosterone, which is given to help with mood and physical changes caused by antiretrovirals, may result in periods of irritability as it reaches peak blood levels. Fluctuations in blood level can be reduced by using a more controlled release form such as a testosterone patch or gel rather than monthly injections. Psychostimulants that are given to help with fatigue or low mood may result in anxiety or sleep problems, and dose reductions or changes in timing of the dose may be necessary.

Alternative medications and treatments are extremely popular for managing the physical and mental health effects associated with HIV infection. It is important to ask about the use of alternative medications and over-the-counter drugs at each visit. Many alternative drugs are either natural stimulants, such as green tea, or have a stimulant-like effect, such as chromium. Patients should be educated on the possible risks, including drug interactions and increased anxiety, so that they may make informed decisions about their use.

PHARMACOTHERAPY OF ANXIETY DISORDERS IN THE HIV-POSITIVE PATIENT

Pharmacotherapy for HIV is a complex and ever-changing field, and psychotropic agents are commonly used to treat anxiety in the HIV-positive population.[16] It is important that psychiatrists collaborate closely with infectious disease specialists in the management of HIV disease and AIDS and their psychological sequelae. Mental health providers should update the current antiretroviral regimen of their patients at each visit and be aware of possible drug interactions between psychotropics and antiretrovirals.

The mainstays of treatment for anxiety disorders are antidepressants, including SSRIs and tricyclic antidepressants, as well as benzodiazepines. Many of the antiretrovirals are potent cytochrome P (CYP) 450 3A4 inhibitors, including indinavir and ritonavir. This increases the risk of supratherapeutic or toxic levels of some anxiolytic drugs, particularly the tertiary tricyclic antidepressants, which are preferentially metabolized by CYP450 3A4. There are also case reports of specific drug interactions of which providers should be aware. In particular, serotonin syndrome has been seen in patients taking ritonavir and fluoxetine, probably due to the ritonavir's inhibition of CYP450 2D6 and 3A4.[17]

Benzodiazepines can be useful in the treatment of anxiety, but they pose the risk of dependence and also may cause or exacerbate cognitive problems in those who are older or have more advanced HIV disease. In particular, several benzodiazepines, including clorazepate, diazepam, estazolam, flurazepam, midazolam, triazolam, and the imidazopyridine zolpidem, are contraindicated with ritonavir because it inhibits their metabolism. The most common benzodiazepines used are lorazepam (0.5 to 1 mg daily to four times daily) or clonazepam (0.25 to 1 mg daily to three times daily). Benzodiazepines appear particularly effective for somatic anxiety symptoms, a rather valuable effect in patients with HIV disease or AIDS, who often suffer from enhanced awareness of bodily sensations and somatic worry.

There are other agents that may be useful in treating anxiety. Choices may include buspirone (10 to 60 mg/day), which affects cognitive symptoms of anxiety over somatic symptoms, and trazodone (25 to 200 mg daily to four times daily)[18] (see also Chapter 16).

BEHAVIORAL TREATMENTS FOR ANXIETY IN HIV-POSITIVE PATIENTS

People cope with the diagnosis of HIV in different, more or less adaptive, manners. Mental health providers should provide empathetic listening and support during the phases of the illness. Education groups and peer support groups can be very helpful in alleviating the anticipatory anxiety about HIV course and treatment. HIV-positive patients who cope with the stress of their diagnosis through strategies other than denial tend to have a slower disease progression.[19]

There are a variety of cognitive-behavioral treatments that have been shown to be effective in managing stress and anxiety in HIV-positive patients. Many of these involve "packages" of self-monitoring, relaxation skills, and cognitive restructuring that are frequently taught in the group setting.[20,21] Individual interpersonal, psychodynamic, or psychoanalytic therapy may also be appropriate for some patients.

For patients who are "triply diagnosed" with HIV, an anxiety disorder, and substance abuse, integrated treatment models have been developed. These models have the advantage of providing coordinated medical, mental health, and substance abuse treatment that may be particularly valuable to those with HIV[1] (see Chapter 35).

It is estimated that about 30% of patients with HIV use nontraditional therapies. Nontraditional behavioral therapies can include acupuncture, visualization, and meditation. Use of these treatments is associated with greater feelings of perceived social support and less hopelessness about the future.[22] This suggests that providers should embrace the use of these therapies as part of the overall treatment of the HIV-positive patient (see Chapter 36).

SUMMARY

Lifetime rates of anxiety disorders in the HIV-positive population are similar to those in the population without HIV infection, but data suggest that the patients with HIV disease have an increased rate of generalized anxiety disorders and current (as opposed to lifetime) anxiety disorders. It is important that providers recognize anxiety disorders in those with HIV because treatment can improve quality of life, decrease disease transmission, and improve health outcomes.

Generally the treatments that are used for other anxiety disorders are appropriate for those who have HIV disease; however, providers need to be aware of the risks of drug interactions between antianxiety and anti-HIV medications. Some HIV-positive patients may also be at greater risk for cognitive effects or substance abuse than the general population. Psychotropic regimens should always be thought of in the context of the antiviral regimen, the stage of HIV disease, and any alternative medications the patient might be taking. In particular, providers should include in their differential diagnoses of anxiety disorders other illnesses that can mimic them, including depression, substance abuse, MCMD, HIV dementia, and delirium.

Behavioral treatments can be a powerful and important aspect of managing anxiety in HIV disease. In addition to decreasing or helping to manage anxiety symptoms, they can provide insight and support for the patient and his or her family system. Alternative treatments such as meditation or visualization should be embraced by the provider, and special interventions are available for those triply diagnosed with HIV, anxiety, and substance abuse.

REFERENCES

1. Klinkenberg WD, Sacks S. HIV/AIDS Treatment Adherence, Health Outcomes and Cost Study Group: mental disorders and drug abuse in persons living with HIV/AIDS. *AIDS Care*. 2004;16(suppl 1):S22–S42.
2. Sewell MC, Goggin KJ, Rabkin JG, Ferrando SJ, McElhiney MC, Evans S. Anxiety syndromes and symptoms among men with AIDS: a longitudinal controlled study. *Psychosomatics*. 2000;41:294–300.
3. Safren SA, Gershuny BS, Hendriksen E. Symptoms of posttraumatic stress and death anxiety in persons with HIV and medication adherence difficulties. *AIDS Patient Care STDS*. 2003;17:657–664.
4. Komiti A, Judd F, Grech P, et al. Suicidal behaviour in people with HIV/AIDS: a review. *Aust N Z J Psychiatry*. 2001;35:747–757.
5. Sherbourne CD, Hays RD, Fleishman JA, et al. Impact of psychiatric conditions on health-related quality of life in persons with HIV infection. *Am J Psychiatry*. 2000;157:248–254.
6. Forstein M. Psychosocial issues in antiretroviral treatment. In: Cournos F, Forstein M, eds. *What Mental Health Practitioners Need to Know About HIV and AIDS*. San Francisco: Jossey-Bass; 2000:17–24.
7. Moreno A, Labelle C, Samet JH. Recurrence of post-traumatic stress disorder symptoms after initiation of antiretrovirals including efavirenz: a report of two cases. *HIV Med*. 2003;4:302–304.
8. Folkman S. Positive psychological states and coping with severe stress. *Soc Sci Med*. 1997;45:1207–1221.
9. Rotheram-Borus MJ, Flannery D, Rice E, Lester P. Families living with HIV. *AIDS Care*. 2005;17:978–987.
10. Koopman C, Gore-Felton C, Azmi N, et al. Acute stress reactions to recent life events among women and men living with HIV/AIDS. *Int J Psychiatry Med*. 2002;32:361–378.
11. Wight RG, Aneshensel CS, LeBlanc AJ. Stress buffering effects of family support in AIDS caregiving. *AIDS Care*. 2003;15:595–613.
12. Smith MY, Egert J, Winkel G, Jacobson J. The impact of PTSD on pain experience in persons with HIV/AIDS. *Pain*. 2002;98:9–17.
13. Brief DJ, Bollinger AR, Vielhauer MJ, et al. HIV/AIDS Treatment Adherence, Health Outcomes and Cost Study Group: understanding the interface of HIV, trauma, post-traumatic stress disorder, and substance use and its implications for health outcomes. *AIDS Care*. 2004;16(suppl 1):S97–S120.
14. Summers J, Zisook S, Atkinson JH, et al. Psychiatric morbidity associated with acquired immune deficiency syndrome-related grief resolution. *J Nerv Ment Dis*. 1995;183:384–389.
15. Kraus RP, Nicholson IR. AIDS-related obsessive compulsive disorder: deconditioning based on fluoxetine-induced inhibition of anxiety. *J Behav Ther Exper Psychiatry*. 1996;27:51–56.
16. Vitiello B, Burnam MA, Bing EG, Beckman R, Shapiro MF. Use of psychotropic medications among HIV-infected patients in the United States. *Am J Psychiatry*. 2003;160:547–554.
17. Cozza KL, Armstrong SC, Oesterheld JR. *Drug Interaction Principles for Medical Practice*. 2nd ed. Washington, DC: American Psychiatric Press; 2003:239–241.
18. Ferrando SJ, Wapenyi K. Psychopharmacological treatment of patients with HIV and AIDS. *Psychiatr Q*. 2002;73:33–49.
19. Leserman J, Petitto JM, Golden RN, et al. Impact of stressful life events, depression, social support, coping, and cortisol on progression to AIDS. *Am J Psychiatry*. 2000;157:1221–1228.
20. Antoni MH, Baggett L, Ironson G, et al. Cognitive-behavioral stress management intervention buffers distress responses and immunologic changes following notification of HIV-1 seropositivity. *J Consult Clin Psychol*. 1991;59:906–915.
21. Najavits LM, Weiss RD, Liese BS. Group cognitive-behavioral therapy for women with PTSD and substance use disorder. *J Subst Abuse Treat*. 1996;13:13–22.
22. Singh N, Squier C, Sivek C, Nguyen H, Wagener M, Yu VL. Determinants of nontraditional therapy use in patients with HIV infection: a prospective study. *Arch Intern Med*. 1996;156:197–201.

CHAPTER 10

Mood Disorders

Pedro Ruiz

Mood disorders are very common; depression constitutes the second most frequently observed illness worldwide. In the United States, depression is observed in about 5.8% of the general population.[1] Among chronically ill persons, the rate of depression is 9.5%. Among patients who suffer from human immunodeficiency virus (HIV) infection or acquired immunodeficiency syndrome (AIDS), the rate of depression is 20% to 35%.[2] Additionally, suicide ideation tends to be present among two thirds of patients who are depressed and the rate of suicide among depressed patients is 10% to 15%. Among patients who have HIV disease or AIDS, however, the suicide rate goes up to 36%.[2]

In a recent meta-analysis conducted on the relationship between HIV infection and risk for depressive disorders, it was found that the frequency of major depressive disorder was nearly two times higher among HIV-positive subjects than among HIV-negative comparison subjects.[3] Among women, the rate of major depressive disorder was found to be four times higher (19.4%) in HIV-seropositive women than in HIV-seronegative (4.8%) women.[4] HIV-infected women were also found to have higher mean depressive symptom scores on the 17-item Hamilton Depression Scale relative to comparison subjects who were HIV-negative.[4] Major depression is one of the most commonly observed psychiatric conditions among persons living with HIV disease or AIDS.

Given the fact that stigma, prejudice, and discrimination are still very high regarding individuals with HIV disease or AIDS, the evaluation and treatment of these patients tend to be delayed because of their fear of discrimination, in its many, varied forms. Additionally, today patients with HIV disease or AIDS live longer because of new treatment discoveries and better understanding of the mechanisms and factors related to this illness; thus the rate of depression has increased in this population. Fortunately, however, treatment approaches for depressive disorders in this population have also improved, as well as become more effective. This chapter presents a clinical review of diagnosis and treatment approaches on the clinical management of mood disorders among patients with HIV disease or AIDS.

DIAGNOSIS AND SYMPTOMS MANIFESTATIONS

The *Diagnostic and Statistical Manual of Mental Disorders (DSM-IV)*[1] diagnostic category of depression is fully applicable to patients with HIV disease or AIDS. With respect to differential diagnosis, however, we must be cognizant of certain psychiatric illnesses that tend to be common in patients with HIV disease or AIDS. Among them are post-traumatic stress disorder (PTSD), primary sleep disorders, mood disorders due to a general medical condition, cognitive disorders, and dementia.[1] For example, among patients with HIV-associated dementia (HAD), symptoms of apathy, social withdrawal, psychomotor slowing, and memory problems may mimic a depressive disorder.[5]

Other than HAD, opportunistic infection illnesses and malignancies may masquerade as depression. The most common are toxoplasmosis, cryptoccocal meningitis, cytomegalovirus (CMV) encephalitis, progressive multifocal leukoencephalopathy (PML), and central nervous system (CNS) lymphoma.[5] Neurotoxic effects of medications that could lead to mood disorders include steroids (mania or depression), interferon (neurasthenia, fatigue syndrome and depression), interlukin-2 (depression), zidovudine (mania or depression), vinblastine (depression); and efavirenz (depression).[2,5] Other medical conditions associated with mood disorders present in patients with HIV disease or AIDS are malnutrition, vitamin deficiencies (specifically B_6 and B_{12}), hypogonadism, Addison's disease, anemia, and hepatic encephalopathy.[2,5]

RISK FACTORS

Patients with HIV disease or AIDS at highest risk for depression are those with a personal or family history of mood disorders, alcoholism, substance use, suicide attempts, or anxiety disorders or current use of alcohol or drugs, exposure to chronic stress, inadequate social support, passive coping style, nondisclosure of HIV status, presence of multiple losses, female gender, advanced illness, or treatment failure or success.[6,7] Among patients with HIV disease, the rate of depression increases 18 months before the diagnosis of AIDS.

TREATMENT MODALITIES

ANTIDEPRESSANTS

As general principles when using antidepressants medications for the treatment of depression among patients with HIV disease or AIDS, clinicians should do the following:

- Educate the patient about depression and the use of antidepressants.
- Start with lower doses of antidepressants and titrate up slowly.
- Use the simplest drug regimens possible.
- Be cognizant of the side effect profile of the antidepressant being used.
- Avoid as much as possible the use of antidepressants with high anticholinergic properties.
- Avoid, if possible, the use of high doses of antidepressants, and monitor carefully the treatment when using high dosages.
- Monitor potential drug–drug interactions
- Be aware that untreated or undertreated major depression may lead to increased utilization of health care services, increased likelihood of unprotected sexual activity, prolonged hospitalization in medical-surgical settings, and poor adherence to both antidepressant and antiretroviral therapy.
- Untreated or undertreated depression also leads to a decrease in the patients' quality of life.
- Untreated and undertreated depression will lead to an increase in the number of suicide attempts and completed suicide.

When entertaining psychopharmacologic interventions for the treatment of depression among patients with HIV disease or AIDS, possible unwanted CNS effects of psychotropic agents must be considered.[2,5] Clinicians should also be aware of the potential for drug–drug interactions between antidepressants and antiviral and primary medical therapies used to treat HIV infection and AIDS.[2,5,8] For example, antidepressant absorption from the gastrointestinal tract may be altered by antiviral agents; alterations in protein binding may influence free drug levels of both medication regimens; activation of the cytochrome P (CYP) 450 isoenzyme system may alter drug levels via induction or inhibitory mechanisms; and the potential use or abuse of addictive substances may also interact with these kinetic and dynamic factors and exert deleterious effects in both the medical and mood-related therapies.

Among the antidepressant drugs used to treat depression in patients with HIV disease or AIDS, the selective serotonin reuptake inhibitors (SSRIs) are the most commonly prescribed.[2] Although SSRIs are all equivalent in the treatment of depression, their different pharmacologic profiles should be carefully considered in the selection of a specific agent for use in patients receiving antiretroviral therapy. Of all the SSRIs, escitalopram and sertraline are the least likely to cause adverse events in patients receiving antiretroviral therapies inclusive of the protease inhibitors. For a full discussion of potential drug–drug interactions between antidepressants and medical therapies, see Chapter 16.

Bupropion can be helpful in withdrawn and anergic patients. Some suggest that it should be avoided in persons with advanced HIV disease, AIDS, or dementia because of its potential for seizures and inducing abnormal involuntary movements.[2] Nefazodone and fluvoxamine are highly protein bound and are inhibitory of the CYP450 3A4 isoenzyme system. Adding them to an established antiviral regimen will likely increase the serum levels of the antivirals and toxicity. Mirtazapine has a low affinity for the CYP450 isoenzyme system, is sedating, and produces weight gain. It is most helpful in the treatment of patients with poor appetite, weight loss, and significant anxiety and insomnia.[2,8]

All the tricyclic antidepressants have proven efficacy in the treatment of depression in the context of HIV disease and AIDS. Nortriptyline, desipramine, doxepin, imipramine, and amitriptyline have been reported useful. However, their anticholinergic burden, α_1 affinity, and interaction with the CYP450 2D6 isoenzyme system greatly increase the risk of significant treatment-related side effects, including cardiac toxicity, undesirable CNS anticholinergic side effects, sedation, and orthostatic hypotension.[2,8] If at all possible, they should be avoided in treating depression in patients with HIV disease or AIDS.

PSYCHOSTIMULANTS

The use of psychostimulants might be indicated in the treatment of depression in patients with HIV disease or AIDS.[9,10] For example, methylphenidate and dextroamphetamine are often useful adjuvants in treatment of depression among medically ill patients, including those with HIV disease or AIDS.[10] Methylphenidate and d-amphetamine have been shown to produce an 85% to 95% positive response in mood symptoms. Psychostimulants can serve to enhance cognition in patients with HIV or AIDS CNS involvement.[10] This effect is independent of their mood-altering effects. Psychostimulants are also helpful in patients who suffer from significant disease-related fatigue.

Psychostimulants must be used with caution, however, in patients who have been or are potentially vulnerable to seizures. Likewise, they should be avoided with patients who are psychotic or potentially vulnerable to psychosis. Their use should also be avoided in patients with history of addictive disorders or who are vulnerable to abuse of addictive substances.[10]

When deciding on whether to use formal antidepressant therapy or psychostimulants, it is useful to rely on antidepressant therapy for patients in the early stages or uncomplicated HIV infection or AIDS; when there is previous personal history of depression; when there is no cognitive impairment or dementia present; and when there is a current or past history of substance abuse or dependence. Use of psychostimulants in depressed patients with HIV disease or AIDS should be reserved for those individuals who have symptomatic disease; whose depression coexists with cognitive impairment or dementia; when significant fatigue is present; and with patients who suffer from secondary mood effects from their cognitive impairments.

HORMONES

Hormonal treatment with testosterone and its derivative dehydroandrosterone (DHEA) have been reported to be helpful in patients with HIV disease or AIDS who also have depression. Patients who are cachectic, with marked fatigue, are the ones most likely to benefit from hormone treatment.[11] Testosterone cypionate in doses up to 382 mg intramuscularly every 2 weeks has been reported to improve mood in 79% of patients. Secondary improvements in energy, stamina, libido, appetite, and weight gain have also been noted. In a separate study, DHEA treatment at 200 to 500 mg per day for 8 to 12 weeks showed a similar mood enhancement in 72% of patients, with corresponding improvements in energy and libido.

PSYCHOTHERAPY

All psychotherapies are effective in the treatment of mood disorders in the context of HIV disease and AIDS. The most common themes in therapy are anger; control issues (decision making related); bereavement; death and dying; illness impact on partners, children, and other relatives; fears (related to rejection, dependency, pain, or dementia); disclosure-related issues; sexuality; spirituality; guilt and regrets; low self-esteem–related issues; self-criticism–related problems; stigma- and discrimination-related issues; and suicide.[2,6]

The available evidence suggests that interpersonal therapy is the most efficacious, but all modalities of therapy should be used in combination with pharmacotherapy to optimize results. No matter the therapeutic intervention used, a psychoeducational framework to address disease management issues, safe sex practices, compliance enhancement, disability, quality of life issues, and effective utilization of community resources is necessary. For a full discussion of psychotherapy issues and their management, refer to Chapter 35.

ELECTROCONVULSIVE TREATMENT

Electroconvulsive treatment has been used successfully in patients with HIV disease and AIDS. For example, it is indicated in these patients who are too medically ill to tolerate full antidepressant doses to achieve remission, those who experience severe suicidality, are psychotic, or are treatment resistant. Electroconvulsive treatment has been reported to increase confusion and even make the patient worse in the presence of coexisting HIV/AIDS-CNS disease.[12,13]

INPATIENT CARE

Inpatient care is recommended in cases in which the patient with HIV-related disease is acutely suicidal, unable to care for self at home, medically frail, or needs to start pharmacotherapy treatment in a controlled environment where clinical and laboratory monitoring can take place. Moreover, when there is a current or past history of manic episodes with rapid cycling characteristics, inpatient care should be considered.[12]

DIAGNOSING MANIA

When diagnosing mania and hypomania in patients with HIV disease or AIDS, *DSM-IV* diagnostic criteria should be used.[1] In the context of HIV disease, the differential diagnostic considerations are extensive. Among them, HAD, psychoneurotoxicities (due to medications such as steroids, all nucleoside antiretrovirals, non-nucleoside reverse transcriptase inhibitors, ganciclovir, sympathomimetics, antidepressants, cocaine, and amphetamines), opportunistic infections (toxoplasmosis, cryptococcal meningitis, and cytomegalovirus [CMV]), and other conditions (CNS lymphoma, neurosyphilis, herpes, and vitamin B_{12} deficiency) must be ruled out before that of a mood disorder with features of mania.[5,13]

TREATMENT OF MANIA

Among the biologic therapies for mania in patients with HIV disease or AIDS, we should consider the full spectrum of psychotropic agents used in bipolar mood disorders.[2,5,8,9,12–14]

LITHIUM CARBONATE

Patients previously treated with lithium for either depression or mania before HIV was diagnosed can continue their regimen. Lithium is devoid of potential for significant drug–drug interactions with antiretrovirals. However, as HIV disease advances and when it progresses to fully developed AIDS, patients may not tolerate lithium as well as previously. Lithium serum levels may fluctuate easily in patients who develop diarrhea, have fever, and have poor fluid intake. Lithium levels must be monitored closely because potential neurotoxicities and other gastrointestinal side effects can adversely affect antiretroviral therapy. The potential for aggravating HIV-related nephropathy exists, and one should be prepared to discontinue lithium in this setting.[2,13,14]

VALPROIC ACID

Like patients who were stable on lithium, those already receiving valproic acid and valproate before HIV is diagnosed should continue their regimen to maintain remission. In patients who develop secondary mania in the context of HIV CNS disease, valproic acid and valproate were found to better control manic symptoms than either lithium or neuroleptics. Its potential for drug–drug interactions and side effect profile even in advanced disease is superior to those of other agents. Coadministration with zidovudine may raise zidovudine levels. Valproate does have a black box warning for causing hepatotoxicity and pancreatitis. Thus, in patients with concomitant liver disease (e.g., hepatitis C), liver function testing and measuring of ammonia must be monitored to avoid added hepatotoxicity. Likewise, care must be taken when valproate is added in patients on antiviral agents that have a propensity to cause pancreatitis. A single report noting increased viral replication with valproate in vivo has never translated into clinically significant changes that would warrant its discontinuation.[2,13,14]

CARBAMAZEPINE AND OXCARBAMAZEPINE

Carbamazepine has a black box warning for aplastic anemia and agranulocytopenia. Although no adverse events have been noted in patients suffering from HIV disease or AIDS, one should carefully monitor patients who are also taking antiviral medications. Plasma levels of carbamazepine may fluctuate due to nonlinear kinetics and autoinduction phenomena. Its affinity for the CYP450 3A4 isoenzyme system raises concern about its use with antiretroviral regimens and protease inhibitors. Thus, it is not particularly useful. Oxcarbamazepine is a weaker inducer of the CYP450 3A4 isoenzyme system and would not be expected to have clinically significant effects on antiretroviral regimens.[2,13,14]

CLONAZEPAM

Clonazepam is often safe and effective as a second or third agent in mania for added stabilization. Most clinicians are cautious when using any benzodiazepine because combination with protease inhibitors may decrease their effectiveness. Nonetheless, clonazepam is a good adjuvant drug for sleep disturbances secondary to acute mania and hypomania.[2,13,14]

GABAPENTIN

Gabapentin has no proven efficacy in mania or hypomania. However, in secondary mania, it is reportedly an effective adjuvant. It is most often used in patients with HIV/AIDS-related neuropathies, and is ideally suited for patients with HIV disease or AIDS because it is not metabolized and has no known interactions with CYP450 inhibitors or inducers. The only drawback is that its clearance is altered by renal impairment and it should be used cautiously in the context of HIV nephropathy.[2,13,14]

LAMOTRIGINE

Although there are no reports as yet on its use in the setting of HIV/AIDS-related mood disorders, lamotrigine had been used in HIV/AIDS-related neuropathies with no significant toxicity. Lamotrigine is mainly metabolized by glucuronidation and less likely to cause potential drug–drug interactions with antiviral regimens.[2,13,14]

TOPIRAMATE

There are no available reports in HIV/AIDS-related mood disorders. Clinically, it may be helpful in the management of impulsivity in the context of HIV/AIDS CNS involvement. However, one should be careful with its associated weight loss. Topiramate is a weak inducer of the CYP450 3A4 isoenzyme system, so it can be used with minimal concern for potential drug–drug interactions with antiviral regimens.[2,13,14]

NEUROLEPTICS

Neuroleptics are useful in the management of manic and hypomanic states. Caution is warranted with traditional neuroleptics (typical neuroleptics) because patients with HIV disease or AIDS are more sensitive to side effects such as extrapyramidal reactions (EPSs) and neuroleptic malignant syndrome (NMS). Low-potency neuroleptics are not benign and can produce severe anticholinergic effects worsening cognitive functions. The atypical neuroleptics have been used without notable sedation, EPRs, or worsening of cognitive impairment. When using atypical antipsychotics for the treatment of mania or hypomania together with antiviral medications, caution is in order because of the potential for drug–drug interactions. To date, the major caution is to avoid coadministration of clozapine with the protease inhibitor ritonavir.[13,14]

SUICIDE AMONG HIV/AIDS PATIENTS WITH MOOD DISORDERS

As in all patients, suicide risk is greatest for individuals with a past personal or family history of psychiatric illness and suicide. The available evidence suggests that people with HIV disease or AIDS are at highest risk early in the course of the illness and late in the disease.

Although the rates of suicide have decreased since the advent of highly active antiretroviral therapy (HAART) to levels comparable to those in other medical illnesses, suicide remains a significant concern and the exploration of suicidal ideation is essential.[2,8,15–17] In the context of depression, psychological factors such as despondency, disillusionment, helplessness, demoralization, and hopelessness may increase the risk of suicide. Psychotherapy with suicidal patients with HIV disease or AIDS that focuses on increasing a sense of control and coping enhancement reduces the risk.[2,8] For a fuller discussion of HIV/AIDS-related suicide and physician-assisted suicide, see Chapters 38 and 40, respectively.

SUMMARY

Mood disorders are the most frequent psychiatric condition associated with HIV disease and AIDS. Mood disorders, including depression and mania, may be secondary to both HIV disease and AIDS complications and the treatment of such illnesses. Suicide risk could be elevated across the trajectory of HIV disease and AIDS, particularly during early stages of HIV infection.

Fortunately, however, multiple effective therapeutic strategies are available today to treat and manage mood disorders in patients with HIV disease and AIDS, as well as other psychiatric conditions in this patient population. Without question, timely treatment of mood disorders in these patients may slow the progression of cognitive impairments and also enhance the quality of life.

Aggressive treatment of any mood disorder or other psychiatric conditions in patients with HIV disease or AIDS should always be offered, because psychiatric disorders profoundly affect patients' decisions regarding their treatment and all other aspects of their lives as well. Hopefully, more research and educational efforts focusing on mood disorders in this patient population will lead to new and better treatment modalities in the near future, as well as enhancement in the overall quality of life of this patient population.

REFERENCES

1. American Psychiatric Association. *Diagnostic and Statistical Manual of Mental Disorders*. 4th ed. (DSM-IV). Washington, DC: American Psychiatric Association; 1994.
2. Ruiz P, Guynn RW, Matorin AA. Psychiatric considerations in the diagnosis, treatment and prevention of HIV/AIDS. *J Psychiatr Pract*. 2000;6:129–139.
3. Ciesla JA, Roberts JE. Meta-analysis of the relationship between HIV infection and risk for depressive disorders. *Am J Psychiatry*. 2001;158:725–730.
4. Morrison MF, Petitte JM, Have TT, et al. Depressive and anxiety disorders in women with HIV infection. *Am J Psychiatry*. 2002;159:789–796.
5. Fernandez F, Maldonado J, Ruiz P. Neuropsychiatric aspects of HIV-I infection. In: Lowinson JH, Ruiz P, Millman RB, Langrod JG, eds. *Substance Abuse: A Comprehensive Textbook*. 4th ed. Philadelphia: Lippincott Williams & Wilkins; 2005:988–1007.
6. Ruiz P. Living and dying with HIV/AIDS: a psychosocial perspective. *Am J Psychiatry*. 2000;157:110–113.
7. Ruiz P, Lile B, Matorin AA. Treatment of a dually diagnosed gay male patient: a psychotherapy perspective. *Am J Psychiatry*. 2002;159:209–215.
8. Cournos F, Forstein MA, eds. *What Mental Health Practitioners Need to Know About HIV and AIDS: New Directions for Mental Health Services*. San Francisco: Jossey-Bass; 2000.
9. Hinkin CH, Castellon SA, Atkinson JH, Goodkin K. Neuropsychiatric aspects of HIV infection among older adults. *J Clin Epidemiol*. 2001;54:544–552.
10. Fernandez F, Levy JK, Ruiz P. The use of methylphenidate in HIV+ patients: a clinical perspective. In: Grant I, Martin A, eds. *Neuropsychology of HIV Infection*. New York: Oxford University Press; 1994:295–309.
11. Rabkin JG, Ferrando SJ, Wagner GJ, Rabkin R. DHEA treatment for HIV+ patients: effects on mood, androgenic and anabolic parameters. *Psychoneuroendocrinology*. 2000;25:53–68.
12. Fernandez F, Ruiz P. Psychiatric aspects of HIV disease. *South Med J.*, 989;82:999–1004.
13. American Psychiatric Association. APA practice guidelines for the treatment of patients with HIV/AIDS. *Am J Psychiatry*. 2000;157:1–62.

14. Bialer PA, Kato K, Latoussakis V. Psychotropic drug interactions with antiretroviral medications. In: Fernandez F, Ruiz P, eds. *Psychiatric Aspects of HIV/AIDS*. Baltimore: Lippincott Williams & Wilkins. 2006:149—160.
15. McKegney FP, O'Dowd MA. Suicidality and HIV status. *Am J Psychiatry*. 1992;149:396–398.
16. Cote T, Biggar R, Dannenberg A. Risk of suicide among persons with AIDS: a national assessment. *JAMA*. 1998;260:1881.
17. Marzuk PM, Tardiff K, Leon AC, et al. HIV seroprevalence among suicide victims in New York City, 1991–1993. *Am J Psychiatry*. 1997;154:1720–1725.

CHAPTER 11

Personality Disorders

Khenu Singh, Herbert Ochitill

Personality is a complex matter, and there is no consensus on how to define it, even in its maladaptive and disordered forms. One thing is clear, however—disordered personality and certain personality traits affect every aspect of the experience of human immunodeficiency virus (HIV) disease and its treatment. Certain personality traits and disorders increase risk behaviors related to both infection and transmission of the HIV virus. Thus certain personality structures, especially borderline and antisocial personality disorders, are significantly more prevalent in HIV-positive individuals. Personality affects the personal meaning of having HIV infection, as well as coping with the illness and its treatment. The patient's experience of caregivers, providers, and others in the interpersonal milieu is also shaped by personality. The larger sociocultural responses to HIV and high-risk subcultures are often experienced in unique ways patients with personality disorder (PD). Personality affects aspects of medical care from compliance with medical care, including potentially life-saving interventions, to the treatment relationship itself. Even seasoned mental health providers struggle with intense, sometimes hateful, countertransference feelings. Clearly, the interface of personality and HIV disease is an area that every practitioner needs to be familiar with, whether medical or psychiatric providers or leaders involved in policy-making and public health systems of care.

MODELS OF PERSONALITY

Most authors consider personality to involve intelligence, temperament, and character with temperament reflecting biologic contributions and character reflecting social and cultural shaping.[1] In regard to maladaptive personality structure, there is some controversy between dimensional and categorical approaches. The *Diagnostic and Statistical Manual of Mental Disorders* (*DSM-IV*) uses categorical constructs with which most clinicians are familiar. However, DSM-V Prelude Project workgroup on personality and relational issues continues to consider the merits of a dimensional approach. *DSM* aside, there are other categorical approaches to disordered personality from the psychoanalytic tradition, including Otto Kernberg's concept of the borderline personality organization, which subsumes the *DSM-IV* borderline, narcissistic, and antisocial personality disorders.

A thorough review of various theories of personality is beyond the scope of this chapter. We review the major temperament and character traits, to provide a conceptual framework and to set the context for studies that reference specific personality traits. Though there are multiple conceptual models, some authors feel these can be reduced to four temperament traits: (a) fearfulness or high harm avoidance, (b) impulsivity or high novelty seeking, (c) social detachment or low reward dependence, and (d) compulsiveness or persistence. The *DSM-IV* personality disorder clusters relate to these four traits in the following manner: cluster A (social detachment or low reward-dependence), cluster B (impulsivity or high novelty-seeking), and cluster C (fearfulness or high harm avoidance).[1]

In addition to temperament, there are three major character dimensions described in the literature: (a) self-directedness, (b) cooperativeness, and (c) self-transcendence.[1] Self-directedness includes the concept of locus of control that has been shown to relate to the extent of involvement with health care.[2] Cooperativeness relates to a sense of being involved in human experience and society and has implications in regard to the interpersonal field, including social support networks and providers. Finally, self-transcendence relates to a sense of being involved in the universe as a whole, expanding the boundaries of self to take on broader life perspectives, and discovering meaning in one's life. This correlates with coping with a chronic illness and the existential issues related to death and dying, issues examined later in this chapter.

Personality models can more broadly be classified as two types: the social-cognitive and the trait-dispositional.[3] The social-cognitive model relates to plans, goals, strategies, and overall narratives that inform behavior and are situated within a larger social context. Neurotic conflict and complex are also included here as significant aspects of personality structure. These social-cognitive or narrative aspects of personality are unique, shaped by particular aspects of relationship and life experience not readily reduced to categorical personality disorders. Trait-dispositional models refer to personality dimensions, as outlined previously. These once competing theories are now considered to be complementary by clinicians and theoreticians in the field of personality.

Thus there are multiple ways to conceptualize both normal and disordered personality—dimensional, categorical, and narrative/social-cognitive approaches are among these. Our focus will be on those personality traits, as well as *DSM-IV* personality disorders that have been described in the literature on HIV and personality and noted in the clinical experience of those working with patients with HIV.

EPIDEMIOLOGIC PERSPECTIVES

Almost by definition, the *DSM* cluster B PDs are associated with an increase in risk-related behaviors. Borderline patients are more impulsive (including impulsive sexual behaviors), and antisocial patients are both more impulsive and less harm-avoidant (i.e., less fearful of consequences). These features suggest an increased prevalence of these personality disorders in HIV-positive samples. This is supported by the literature, which shows a higher rate of PD in HIV-positive individuals, with the largest constituents being the cluster B PDs, especially borderline (BPD) and antisocial (ASPD).[4,5] As we know from clinical practice, comorbidities are common between various Axis II PDs, yet this is not a feature mentioned in the HIV-related studies reviewed. Also, studies offer little about the prevalence and experience of individuals with other PDs, traits, and styles and how these relate to infection with HIV.

DIAGNOSIS OF PERSONALITY DISORDER IN THE HIV-POSITIVE POPULATION

Clinical experience of HIV care providers reveals that though they describe the "difficult" patient, they have a hard time diagnosing PD or maladaptive personality traits. Mental health clinicians also may struggle in making PD diagnoses, because diagnosis can be complicated by numerous factors in the HIV-positive population, including drug-using and gay subcultures. In gay and drug-using patients, there are also barriers to contacting family members and other individuals, who ordinarily can provide useful longitudinal history helpful in assessing the patient's personality structure. Often, stabilization of drug addiction is necessary before a firm diagnosis can be made.

There are specific challenges of diagnosing *DSM-IV* BPD in the gay context, raising questions such as: (a) rating sexual impulsivity within certain gay lifestyles, where contact may move quickly to sexual acts; (b) assessing impulsive substance use in the gay club culture, where it may be more a cultural norm; and (c) assessing instability of self-image, which can be a consequence of the difficult coming-out process for gay and bisexual individuals.[6] Initially, these specific high-risk behaviors can be targeted; often, more sustained and longitudinal contact with the patient allows accurate assessment of underlying personality disorder and maladaptive traits.

HIV-related cognitive disorder may decrease memory and affect self-appraisal, impeding diagnostic assessment. Patients with active legal entanglements and extensive drug histories may minimize or deny their legal history or drug use, masking historical facts useful for diagnosis. They may also limit access to useful sources of collateral history out of similar fears. Relational ties may have declined so severely that no access to collateral sources is possible. Gay patients with HIV may be estranged from their families, sometimes rejected by them after coming out or disclosing their HIV infection status. Even when these patients are still connected with them, they may resist provider contact with family members and other sources of collateral history out of shame and concern for stigmatization, fearing disclosure of their HIV status, drug use, or gay lifestyle.

PERSONALITY, MALADAPTIVE BEHAVIOR, AND ILLNESS RESPONSE

PERSONALITY AND HIGH-RISK BEHAVIORS

The main HIV transmission categories relate to high-risk sexual and drug-related behaviors, behaviors that are increased in certain PD populations. The *DSM* ASPD and BPD, as well as the traits of high novelty-seeking (high impulsivity) and low harm avoidance (low fearfulness), have been linked with high-risk behaviors. As well, with narcissistic pathology, low self-esteem and defensive grandiosity can reduce the perceived risk of infection and thus the barrier to high-risk behavior.

When compared to non–PD controls at risk for HIV infection, patients with ASPD have been shown to have increased needle-sharing, decreased needle-cleaning, more needle-sharing partners, and higher self-reported rates of intravenous drug use. These patients have a larger number of sexual partners, higher rates of prostitution, and higher rates of risky sexual behavior, including anal sex.[5] Thus, not only are these patients at high risk for infection, with multiple sexual and needle-sharing partners, as well as higher rates of prostitution, they also pose a significant risk to others in the community.

In studies of personality traits, novelty-seeking has been related to high-risk sexual behavior. Novelty-seeking was related to high-risk sexual behaviors, including number of sex partners or frequency of unprotected sexual intercourse—through its correlation with alcohol use in gay and bisexual men, this further and promotes high-risk sexual behaviors.[7]

The highest transmission category for women does not relate to intravenous drug use or same-sex sexual activity, but to heterosexual sexual activity. Women with narcissistic spectrum pathology who have low self-esteem sometimes try to bolster this low sense of self by adopting a rescuing role with drug-abusing HIV-positive males, which gives them a sense of narcissistic gratification (by feeling like heroic martyrs) and is a response to an extremely rigid and self-deprecating ego ideal. These factors are proposed to make sense of those seronegative women who sustain relationships with HIV-infected partners, placing themselves at high risk.[6]

PERSONALITY AND PSYCHOLOGICAL EXPERIENCE OF INFECTION

HIV infection is a significant life experience for anyone affected. There is the specific impact of HIV disease and related medical sequelae, as well as the complex experience of dealing with a chronic illness. Issues can arise in relation to the patient's self-perception and the response from family, friends, and the larger society of which they are part. There are existential questions in regard to meaning and death. This experience is unique for everyone dealing with HIV disease, yet there are particular issues that are common with patients with PD.

Patients with narcissistic pathology and with other disorders of the self, including BPD, can experience the diagnosis of serious illness most intensely. For those using primitive defenses, especially splitting, this may contribute to increased denial of illness and medication nonadherence. Because AIDS affects various systems of the body, including visible and stigmatizing AIDS-specific lesions such as Kaposi's sarcoma, this can be especially fragmenting for those with preexisting narcissistic vulnerabilities. To illustrate, a colleague described a patient who had severe narcissistic pathology and developed visible Kaposi's lesions during the progression of his HIV disease. The resulting narcissistic injury was so fragmenting that he committed suicide.

Like a child, the very ill individual yearns for omniscient and omnipotent caregivers to fulfill idealized self-object needs.[8] For patients who experienced prior abuse, they may vacillate between help-seeking and help-rejecting behaviors. This reflects primitive aspects of the psyche acting to prevent patients from being retraumatized as they were by their early attachment figures.[9] Thus, as self-object ties are disrupted, the resulting destabilization of the self can be experienced as a recapitulation of the inadequate early environment. In these states of heightened dependency, there can be a triggering of old fears of being neglected/abandoned, mistreated/abused, or even narcissistically used by caregivers who need the child to be sick and dependent. A failure of the early self-object environment may be rationalized as a fault of the patient, such that AIDS can even be experienced as a "just retribution for being fundamentally bad."[8]

For patients with personality disorder, HIV infection can reactivate other intrapsychic conflicts related to early traumatic childhood experience. Fears of separation and annihilation can be triggered in relation to early environmental deprivation, abandonment, loss, and unprocessed grief, all which are more common in patients with severe PD. The HIV infected patient can play out the persecutor-victim object-relational dyads common to patients with borderline personality organization and those with histories of severe trauma.[6] HIV-positive patients can also experience themselves as persecutor because they can infect others and subsequently feel guilty. The potential stigma around HIV is one more element in a persecutory environment perceived by patients with the object-relations of borderline personality organization.[6]

PERSONALITY, COPING, AND SELF-TRANSCENDENCE

HIV infection often heightens one's sense of mortality; in addition to the suffering, or perhaps because of it, there is the potential for growth of self-transcendence.[10] This echoes Jung's notion of the potential for transformation and even growth through experiences of suffering, including illness. Self-transcendence involves an expansion of one's boundaries to larger perspectives and is accomplished through introspective activities, concern and involvement with others' activities, and integrating one's experiences to make or discover meaning in the present circumstance. In the setting of HIV disease, self-transcendence has been associated with increased self-worth, a sense of increased strength, improved life satisfaction, and a deeper sense of themselves and others. In one sample of 46 HIV-positive individuals, quality of life, as measured by a quality of life index (QLI) positively correlated with measures of self-transcendence, as measured by the self-transcendence scale (STS).[10] These studies suggest that self-transcendence can be a protective personality factor of significance for HIV-positive patients. Providers and therapists who are comfortable with transpersonal issues can be particularly useful in nurturing self-transcendence. Otherwise, referrals for pastoral or spiritual guidance can be considered.

PERSONALITY AND TREATMENT ADHERENCE

Adherence is a critical issue because partial adherence can select for medication-resistant HIV viral strains. Thus, in addition to the consequences of untreated HIV infection for any given individual, there is also a risk of transmission of resistant virus within sexual relationships and drug-related social networks. In a study looking at medication adherence in 107 HIV-positive methadone maintenance patients with at least one psychiatric diagnosis and one substance-abuse diagnosis, the rate of BPD was 37% and of ASPD 56%.[11] There was significantly decreased medication adherence in the BPD group. The investigators also looked at employment/support, alcohol use, drug use, legal status, and family/social issues and found that only the family and social indices were related to HIV treatment adherence. They suggested that the BPD itself contributed to this finding through its association with social and relational instability. Our clinical experience supports these findings, with adherence most problematic with patients with ASPD and BPD.

PERSONALITY DISORDER AND AXIS I DIAGNOSES

HIV-positive patients with PD have been shown to have higher levels of psychiatric symptoms and to be at increased risk for developing Axis I disorders compared with HIV-positive patients without PD.[12] If, with further work, patients with PD and HIV disease prove more likely to develop Axis I psychiatric disorders than their HIV-positive counterparts who do not have PD, this would provide further impetus to treat PD and assess for treatable Axis I disorders.

TREATMENT CONSIDERATIONS AND IMPLICATIONS

In treatment, flexibility and intuition coexist with the precepts and principles of empirically supported treatments, whether psychoanalytic or cognitive-behavioral. Each treatment, in its focus and approach over time, changes in response to the needs of the individual patient. Though forms of treatment are considered individually, there are often elements that need to be coordinated within an optimally effective therapeutic program. Such a program typically includes individual psychotherapy, regular group treatment, chemical dependency treatment, and routine contact among therapists and providers for consultation.

First, we briefly consider treatment perspectives that relate to personality dimensions. The remaining sections on treatment focus on individual and group therapies of borderline and narcissistic disorders. There are no well-established treatment approaches for ASPD, though some have argued for certain forms of ASPD to be considered on the spectrum of narcissistic personality disorder and that individual psychotherapeutic approaches can be effective for the milder variants of ASPD.

In regard to high novelty-seeking, these individuals tend to seek rewards and are less attuned to avoiding consequences. Three treatment approaches have been suggested: (a) reframing consequence avoidance in terms of reward attainment, (b) appealing to people's cognitive side, and (c) developing a written treatment plan.[13]

The character dimension of self-transcendence has been shown to have a positive impact on coping and quality of life. Cultivation of self-transcendence includes assuming an attitude of acceptance, developing a practice of introspection and meditation, using bibliotherapy with spiritually themed books, becoming involved with support groups or volunteer organizations, and becoming involved with spiritual or religious groups. Also, there are psychotherapeutic approaches, including existential, Jungian, and transpersonal therapies, which attempt to cultivate what has been called a "quest narrative," in which the suffering is looked at as necessary for development.[14] These more adaptive narratives tend to include spiritual experiences and value community service and involvement. They are in contrast to the less adaptive narratives in more common use by patients with personality disorder: "restitution narratives," which minimize the experience of illness and limit the patient's responsibility to taking medications to "get well," and "chaos narratives," in which the patient experiences a loss of control and expects terrible things to continue happening without any order or meaning.[14]

COUNTERTRANSFERENCE ISSUES

Patients with BPD organization can evoke intense affects in the countertransference, through their intense oscillations between idealization and devaluation, through their often rageful and stormy interpersonal styles, and through projective identification. If not addressed, these elements can lead to fractured treatment alliances in which the therapist burns out or unconsciously colludes with treatment-interfering behavior, possibly provoking the patient's exit from treatment.

Although psychotherapists may be skilled at dealing with their own responses, these patients are seen by other providers in various health care settings. Mental health providers play an important role in identifying and managing provider responses to patient splitting toward health care staff. Multidisciplinary meetings and regular communication among providers can facilitate coordination. Providers need to acknowledge their angry and even hateful feelings toward these patients, to reduce guilt and secondary anxiety that may lead to avoidance and distancing from these patients.

INDIVIDUAL PSYCHOTHERAPY

The patient's life history, personality structure, and current life context determine the extent to which the individual's psychological balance and sense of self are threatened by the HIV infection. It is important to provide the individual psychological space to explore potential recapitulations of earlier traumas and unresolved conflicts and also to explore fantasies of disease, death, and HIV-related fears and worries. It is also important to differentiate between neurotic anxiety that relates to these unconscious conflicts and existential anxieties.[6] The psychotherapeutic relationship can be a crucial space in which experience is held, metabolized, and digested. It is vital in its provision of self-object functioning, which includes experiences of feeling soothed, strengthened, validated, and acknowledged by the other. This space can help alleviate separation anxiety, address fears of loss and death, and facilitate mourning.[6] It can also provide hope and help maintain the dying person's sense of self.

The psychotherapeutic frame may need to be expanded to include hospital or home visits, couples and family work, and communicating with the medical providers.[8] Treatment recommendations from a self-psychological perspective[8] are based on the three types of self-object needs: (a) mirroring needs (the need to feel understood, accepted, and appreciated), (b) twinship or alter-ego needs (the need to be involved with other beings like themselves), and (c) idealizing needs (the need to be experienced in relation to one who is admired and respected). Although these recommendations are not all exclusive to patients with personality disorder, they often are intensified in these individuals.

Regarding mirroring needs, the therapist can provide a critical role as a validating, sustaining self-object; this can heal the patient's negative self-image and help restore self-esteem. Various losses and narcissistic injuries need to be interpreted, and self-object transferences related to early attachment figures need to be worked through.[8] It can be helpful to interpret the self-object needs that sexuality and drug use fulfilled, including attention, approval, and confirmation of worth. This can be followed by exploration of safer and drug-free ways of meeting these needs.[8] Outside of the therapeutic relationship, there is a need to help the person with AIDS build a supportive relational network, both by strengthening previous relationships and creating new ones. These all have the potential to provide needed mirroring and self-object functions.

Regarding alter-ego or twinship needs, in addition to working through the patient's shame, which often leads to isolation, there is often a need for family and couples work to address their fears and rejection.[8] The patient can be directed to community initiatives, which can be stabilizing and provide a supportive alter-ego milieu; these can include political and activist organizations, self-help groups, yoga and meditation groups, 12-step recovery groups, and other support groups.[8]

Finally, we consider idealizing needs: there is often a developmental need for some idealization, as well as a need to work through the client's inevitable disappointment in those providers who were supposed to provide idealized self-object needs. The therapist can repair disruptions with providers critical for the patient's medical treatment. Establishing or reconnecting with spirituality can provide a powerful idealized self-object function. If the patient's spiritual orientation allows viewing the body as only a vehicle for something transcendent, this can also make physical death less threatening.[8]

Dialectical behavior therapy (DBT) draws from standard cognitive-behavioral therapy and incorporates mindfulness and the notion of dialectics. DBT is a four-stage target system: (a) pretreatment targets of commitment; (b) first-stage targets of stability, connection, and safety; (c) second-stage targets of exposure and processing the past, and (d) third-stage targets of individual goals. The main components of treatment include a weekly 60-minute individual therapy and 90-minute skills group. There is a modification of DBT for the triply diagnosed,[15] which includes a stage-two modification that focuses on HIV-adherence behaviors including taking medications as prescribed, monitoring T cell and viral load counts, attending primary care appointments, and attending substance abuse counselor appointments. Diary cards are used to track target behaviors and the use of DBT skills. There are also modifications to the skills, including the development of methadone clinic–relevant skills, including mindfulness in the dosing line, as well as application of interpersonal effectiveness skills, distress tolerance skills of "radical acceptance," and the emotion-regulation skill of "acting opposite," all with the goal of increasing the patient's effectiveness in the methadone clinic setting. There is a "DBT Path to Adherence," which applies standard DBT skills to adherence-related issues, which is broken into two parts. Part I, "Clarifying the Recommended Treatment Regimen," explicitly looks at clarifying elements of treatment, whether treatment is being followed, barriers to treatment, environmental contingencies, fears of treatment, and side effects of treatment. Part II, "Following the Recommended Treatment," looks at specific ways of promoting adherence, including promoting positive health beliefs, making a self-management plan, structuring the environment for adherence, and enlisting the help of friends, family, and providers.

Finally, there are other empirically supported treatment approaches for BPDs that can be considered, including Transference-Focused Psychotherapy; Psychodynamic Partial Hospitalization, and its more recent offshoot, Mentalization-Based Therapy; and, finally, Supportive Therapy for Borderline Patients. Given the chronicity of personality dysfunction and the course of HIV illness, individual psychotherapy should be considered an extended treatment for many patients.

GROUP PSYCHOTHERAPY

Groups are an important part of substance-abuse treatment, and peer-support interventions have been developed for HIV-prevention interventions. In the presence of PD, group approaches are usually combined with individual treatment. Conventional group work tends to exclude active substance users and those with ASPD from sessions for those with BPD.

A psychodynamic group therapy with HIV-positive patients with PD has been described.[6] The experience of belonging in a group can be a critical process toward building a sense of self, because many patients with PD had either absent parental figures or extremely narcissistic parental figures, with the children just narcissistic extensions of the parent figure. It can be important to not interpret this process, but to allow it to unfold first, perhaps later to be interpreted. These groups, even when positive, can be such a new experience for these patients that it can be frightening and induce defensive reactions. A patient may act out by not showing for a group; this can be framed as a communication that permits an increased awareness for other members of the group, who may share such fears of intimacy. Initially, there is a regressed stage in the group process, which provides an omniscient and idealized self-object function and the experience of being as one with the group. After this phase, the patients need to work on passing into a phase of healthy individuation, a spiraling process of change. The overall group process in terms of allowing repair of the pathway to narcissistic development ("the grandiose self") and also an opportunity to integrate split internal object-relational dyads (i.e., representations of self and other, linked by affect).[6]

PSYCHOPHARMACOLOGY

Given that many personality disorders often have comorbid Axis I *DSM* diagnoses, including mood and anxiety disorders, these need to be identified and treated. With regard to drug-treatment of PD, BPD has substantial evidence supporting the use of psychoactive medications. As described in the American Psychiatric Association (APA) treatment guidelines for BPD,[16] there are three core symptom areas: (a) affective dysregulation, (b) impulsive-behavioral dyscontrol, and (c) cognitive-perceptual disturbances. Affective dysregulation includes mood lability, rejection sensitivity, inappropriate anger and temper outbursts, and "mood crashes"; selective serotonin reuptake inhibitors (SSRIs) or related antidepressants such as venlafaxine are recommended as initial treatment. For severe behavioral dyscontrol, low-dose neuroleptics can be considered. Mood stabilizers such as lithium, divalproex sodium, and carbamazepine are second-line options, though studies are limited. Impulsive-behavioral dyscontrol includes impulsive aggression, self-mutilation, or self-damaging behavior. SSRIs are again the treatment of choice, with low-dose neuroleptics considered for severe behavioral dyscontrol. Lithium, divalproex sodium, and carbamazepine are additional second-line agents. Finally, cognitive-perceptual symptoms include suspiciousness, referential thinking, illusions and hallucination-like symptoms, as well as depersonalization. Low-dose neuroleptics are the treatment of choice for these symptoms.

OTHER INTERVENTIONS AND CONSIDERATIONS

In preliminary data presented at the 2004 APA meeting, Zanarini described a randomized control trial, not specific for HIV-infected persons, that examined psychoeducation for BPD, reportedly demonstrating decreased impulsivity and relationship dysfunction with psychoeducational intervention. Defining the disorder and related behaviors may create more observing ego, improving affective regulation and behavioral control. Related psychoeducational material is available, which can augment other treatment approaches for BPD, including, *Lost in the Mirror: An Inside Look at Borderline Personality Disorder*, by Richard Moskovitz and *Borderline and Beyond: Workbook and Personal Journal*, by Laura Paxton.[17,18]

HEALTH CARE POLICY

These patients are at high risk of infecting others and thus place a significant burden on the health care system through their own illness, that of people they infect, and the increased cost associated with poor adherence and repeated emergency department visits and hospitalizations. Effort needs to be put into screening for BPD and ASPD in relevant settings, such as drug treatment programs, prisons, and so on. Patients with ASPD do respond to HIV prevention interventions, though with an attenuated response.[19] Prevention intervention programs need to be implemented that target these high-risk individuals. Available and effective treatments for these PDs should be applied, with the cost of such programs weighed against the larger economic burden related to HIV disease and AIDS in these high-risk and often poorly adherent individuals.

SUMMARY AND FUTURE RESEARCH DIRECTIONS

Although patients with PD and high-risk personality traits are more likely to develop HIV disease, and are disproportionately represented in those with HIV, the literature is relatively sparse. Most aspects of the complicated interface of personality and HIV risk, infection, and illness course need further investigation. Treatment adherence in this setting needs more careful study; as this is further fleshed out, interventions that target adherence need to be developed and tested. The recent modification of DBT, which targets HIV-related adherence, is a good step, albeit one that has not yet been validated or shown to increase adherence in controlled trials. The areas of coping and spiritual transcendence also need to be investigated in more detail in this population, to help shape interventions that improve quality of life for these individuals. Psychotherapies targeting patients with BPD or ASPD in HIV-positive individuals need to be further researched. Comparative and combined treatment approaches to single and comorbid conditions require study. Finally, prevention and risk reduction strategies that target these patients need to be developed and tested.

REFERENCES

1. Cloninger CR, Svrakic DM. Personality disorders. In: Sadock BJ, Sadock VA, eds. *Kaplan and Sadock's Comprehensive Textbook of Psychiatry*. 7th ed. Philadelphia: Lippincott Williams & Wilkins; 2000:1723–1764.
2. Strickland BR. Internal-external expectancies and health-related behaviors. *J Consult Clin Psychol*. 1987;46:1192–1211.
3. Trobst KK, Wiggins JS, Costa PT, et al. Personality psychology and problem behaviors: HIV risk and the five-factor model. *J Pers*. 2000;68:1233–1252.
4. Perkins DO, Davidson EJ, Lesserman J, et al. Personality disorder in patients infected with HIV: a controlled study with implications for clinical care. *Am J Psychiatry*. 1993;150:309–315.
5. Brooner RK, Greenfield L, Schmidt CW, et al. Antisocial personality disorder and HIV infection among intravenous drug abusers. *Am J Psychiatry*. 1993;150:53–58.
6. Visintini R, Campanini E, Ama A, et al. HIV infection, personality structure, and psychotherapeutic treatment. In: Derksen J, Cesare M, Herman G, eds. *Treatment of Personality Disorders*. Dordrecht, The Netherlands: Kluwer Academic Publishers; 1999.
7. Hoyle RH, Fejfar MC, Miller JD. Personality and sexual risk taking: a quantitative review. *J Pers*. 2000; 68:1203–1231.
8. Cohen J, Abramowitz S. AIDS attacks the self: a self psychological exploration of the psychodynamic consequences of AIDS. In: Goldberg A, ed. *The Realities of Transference: Progress in Self Psychology*. Vol 6. Hillsdale, NJ: Analytic Press; 1990.
9. Kalsched D. *The Inner World of Trauma: Archetypal Defenses of the Personal Spirit*. London: Routledge; 1996.
10. Mellors MP, Riley TA, Erlen JA. HIV, self-transcendence, and quality of life. *J Assoc Nurs AIDS Care*. 1997;8:59–69.

11. Palmer NB, Salcedo J, Miller AL, et al. Psychiatric and social barriers to HIV medication adherence in a triply diagnosed population. *AIDS Patient Care and STD's*. 2003;17:635–644.
12. Johnson JG, Williams JBW, Goetz RR, et al. Personality disorders predict onset of Axis I disorders and impaired functioning among homosexual men with and at risk of HIV infection. *Arch Gen Psychiatry*. 1996;53:350–357.
13. Treisman GJ, Angelino AF, Hutton HE. Psychiatric issues in the management of patients with HIV infection. *JAMA*. 2001;286:2857–2864.
14. Ezzy D. Illness narratives: time, hope and HIV. *Soc Sci Med.* 2000;50:605–617.
15. Wagner EE, Miller AL, Greene LI, et al. Dialectical Behavior Therapy for substance abusers adapted for persons living with HIV/AIDS with substance use diagnoses and borderline personality disorder. *Cogn Behav Pract*. 2004;11:202–212.
16. American Psychiatric Association practice guidelines for the treatment of patients with borderline personality disorder. *Am J Psychiatry*. 2004;158(10 suppl):1–52.
17. Moskovitz RA. Lost in the Mirror: An Inside Look at Borderline Personality Disorder. Dallas, TX: Taylor Publishing Company; 2001.
18. Paxton L. Borderline and Beyond: Workbook and Personal Journal. New York: White Tiger Press; 2001.
19. Compton WM, Cottler LB, Ben-Abdallah A, et al. The effects of psychiatric comorbidity on response to an HIV prevention intervention. *Drug Alcohol Depend*. 2000;58:247–257.

CHAPTER **12**

Cognitive Disorders

Angela M. McBride, Francisco Fernandez

Cognitive difficulties and complaints are common in human immunodeficiency virus (HIV) disease. Symptomatic individuals with HIV infection have been shown to experience greater cognitive impairment than those without HIV infection or those with HIV infection who are asymptomatic. Assessment of cognitive functioning in individuals with HIV disease is an important aspect of the diagnostic and treatment process. It may assist the clinician in choosing appropriate psychotherapeutic interventions, as well as providing systematic assessment of change over time. This chapter provides an overview of the various degrees of cognitive deficits associated with HIV disease, as well as how these deficits are commonly classified. It also summarizes results of studies that reveal how cognitive domains are differentially affected as the disease progresses. In addition to neuropathologic changes affecting cognitive function, individuals with HIV disease are at greater risk for affective disorders and have more cognitive complaints, which are related in some degree to neuropsychological test performance. Methods of assessment are discussed, including the use of test batteries and the use of clinical ratings in characterizing the course of the disease. This chapter also examines the impact of cognitive disorders due to HIV in some special populations, including children, older adults, and individuals with comorbid substance abuse disorders.

CHARACTERISTICS OF COGNITIVE DISORDERS

The stages of disease progression in terms of cognitive functioning are typically classified into three groups, using the system developed by the American Academy of Neurology[1]: (a) neuropsychological deficit (below-expected performance in one domain) or neuropsychological impairment (impairment in two or more cognitive domains), (b) minor cognitive motor disorder (MCMD; neuropsychological impairment with mild functional impairment) (Table 12.1), and (c) HIV-associated dementia (HAD; involves marked cognitive and functional impairment sufficient to interfere with daily life, of at least 1 month's duration) (Table 12.2). Although these terms are widely used throughout the literature, there is as yet no consensus as to the best system of measurement.

A meta-analysis of 41 primary studies of neuropsychological test performance (8,616 total participants) revealed that overall, disease progression was accompanied by increasingly larger effect sizes between control (seronegative), asymptomatic, symptomatic, and patients with

TABLE 12.1 Criteria for Clinical Diagnosis of HIV-Associated Minor Cognitive Motor Disorder

1. Cognitive/motor/behavioral abnormalities (each of the following)
   a. At least two of the following present for at least 1 month
      (1) Impaired attention or concentration
      (2) Mental slowing
      (3) Impaired memory
      (4) Slowed movements
      (5) Incoordination
      (6) Personality change, irritability or emotional lability
   b. Acquired cognitive/motor abnormality verified by clinical neurologic examination or neuropsychological testing (e.g., fine motor speed, manual dexterity, perceptual motor skills, attention/concentration, speed of processing information, abstraction/reasoning, visuospatial skills, memory/learning, or speech/language)
2. Disturbance from No. 1 causes mild impairment of work or activities of daily living.
3. Does not meet criteria for HIV-1-associated dementia complex or HIV-1-associated myelopathy.
4. No evidence of another etiology, including active CNS opportunistic infection or malignancy, severe systemic illness, active alcohol or substance use, acute or chronic substance withdrawal, adjustment disorder, or other psychiatric disorders.
5. HIV seropositivity (ELISA test confirmed by Western blot, polymerase chain reaction, or culture).

TABLE 12.2 Criteria for Clinical Diagnosis of HIV-Associated Dementia

A. HIV-1–associated dementia complex
   Each of the following:
   1. Acquired abnormality in at least two of the following cognitive abilities for at least one month: attention/concentration, speed of processing information, abstraction/reasoning, visuospatial skills, memory/learning, and speech/language.

      Cognitive dysfunction causing impairment of work or activities of daily living, should not be attributable solely to severe systemic illness.
   2. At least one of the following:
      a. Acquired abnormality in motor function or performance verified by clinical examination, neuropsychological testing or both.
      b. Decline in motivation or emotional control or change in social behavior.
   3. Absence of clouding of consciousness during a period long enough to establish the presence of No. 1.
   4. No evidence of another etiology, including active central nervous system opportunistic infection or malignancy, other psychiatric disorders (e.g., depression), active alcohol or substance use, or acute or chronic substance withdrawal.
   5. HIV seropositivity (ELISA test confirmed by Western blot, polymerase chain reaction, or culture).

AIDS, respectively.[2] Differences between the asymptomatic and control (seronegative) groups were present, but small (<0.2 standard deviations), whereas larger effect sizes were noted between both the symptomatic groups and groups with AIDS compared to control subjects. In later stages of the disease, motor deficits were most prominent, with deficits also present in problem-solving and other executive functions, rate of information processing, expressive language, memory, and, to a lesser degree, attention and concentration. The progression of cognitive decline followed a frontal-subcortical pattern initially, with the areas of greatest deficit early in the disease (motor and executive functions) being those subserved by these brain regions and neural circuits. In later stages of the disease, abilities such as memory and visuospatial skills, which are less dependent on frontal-subcortical circuitry, also declined. Notably, there was a high degree of variability among the studies included in this quantitative review. One factor suggested by the authors relates to test specificity; to the extent that some instruments measure more than one discrete domain of cognitive functioning, results of analyses using these instruments varied. Another issue is the method of categorization of individuals by disease stages and failure to consistently account for the wide range of psychosocial variables that may affect test performance, such as demographic characteristics including age and education, the presence of affective disorders, and differences in medical comorbidity and substance use history.

Results of an 8-year longitudinal study in which participants underwent neuropsychological evaluation at 6-month intervals were largely consistent with the above meta-analysis, also revealing a decline in cognitive function with HIV disease progression.[3] Of the five functional domains assessed (fine motor speed, attention, verbal memory, executive functioning, and information processing speed), fine motor speed and information processing speed showed the most significant decline over time, and this decline became increasingly prominent as individuals developed AIDS-defining illnesses.

COURSE AND PROGRESSION OF COGNITIVE DECLINE

Persons with HIV-related cognitive impairment typically show fluctuation in cognitive signs and symptoms. There can be stable deficits without progression. Some individuals will experience only episodic worsening that may or may not be associated with somatic changes associated with active systemic disease. Other individuals will experience more rapid progression associated with advanced central nervous system (CNS) disease. The group with rapid progression and deterioration of CNS function also has more advanced symptomatic HIV disease and fully developed AIDS. No matter which group, cognitive impairment is not a benign condition. Psychosocial dysfunction, diminished quality of life, poor treatment compliance, and decreased survival are associated with all types of cognitive impairment.[4] Although progression of cognitive impairment is typically idiosyncratic, some reports suggest that it can be predicted by HIV ribonucleic acid (RNA) in the cerebrospinal fluid (CSF).[5]

ASSESSMENT AND NEUROPSYCHOLOGICAL TESTING

The 2002 meta-analysis by Reger et al.[2] includes a list of all the neuropsychological tests employed in the 41 studies cited.[2] These are categorized by cognitive domain and show the percentage of primary studies in which each measure was used. To a large degree, these overlap with the National Institute of Mental Health's core neuropsychological battery employed in the assessment of patients with HIV-1[6] (Table 12.3).

In addition to the cognitive domains of attention/concentration, executive functioning (including abstraction and problem solving), information-processing speed, language/verbal abilities, visuospatial/visuoconstruction skills, and both visual and verbal memory, many studies also include measures of overall intellectual abilities, motor skills, and psychiatric symptoms, particularly those related to anxiety and affective disorders.

Differences between asymptomatic and symptomatic groups have been more frequently observed when comprehensive test batteries were administered compared to briefer batteries or screening instruments.[7] Clinical ratings have also been shown to be of value in assessing the presence and degree of neuropsychological impairment.[8] In contrast to data analysis with an emphasis on mean differences between groups, clinical ratings provide a closer picture of

TABLE 12.3 | NIMH Neuropsychological Battery

A. Indication of premorbid intelligence
  1. Vocabulary (WAIS-R)
  2. National Adult Reading Test (NART)
B. Attention
  1. Digit Span (WMS-R)
  2. Visual Span (WMS-R)
C. Speed of processing
  1. Sternberg Search Task
  2. Simple and Choice reaction Time
  3. Paced Auditory Serial Addition test (PASAT)
D. Memory
  1. California Verbal Learning Test (CVLT)
  2. Working Memory test
  3. Modified Visual Reproduction test
E. Abstraction
  1. Category Test
  2. Trail Making Test, Parts A and B
F. Language
  1. Boston Naming Test
  2. Letter and category fluency test
G. Visuospatial
  1. Embedded Figures test
  2. Money's Standardized Road-Map Test of Direction Sense
  3. Digit Symbol Substitution
H. Construction abilities
  1. Block Design test
  2. Tactual Performance Test
I. Motor abilities
  1. Grooved Pegboard
  2. Finger Tapping test
  3. Grip Strength
J. Psychiatric assessment
  1. Diagnostic Interview Schedule (DIS)
  2. Hamilton Depression Scale
  3. State-Trait Anxiety Inventory
  4. Mini-Mental State Examination

individual profile differences across domains. This is particularly effective for the study of individuals with HIV infection, who, at least early in the disease course, show relatively mild and diverse types of neuropsychological deficits. Using the process advocated in some studies, clinical ratings are made by grouping scores from tests according to the cognitive domain measured, and then rating each domain on a scale of 1 (above average) to 9 (severe impairment).[9] This method showed very strong inter-rater reliability on ratings of severity of impairment across domains, but was less effective in making neurocognitive diagnoses, possibly because of issues related to comorbidity and other risk factors.[8] Used as a method of summarizing neuropsychological test results, global deficit scores have been shown to have strong positive predictive value for neuropsychological impairment. A cut point of 0.50 or greater was determined to produce maximum sensitivity and specificity for classification of impairment.[10]

COGNITIVE COMPLAINTS

Because a major source of information about the patient's cognitive and functional abilities is the patient's self-report, it is important to understand the contribution of affective disorders and medical symptoms to the cognitive complaints of patients. The use of structural equation modeling allows for analysis of the complex interaction of these variables. Results from a study of 160 adults with HIV infection showed that neuropsychological performance was predicted by cognitive complaints, independent of the effect of depression and medical symptoms on these complaints, and neuropsychological test performance showed an inverse relationship with degree of cognitive complaints.[11] Although affective and medical symptoms were related to cognitive complaints, their influence on these complaints revealed an indirect, and small, relationship with test scores. Depression among individuals with HIV infection was not a significant factor in neuropsychological test performance; the same was true for medical symptoms. However, research also suggests that there may be a link between symptoms of depression and performance on measures of attention, executive function, and information processing.[3]

TEST PERFORMANCE AND FUNCTIONAL ABILITIES

In the largest study of its kind to date, 267 HIV-positive individuals received comprehensive evaluations of neuropsychological functioning, medical status, and assessment of functional abilities, including laboratory measures of a variety of instrumental activities of daily living (IADL).[12] A comparison of group test performance revealed that individuals classified as having abnormal neuropsychological functioning, requiring at least mild impairment in two or more cognitive domains, performed significantly worse on laboratory measures of daily functional abilities. The domains most strongly correlated with failure on the functional measures included abstraction and executive functioning, learning, attention and working memory, and verbal abilities. This suggests that neuropsychological impairment is related to functional deficits, further emphasizing the importance of objective cognitive assessment in addition to measures of cognitive complaints and other self-report measures.

SPECIAL POPULATIONS

INFANTS AND CHILDREN

HIV infection among infants and children presents the clinician with a unique set of issues. The vast majority (91%) of cases of pediatric HIV infection result from vertical (mother-to-fetus/infant) transmission.[13] Unlike horizontal transmission, vertical transmission of HIV may result from prenatal exposure, which affects cognitive development in utero. The disease may also be transmitted during the birth process or through breast feeding. Mothers of infants born HIV-positive may have had comorbid substance dependence, lower levels of education, and poorer prenatal care than those without HIV. Thus it is important to consider prenatal and environmental factors when assessing cognitive function in infants and children.[14] Overall cognitive functioning among infants with HIV infection is delayed compared to those with similar demographic characteristics who are HIV-negative. However, differences in specific neurocognitive domains before 24 months of age are largely unknown, due to the inability to administer measures that rely on verbal responses or understanding of language. Studies of school-age children have been more inconclusive, with some studies showing no cognitive impairment. In addition, children with HIV disease do not show a common pattern of affected areas of cognitive function.[14] Deficits in attention, particularly sustaining attention, may be present in later stages of the disease. In addition, expressive language, visuospatial and verbal memory, cognitive flexibility, and visual scanning and perception may be affected[13]; however, further longitudinal research with appropriate control groups is needed.

OLDER ADULTS

Recent data from the Hawaii Aging with HIV Cohort (n = 202) indicated that older individuals (>50 years) were 3.26 times more likely than younger adults (aged 20 to 39) to be diagnosed with HIV-associated dementia (HAD), after controlling for factors including education, race, degree of depressive symptoms, comorbid substance dependence, and disease markers, including viral load and CD4 lymphocyte count.[15] A trend toward more severe dementia among older adults was also noted. Although the reasons for increasing HAD in older age have not yet been determined, the authors suggest the contribution of multiple factors. These include comorbid illnesses, degenerative CNS disease mechanisms, and degree of immunosuppression present before the advent of highly active antiretroviral therapy (HAART).

Compared to results in older adults with HIV disease, in younger adults with HIV disease results to date from an ongoing study indicate that some domains of functioning, such as reaction time, are more impaired in younger adults.[16] However, other cognitive domains, such as memory retrieval and learning, showed impairment that was independent of age.

SUBSTANCE USERS

A 4.5-year longitudinal study of intravenous drug users indicated that, compared to seronegative intravenous drug users, no significant differences in neuropsychological test performance were present among HIV-positive individuals who did not have AIDS; this held true even after controlling for education and practice effects from repeated testing every 6 months.[17] However, a mild decline in performance was observed among individuals with clinical symptoms resulting from HIV or AIDS-related illness. This decrease was more prominent on measures of motor skills and psychomotor speed. These data do not indicate that use of intravenous drugs contributes to an increased rate of cognitive decline. The test performance of individuals who have become symptomatic is also likely affected by factors including fatigue, side effects of medication, disturbances of sleep, and the stress of living with a chronic illness.[17]

NEUROIMAGING

Imaging, by both computed tomography (CT) and magnetic resonance imaging (MRI), is most useful to demonstrate pathologic processes such as primary tumors, opportunistic infections, and other processes involved in the differential diagnostic process of an altered mental status and are treatable complications of HIV-1 infection.[18] For HIV-related changes such as atrophy and some aspects of white matter involvement, MRI is superior to CT.[19] MRI has not proven useful in depicting structural correlates of cognitive impairment in otherwise neurologically asymptomatic HIV infection. Volumetric reductions in cerebral gray and white matter in neurologically symptomatic patients were reported by MRI.[20] MRI using diffusion tensor imaging (DTI) to study HIV-related white matter abnormalities such as white matter pallor has been found useful in distinguishing between HIV-1-infected patients and normal control subjects.[21] These white matter changes are reported as reversible with HAART.[22]

Functional imaging of the nervous system, such as positron emission tomography (PET),[23] single photon emission computed tomography (SPECT),[24] magnetic resonance spectroscopy (MRS),[25] functional magnetic resonance imaging (fMRI),[26] and regional cerebral blood flow (rCBF),[27] all have shown regional functional abnormalities in HIV disease. These imaging modalities have established themselves as sensitive to different aspects of functioning: PET reflects metabolism; SPECT, fMRI, rCBF reflect brain perfusion; and MRS reflects biochemical function and dysfunction.

PET-detected subcortical hypermetabolism in basal ganglia and thalamus can be seen early in the course of CNS disease, followed by regional and then general hypometabolism as the disease progresses.[28] PET scanning may be used in monitoring the effects of antiviral treatment. PET studies have noted reversal of focal cortical abnormalities of glucose metabolism after the AIDS dementia complex was treated with zidovudine.[28]

SPECT scanning also is useful in delineating brain cortical and subcortical perfusion changes in association with neurologic and neuropsychological studies. One study demonstrated correlations with gross neurologic impairments but not with neuropsychological deficits.[24]

MRS using a quantitation of choline-to-creatine signals ratio has been suggested to characterize neuronal dysfunction. This ratio was determined to increase with cellular membrane turnover.[29] The *N*-acetyl aspartate–to–creatine ratio[29] and phosphocreatine[30] concentration also were found to decrease in relation to neuronal dysfunction. MRS studies reveal an increase in choline and reductions in *N*-acetyl aspartate. These findings have been correlated with severity of cognitive changes, severity of dementia, CD4 cell count, and both plasma and CSF viral load.[31] With antiretroviral treatment, these MRS changes can normalize over time.[32] Proton MRS may be a useful way to follow patients from the neurologically asymptomatic stage through the spectrum of cognitive impairment, HIV-associated MCMD, and HAD.[33] It may provide an early marker of neuronal dysfunction before irreversible damage to the CNS occurs.

SUMMARY

HIV infection is associated with progressive cognitive decline, ranging from neuropsychological deficit/impairment, to MCMD, and, in later stages, HAD. Although consensus has yet to be developed regarding the extent and nature of cognitive deficits among asymptomatic individuals with HIV infection, the use of comprehensive test batteries and clinical ratings to characterize individual profiles allows for enhanced detection of subtle areas of decline. Early areas of deficit include motor speed, information-processing speed, and executive functions, whereas individuals who develop HAD show a wide range of neuropsychological impairment, including deficits in memory, language, and visuospatial skills. Given the complex relationship of psychosocial factors with neuropsychological test performance, it is essential when assessing neuropsychological status in this population to consider factors such as age, cohort effects, medication regimens, educational attainment, and comorbid substance use.

REFERENCES

1. American Academy of Neurology AIDS Task Force. Nomenclature and research case definitions for neurologic manifestations of human immunodeficiency virus-type 1 (HIV-1) infection. *Neurology*. 1991;41:778–785.
2. Reger M, Welsh R, Razani J, et al. A meta-analysis of the neuropsychological sequelae of HIV infection. *J Int Neuropsychol Soc*. 2002;8:410–424.
3. Baldewicz TT, Leserman J, Silva SG, et al. Changes in neuropsychological functioning with progression of HIV-1 infection: results of an 8-year longitudinal investigation. *AIDS Behav*. 2004;8:345–355.
4. Ellis RJ, Deutsch R, Heaton RK, et al. Neurocognitive impairment is an independent risk factor for death in HIV infection. *Arch Neurol*. 1997;54:416–424.
5. Ellis RJ, Moore DJ, Childers ME, et al. Progression to neuropsychological impairment in human immunodeficiency virus infection predicted by elevated cerebrospinal fluid levels of human immunodeficiency virus RNA. *Arch Neurol*. 2002;59:923–928.
6. Butters N, Grant I, Haxby J, et al. Assessment of AIDS-related cognitive changes: recommendations of the NIMH Workshop on Neuropsychological Assessment Approaches. *J Clin Exp Neuropsychol*. 1990;12:963–978.
7. Grant I, Marcotte TD, Heaton RK, et al. Neurocognitive complications of HIV disease. *Psychol Sci*. 1999;10:191–195.
8. Woods SP, Rippeth JD, Frol AB, et al. Interrater reliability of clinical ratings and neurocognitive diagnoses in HIV. *J Clin Exp Neuropsychol*. 2004;26:759–778.
9. Heaton RK, Grant I, Butters N, et al. The HNRC-500: neuropsychology of HIV infection at different disease stages. *J Int Neuropsychol Soc*. 1995;1:231–251.
10. Carey CL, Woods SP, Gonzalez R, et al. Predictive validity of Global Deficit Scores in detecting neuropsychological impairment in HIV infection. *J Clin Exp Neuropsychol*. 2004;26:307–319.

11. Carter SL, Rourke SB, Murji S, et al. Cognitive complaints, depression, medical symptoms, and their association with neuropsychological functioning in HIV infection: a structural equation model analysis. *Neuropsychology*. 2003;17:410–419.
12. Heaton RK, Marcotte TD, Rivera Mindt M, et al. The impact of HIV-associated neuropsychological impairment on everyday functioning. *J Int Neuropsychol Soc*. 2004;10:317–331.
13. Woulters PL, Brouwers P, Perez LA. Pediatric HIV infection. In: Brown RT, ed. *Cognitive Aspects of Chronic Illness in Children*. New York: Guilford; 1999:105–141.
14. Pulsifer MB, Aylward EH. Human immunodeficiency virus. In: Yeates KO, Ris DM, Taylor GH, eds. *Pediatric Neuropsychology: Research, Theory and Practice*. New York: Guilford Press; 2000;381–402.
15. Valcour V, Shikuma C, Shiramizu B, et al. Higher frequency of dementia in older HIV-1 individuals. *Neurology*. 2004;63:822–827.
16. Wilkie FL, Goodkin K, Khamis I, et al. Cognitive functioning in younger and older HIV-1-infected adults. *J Acquir Immune Defic Syndr*. 2003;33:S93–S105.
17. Selnes OA, Galai N, McArthur JC, et al. HIV infection and cognition in intravenous drug users: Long-term follow-up. *Neurology*. 1997;48:223–230.
18. McArthur JC, Brew BJ, Nath V. Neurological complications of HIV infection. *Lancet Neurol* 2005;4:543–555.
19. Dooneief G, Bello J, Todak G, et al. A prospective controlled study of magnetic resonance imaging of the brain in gay men and parenteral drug users with human immunodeficiency virus infection. *Arch Neurol*. 1992;49:38–43.
20. Jernigan TL, Archibald S, Hesselink JR, et al. Magnetic resonance imaging morphometric analysis of cerebral volume loss in human immunodeficiency virus: the HNRC group. *Arch Neurol*. 1993;50:250–255.
21. Filippi CG, Ulug AM, Ryan E, et al. Diffusion tensor imaging of patients with HIV and normal appearing white matter on MR images of the brain. *Am J Neuroradiol*. 2001;22:272–283.
22. McArthur JC, Brew BJ, Nath A. Neurological complications of HIV infection. *Lancet Neurol*. 2005;4:453–455.
23. Hinkin CH, van Gorp WG, Mandelkern MA, et al. Cerebral metabolic change in patients with AIDS: report of a six-month follow-up using positron-emission tomography. *J Neuropsychiatry Clin Neurosci*. 1995;7:1880–1887.
24. Sacktor N, Van Heertum RL, Dooneief G, et al. A comparison of cerebral SPECT abnormalities in HIV-positive homosexual men with and without cognitive impairment. *Arch Neurol*. 1995:52:1170–1173.
25. Jernigan TL, Archibald S, Hesselink JR, et al. Magnetic resonance imaging morphometric analysis of cerebral volume loss in human immunodeficiency virus: the HNRC group. *Arch Neurol*. 1993;50:250–255.
26. Navia BA, Gonzalez RG. Functional imaging of the AIDS dementia complex and the metabolic pathology of the HIV-1-infected brain. *Neuroimaging Clin North Am*. 1997;7:431–445.
27. Schielke E, Tatsch K, Pfister HW, et al. Reduced cerebral blood flow in early stages of human immunodeficiency virus infection. *Arch Neurol*. 1990;47:1342–1345.
28. Brunetti A, Berg G, Di Chiro G, et al. Reversal of brain metabolic abnormalities following treatment of AIDS dementia complex with 3′-azido-2′,3′-dideoxythymidine (AZT, zidovudine): a PET-FDG study. *J Nucl Med*. 1989;30:581–590.
29. Chong WK, Sweeney B, Wilkinson ID, et al. Proton spectroscopy of the brain in HIV infection: correlation with clinical, immunologic, and MR imaging findings. *Neuroradiology*. 1993;188:119–124.
30. Deicken RF, Hubesch B, Jensen PC, et al. Alterations in brain phosphate metabolite concentrations in patients with human immunodeficiency virus infection. *Arch Neurol*. 1991;48:203–209.
31. Chang L, Ernst T, Leonido-Yee M, et al. Cerebral metabolic abnormalities correlate with clinical severity of HIV-1 cognitive motor complex. *Neurology*. 1999;52:100–108.
32. Chang L, Witt M, Eric M, et al. Cerebral metabolite changes during the first nine months after HAART [abstract]. *Neurology*. 2001;26:474.
33. Cecil KM, Lenkinski RE. Proton MR spectroscopy in inflammatory and infectious brain disorders. *Neuroimaging Clin North Am*. 1998;8:863–880.

CHAPTER **13**

Psychotic Disorders

Ewald Horwath, Francine Cournos

The association between psychotic disorders and human immunodeficiency virus (HIV) infection is complex. Psychotic disorders may precede HIV infection, a common etiologic factor may predispose to both HIV infection and psychosis, or HIV infection may play an etiologic role, either directly or indirectly, in the development of the psychosis. A solid understanding of the complex relationship between HIV and psychosis allows for better evaluation and more effective treatment for psychotic patients at risk for or infected with HIV.

PSYCHOTIC DISORDERS THAT PRECEDE HIV INFECTION

Persons with severe and persistent mental illness, most of whom have psychotic disorders, are at risk to develop comorbid HIV infection and acquired immunodeficiency syndrome (AIDS). Published studies show that people with severe mental illness frequently engage in sexual and drug use behaviors that place them at risk for HIV infection and that they have substantial rates of HIV seropositivity, varying from 3% to 23%.[1-3] The most common Axis I psychiatric diagnoses in this population are schizophrenia, schizoaffective disorder, and bipolar disorder, all of which have been shown to be highly comorbid with alcohol or other substance use disorders, which in turn strongly correlate with the likelihood of HIV infection.

Substance use alone can predispose people to both psychosis and HIV infection. Substances that can cause psychotic symptoms include amphetamines, methamphetamine (crystal meth), cannabis (especially high-dose forms such as hashish), cocaine (especially when smoked as crack, free-based, or injected intravenously), hallucinogens, phencyclidine (angel dust, PCP), and inhalants. Withdrawal from alcohol, sedative/hypnotics (especially barbiturates), and opiates can also produce psychotic symptoms. Substance use is often accompanied by unsafe sexual activities and/or use of nonsterile works for drug injection, activities that link these disorders to risk for HIV infection.

A growing literature documents the usefulness of HIV prevention and harm reduction techniques in reducing the acquisition of HIV infection in these populations, but evidence suggests that access to prevention services remains low in these groups.[4]

ETIOLOGY AND PRESENTATION OF NEW-ONSET PSYCHOTIC DISORDERS

Psychosis is more common among people with HIV infection than it is in the general population. Factors that may be associated with the onset of psychosis in HIV-positive people include the direct effects of HIV on the central nervous system (CNS), CNS opportunistic infections, CNS neoplasms, severe systemic illness, medical treatments, substance use disorders, and the psychological stresses of HIV infection, including deteriorating health and functional impairment.[3] Symptoms of mania may or may not accompany these psychotic episodes. (For discussion of mania and its treatment, see Chapter 10.)

Several studies have evaluated small samples of HIV-positive subjects with and without psychotic symptoms. One study examined 20 HIV-infected psychotic men who had noniatrogenic psychosis without delirium, current substance abuse, or previous psychotic episodes and compared them with a group of 20 nonpsychotic HIV-infected men matched to the psychotic subjects with respect to age, race, years of education, and stage of HIV infection. The psychotic men differed from the nonpsychotic comparison group in having significantly higher rates of past stimulant and sedative/hypnotic abuse or dependence and, at follow-up, a higher rate of mortality. On autopsy three of the psychotic subjects had high HIV burdens in their brains and three had no detectable virus. The authors concluded that new-onset psychosis may be, at least in some cases, a manifestation of HIV-associated encephalopathy.[5]

Another study in an outpatient clinic compared 12 HIV-positive patients with new-onset psychosis to 15 matched nonpsychotic subjects, with a 2-year follow-up for 22 of the patients. The HIV-seropositive patients with new-onset psychosis more often had a positive past psychiatric history, no antiretroviral therapy, and a lower global cognitive performance than did the nonpsychotic HIV-seropositive patients. The authors concluded that antiretroviral therapy may play a preventive role for psychosis in some vulnerable patients.[6]

A third study evaluated 26 patients admitted to the hospital with HIV-associated psychosis and compared those who had opportunistic infections or metabolic encephalopathy to those without these conditions.[7] The 13 patients with CNS opportunistic infections or with metabolic encephalopathy related to pulmonary, hepatic, or renal failure were defined as having "secondary psychosis," and the other 13 patients were diagnosed with "primary psychosis" because they had no HIV-related CNS disease or acute metabolic disorder. Those patients with secondary psychosis were more likely to show disorders of consciousness, orientation, attention, and memory than those with primary psychosis.

The authors subdivided the secondary psychosis group on the basis of whether the patient had a focal brain lesion, defined as a space-occupying lesion visible on computed tomography (CT) scan. Six patients had a focal brain lesion, diagnosed as cerebral toxplasmosis ("lesional" secondary psychosis), and the remaining 7 had no space-occupying lesion ("nonlesional" secondary psychosis). When the lesional and nonlesional secondary psychosis groups were considered separately and compared with the primary psychosis group, only the scores on consciousness, orientation, attention, and memory for the nonlesional patients were significantly higher than those for the primary patients. All of the nonlesional psychotic patients died within a short time (mean = 31 days); patients in the focal brain lesion group recovered from their psychotic episode with antipsychotic treatment, but died months later (mean = 158 days), similar in course to the primary psychotic group (mean survival 160 days). The authors concluded that psychotic symptoms in some HIV-seropositive patients are related to the systemic and cerebral complications of HIV infection, and given the difference between the groups in mean survival time, that the distinction between lesional secondary, nonlesional secondary, and primary psychosis may have important prognostic value.[7]

A common clinical feature noted in new-onset psychosis in HIV-infected patients is the acute or subacute onset of symptoms, including delusions, hallucinations, bizarre behavior, and mood or affective disturbances, accompanied by memory disturbance or cognitive impairment. Some patients, especially those with an abnormal CT image and electroencephalogram at the time of presentation with psychosis, tend to have a relatively rapid deterioration in cognitive and medical status.[8]

The following case provides an example of a psychotic episode occurring along with HIV-associated dementia in a patient with typical radiologic findings of dilated lateral ventricles and hypodensity of the subcortical white matter, but no other evidence of CNS disease.

A 33-year-old African-American woman with AIDS and a history of cocaine abuse and heroin dependence presented to an emergency room with altered mental status and inability to care for herself in the community. Her CT scan showed prominent dilated lateral ventricles and hypodensity of the subcortical white matter, with no focal intracranial lesions. Cerebrospinal fungal, acid-fast bacillus, and bacterial cultures and cryptococcal antigen were negative. Her CD4 count was 160 cells/ml, hemoglobin was 9 g/dl, and hematocrit was 27 ml/dl. The urine toxicology was positive for cocaine. Although she was alert, she had profound poverty of speech and answered questions with one- or two-word responses. She was able to state her name, but could not identify the hospital, city, date, month or year. She reported auditory hallucinations of frightening voices, often appeared quite frightened, and intermittently picked at her clothing. Her behavior included occasional agitation and piercing screams for no apparent reason. She could not ambulate. The hallucinations, picking behavior, and agitation resolved with the addition of quetiapine up to 150 mg/day in divided doses. The cognitive and motor impairment persisted even after several months of highly active antiretroviral therapy (HAART), at which time the CD4 count was 506 cells/ml and the viral load was less than 75 copies/ml.

In this case the psychosis responded to treatment with an atypical antipsychotic, but the dementia did not improve in response to an otherwise effective course of antiretroviral therapy.

Several authors have reported new-onset cases of psychosis in HIV-infected individuals in the absence of concurrent substance use, iatrogenic causes, CNS opportunistic infection, CNS neoplasm, or detectable cognitive impairment. It is possible that new-onset psychotic symptoms also may occur as a manifestation of HIV-associated encephalopathy in the absence of frank HIV-associated dementia.[3] One author has hypothesized, on the basis of a review of 14 cases of mania in the English language literature, that AIDS-related mania and agitated psychosis may be related to increased intracellular free calcium.[9] On the other hand, because teenagers and young adults are the age-groups at greatest risk for HIV infection, as well as for the onset of a major mental illness, the two disorders may also co-occur entirely independently of one another.

PSYCHOTIC DISORDER ASSOCIATED WITH HIV-RELATED MEDICAL CONDITIONS

Mental status may be altered by CNS opportunistic diseases, including cerebral toxoplasmosis, cryptococcal meningitis, herpes encephalitis, progressive multifocal leukoencephalopathy (PML), neurosyphilis, tuberculous meningitis, and CNS neoplasms, such as lymphoma or Kaposi's sarcoma. An acute mental status change may also be the presenting sign of systemic illness such as diarrhea, dehydration, electrolyte disturbances, fever, pneumonia, and septicemia. Although psychosis is not the most common psychiatric problem seen in these conditions, it can accompany any of them.

A number of clinical reports describe individual cases of psychosis that presented as a manifestation of opportunistic infection, including a case of tuberculous meningitis that presented as paranoid psychosis and a case of catatonia that presented as a manifestation of progressive multifocal leukoencephalopathy (PML), a slowly progressive viral CNS infection often seen in association with HIV disease. In another case, paranoid psychosis was the first presentation of AIDS in a patient who succumbed to septicemia within 2 weeks of diagnosis.

Schwartzman et al.[10] reported an association between psychosis and the intrathecal production of antibodies to *Bartonella henselae*, a gram-negative bacterium, in a patient with AIDS. These data are consistent with previous observations that neuropsychiatric disorders in HIV disease may be associated with exposure to *B. henselae*. The nature of such an association remains to be determined.

Crichton and Lewis[11] reported a case of Capgras' syndrome, the delusion that a particular person is an impostor or double, as part of an acute confusional state resulting from an opportunistic infection. Neuropsychological testing of the affected patient suggested nondominant hemisphere dysfunction with impaired facial recognition, and CT scan showed a right parietal lesion, which resolved at the same time as the psychosis improved.

PSYCHOSIS ASSOCIATED WITH SUBSTANCE ABUSE OR DEPENDENCE

Diagnosis of a substance-induced psychotic disorder should be considered in HIV-infected people who use alcohol or other drugs and develop psychotic symptoms during or within 1 month of substance-related intoxication or withdrawal.

An Australian study of 1,245 injection drug users found that over half of daily amphetamine injectors had shared injecting equipment in the past several months and that approximately one third were injecting on a daily basis, a pattern of use that increases the risk of experiencing an amphetamine-induced psychosis. These findings suggest that amphetamine injection may be a shared risk factor for the development of HIV infection and psychotic symptoms in those persons who inject frequently and share injecting equipment.[12]

PSYCHOSIS AS A COMPLICATION OF MEDICAL TREATMENT

A variety of medications used to treat HIV-infection, AIDS, or the medical complications of AIDS can cause mental status changes, including psychotic symptoms. Among antiretroviral drugs, the non-nucleoside reverse transciptase inhibitor (NNRTI) efavirenz has most often been associated with neuropsychiatric side effects. Efavirenz is frequently used in initial antiretroviral regimens because of the effectiveness and durability of patients' responses to it.

Clinical trials report that as many as 50% of patients taking efavirenz experienced some type of CNS side effect, although most of these were mild and transient. Vivid dreams, insomnia, and mood symptoms are among the commonly reported adverse effects,[13] although hallucinations and acute psychosis have also been reported.

In the following case a man experienced a dramatic and severe psychotic episode associated with efavirenz treatment.

> B is a 43-year-old African-American man who was diagnosed HIV-seropositive in 1995. His first HAART regimen was started in 1997 and included efavirenz. After 1 week of treatment, he developed acute confusion and disorganized thinking, which persisted for 1 to 2 weeks and resolved after efavirenz was discontinued. He then started a new HAART regimen that did not contain efavirenz. In June 2003, he had an episode of major depression that responded well to treatment with sertraline 100 mg/day. In November 2003, he was switched back to an efavirenz-based HAART regimen in response to an increasing viral load. Within several days, he experienced the onset of auditory hallucinations, paranoia, disorganized thinking, headache, and a detached

feeling. It was recognized that the symptoms occurred after starting efavirenz and the drug was discontinued; the psychotic episode resolved.

This case represents an adverse reaction that is more acute and severe than is typical, but it is of interest because in each instance the acute psychotic symptoms occurred when the patient was challenged with efavirenz and resolved when it was discontinued.

Puzantian et al.[14] reported that a variety of CNS adverse effects occur more frequently in patients treated with an efavirenz-based antiretroviral regimen compared to those on a nelfinavir-based cocktail. Among the reported side effects, hallucinations and agitation occurred in less than 5% of patients treated with efavirenz, but in none of the subjects on nelfinavir.

Foster et al.[15] reported a case of acute paranoid psychosis associated with antiretroviral treatment in a 37-year-old woman who developed persecutory delusions and auditory hallucinations of the voice of God approximately 1 month after the commencement of a regimen of abacavir, nevirapine, and Combivir. The psychotic episode resolved after HAART was stopped and low-dose antipsychotic treatment was started. It is interesting that she was restarted on Combivir and nevirapine (but not abacavir) after 3 months, but experienced no further psychotic symptoms.

Other drugs commonly associated with mental status changes include corticosteroids, some antibacterials (e.g., dapsone, sulfadiazine), antiviral agents (e.g., acyclovir, ganciclovir), antifungal agents (e.g., amphotericin B), and antineoplastic agents (e.g., vincristine, methotrexate, procarbazine). Cases of psychosis have been described following the initiation of many of these medications.

Psychosis has been reported in patients being treated with corticosteroids for HIV-associated nephropathy and *Pneumocystis jeroveci carinii* pneumonia (PCP) and as a result of treatment with dapsone, an antibacterial used in the prophylaxis of PCP in HIV-infected patients.

In another report, a patient with AIDS who had no known psychiatric history developed nightmares, visual hallucinations, and severe agitation following a 2-week course of ganciclovir therapy for an exacerbation of cytomegalovirus retinitis.[16] The psychotic symptoms resolved after haloperidol administration and ganciclovir withdrawal and reappeared when the same regimen was reinstituted. Encephalopathy and psychosis have also been reported in association with sulfadiazine treatment in two patients with AIDS and CNS toxoplasmosis, and buspirone-induced psychosis has been reported in an HIV-infected man.

TREATMENT OF HIV-ASSOCIATED PSYCHOSIS

When a psychotic episode occurs in the context of HIV infection, it is essential to perform a thorough differential diagnosis with the initial goal of detecting the presence of life-threatening medical problems. We have already discussed various common medical conditions that may cause psychotic symptoms, sometimes in conjunction with delirium, dementia, mood disorder, or other psychiatric symptoms. At the same time, in many cases, the clinician will need to initiate treatment of the psychotic symptoms before potential medical causes have been fully evaluated and treated. This is necessary when psychotic agitation, severe paranoia, disorganization, violence, or menacing behavior threaten to disrupt the medical evaluation, cause injury to the patient or others, or otherwise seriously impair the patient's well-being. In these situations, symptomatic treatment of the psychotic disorder is indicated while the medical workup is being done.

Studies focused on the treatment of HIV-associated psychosis are sparse.[3] However, a review of the available literature and our own experience suggest several useful guidelines.

Antipsychotic medications remain effective treatments even in the presence of advanced HIV disease and cognitive disturbances.[3] Treatment modifications are often necessary, however, because patients are more sensitive to the side effects of antipsychotics and because patients are frequently taking multiple other medications that pose a risk for drug interactions or overlapping toxicities.

The extrapyramidal side effects of first-generation antipsychotics (or neuroleptics) are particularly problematic, and case reports document the risk of neuroleptic malignant syndrome and the possibility of relatively rapid-onset tardive dyskinesia when patients with AIDS are exposed to these medications.[3] Because HIV affects subcortical brain structures, such as the basal ganglia, Parkinsonian symptoms may occur spontaneously, and the added effect of a first-generation neuroleptic may precipitate Parkinsonian symptoms that do not reverse even after the neuroleptic is withdrawn and treatment for the Parkinsonian symptoms is initiated.[3] For these reasons, second-generation or atypical antipsychotics are better tolerated by HIV-infected patients, as evidenced by our own clinical experience and by two reports of 30 combined patients who received risperidone, one report of four patients who received remoxipride, and another of four patients who received molindone.[3,17]

Second-generation antipsychotics are better tolerated than first-generation neuroleptics. The epicenter of the AIDS pandemic is in sub-Saharan Africa, where neuroleptics are often the only affordable or available medications.[18] At least one study has found that standard neuroleptics can be used without severe extrapyramidal side effects in advanced HIV infection. This study was conducted in hospitalized patients with AIDS, some of whom were randomly assigned to chlorpromazine or haloperidol for treatment for delirium.[19] Using very low doses of neuroleptic, that is, average maintenance doses of 36 mg/day for chlorpromazine and 1.4 mg/day for haloperidol, the authors reported that "no clinically significant medication-related side effects were noted." The study is consistent with the rest of the literature in stressing the importance of treating patients with advanced HIV infection with the lowest possible effective dose when using a typical neuroleptic.

In chronically ill HIV-positive people, a conservative dosing strategy is indicated for all antipsychotic medications due to the sensitivity to side effects, medical fragility, and large medication burden of these patients. In addition, the initiation of any psychotropic medication should be done with consideration of the risk of drug interactions and overlapping toxicities with the many other medications prescribed to these patients.

In our clinical experience, each of the available atypical antipsychotics—risperidone, olanzapine, quetiapine, ziprasidone, aripiprazole, and clozapine—is effective and well tolerated in treating patients with AIDS. The choice of a specific antipsychotic needs to be guided by the individual clinical situation.

A common presenting complaint is the onset of agitation, visual hallucinations, and behavioral dyscontrol, often at night, in a patient with HIV-associated dementia or MCMD. The visual hallucinations may be subtle (e.g., shadows in the periphery, indistinct sounds or whispers, or a tap on the shoulder) or quite striking and bizarre (e.g., a visual image of a brightly colored figure or a demonic creature). In patients with psychotic symptoms such as these, quetiapine at a starting dose of 25 to 50 mg at bedtime is very useful in treating insomnia and agitation. If higher doses are needed to treat hallucinations and behavioral dyscontrol, the dose can be titrated upward at 25 to 50 mg/day until the desired response is achieved. Quetiapine is well tolerated because it tends not to cause extrapyramidal or anticholinergic side effects. Caution is required at higher doses, especially in fluid-depleted patients (e.g., due to persistent diarrhea), because quetiapine may cause orthostatic hypotension in these circumstances.

For patients who do not require sedation or cannot tolerate the orthostatic blood pressure changes with quetiapine, positive treatment responses have been observed with risperidone, olanzapine and aripiprazole. In a case report, Meyer et al.[20] highlighted the differential sensitivity to risperidone and olanzapine in an HIV-infected patient who had extrapyramidal side effects (tremor) with typical antipsychotics and risperidone, and later developed a dose-dependent akathisia when treated with olanzapine 10 to 15 mg/day. The akathisia responded to dose reduction and the addition of a β-adrenergic blocker.

Several reports have called attention to the need to be aware of potential drug interactions with atypical antipsychotics. Jover et al.[21] reported the case of a 48-year-old man with AIDS, who was treated for mania with risperidone 3 mg twice daily and developed a reversible coma after two doses of risperidone. The coma resolved with discontinuation of the risperidone and, in the absence of any evidence of another physiologic or infectious cause, the authors suspected a drug interaction between risperidone and the antiretroviral drugs ritonavir and indinavir.

As this case suggests, the risk for potentially clinically significant drug interactions between antipsychotics and antiretrovirals is highest for the protease inhibitor ritonavir. Ritonavir causes strong inhibition of the cytochrome P450 3A4 isoenzyme and moderate inhibition of the 2D6 isoenzyme. These two isoenzymes are involved in the metabolism of many psychotropic drugs, including the antipsychotics. Other protease inhibitors are also inhibitors of these enzymes, but to a lesser extent.

Most HIV-infected patients with new-onset psychosis or psychosis secondary to cerebral or metabolic disorders require only short-term treatment with antipsychotic drugs. However, in those patients who require longer term or maintenance treatment, the adverse metabolic effects of the atypical antipsychotics should be considered. There is growing awareness that atypical antipsychotics, like the protease inhibitors, can increase the risk for metabolic syndrome, abnormal lipid profiles, and diabetes mellitus, although the degree of risk varies between the different atypical agents. Generally, clozapine and olanzapine are associated with the highest risk for weight gain and metabolic syndrome, risperidone and quetiapine are considered moderate risk factors, and aripiprazole and ziprasidone cause little weight gain or other metabolic disturbance. For patients taking atypical antipsychotics for long periods, the likelihood of contributing to metabolic syndrome, lipid abnormalities, and diabetes should be one factor in choosing an antipsychotic drug, especially in those patients who are also taking protease inhibitors.

Patients who require long-term management for chronic psychotic disorders may also benefit from psychosocial interventions that have been developed for this population. These interventions include supportive psychotherapy, case management, family therapy, day programming, residential care, outreach, assistance with medication adherence, treatment for comorbid substance use, and HIV prevention interventions. Integration and coordination of treatment are very important for these complex patients.

SUMMARY

Many factors are associated with psychosis in HIV-infected people. Although some cases may strongly implicate a single etiologic cause, an overview of the literature suggests that the pathophysiology of psychosis in HIV infection is complex and that a multifactorial etiology of psychotic symptoms is quite likely.[5] Regardless of the etiology, psychosis represents a serious complication in the course of HIV infection and always merits a careful differential diagnosis. Psychosis in advanced HIV disease usually responds well to antipsychotic treatment, but lower doses of medication and attention to side effects and toxicities are necessary. It is also important to remember that patients with psychotic illnesses are at increased risk of acquiring or transmitting HIV, and prevention strategies are an important part of an integrated approach to this population.

REFERENCES

1. Cournos F, McKinnon K. HIV seroprevalence among people with severe mental illness in the United States: a critical review. *Clin Psychol Rev.* 1997;17:259–269.
2. Rosenberg SD, Goodman LA, Osher FC. Prevalence of HIV, hepatitis B, and hepatitis C in people with severe mental illness. *Am J Public Health.* 2001;91:31–37.

3. McDaniel JS, Chung JY, Brown L, et al. Practice guidelines for the treatment of patients with HIV/AIDS. *Am J Psychiatry*. 2000;157:1–62.
4. Cournos F, McKinnon K, Wainberg ML. What can mental health interventions contribute to the global struggle against HIV/AIDS? *World Psychiatry*. 4:135–141, 2005.
5. Sewell DD, Jeste DV, Atkinson JH, et al. HIV-associated psychosis: a study of 20 cases. *Am J Psychiatry*. 1994;151:237–242.
6. DeRonchi D, Faranca I, Forti P, et al. Development of acute psychotic disorders and HIV-1 infection. *Intl J Psychiatry Med*. 2000;30:173–183.
7. Alciati A, Fusi A, Monforti AD, et al. New-onset delusions and hallucinations in patients infected with HIV. *J Psychiatry Neurosci*. 2001;26:229–234.
8. Harris MJ, Jeste DV, Gleghorn A, Sewell DD. New onset psychosis in HIV-infected patients. *J Clin Psychiatry*. 1991;52:369–376.
9. El-Mallakh RS. Mania in AIDS: clinical significance and theoretical considerations. *Int J Psychiatry Med*. 1991;21:383–391.
10. Schwartzman WA, Patnaik M, McCutchan JA. Prevalence of CSF *Bartonella henselae* antibodies in HIV+; psychosis. *2nd. Natl Conf Hum Retroviruses Relat Infect*. Jan 29-Feb 2, 1995, p. 78.
11. Crichton P, Lewis S. Delusional misidentification, AIDS and the right hemisphere. *Br J Psychiatry*. 1990;157:608–610.
12. Hall W, Darke S, Ross M, Wodak A. Patterns of drug use and risk-taking among injecting amphetamine and opioid drug users in Sydney, Australia. *Addiction*. 1993;88:509–516.
13. Fumaz CR, Munoz-Moreno JA, Molto J, et al. Long-term neuropsychiatric disorders on efavirenz-based approaches: quality of life, psychologic issues, and adherence. *J Acquir Immune Defic Syndr*. 2005;38:560–565.
14. Puzantian T, et al. 41st Infectious Disease Society of America Annual Meeting. Chicago, Ill, October 24-27, 2002. Abstract 481.
15. Foster R, Olajide D, Everall IP. Antiretroviral therapy-induced psychosis: case report and brief review of the literature. *HIV Med*. 2003;4:139–144.
16. Chen JL, Brocavich JM, Lin AY. Psychiatric disturbances associated with ganciclovir therapy. *Ann Pharmacother*. 1992;26:193–195.
17. Fernandez F, Levy JK. The use of molindone in the treatment of psychotic and delirious patients infected with the human immunodeficiency virus: case reports. *Gen Hosp Psychiatry*. 1993;15:31–35.
18. Cournos F, Wainberg M, Horwath E. *Psychiatric Care in Anti-retroviral (ARV) Therapy*. Field Test Version. Geneva: World Health Organization, 2005.
19. Breitbart W, Marotta R, Platt M, et al. A double-blind trial of haloperidol, chlorpromazine and lorazepam in the treatment of delirium in hospitalized AIDS patients. *Am J Psychiatry*. 1996;153:231–237.
20. Meyer JM, Marsh J, Simpson G. Differential sensitivities to risperidone and olanzapine in a human immunodeficiency virus patient. *Biol Psychiatry*. 1998;44:791–794.
21. Jover F, Cuadrado JM, Andreu L, Merino J. Reversible coma caused by risperidone-ritonavir interaction. *Clin Neuropharmacol*. 2002;25:251–253.

CHAPTER **14**

Substance Use Disorders

Stephen J. Ferrando, Steven L. Batki

The connection between human immunodeficiency virus (HIV) and substance use has been recognized since the early stages of the epidemic. In the United States, it is estimated that more than 800,000 persons have been diagnosed with acquired immunodeficiency syndrome (AIDS).[1] Men who have sex with men (MSM) and injection drug users (IDUs) have been the predominant HIV risk groups. Of men living with AIDS, 32% were IDUs or MSM who were also IDUs.[1] Women, ethnic minority groups, and children have been particularly hard hit by injection drug–related and heterosexual transmission of HIV. Since the epidemic began, 57% of AIDS cases among women have been attributed to injection drug use or sex with partners who inject drugs. Of new AIDS cases reported in 2000, IDU-associated AIDS accounted for 26% of cases among African American and 31% among Hispanic adults and adolescents, compared with 19% of all cases among whites.[1] Noninjection drugs, such as crack cocaine, and alcohol are also associated with HIV risk via unsafe sexual behaviors.[2]

Practitioners in HIV treatment settings routinely face the clinical problems associated with substance use disorders. The treatment of individuals with the "triple diagnosis" of HIV, substance abuse, and psychiatric disorders has multiple levels of complexity, including ongoing substance use, increased psychological distress, and potentially poor adherence to medical treatment regimens. These co-occurring disorders may be associated with greater morbidity and mortality and have led to the development of integrated HIV, drug abuse, and psychiatric treatment services.[3]

In this chapter, we begin by reviewing the potential association between substance use, psychiatric disorders, and HIV risk behaviors. We then discuss the prevalence of psychiatric and substance use disorders among HIV-infected individuals in various treatment settings and research cohorts. Next, we discuss the medical, psychiatric, and substance abuse treatment of individuals with a triple diagnosis of psychiatric disorder, substance use, and HIV infection.

SUBSTANCE USE, PSYCHIATRIC DISORDERS, AND HIV DISEASE: SCOPE OF THE PROBLEM

Evidence for a connection between psychiatric disorders, substance use, and HIV can be derived from four sources: (a) data concerning HIV risk behaviors of individuals with psychiatric and/or substance use disorders, (b) HIV seroprevalence studies in psychiatric and substance abuse treatment settings, (c) clinical samples of patients with HIV in various treatment settings, and (d) cohort studies of psychopathology among homosexual/bisexual men and IDUs with HIV infection.

HIV RISK BEHAVIORS OF INDIVIDUALS WITH PSYCHIATRIC AND SUBSTANCE USE DISORDERS

Injection and noninjection drug use, as well as alcohol use, are associated with HIV risk behaviors.[4] Both psychiatric inpatients and outpatients have revealed high rates of HIV risk behaviors associated with substance use.[5] For example, Cournos et al.[5] found that 44% of inpatients with schizophrenia were sexually active in the previous 6 months, more than half of whom had multiple sexual partners. Among the sexually active group, consistent condom use was infrequent, nearly half used alcohol or drugs during sex, and half had exchanged sex for money or drugs.[5]

To date, evidence that presence of a dual diagnosis confers higher risk for HIV infection than presence of a substance use or psychiatric disorder alone is largely indirect. An inferential link between dual diagnosis and HIV risk can be derived from the knowledge that psychiatric and substance use disorders frequently co-occur, that injection and noninjection drug use are known risk factors for HIV infection, and that psychiatric symptoms may magnify HIV risk by producing impaired knowledge, judgment, and interpersonal skills regarding sexual and drug use behavior.[6]

HIV SEROPREVALENCE IN PSYCHIATRIC AND SUBSTANCE ABUSE TREATMENT SETTINGS

Among drug users entering treatment, the prevalence of HIV varies greatly by geographic region and ranges from 0 to 35%.[7] Among psychiatric patients, studies in the United States—mostly from the New York City area—using discarded blood samples, revealed rates of HIV infection between 4.0% and 22.9% among inpatients.[8] Factors associated with HIV-positive serostatus in studies of psychiatric inpatients have included younger age, ethnic minority status, poor reality testing, hypersexuality, childhood and adult sexual victimization, and homelessness, but the most prevalent risk factors have consistently been homosexual/bisexual activity among men and history of injection drug use.[8] Males and females in these studies have generally had equal HIV infection rates. Information on specific psychiatric and substance use disorders, and their combinations, has been limited in these studies.

PSYCHOPATHOLOGY AND SUBSTANCE ABUSE IN CLINICAL SAMPLES OF PATIENTS WITH HIV

The triple diagnosis of HIV infection, psychiatric disorder, and substance use disorder is commonly described in studies of HIV-positive patients seen in integrated methadone maintenance treatment (MMT) programs and HIV medical clinics. Clinical samples of IDUs with HIV infection entering MMT reveal high rates of prior psychiatric morbidity, current distress, and suicidal ideation. Further, while in MMT, up to 80% of these patients require psychiatric consultation for the treatment of depression, psychotic symptoms, anxiety, insomnia, cognitive impairment, and behavioral disinhibition, often with concurrent substance abuse (cocaine, amphetamine, alcohol, and/or sedative-hypnotics).[9]

Reports describing HIV-positive patients seen in specialized HIV medical clinics document the frequent occurrence of psychiatric and substance use disorders, which complicate the manifestations and treatment of HIV infection. Lyketsos et al.[10] found that more than 50%

of individuals in their HIV clinic had a psychiatric diagnosis, most of them had a concurrent psychiatric and substance use disorder, and those with a triple diagnosis had the highest mean scores on the Beck Depression Inventory (BDI) and the General Health Questionnaire compared to individuals with no diagnosis or a psychiatric or substance use disorder alone. The collective data from clinical studies underscore the importance of psychiatric and substance abuse screening in HIV medical clinics.

PSYCHOPATHOLOGY AND SUBSTANCE ABUSE IN RESEARCH COHORTS

Data derived from controlled studies of mostly asymptomatic HIV-positive gay men have shown very high lifetime rates and generally much lower current rates of major depressive, drug use, and alcohol use disorders.[11] In recent years, there have been resurgences of HIV risk behavior among young gay men and men of color in association with the use of methylenedeoxymethamphetamine (MDMA, "Ecstasy") and methamphetamine.

In a cross-sectional study of psychopathology among IDUs with HIV infection, Lipsitz et al.[12] reported relatively high rates of current depressive disorders among both male and female IDUs. The rates of current depressive disorders they found were comparable to those found in in-treatment IDU populations studied before the HIV epidemic, but much higher than the rates found in studies of homosexual men.[11] When these investigators compared rates of current depressive disorders among HIV-positive IDUs versus HIV-negative IDUs, HIV-positive men (but not HIV-positive women) were more depressed than their HIV-negative counterparts. Longitudinal follow-up of this cohort over 3 years revealed that HIV serostatus and baseline major depressive disorder (MDD) independently predicted persistent or recurrent episodes of MDD after sociodemographic and other factors were controlled statistically.[13]

Personality disorders are associated with substance abuse, HIV risk behavior, distress, and maladaptive coping with HIV infection. In a study of individuals from various risk groups presenting for HIV testing and counseling, Jacobsberg et al.[14] found higher rates of antisocial personality disorder among individuals who were seropositive compared with those who were seronegative. Among 100 IDUs tested for HIV, individuals with antisocial personality disorder (ASPD), 36% engaged in more needle sharing with more drug use partners than IDUs without ASPD.

Cognitive dysfunction is an important aspect of psychopathology in HIV infection. Studies on neuropsychological performance in HIV-positive drug and alcohol users reveal that up to 88% of patients have impairment in one or more cognitive domains.[15] In comparing asymptomatic HIV-positive IDUs with HIV-negative IDUs, investigators found that drug use is a more important factor in producing neuropsychological impairment than HIV itself. In addition to drug use, independent predictors of poor neuropsychological test performance among HIV-positive IDUs include HIV viral load, low educational attainment, and premorbid medical and psychiatric problems.[15] Furthermore, increasing evidence suggests that individuals with HIV and comorbid methamphetamine, cocaine, heroin, or alcohol abuse may experience more rapid deterioration in cognitive function than individuals without such comorbidity.[16] This may be due to the propensity for HIV and these substances to induce neuropathologic changes in striatal and other dopaminergic systems.

MEDICAL ASPECTS OF HIV INFECTION IN SUBSTANCE USERS

COMMON HIV-ASSOCIATED AND OTHER MEDICAL PROBLEMS IN SUBSTANCE USERS

The course and complications of HIV disease may be different for substance users than individuals in other HIV risk groups. Once substance users enter medical treatment, the secondary complications of continued drug and alcohol use (e.g., decreased self-care, pneumonia, skin abscesses, sexually transmitted diseases) and behavioral disturbances secondary to psychiatric distress or disorders may complicate the course and treatment of HIV infection. Longitudinal epidemiologic evidence suggests that alcohol and illicit drug use accelerates progression of HIV infection.[17]

Severe bacterial infections, including pneumonias, endocarditis, and sepsis are common in IDUs and may be mistaken for other complications of HIV disease (e.g., bacterial pneumonia may be presumed secondary to *Pneumocystis jiroveci* (formerly *carinii*) infection (i.e., PCP). In addition, *Mycobacterium tuberculosis* (TB), including drug-resistant strains, may be seen in drug users with HIV and homeless individuals living in shelters; however, the incidence of TB has declined in epicenter cities in the United States, likely because of better HIV treatment and TB control strategies.[18] Primary sexually transmitted diseases are common among IDUs with HIV infection because many HIV-infected drug users continue to practice unsafe sex and risky drug use practices.[19] In addition, reactivation of old infections, such as with the development of neurosyphilis, may occur in drug users with advanced immunosuppression and may be difficult to diagnose because of the broad differential diagnosis for encephalopathy (see Chapters 12 and 19).

Hepatitis C virus (HCV) infection is increasingly recognized as a significant comorbid condition that affects the clinical outcome of patients with substance use disorders and HIV disease. Coinfection is common because both HIV and HCV share routes of transmission, notably injection.[7] HIV is a risk factor for accelerating the course of HCV, and HCV can worsen the outcome of HIV disease. HCV treatment involves the use of interferon alpha, which is associated with numerous neuropsychiatric adverse effects, most notably the onset or exacerbation of depression and other dysphoric symptoms. These psychiatric adverse effects can be successfully treated with antidepressant medications such as selective serotonin reuptake inhibitors (SSRIs).[20,21] Alcohol use is a highly significant cofactor in further increasing the morbidity and mortality associated with HCV infection, making abstinence from alcohol an important treatment goal in the individual with HCV infection.

MEDICAL TREATMENT OF SUBSTANCE USERS WITH HIV INFECTION

Because of the medical complications and barriers to medical care for HIV-infected substance users with and without psychiatric morbidity, innovative models of care delivery are needed. Primary medical care provided on-site may be an especially relevant model for opioid-dependent IDUs in MMT, because it may allow easier access to treatment. Some investigators have shown that such on-site medical care, compared to off-site referral, can improve the utilization of health care services by HIV-infected drug users.[22] Some MMT programs with on-site medical care may directly dispense antiretroviral or antituberculosis medications daily to drug users with HIV as a means of increasing adherence.[23] For HIV-infected drug users not in MMT, some urban HIV medical clinics provide on-site psychiatric and drug abuse treatment, which assists individuals in adhering to medical care.[10] However, these comprehensive services are not always available, especially in smaller, nonepicenter cities. In settings where medical, substance abuse, and psychiatric treatment may be split, intensive case management services delivered by individuals with some substance abuse and/or psychiatric training may help to coordinate care and increase the likelihood that individuals will adhere to their medical treatment.

Adherence to antiretroviral treatment is adversely affected by both substance use and psychiatric disorders. Interventions that appear to increase the likelihood of adherence among substance users with HIV disease include peer-driven support systems, on-site dispensing of HIV medications in substance abuse treatment programs, and individual medication management programs.[24]

The treatment of pain is an important issue for the substance user with HIV infection or AIDS. Clinicians in substance abuse treatment programs and medical doctors are often concerned about opioid-seeking behavior among drug users and may be hesitant to prescribe opioids for pain complaints. Breitbart and Dibiase[25] did not find an increased number or intensity of pain complaints or opioid analgesic use among HIV-positive substance users compared to individuals in other HIV risk groups. They point out that it is the actively using drug user who is most problematic to treat, but that individuals with extended sobriety or on MMT are often treated without difficulty. Generally, if opioids are necessary, long-acting agents (e.g., sustained-release morphine) are helpful in providing stable opioid analgesic levels without the sensation of intoxication produced by shorter acting agents. Methadone-maintained patients should receive appropriate opioid analgesia over and above their usual methadone dose, because methadone alone does not provide appropriate analgesia for these patients. It is also important to keep in mind that substance users with AIDS may require chronic opioid analgesics in the late stages of illness for complications such as peripheral neuropathy. When possible, the patient and medical and substance abuse treatment clinicians should collaborate in pain management, because this may optimize pain control and ease concerns about opioid abuse.

PSYCHIATRIC TREATMENT OF SUBSTANCE USERS WITH HIV INFECTION

Psychiatric treatment of individuals with a triple diagnosis may be complicated by the same factors that may affect access to medical care. When drug users discover their HIV-positive status, they may react with higher and more sustained levels of distress than individuals in other risk groups, and their continued or heightened drug use in combination with depression may increase ongoing high-risk sexual activity.[26] The provision of HIV testing and counseling of drug users in treatment centers or where referral to substance abuse treatment and ongoing counseling are readily available allows the issues of distress, risk reduction, and relapse to be addressed.

The diagnosis and psychiatric treatment of HIV-infected drug users may be complicated by multiple factors that can produce neuropsychiatric disturbance in these patients. These include long-term and acute effects of alcohol and drugs of abuse, use of methadone, and past history of head trauma.[9] HIV-associated opportunistic infections of the central nervous system (CNS) may cause neuropsychiatric disturbances.[27] Finally, HIV itself may be associated with cognitive, motor, and behavioral abnormalities both early and late in the course of HIV infection, progressing from HIV-associated minor cognitive motor disorder (MCMD) to HIV-associated dementia (HAD).[27] Early cognitive/motor deficits are subtle, with impaired attention, concentration, and short-term memory and reduced psychomotor speed. Only later, with severe immunosuppression and AIDS, does a frank dementia develop, with global cognitive impairment, apathy, other behavioral disturbances (including psychosis and mania), and movement disorders. Neuropathologically, HAD has been associated with periventricular white matter, subcortical gray, thalamic, and basal ganglia abnormalities, consistent with the neuropsychiatric manifestations of the disorder. Clinical neuropsychiatric and neuropsychological assessment and brain imaging should be available to drug users with HIV disease to characterize the nature of cognitive deficits and help distinguish the multiple factors that may be responsible for these deficits. Serial assessments are helpful, especially in differentiating the acute effects of drugs and alcohol from other sources of cognitive dysfunction. Fortunately, combination antiretroviral treatment may significantly benefit neuropsychological function.[27]

Both psychotherapeutic and psychopharmacologic treatments may be necessary for drug users with HIV disease. In terms of psychotherapeutic treatment, support groups can help reduce social isolation, support sustained risk reduction behaviors, and educate about the basics of health care for HIV disease. Attendance at self-help groups can also be quite helpful, though patients should be steered toward meetings where discussion of HIV, psychiatric symptoms, methadone, and other psychotropic medications will be accepted. These may be difficult to find, and patients should be encouraged to try a number of meetings in order to find a "good fit." In drug abuse treatment programs, counselors can provide supportive psychotherapy, though patients with severe psychiatric disorders, including HIV- and drug-associated neuropsychiatric disturbances, may require psychiatric consultation and treatment.

There are relatively few specific data on the safety or efficacy of psychopharmacologic treatment of psychiatric disorders in drug users with HIV infection, because drug users have generally been excluded from psychotropic medication trials.[3] For most treatments, available recommendations are based on studies that have involved HIV-infected patients who were not drug users.[28] In general, psychopharmacologic treatment of drug users with HIV infection is guided by three main issues: safety, abuse liability, and compliance. A stepwise, hierarchical approach to the pharmacologic treatment of psychiatric disorders in drug users with HIV has been proposed, to reduce possible risks associated with these medications.[3]

For treatment of depression, the SSRIs are preferred because of their lack of anticholinergic and antiadrenergic side effects and lethality on overdose.[28] In HIV-infected, cocaine-dependent patients on MMT, fluoxetine, in doses up to 40 mg/day, was well tolerated and associated with improvements in ratings of both depression and cocaine use. Although tertiary amine tricyclic antidepressants (e.g., imipramine) may be helpful for HIV-associated depression, anxiety, and insomnia and as adjuvant analgesics in lower doses, long-term treatment is hampered by adverse effects of these medications[28]; thus many clinicians choose less-sedating secondary amines, such as desipramine. The psychostimulants dextroamphetamine and methylphenidate are generally safe and rapidly effective in the late stages of HIV infection and AIDS for the treatment of apathy, fatigue, and cognitive impairment,[29] although these medications may carry considerable abuse liability if used to treat drug users in earlier stages of HIV disease.

The treatment of anxiety and insomnia in the HIV-infected drug and alcohol user is particularly problematic because of abuse liability associated with benzodiazepines and other sedative-hypnotics.[28] It is best to initiate pharmacotherapy for anxiety disorders with a medication that has little or no abuse liability, such as the SSRIs or buspirone. An open trial of buspirone in doses of 30 to 40 mg/day in HIV-infected drug users found that the majority of patients showed improvement in anxiety levels, with few adverse effects.[30] Other useful non-addicting agents for the treatment of anxiety and insomnia include hydroxyzine, trazodone, and atypical neuroleptic medications such as quetiapine, olanzapine, and risperidone.

Manic syndromes have been reported to be a manifestation of HIV infection in the CNS, though it is not uncommon to encounter HIV-infected drug and alcohol users with bipolar spectrum disorders and characteristic mood instability.[9] The diagnosis of mania and mood instability in drug users is complicated by the possibility of concurrent stimulant use, sedative or alcohol withdrawal, sorting out past history suggestive of mania, and comorbidity with personality disorders. Treatment of HIV-associated mania in drug users is complicated by the toxicity of mood stabilizers, particularly lithium (neurotoxicity) and carbamazepine (blood disorders and induction of antiretroviral metabolism).[28] Divalproex sodium is often chosen as a treatment for HIV-associated mania because it is the best tolerated of the mood stabilizers; however, there has been some concern over its use because of in vitro evidence that this drug may stimulate HIV replication.[28] More recently, the atypical neuroleptics, such as olanzapine, have been used to treat HIV-associated mania, particularly in patients less likely to adhere to serum level monitoring of other mood stabilizers.

The diagnosis and treatment of psychosis in the HIV-infected drug or alcohol user is also complicated by concurrent drug use and withdrawal, difficulty in sorting out a past history of psychosis, delirium related to acute medical illness, and the increased risk of anticholinergic and antiadrenergic effects, extrapyramidal symptoms (EPS), and neuroleptic malignant syndrome (NMS) in HIV-infected patients. As in the treatment of mania, atypical neuroleptic agents such as risperidone and olanzapine may be useful for HIV-associated psychosis and mania because of their relatively low incidence of EPS.[28]

TREATMENT OF SUBSTANCE USE DISORDERS IN HIV-INFECTED PATIENTS

The treatment of substance use disorders is an important aspect of the overall care of HIV-infected substance users. It improves their quality of life and reduces the risk of their spreading HIV infection to others. As previously discussed, substance abuse treatment can also serve as a mechanism for providing primary medical and psychiatric care for the HIV-infected patient. Alcohol and drug abuse treatment settings range in intensity from outpatient to inpatient and vary widely in their ability to manage psychiatric problems. Treatment has acute and non-acute phases and includes pharmacologic and psychosocial modalities.

The initial phase of treatment focuses on detoxification, which may require brief inpatient treatment, particularly for severe alcohol withdrawal.[31] Alcohol and sedative withdrawal in the HIV-infected patient can be managed with benzodiazepines, generally at the same dosages as in noninfected patients, except in the later stages of HIV illness, in which patients may require smaller doses because of serious physical debility. Methadone is generally helpful for management of acute opioid withdrawal symptoms, both on an inpatient and outpatient basis.[31]

After patients are medically stabilized and no longer require detoxification, the goals of treatment ideally include maintenance of abstinence and rapid remission of relapses. Several weeks of abstinence provides an opportunity to evaluate psychiatric and cognitive symptoms, which, when treated, may increase substance abuse treatment retention.[3] Substance abuse treatment is usually provided on an outpatient basis, although residential therapeutic communities may be indicated for HIV-infected patients with more severe, refractory substance use disorders.

Outpatient treatments for drug abuse include drug-free programs that are most often used for those who are dependent on stimulants, alcohol, multiple drugs, and opioids (but who are not candidates for methadone treatment). Because of the high prevalence of HIV infection, outpatient programs are increasingly equipped to address HIV risk reduction and emotional sequelae of HIV infection. Self-help programs, such as Alcoholics Anonymous and Narcotics Anonymous are generally encouraged as part of outpatient treatment, and groups have formed that openly encourage participation by those with HIV infection. As part of outpatient treatment programs, adjunctive pharmacologic treatments, such as aversive and anticraving agents, may be used for the HIV-infected substance user who is likely to comply with such treatment.[31] These include disulfiram and acamprosate for alcohol dependence and naltrexone for alcohol and opioid dependence. Naltrexone is, however, contraindicated in patients with late-stage AIDS who require opioid analgesics for pain control.

Although outpatient drug-free programs compose the bulk of substance abuse treatment, pharmacologic maintenance treatments play a particularly important role in the long-term management of injection opioid users with HIV infection. The pharmacologic maintenance treatment of greatest applicability to HIV-infected injection drug users is MMT.[3] Because the majority of opioid-using patients are at risk for resuming injection drug use after methadone is discontinued, it is recommended that HIV-infected, opioid-dependent patients be offered long-term MMT. Standard doses of methadone can be used—generally 60 mg/day—and can be maintained even when the patient with HIV disease or AIDS is acutely ill and requires additional analgesia, though at times dosage must be lowered based on the degree of the patient's physical debility. The dosage of methadone may be affected by some important interactions with other medications used in HIV disease. For example, the antiretrovirals ritonavir and nevirapine and the antibiotic rifampin may significantly enhance the elimination of methadone and could induce opioid withdrawal symptoms.[28] Thus close monitoring of opioid withdrawal symptoms and serum methadone levels may be warranted when initiating these drugs in methadone-maintained patients.

MMT is particularly effective for opioid-dependent patients with HIV infection because it affords nearly daily contact and provides a stable setting for the provision of medical and psychiatric care. Despite some concerns about the potential for opioids (including methadone) to depress immune function, studies of IDUs have found that MMT is associated with normalization of alterations in immune function associated with intravenous heroin use[32] and with reduction in serum neopterin levels (a predictor of progression to AIDS), so long as MMT patients do not continue to use heroin. Furthermore, MMT is protective against the spread of HIV[33] and may have some efficacy in slowing the progression of HIV disease.[34]

Drug abuse treatment of patients with HIV disease requires more flexibility than is customary in traditional substance abuse treatment programs.[3] This flexibility is required because of medical and psychiatric comorbidity and the potential for relapse when HIV-infected substance users are out of treatment. The latter raises personal and public health concerns because of the potential for high-risk drug use and sexual behavior and is consistent with other approaches based on the concept of harm reduction.[35] Physical illness, depressed mood, hopelessness, and suicidal ideation may erode motivation to succeed in drug abuse treatment. Consequently, depressed or medically ill patients with HIV disease need more assistance in reducing or stopping drug use compared to others who are more physically and psychologically healthy.

HIV RISK REDUCTION INTERVENTIONS

Reducing the risk of transmitting HIV infection is a public health priority, and it is crucial that risk reduction interventions be delivered to individuals with or at high risk for HIV infection. The concept of harm reduction has been advanced as a useful overarching strategy in approaching HIV prevention in drug users.[35] The basic assumption behind harm reduction is that the harmful consequences of drug use (i.e., HIV transmission) can be reduced through various interventions. Harm reduction realistically assumes that a certain percentage of individuals will continue to use drugs and that the vast majority will not abstain from sexual activity, and thus encourages strategies that reduce the risk of these activities. Harm reduction strategies employ multiple, sometimes simultaneous interventions, including MMT, provision of sterile syringes, syringe exchange, syringe cleaning education (with bleach distribution), and education on safer sex practices (with condom distribution). Syringe exchange programs not only provide a mechanism for IDUs to obtain clean injection equipment, but also for them to receive safe sex and drug use education, to obtain condoms, and to be encouraged to seek HIV testing and counseling, along with medical and drug abuse treatment.

The National Institute on Drug Abuse (NIDA)[36] published a summary of research-based findings on prevention interventions. The approach recommended by NIDA stresses community-based outreach, education, and sterile syringe access.

Individuals with psychiatric disorders, especially severe disorders, pose special challenges in HIV risk education and have been shown to respond less well to HIV prevention efforts.[37] For many reasons (including thought disorder, impaired reality testing, inattention, poor concentration, impulsivity, helplessness, impaired judgment, low motivation, and poor social skills), they may have difficulty absorbing, retaining, and implementing safe sex and drug use practices. It is necessary to first treat the underlying psychiatric and substance use disorder. Then, risky behavior can be assessed. McKinnon et al.[38] found that the Sexual Risk Behavior

Assessment Schedule developed for IDUs and adapted for a psychiatric population had high test-retest reliability for sexually active psychiatric inpatients and did not exacerbate psychiatric symptoms. Interventions should be tailored to individuals based on their level of HIV knowledge, risk, and manifestations of their psychopathology. For example, individuals with poor social skills and depression may benefit from education plus assertiveness training, while those with impaired attention and concentration may benefit from multimedia presentation of educational material and an active "role-playing" approach to learning to manage various potentially risky situations. One pilot HIV prevention study with psychiatric inpatients, most of whom had comorbid substance use disorders, used a 7-week, multifaceted group approach that relied heavily on topical discussion, role-playing, and assertiveness training.[39] The group was well-received and well-tolerated and was supplemented by individual counseling to cover topics that patients were reluctant to discuss in a group setting. Whatever the approach, risk reduction efforts for individuals with substance use and psychiatric disorders require repetition and reinforcement, because their efforts to reduce risk may attenuate over time.

SUMMARY AND FUTURE DIRECTIONS

Several areas of future research are relevant to HIV infection in individuals with drug use and psychiatric disorders. The first is primary HIV disease prevention. In this area, it is necessary to continue to target specific risk reduction interventions to meet the needs of an ever-broadening population that may be vulnerable to HIV transmission. This includes women, individuals in ethnic minority groups, adolescents, and individuals with different types of psychiatric disorders. Related to this is the need to continue to develop and test harm reduction strategies in terms of their ability to reduce HIV transmission and to make these interventions more acceptable to society at large. The second area for future research is secondary prevention of HIV disease progression. The course of HIV disease in drug users, and particularly in women and ethnic minorities infected directly or indirectly via drug use, needs to be better characterized so that medical interventions can be specifically tailored to meet the needs of these individuals. Further, innovative service delivery mechanisms need further development and testing, particularly those that can integrate a broad array of services, including medical, psychiatric, and drug abuse treatment. However, a necessary feature of enhanced service delivery mechanisms are strategies to increase access, appropriate utilization, and compliance with medical treatment for HIV infection, because these issues are most likely to affect HIV disease progression in drug users.

REFERENCES

1. Centers for Disease Control and Prevention. HIV/AIDS surveillance report. Year-end ed. December, 2001. Available at: http://www.cdc.gov/hiv/stats/hasr1302.htm. Accessed November 2, 2005.
2. Woody GE, Donnell D, Seage GR, et al. Non-injection substance use correlates with risky sex among men having sex with men. Data from HIVNET. *Drug Alcohol Depend.* 1999;53:197–205.
3. Center for Substance Abuse Treatment; Batki SL, Selwyn P. Consensus Panel Co-Chairs. *Substance Abuse Treatment for Persons with HIV/AIDS.* Washington, DC: US Government Printing Office; 2000. US Dept. of Health and Human Services Publication No. (SMA) 00–3410.
4. Centers for Disease Control and Prevention: Revised guidelines for HIV counseling, testing, and referral. *MMWR Morbid Mortal Wkly Rep.* Nov 2001. Available at: http://www.cdc.gov/mmwr/preview/mmwrhtml/rr5019a1.htm. Accessed November 2, 2005.
5. Cournos F, Guido JR, Coomaraswamy S, et al. Sexual activity and risk of HIV infection among patients with schizophrenia. Am J Psychiatry. 1994;151:228–32.
6. McMahon RC, Malow RM, Penedo FJ. Psychiatric symptoms and HIV risk in MMPI-2 cluster subgroups of polysubstance abusers in treatment. *J Addict Disord.* 2001;20:27–40.
7. Sorensen JL, Masson CL, Perlman DC. HIV/hepatitis prevention in drug abuse treatment programs: guidance from research. *Sci Pract Perspect.* 2002;1:4–11.
8. Judd F. HIV/AIDS and the severely mentally ill. *Prim Psychiatry.* 1999;6:37–46.
9. Batki SL, Ferrando SJ, Manfredi LB, et al. Psychiatric disorders, drug use, and medical status in 84 injection drug users with HIV disease. *Am J Addict.* 1996;5:249–258.
10. Lyketsos CG, Hanson A, Fishman M, Mc Hugh PR, Treisman GJ. Screening for psychiatric morbidity in a medical outpatient clinic for HIV infection: the need for a psychiatric presence. *Int J Psychiatry Med.* 1994;24:103–113.

11. Rabkin JG, Ferrando SJ, Jacobsberg LB, Fishman B. Prevalence of psychiatric disorders in an AIDS cohort: a controlled study. *Compr Psychiatry.* 1997;38:146–154.
12. Lipsitz JD, Williams JBW, Rabkin JG, et al. Psychopathology in male and female intravenous drug users with and without HIV infection. *Am J Psychiatry.* 1994;151:1622–1668.
13. Johnson JG, Rabkin JG, Lipsitz JD, Williams JB, Remien RH. Recurrent major depressive disorder among human immunodeficiency virus (HIV)-positive and HIV-negative intravenous drug users: findings of a 3-year longitudinal study. *Compr Psychiatry.* 1999;40:31–34.
14. Jacobsberg L, Frances A, Perry S. Axis II diagnosis among volunteers for HIV testing and counseling. *Am J Psychiatry.* 1995;152:1222–1224.
15. Margolin A, Avants SK, Warburton LA, Hawkins KA. Factors affecting cognitive functioning in a sample of human immunodeficiency virus-positive injection drug users. *AIDS Patient Care STDs.* 2002;16:255–257.
16. Nath A, Hauser KF, Wojna V, et al. Molecular basis for interactions of HIV and drugs of abuse. *J Acquir Immune Defic Syndr.* 2002;2(suppl 31):S62–S69.
17. Kapadia F, Cook JA, Cohen MH, et al. The relationship between non-injection drug use behaviors on progression to AIDS and death in a cohort of HIV seropositive women in the era of highly active antiretroviral therapy use. *Addiction.* 2005;100:990–1002.
18. Geng E, Kreiswirth B, Driver C, et al. Changes in the transmission of tuberculosis in New York City from 1990 to 1999. *N Engl J Med.* 2002;346:1453–1438.
19. Santibanez SS, Garfein RS, Schwartzendruber A, et al. Prevalence and correlates of crack-cocaine injection among young injection drug users in the United States, 1997–1999. *Drug Alcohol Depend.* 2005;77:227–233.
20. Gleason OC, Yates WR, Isbell MD, Philipsen MA. An open-label trial of citalopram for major depression in patients with hepatitis C. *J Clin Psychiatry.* 2002;63:194–198.
21. Kraus MR, Schafer A, Faller H, Csef H, Scheurlen M. Paroxetine for the treatment of interferon-alpha-induced depression in chronic hepatitis C. *Ailment Pharmacol Ther.* 2002;16:1091–1099.
22. Soto TA, Bell J, Pillen MB, et al. Literature on integrated HIV care: a review. *AIDS Care.* 2004;16(suppl 1):S43–S55.
23. Lucas GM, Weidle PJ, Hader S, Moor SD. Directly administered antiretroviral therapy in an urban methadone maintenance clinic: a nonrandomized comparative study. *Clin Infect Dis.* 2004;38:S409–S413.
24. Sorensen JL, Mascovich A, Wall TL, et al. Medication adherence strategies for drug abusers with HIV disease. *AIDS Care.* 1998;10:297–312.
25. Breitbart W, Dibiase L. Current perspectives on pain in AIDS. *Oncology.* 2002;16:818–29, 834–835.
26. Kelly JA, Murphy DA, Bahr R, et al. Factors associated with severity of depression and high-risk sexual behavior among persons diagnosed with human immunodeficiency virus (HIV) infection. *Health Psychol.* 1993;3:215–219.
27. Ferrando SJ. Diagnosis and treatment of HIV-associated neurocognitive disorders. *New Direct Mental Health Serv.* 2000;87:25–35.
28. Ferrando SJ, Wapenyi K. Psychopharmacological treatment of patients with HIV and AIDS. *Psychiatr Q.* 2002;73:33–49.
29. Breitbart W, Rosenfeld B, Kaim M, Funesti-Esch J. A randomized, double-blind, placebo controlled trial of psychostimulants for the treatment of fatigue in ambulatory patients with human immunodeficiency virus disease. *Arch Intern Med.* 2001;161:411–420.
30. Batki SL. Buspirone in drug users with AIDS or AIDS-related complex. *J Clin Psychopharmacol.* 1990;10(suppl 3):111S–115S.
31. American Psychiatric Association Work Group on Substance Use Disorders. Practice guideline for the treatment of patients with substance use disorders: alcohol, cocaine, opioids. *Am J Psychiatry.* 1995;152(suppl 11):1–59.
32. Novick DM, Ochshorn M, Ghali V, et al. Natural killer cell activity and lymphocyte subsets in parenteral heroin abusers and long-term methadone maintenance patients. *J Pharmacol Exp Therapeut.* 1989;250:606–610.
33. Metzger DS, Woody GE, McLellan AT, et al. Human immunodeficiency virus seroconversion among intravenous drug users in- and out-of-treatment: an 18-month prospective follow-up. *J Acquir Immune Defic Syndr.* 1993;6:1049–1056.
34. Weber R, Ledergerber B, Opravil M, Siegenthaler W, Luthy R. Progression of HIV infection in misusers of injected drugs who stop injection or follow a programme of maintenance treatment with methadone. *Br Med J.* 1990;301:1362–1365.
35. Des Jarlais DC, Friedman SR, Ward TP. Harm reduction: a public health response to the AIDS epidemic among injection drug users. *Annu Rev Public Health.* 1993;14:413–450.
36. National Institute on Drug Abuse. Principles of HIV prevention in drug-using populations: a research-based guide. Rockville, Md: National Institute on Drug Abuse; 2002. NIH Publication No 02–4733.
37. Compton WM, Cottler LB, Ben-Abdallah A, Cunningham-Williams R, Spitznagel EL. The effects of psychiatric comorbidity on response to an HIV prevention intervention. *Drug Alcohol Depend.* 2000;58:247–257.
38. McKinnon K, Cournos F, Meyer-Bahlburg HFL, et al. Reliability of sexual risk behavior interviews with psychiatric patients. *Am J Psychiatry.* 1993;150:972–974.
39. Meyer I, Cournos F, Empfield M, Agosin B, Floyd P. HIV prevention among psychiatric inpatients: a pilot risk-reduction study. *Psychiatric Q.* 1992;63:187–197.

CHAPTER **15**

Sleep Disorders

Carlos A. Santana, Francisco Fernandez

Sleep disorders are common in human immunodeficiency virus (HIV) disease. Disturbance of sleep may contribute to the fatigue and excessive disability associated with HIV infection. Insomnia is underdiagnosed in HIV disease, and clinicians need to be more aware of the high prevalence of insomnia in HIV-seropositive patients. HIV-positive individuals often contend with a number of psychological stressors and social challenges, such as financial concerns, impaired autonomy, social stigma, multiple bereavements, and numerous other psychosocial stressors. Even with the discovery of newer medications, they must also cope with the complex psychosocial demands of their chronic illness and its treatment. These types of recurrent stressors may affect their sleep and their immune status.

Health care providers need to consider the factors that contribute to impaired sleep in developing effective care for HIV-infected individuals with sleep disturbance. In the context of a chronic illness such as HIV infection, achieving the balance of sleep and wakefulness can be difficult yet crucial.

CHARACTERISTICS OF NORMAL SLEEP

Although sleep appears to be simply a body and mind at rest, it is actually a dynamic and complex physiologic state necessary for survival. Normal sleep is characterized by behavioral and physiologic changes, as well as two distinct sleep states—rapid eye movement (REM) and non–rapid eye movement (NREM). Through the course of a night, people cycle between NREM and REM sleep via an ultradian rhythm, with most sleep spent in NREM. Despite being highly regulated, sleep is fragile and its stages and duration may be affected by multiple factors, such as age, drugs, temperature, and medical and psychiatric disease. Variations in nighttime sleep affect subsequent sleep periods and daytime function.

During sleep, a person's response to or engagement in his or her surroundings is diminished but not completely absent. This reduced consciousness coupled with rapid reversibility distinguishes sleep from death, coma, and hibernation.

Activity in the parasympathetic nervous system is increased during most of sleep, while sympathetic nervous system activity is similar to that of wakefulness, except for periods of REM sleep. Breathing becomes irregular and even periodic in sleep. Control of body temperature is altered; during NREM sleep, body temperature is set and maintained at a lower temperature than during wakefulness. Temperature control seizes almost entirely during REM sleep.

NREM AND REM SLEEP

During sleep, a person alternates between NREM and REM sleep.[1] This NREM-REM cycle is hypothesized to be controlled by an ultradian process that lasts approximately 90 to 120 minutes. The NREM-REM cycle occurs 3 to 6 times per night in normal nocturnal sleep, with biologic sleep needs being about 8 hours on average.

During NREM sleep, cognitive activity is typically fragmented and body activity periodically occurs as a person moves through the four stages of NREM sleep, each of which is defined along electroencephalographic measures. Stage 1 lasts for 1 to 7 minutes, occurs primarily at the onset of sleep, and serves as a transitional stage throughout sleep. After stage 1 a person enters stage 2, which last 1 to 25 minutes. During stage 2, sleep spindles and k complexes occur periodically. As stage 2 progresses, high-voltage, slow-wave activity increases to the point of becoming stage 3. In the first sleep cycle the duration of stage 3 lasts only a few minutes, with the onset of stage 4 occurring as high-voltage, slow-wave activity continues to increase. When high-voltage, slow-wave activity accounts for more than 50% of the electroencephalogram (EEG), a person has entered stage 4 and stays there for 20 to 40 minutes in the first sleep cycle. Stages 3 and 4 are sometimes referred to collectively as slow-wave, delta, or deep sleep.

Unlike in NREM sleep, during REM sleep the brain exhibits fast encephalographic activity, with the body almost paralyzed except for a few muscle twitches. Thus encephalographic activation, skeletal muscle atonia, bursts of autonomic activity, and episodes of REM characterize REM sleep. The first one third of sleep is spent primarily in NREM stages 3 and 4, and the last one third is spent primarily in REM. Although a sleeping person cycles between NREM and REM every 1.5 to 2 hours, the time spent in these different sleep states is not equal. Most (75% to 85%) of sleep is spent in NREM sleep; the other 20% to 25% of sleep is REM.

DETERMINANTS OF SLEEP

In the brain, sleep and wakefulness are controlled via the hypothalamus through the ventrolateral preoptic nucleus (VLPO) and the posterior lateral hypothalamus, respectively. Within the hypothalamus the VLPO has been identified as containing γ-aminobutyric acid (GABA) and galanin neurons, which are necessary for normal sleep.[2] During sleep, the VLPO neurons have been found to fire twice as much as in the awake state. In animals with lesions in the VLPO cluster, duration of sleep was diminished by about 50%.[2]

Wakefulness appears to be mediated by hypocretin (also termed orexin) neurons contained in the posterior lateral hypothalamus. These neurons appear to inhibit the VLPO neurons, thereby establishing a feedback loop that offers two stable patterns, wakefulness and sleep. If either set of neurons fail to fire at its normal rate, instability occurs, with insomnia and/or daytime sleepiness. Hypocretin was discovered in 1998, and its role in sleep and narcolepsy was identified in 2001. As of yet, undiscovered transmitters are undoubtedly involved in sleep control. Most individuals with narcolepsy and cataplexy exhibit about a 90% decrease in the number of hypocretin cells.[3]

INSOMNIA

Insomnia is a pervasive condition with various causes, manifestations, and health consequences. Regardless of the initial cause, or event that precipitates insomnia, it is perpetuated into a chronic condition through learned behaviors and cognitions that foster sleeplessness.

Insomnia comprises various manifestations of sleep disturbances and has numerous origins. For some patients, insomnia consists of inadequate sleep duration at night, whereas others experience poor sleep efficiency or poor sleep quality. Complaints from patients with insomnia include difficulties falling or staying asleep during the night, an inability to fall asleep again after nighttime arousals, and awakening too early in the morning.

Insomnia may be acute or chronic and primary or secondary. Acute insomnia usually lasts less than 1 month and is often directly attributable to known causes, such as jet lag, medications, or poor sleep environment. Insomnia that lasts 1 to 6 months is considered short term or subacute. Chronic insomnia generally lasts more than 6 months and may be recurrent over many years. Primary or intrinsic insomnia is a condition autonomous from other disorders and may be idiopathic. Secondary or extrinsic insomnia is caused by other medical or psychiatric disorders, alcohol or drug dependence, sleep-induced respiratory disorders, movement disorders, circadian rhythm sleep disorders, environmental factors, or parasomnias.[4]

When assessing the patient with sleep disorder, we should start with the simple questions: is your sleep restorative and does sleep or fatigue intrude in your daily activity. We should then establish the duration of the sleep problem and determine whether another condition might be the cause of the sleep complaint, modifies a sleep complaint, or affects possible treatments. Because common sleep disorders are frequently secondary to underlying causes, treatment should be directed at underlying medical, psychiatric, pharmacologic, psychosocial, or other disorders.

The evaluation of chronic sleep complaints should include the following:

1. A detailed history exploring predisposing, precipitating, and perpetuating factors
2. A detailed review of difficulties in falling asleep, maintaining sleep, and awakening early
3. Timing of sleep and wakefulness in a 24-hour day
4. Evidence of excessive daytime sleepiness and fatigue
5. Bedtime routines, sleep settings, preoccupations, anxiety, beliefs about sleep and sleep loss, and fears about consequences of sleep loss
6. Medical and neurologic history and examination, routine laboratory examinations
7. Social and occupational history and level of physical activity
8. A self-report 2-week sleep–wake diary
9. Careful assessment of the use of prescription, nonprescription, and illegal drugs and alcohol and caffeine intake
10. Careful evaluation of any pain complaint
11. Interview with bed partners or persons who observe the patient during sleep, if possible

INSOMNIA IN HIV INFECTION AND POLYSOMNOGRAPHIC CHANGES

The early clinical reports of HIV infection highlighted sleep disturbances as a prominent complaint.[5] Insomnia has been described in all stages of reported HIV illness and may lead to chronic fatigue, reduced physical and social function, and an overall reduction of quality of life.[6] A number of studies have reported on factors thought to contribute to the development of insomnia in people with HIV disease and acquired immunodeficiency syndrome (AIDS). Early investigations were primarily laboratory based, analyzing sleep architecture through the use of polysomnography and with a focus on biologic correlates, in particular central nervous system (CNS) manifestations of HIV infection and altered immune response. This emphasis has subsequently shifted, with epidemiologic studies evaluating subjectively reported insomnia and its associations. As well as the direct effects of HIV infection on sleep, some studies have considered the effects of other variables, including antiretroviral medication, psychiatric illness, and drug and alcohol use.

The most frequently reported change in the sleep profile of HIV-positive subjects has been a significant increase in slow-wave sleep (SWS), particularly during later sleep cycles.[7] It has been suggested that changes in SWS may be dependent on illness progression, although other factors such as age, psychiatric illness, and use of psychotropic medication are potential confounders. One case control study found that CD4 count was a determining factor.[8] Uncontrolled studies suggested an increase in the number of REM periods in HIV-positive subjects, with a reduction in their duration.[9]

Rubinstein and Selwyn[10] found that in 10% of their sample with cognitive impairment, reports of insomnias were universal, and multivariate analysis found that cognitive impairment was the best predictor of insomnia, suggesting an effect of CNS infiltration. A significant association has also been reported with reduced CD8 cells,[11] suggesting that psychological morbidity may influence CD8 count by its effect on sleep quality. Norman et al.[7] proposed that a possible explanation for the observed relationship between HIV infection and sleep disorders may lie in the relationship between immune mediators and sleep. Elevated levels of interferon, tumor necrosis factor, and interlukin-1 have been detected in HIV-seropositive patients.[5] These substances have been shown to affect sleep physiology by enhancing SWS, thereby disrupting normal REM and NREM sleep cycles.

However, whether sleep disruptions experienced by this population are primarily due to immune dysregulation, virus progression, infection, fatigue, depression, stress, side effects of drugs, rigid medication administration times that interfere with normal sleeping hours, other factors, or their cumulative effects remains largely unknown.

ANTIRETROVIRAL THERAPY

The introduction of highly active antiretroviral therapy (HAART) was accompanied by a dramatic decrease in HIV-associated morbidity and mortality. The goal of HAART is to keep the virus at bay by minimizing its level in the bloodstream and thereby decreasing its affect on the immune system. Unfortunately, the immune system and blood circulation are not the only sites in which the virus resides. Early in its course, HIV also has the ability to penetrate the CNS. As a result, psychiatric and neurologic symptoms may be evident despite the absence of an opportunistic infection. In addition, HAART therapy may be associated with certain psychiatric side effects, including interactions with psychotropic medications. Living with HIV and maintenance therapy with HAART is now the norm rather than the exception for HIV-infected patients. However, the drugs included in HAART may be associated with side effects that become severe enough to require treatment modification or even cessation.

Frequent reports of neuropsychiatric complications associated with the non-nucleoside reverse transcriptase inhibitor efavirenz have been the subject of particular scrutiny. Nuñez et al.[12] found a significant difference in case-controlled comparison of insomnia in 51 patients taking efavirenz. A further trial of an antiretroviral regimen including efavirenz versus a protease inhibitor–containing regimen in 100 patients found that 35% of those prescribed efavirenz reported difficulty sleeping compared with 4% in the protease inhibitor group. Patients receiving efavirenz frequently report vivid dreams, difficulty falling asleep, and numerous night awakenings shortly after starting therapy. These symptoms usually appear within the first month of treatment and may be self-limiting, but they often persist for 3 months or longer and disrupt the patient's quality of life.[12]

PSYCHIATRIC DISORDERS

Insomnia is a well-recognized feature of psychological morbidity, and given the prevalence of anxiety and depression reported in HIV infection, it is not surprising that psychiatric disorders are associated with sleep disturbance in this group. Depression is the most common psychiatric disorder for which HIV-infected individuals seek treatments. Lifetime rates of major depression in at-risk cohorts are as high as 22% to 45%.[13] Rates of current depression among HIV-infected patients are at least twice those of the general population. The prevalence rate of current major depression found in studies utilizing structured diagnostic interviews ranges from 4% to 14%, depending on the setting of the risk groups studied. However, these rates may exceed 50% in those seeking psychiatric treatment.

Rabkin et al.[14] in a longitudinal study of 173 HIV-infected men with symptomatic illness assessed semiannually after the initiation of HAART observed a statistically significant, but clinically modest reduction in measures of depression and hopelessness in the sample as a whole. As can be expected, there is a significant association between a diagnoses of major depression and complaints of insomnia.

Anxiety and depression are often comorbid. As with depression, anxiety presents predominantly with somatic symptoms, so the differential diagnostic considerations are central to the context of HIV disease.

ALCOHOL AND SUBSTANCE INDUCED SLEEP DISORDER

Substance abuse disorders figure prominently in the differential diagnosis and management of HIV disease. The treatment of individuals with the triple diagnosis of HIV infection, substance abuse, and psychiatric disorder has multiple levels of complexity, including potentially poor adherence to medical treatment regimens. Although alcohol and illicit drugs are recognized as having a disruptive effect on sleep, few studies have considered their effect in people with HIV disease. Cocaine, amphetamines, caffeine, and nicotine can all have a negative effect on sleep. Addressing the substance-related disorder through different treatment modalities, including counseling, detoxification, group therapy, 12-step program, or drug rehabilitation facility is critical.

PAIN WITH SLEEP COMPLAINTS

Acute pain will cause arousal during sleep and should be treated aggressively with analgesics. Most of these medications have both analgesic and soporific effects; therefore hypnotics are usually not needed.

Medications to treat chronic pain with sleep disturbance include opioid analgesics, hypnotics, muscle relaxants, sedating antidepressants, and anticonvulsants. It is often difficult to determine whether the reduction in sleep disturbance should be attributed to the direct sedating effect of a medication or to a true reduction in the mechanism in which pain may interfere with sleep. Chronic pain that disturbs sleep in HIV-infected patients should be aggressively treated with longer-acting opioids. There is some evidence that light exercise should be encouraged for patients with chronic pain and sleep disturbance. Unfortunately, many chronic pain sufferers cannot even begin a program of light exercise because their symptoms are so disabling.

Cognitive-behavioral therapy is also used to treat chronic pain with sleep complaints. A variety of methods may be involved, including progressive muscle relaxation, guided imagery, biofeedback, stimulus control, hypnotherapy, and restriction of time in bed. These methods have been used to manage chronic insomnia, but may help to manage pain if a sleep disturbance is exacerbating the pain.

CURRENT TREATMENT PRACTICES

Despite the existence of several treatment options for insomnia, people who experience sleep difficulties usually start with passive strategies. Many people with insomnia report that they do nothing except lie in bed, tossing and turning, waiting for sleep to come. The next step for most is self-medication with alcohol, over-the-counter sleep aids, or natural herbal dietary supplements. If people with insomnia eventually seek medical help for their condition, they are generally prescribed a hypnotic drug. However, nonpharmacologic treatments such as behavioral and psychological interventions should be considered. Hypnotics may be contraindicated by the use of other medications in patients with high susceptibility to substance abuse or addiction.

Cognitive-behavioral therapy for insomnia targets factors that perpetuate insomnia over time.[7] The first step of cognitive-behavioral therapy is to modify poor sleep habits. People with chronic insomnia often not only maintain maladaptive sleep habits but also engage in a fairly irregular sleep schedule. An important first step is to regulate sleep–wake schedules. Faulty beliefs and attitudes about sleep also must be corrected through information and education.

Although sleep disturbances are usually caused by an initial stressor or illness, true insomnia is generally the result of maladaptive behaviors that continue beyond the original precipitating event. Stimulus control consists of the following seven simple instructions that help the patient reassociate sleep stimuli with proper behavior and encourage the establishment of a consistent sleep–wake schedule:

1. Go to bed only when sleepy. Extra time spent in bed only heightens arousal by causing more intrusive thoughts, worry, and frustration about the inability to sleep.
2. Use the bed or bedroom only for sleep. Associating this setting with only sleep will help prompt sleepiness.
3. Get out of bed when unable to sleep. If the patient is unable to fall asleep after 15 minutes spent in bed, he or she should go to another room and engage in some quiet activity (reading, watching TV, listening to the radio).
4. Arising at the same time every morning will help reestablish synchronized circadian rhythms.
5. Do not nap during the day because it will only perpetuate the cycle of irregular circadian rhythms and make it difficult to fall asleep at the desired bedtime.
6. Avoid large meals before bedtime.
7. Practice evening relaxation techniques, such as meditation.

Cognitive-behavioral therapy shows the patient with chronic insomnia how to identify behavioral and psychological factors over which the patient can exercise some control. In general, this form of therapy helps to change the underlying ideas that perpetuate insomnia.

Sleep hygiene can address some of the factors that play a large role in sleep disturbances. Caffeine and all stimulants should be avoided after dinner. Avoid smoking near bedtime and upon waking at night. Do not drink alcohol in the late evening, and do not exercise close to bedtime. Regular exercise in the late afternoon or early evening may deepen sleep. Also, minimize noise, light, and excessive temperatures.

Cognitive-behavioral therapy offers a safe, effective alternative to pharmacologic treatment and has shown success as an augmentation of hypnotic drug treatment. Sleep diaries play a vital role in the assessment and treatment of insomnia, providing valuable information to both the patient and physicians.

PHARMACOLOGIC TREATMENTS

Before starting pharmacologic therapy, all possible causes of insomnia should be examined. Before selecting a specific hypnotic the clinician should consider the pharmacologic properties, side effect profiles, and patient's medical history, including the history of sedative hypnotic use. A useful initial approach to the patient with insomnia is to consider the duration of the complaint. The duration of insomnia not only suggests its cause but also provides some guidance of how to best use hypnotics. The most appropriate use of drugs is in patients whose sleep disturbance is clearly causing some daytime dysfunction. It is always helpful to start with the lowest dose of hypnotic possible and to try to avoid daily use. The most important pharmacologic properties to consider when selecting a hypnotic for treatment are how quickly it acts and how long the effects will last.

SEDATIVE-HYPNOTICS

Barbiturates

The main effects of barbiturates are sedation, sleep induction, and anesthesia. Barbiturates decrease sleep latency; however, they slightly increase fast electroencephalographic activity during sleep. Stages 3 and 4 generally decrease REM, sleep latency is prolonged, and both the total time spent in REM sleep and the number of REM cycles are diminished. Tolerance and dependence occur rapidly as a result of both pharmacokinetics and pharmacodynamic factors. The risks of barbiturates outweigh their benefits, and they should be avoided in HIV-infected patients.

Barbiturates compare poorly with benzodiazepines and have life-threatening withdrawal reactions. Abrupt discontinuation after high dosage is likely to induce convulsions and delirium. Barbiturates may increase the activity of hepatic microsomal enzymes 2- to 3-fold.

Benzodiazepines

Most of the benzodiazepines available were selected for their high anxiolytic potential. Nevertheless, all benzodiazepines have sedative-hypnotic properties to various degrees, and some compounds that facilitate sleep are used as hypnotics.

Benzodiazepines are powerful potentiators of GABA. They are generally absorbed rapidly and completely, and because they are also very lipophilic they penetrate rapidly into the brain.

The hypnotic effects of benzodiazepines have been suggested to result from the modulatory effects of the GABAergic system on the raphe and locus ceruleus monoaminergic projections. Most benzodiazepines decrease sleep latency, and all benzodiazepines increase time spent in stage 2 sleep. Stages 3 and 4 are suppressed, and the decrease in stage 4 sleep is accompanied by reduction in nightmares. Most benzodiazepines increase REM latency.

The most frequently prescribed hypnotics are flurazepam (Dalmane), quazepam (Doral), estazolam (ProSom), temazepam (Restoril), and triazolam (Halcion). Typically, benzodiazepine-hypnotics with short to intermediate half-lives are preferred. Lorazepam, temazepam, and triazolam are the most commonly prescribed. These hypnotics bypass the hepatic oxidative pathways and are theoretically safest to prescribe in patients receiving protease inhibitors (ketoconazole, itraconazole, macrolide antibiotics, and any other drugs that inhibit the cytochrome P [CYP] 450 3A4 isoform). All three disrupt sleep architecture. It is best to use the benzodiazepines after two or three consecutive nights of poor sleep. When insomnia is severe and refractory to nonpharmacologic approaches, any of these three benzodiazepines could be prescribed for bedtime. These medications should be avoided in the middle of the night or in combination with alcohol.

Short-acting benzodiazepines are specifically associated with rebound insomnia, daytime anxiety, and early morning wakefulness. Lorazepam and triazolam have been associated with amnesia. Alprazolam, triazolam, estazolam, and midazolam should be specifically avoided in patients receiving protease inhibitors. Habituation is common, as well as tolerance and physical dependence, with marked withdrawal syndrome, which can be life threatening. Estazolam (ProSom) is another triazolobenzodiazepine similar to Halcion, except it has a longer half-life. As with other triazolobenzodiazepines, it should be avoided with protease inhibitors.

Quazepam (Doral) is a selective benzodiazepine receptor agonist with a long half-life and hangover effect. It should be avoided because of its longer half-life.

Nonbenzodiazepine Hypnotics

Zolpidem (Ambien) is a nonbenzodiazepine sedative hypnotic. Although chemically unrelated to other hypnotics such as the benzodiazepines or barbiturates, zolpidem does share some pharmacologic actions with these drugs. It interacts with the GABA benzodiazepine reception complex by binding to the omega-1 receptor. Although not absolute, the relative selectivity of zolpidem for the type 1 omega receptor subtype may explain its lack of anxiolytic, muscle relaxant, and anticonvulsant effects at normally prescribed hypnotic dosages. Sleep studies in animals and humans indicate that zolpidem normally preserves deep sleep (stages 3 and 4) and that any minor changes in REM sleep occur only inconsistently. As with benzodiazepines, flumazenil, a benzodiazepine antagonist, can antagonize the sedative actions of zolpidem. The mean half-life in healthy patients is 2.2 hours. Zolpidem's half-life is significantly increased to an average of 9.9 hours, necessitating dosage reductions in the hepatically impaired.

Zolpidem is primarily a substrate of CYP3A4, an isoenzyme of the CYP450 system. Clinically significant interactions may be considered with concurrent use of CYP3A4 inhibitors and inducers. Nevirapine (Viramune) might decrease the plasma concentration of certain highly metabolized sedatives and hypnotics as a result of induction of CYP450 enzymes, including zolpidem. Delavirdine (Rescriptor) and Ritonavir (Norvir) are potent inhibitors of CYP450 3A4 and are expected to inhibit zolpidem CYP3A4 metabolism, leading to large increases in zolpidem plasma concentrations. Excessive sedation and possible respiratory depression can occur. Zolpidem has no active metabolites and appears to be safer than the benzodiazepines. Dose-dependent side effects overlap with those of the benzodiazepines, except there is no evidence for acute withdrawal syndrome. It should be used with caution in neurologically symptomatic patients. Zolpidem is safe in patients with renal impairment. The usual dosage of zolpidem is 5 to 10 mg at bedtime.

Zaleplon (Sonata) is a short-acting, nonbenzodiazepine sedative hypnotic. It belongs to a new class of drugs known as pyrazolopyrimidines. Zaleplon possesses anticonvulsant, anxiolytic, hypnotic, and muscle relaxant properties. It has been shown to decrease the time to sleep onset compared to zolpidem, and it has a faster onset of action and a shorter elimination half-life.

Zaleplon is an agonist at type 1 benzodiazepine (BZ1 or omega 1) receptors on the GABA-A/chloride ion channel complex within the CNS. Zaleplon is administered orally and has extensive first-pass metabolism. The onset of action is approximately 30 minutes, and the duration of action is about 4 hours. Zaleplon is primarily metabolized by aldehyde oxidize to form 5-oxo-zaleplon. To a lesser extent, zaleplon is metabolized by the hepatic isoenzyme CYP3A4 and all its metabolites are inactive. Antiretroviral protease inhibitors may increase the levels of zaleplon, although clinical data do not exist and this interaction is not expected to require routine zaleplon dosage adjustment. The usual recommended dosage for zaleplon is 5 to 20 mg at bed time.

Eszopiclone (Lunesta), a nonbenzodiazepine hypnotic agent that is a pyrrolopyrazine derivative of the cyclopyrrolone class, was just recently introduced into the market. This medication is rapidly absorbed, with a time to peak concentration of approximately 1 hour and an elimination half-life of approximately 6 hours. It is weakly protein bound, so it should not be affected by drug interactions caused by protein binding.

Eszopiclone is metabolized by CYP3A4 and CYP2E1 via demethylation and oxidation. Eszopiclone is not expected to alter the clearance of drugs metabolized by common CYP450 enzymes. Inhibitors of CYP3A4 will result in an increase in the levels of eszopiclone. Clinical experience with eszopiclone in patients with concomitant illness is limited. The recommended dosage for eszopiclone is 1 to 3 mg before bedtime.

Antidepressants

Tricyclic antidepressants (TCAs) have variable sedative-hypnotic effects. Amitriptyline and doxepin are the most frequently prescribed. TCAs suppress REM sleep, and their sedating properties correlate with their antihistaminic effect.

Trazodone (Desyrel) has little anticholinergic effect and no effect on seizure threshold, making it preferable to doxepin or amitriptyline. There is no reported development of tolerance, addiction, or abuse. Priapism (including clitoral priapism) has been reported, although rare, in some patients. Trazodone is a substrate of CYP2D6 and CYP3A4.

Coadministration with inhibitors of this enzyme may lead to substantial increases in trazodone plasma concentration, with the potential for adverse effects. CNS depressants should be used cautiously in patients receiving trazodone because of additive CNS depressant effect, including possible respiratory depression or hypotension. Delaviridine (Rescriptor), a potent inhibitor of CYP2D6, might decrease the metabolism of trazodone. Indinavir (Crixivan) may also lead to an increase in trazodone plasma concentration. Ritonavir (Norvir) can decrease trazodone clearance significantly. The usual treatment dosage for insomnia is 25 to 200 mg before bedtime.

Mirtazapine (Remeron) has sedating and appetite stimulating effects. At low doses of 7.5 to 15 mg it may help patients with severe insomnia. Mirtazapine is not a potent inhibitor of CYP450. There are no clinically significant pharmacokinetic interactions with medications metabolized by CYP enzymes. It has a relatively low affinity for CYP450 isoform, so it is theoretically safe to combine with protease inhibitors.

Nefazodone (Serzone) has specific restorative effects on sleep architecture without causing sedation. Monitoring of liver function is essential if this medication is prescribed. In general, nefazodone is not recommended for use with triazolam or alprazolam. Nefazodone inhibits the hepatic CYP3A4 isoenzyme and substantially increases the plasma concentrations of these drugs.

Antiretroviral agents may interact with nefazodone. Nefazodone inhibits the metabolism of efavirenz (Sustiva) and nevirapine (Viramune) through inhibition of the CYP3A4 isoenzyme. Ritonavir (Viracept) and delaviridine (Rescriptor) are potent inhibitors of nefazodone metabolism.

Antihistamine

Hydroxyzine (Atarax) is preferred over diphenhydramine (Benadryl) in HIV disease. It has a minimal anticholinergic effect, therefore is less likely to induce or aggravate HIV-related cognitive impairment.

Chloral Hydrate

Chloral hydrate is a CNS depressant that is extensively metabolized by the liver. It should be used with caution in patients with hepatic disease or severe or moderate renal impairment. Adverse CNS effects during chloral hydrate therapy include sleep walking. Patients receiving chloral hydrate may develop tolerance, and symptoms of dependence are similar to those of chronic alcoholism. Sudden withdrawal may produce delirium tremens and hallucinations in patients physically dependent on chloral hydrate. It offers no advantages in patients with HIV disease over benzodiazepines and generally should be avoided.

SUMMARY

Quality of life issues are becoming more important for persons living with HIV disease. As HIV disease becomes increasingly chronic, with longer life spans predicted for persons who receive optimal medical monitoring and management, there should be further research to identify the degree to which health status can be improved by improvements in sleep and overall well-being.

There is evidence that insomnia is associated with substantial functional impairment and greater use of health care services independent of the effects of medical comorbidity or psychiatric disorder. Further research can help to determine whether insomnia adds significantly to the burden of disability in HIV disease and AIDS, particularly in otherwise asymptomatic patients. Psychological morbidity is a major determinant of insomnia in asymptomatic infection, but the role of a number of variables such as immune dysregulation, virus progression, and adverse drug effects deserve further study. Epidemiologic studies would be of value in clarifying these questions, particularly in samples representing the changing demographic of the seropositive population.

A high proportion of patients receiving sleep medications or other techniques to enhance sleep report benefits. This suggests that clinicians need to be more aware of the high prevalence of insomnia in HIV-seropositive patients while at the same time addressing adequate symptom relief. The impact of insomnia on functioning and quality of life also merits further attention.

REFERENCES

1. Carskadon M, Dement W. Normal human sleep: an overview. In: Kryger MH, Roth T, Dement WC, eds. *Principles and Practices of Sleep Medicine*. 3rd ed. Philadelphia: WB Saunders; 2000:15–25.
2. Saper CB, Chou TC, Scammell TE. The sleep switch: hypothalamic control of sleep and wakefulness. *Trends Neurosci*. 2001;24:726–731.
3. Thannickal TC, Moore RY, Nienhuis R, et al. Reduced number of hypocretin neurons in human narcolepsy. *Neuron*. 2000;27:469–474.
4. Morin CM, Espie CA. *Insomnia: A Clinical Guide to Assessment and Treatment*. New York: Kluwer Academic/Plenum Publishers; 2003.
5. Norman SE, Resnick L, Cohn MA, et al. Sleep disturbances in HIV-seropositive patients. *JAMA*. 1988;260:922.
6. Simon GE, VonKorff M. Prevalence, burden, and treatment of insomnia in primary care. *Am J Psychiatry*. 1997;154:1417–1423.
7. Norman S, Shaukat M, Nay KN, Cohn M, Resnick L. Alterations in sleep architecture in asymptomatic HIV seropositive patients. *Sleep Res*. 1987;16:494.
8. White JL, Darko DF, Brown SJ, et al. Early central nervous system response to HIV infection: sleep distortion and cognitive-motor decrements. *AIDS*. 1995;9:1043–1050.
9. Norman SE, Chediak A, Kiel M, Gazeroglu H, Mendez A. HIV infection and sleep: follow up studies. *Sleep Res*. 1990;19:339.
10. Rubinstein ML, Selwyn PA. High prevalence of insomnia in an outpatient population with HIV infection. *J Acquir Immun Defic Syndr Human Retrovirol*. 1998;19:260–265.
11. Cruess DG, Antoni MH, Gonzalez J, et al. Sleep disturbance mediates the association between psychological distress and immune status among HIV-positive men and women on combination antiretroviral therapy. *J Psychosom Res*. 2003;54:185–189.
12. Nuñez M, de Requena DG, Gallego L, et al. Higher efavirenz plasma levels correlated with development of insomnia. *J Acquir Immune Defic Syndr Human Retrovirol*. 2001;28:399.
13. Penzak SR, Reddy YS, Grimsley SR. Depression in patients with HIV infection. *Am J Health Syst Pharm*. 2000;57:376–386.
14. Rabkin JG, Ferrando SJ, Lin SH, Sewell M, McElhiney M. Psychological effects of HAART: a 2 year study. *Psychosom Med*. 2000;62:413–422.

SECTION IV

Medical Comorbidity

CHAPTER 16

Psychotropic Drug Interactions with Antiretroviral Medications

Philip A. Bialer, Kyle S. Kato, Vassilios Latoussakis

With the Food and Drug Administration (FDA) approval and release of saquinavir in December of 1995, and the subsequent approval and release of two more protease inhibitors in early 1996, the age of highly active antiretroviral therapy (HAART) transformed the medical management of patients with human immunodeficiency virus (HIV) infection and acquired immunodeficiency syndrome (AIDS). The early 1990s also brought a more complete understanding of the way medications were metabolized, particularly the process of oxidative metabolism by the cytochrome P (CYP) 450 enzyme system. When reports of serious interactions between two relatively benign medications such as erythromycin and terfenadine surfaced, the importance of more complete knowledge of the pharmacokinetics of commonly used medications became clear. Possibly for more than any other type of patient, the practitioner treating those with HIV infection or AIDS needs to be very aware of the potential for drug–drug interactions because of the large number of medications often prescribed by multiple providers that these patients could be taking. This chapter examines the drug–drug interactions, reported and potential, that are most likely to be encountered by patients being dually treated for HIV and mental health problems.

BASIC PHARMACOLOGY

To fully understand how drugs interact, it will be helpful to review some basic pharmacologic principles and mechanisms. First, the clinician must differentiate between pharmacodynamic and pharmacokinetic interactions. Pharmacodynamic interactions refer to one drug's influence on another drug's effect at the intended receptor site. For example, the opioid agonist methadone blocks the effects of administered heroin by occupying all available opioid receptors. Pharmacokinetic interactions refer to the effect of one drug on the movement throughout the body of another drug—meaning absorption, distribution, metabolism, or excretion of the drug. Although drug–drug interactions affecting any of these steps can produce serious results, there has been increasing attention on interactions involving drug metabolism; this chapter focuses primarily on these interactions.

Phase I metabolism, in which drugs are oxidized, is mainly mediated by the CYP450 system. Although most drugs are inactivated during this process, some have pharmacologically active metabolites and some prodrugs must be oxidized before they become active. There are over 40 CYP450 enzymes found in humans that may be involved in metabolizing both endogenous and exogenous materials, but only 6 of these enzymes are responsible for 90% of drug metabolism: 1A2, 3A4, 2C9, 2C19, 2D6, and 2E1. After oxidation, some drugs may be excreted in the bile or feces, but most undergo phase II metabolism or conjugation for excretion in the urine. Glucuronidation accounts for most phase II metabolism and is mediated by uridine 5'-diphosphate glucuronosyltransferase (UGT) enzymes. As with CYP450 enzymes, there are many UGTs, but UGT2B7 accounts for the majority of glucuronidation. Some drugs, such as lorazepam, oxazepam, temazepam, lamotrigine, valproate, nonsteroidal anti-inflammatory agents, most opiates, and zidovudine are primarily metabolized by UGT enzymes without undergoing any oxidation. CYP450 enzymes and UGTs are found throughout the body, but primarily in the liver and gut wall.[1]

Some drug–drug interactions occur when the metabolic process is either inhibited or induced. Metabolic inhibition leads to a prolonged pharmacologic effect and may lead to drug toxicity. In the case of a prodrug that must be metabolized to be effective, inhibition may have an opposite effect and lead to inactivity. Inhibition usually occurs when two drugs have an affinity for a particular metabolic enzyme, with the more tightly bound drug inhibiting the other, and occurs fairly quickly. Metabolic induction usually involves the synthesis of more metabolic proteins, making more sites available for metabolism and thus increasing the rate of drug inactivation. The induction process takes longer to occur than inhibition and may lead to subtherapeutic levels of a drug. For patients on HAART, this can have an extremely negative impact if subtherapeutic levels of one drug allow for the development of viral drug resistance. Both phase I and phase II enzymes can be inhibited or induced.[1]

TAKING A DRUG HISTORY

In approaching a patient with respect to drug–drug interactions, the first step is to determine all of the medications that a person is taking. This includes prescriptions drugs, over-the-counter medications, supplements, alternative medications, nonprescription psychoactive substances, and foods. Because these patients may be taking a large number of medications, they are not always fully aware of all the names and dosages, so it is helpful to have them bring their medications to the office and/or get corroborating information. In addition to antiretrovirals, patients with HIV disease or AIDS are most often taking additional medications for intercurrent infections and other medical problems, prophylaxis against opportunistic infections, and nutritional supplements or herbal remedies; any one of these may have potential interactions with psychotropics. A large proportion of patients in this population also have past and current histories of substance use, and some illicit drugs can have potentially serious interactions with AIDS medications and psychotropics. One should try to obtain this information in a nonthreatening way so the patient can be educated about these dangers.

PROTEASE INHIBITORS

All protease inhibitors (PIs) are metabolized primarily by CYP3A4, and all PIs can competitively inhibit 3A4 metabolism to some degree.[2] However, ritonavir is by far the most potent inhibitor of 3A4 among the PIs and has caused the most concern about potential drug–drug

TABLE 16.1	Antiretrovirals: Metabolism, CYP450 Enzyme Inhibition, and Induction		
Drug	**Metabolism Site(s)**	**Enzyme(s) Inhibited**	**Enzyme(s) Induced**
Protease Inhibitors			
Amprenavir (Agenerase)	3A4	3A4[b]	None known
Indinavir (Crixivan)	3A4	**3A4**[a]	None known
Lopinavir/ritonavir (Kaletra)	3A4	**3A4**,[a] 2D6[1]	3A4, UGT (phase II)
Nelfinavir (Viracept)	3A4, 2C19	3A4,[c] 1A2, 2B6[1]	?2C9
Ritonavir (Norvir)	3A4, 2D6[2]	**3A4**,[a] **2D6**,[a] **2C9**,[a] **2C19**,[a] 2B6[1]	**3A4**,[a] 1A2,[b] 2C9,[b] 2C19, UGT
Saquinavir (Invirase)	3A4	3A4[c]	None known
Non-nucleoside Reverse Transcriptase Inhibitors (NNRTIs)			
Delavirdine (Rescriptor)	3A4, 2D6, 2C9,[2] 2C19[2]	**3A4**,[a] 2C9,[1] 2C19,[1] 2D6[1]	None known
Efavirenz (Sustiva)	3A4, 2B6	**3A4**,[a] 2C9,[1] 2C19,[1] 2B6[1]	3A4,[b] 2B6[c]
Nevirapine (Viramune)	3A4, 2B6	None known	3A4,[b] 2B6[b]
NRTIs			
Abacavir (Ziagen)	Alcohol dehydrogenase, UGT	None known	None known
Didanosine (ddI, Videx)	Purine nucleoside phosphorylase	Unknown	Unknown
Emtricitabine (Emtriva)	Full recovery in urine and feces	None known	None known
Lamivudine (3TC, Epivir)	Minimal metabolism	None known	None known
Stavudine (d4T, Zerit)	Not yet known	None known	None known
Tenofovir (Viread)	Renal	1A2[a]	None known
Zalcitabine (ddC, Hivid)	Renal		
Zidovudine (AZT, Retrovir)	UGT 2B7, CYP450 b5		None known

[1]Inhibited in vitro.
[2]Minor pathway.
[a]Potent (**bold** type).
[b]Moderate.
[c]Mild.
This table was adapted from two tables by the same authors. Reprinted with permission from *Concise Guide to Drug Interaction Principles for Medical Practice: Cytochrome P450s, UGTs, P-Glycoproteins*, 2e (Copyright 2003). Washington, DC: American Psychiatric Publishing, Inc.; and *Psychosomatics*, Washington, DC: American Psychiatric Publishing; 2004.

interactions (Table 16.1). The triazolobenzodiazepines alprazolam, midazolam, and triazolam are metabolized by 3A4, and coadministration with ritonavir can lead to higher serum levels of these drugs, with resulting oversedation and respiratory distress. Other psychotropics that are substrates for 3A4 include trazodone, fluvoxamine, and nefazodone, and coadministration of these drugs with ritonavir can result in toxicity. After several weeks, ritonavir can also induce 3A4 metabolism and actually decrease the efficacy of the psychotropic medications already mentioned.

Ritonavir is also a moderately potent inhibitor of CYP2D6, which is the primary metabolic enzyme for many psychotropic medications. Therefore it is necessary to monitor serum tricyclic antidepressant levels in patients taking both of these drugs and to monitor carefully for side effects in patients taking selective serotonin reuptake inhibitors (SSRIs) and most neuroleptics. Ritonavir also inhibits 2C9 and 2C19 and induces 1A2, 2C9, and 2C19 (Table 16.1). Ritonavir can have multiple effects on the CYP450 enzyme system, so it is imperative to review the specific contraindications and warnings for any patient taking this medication before prescribing additional medications. The clinician must also remember that Kaletra is composed of lopinavir and ritonavir, although the lower dose of ritonavir in this formulation may preclude some of the potential drug–drug interactions. Similarly, ritonavir must always be given along with the newly approved tipranavir so the same cautions and contraindications apply for this drug.

Because all of the PIs are CYP3A4 substrates, medications that inhibit or induce this enzyme can also cause potentially serious interactions (Table 16.2). Nefazodone is a potent CYP3A4 inhibitor and can result in PI toxicity. Carbamazepine, phenobarbital, St. John's wort, and phenytoin are inducers of 3A4 and can potentially decrease PIs to subtherapeutic serum levels. Chronic alcohol use can also induce CYP3A4.

NON-NUCLEOTIDE REVERSE TRANSCRIPTASE INHIBITORS

The non-nucleotide reverse transcriptase inhibitors (NNRTIs) bind directly and noncompetitively to the reverse transcriptase enzyme to inhibit it and prevent viral replication. They are commonly a component of HAART. Delavirdine may be the least used of the NNRTIs, but it is important to know that it is a potent inhibitor of CYP3A4, 2C9, 2C19, and 2D6 and can interact with many of the same medications as ritonavir. Nevirapine is more commonly used and induces 3A4.[3] Case reports and clinical experience have demonstrated an increased rate of metabolism of methadone among patients taking nevirapine, requiring an upward adjustment of the methadone dose.[4] Efavirenz has more complex effects on the CYP450 system by both inhibiting and then inducing 3A4. It also has some inhibitory effects on 2C9, 2C19, 2D6, and 1A2, resulting in a drug interaction profile similar to that of ritonavir (Table 16.1). Patients on methadone maintenance taking efavirenz may also need their dose adjusted upward.

NUCLEOSIDE REVERSE TRANSCRIPASE INHIBITORS, FUSION INHIBITORS

These nucleoside reverse transcriptase inhibitors (NRTIs) are analogs of the nucleotide building blocks of DNA and RNA and inhibit the reverse transcriptase enzyme by being incorporated into the viral DNA at a key point, thus preventing viral replication. None of these drugs are metabolized by the CYP450 system, but they undergo metabolism by intracellular enzymes and/or glucuronidation. Zidovudine (AZT) is metabolized by UGT2B7, and some UGT inhibitors, such as valproate and methadone, have been reported to increase serum levels of AZT, resulting in toxicity. Otherwise, there do not appear to be any other potential interactions between this class of drugs and psychotropic medications. The fusion inhibitor enfuvirtide also has no significant CYP450 or UGT interactions.

TABLE 16.2 Psychotropic Medications That Are Potent Inhibitors or Inducers of CYP3A4	
3A4 Inhibitors	**3A4 Inducers**
Nefazodone	Carbamazepine
Fluvoxamine	Phenytoin
	Phenobarbital
	St. John's wort

OTHER MEDICATIONS USED IN HIV TREATMENT

Although it is not within the scope of this chapter to examine the drug–drug interactions of all the possible medications a patient with HIV disease or AIDS could be taking, there are a few instances in which special precautions should be taken. Given for intercurrent infections such as community-acquired pneumonia, clarithromycin (Biaxin) is a potent CYP3A4 inhibitor and can cause increased serum levels of many of the same medications as ritonavir, such as the triazolobenzodiazepines. Azithromycin (Zithromax) is a mild CYP3A4 inhibitor and can probably be used safely with most psychotropics. Patients may be taking antifungal agents for oral thrush. Of these, both ketoconazole (Nizoral) and itraconazole (Sporanox) are potent CYP3A4 inhibitors. Ketoconazole (Diflucan) has moderate 3A4 inhibition activity, so psychotropics metabolized by this enzyme should be used in lower doses or not at all. Patients with HIV disease or AIDS may be at higher risk for the development of tuberculosis. Two antituberculosis drugs, rifampin and rifabutin, are potent CYP3A4 inducers that may result in lower serum levels of psychotropics metabolized by 3A4 when these drugs are coadministered. Of particular concern would be withdrawal reactions among patients taking methadone.

Fortunately, most of the other nonantiretroviral medications that patients with HIV disease and AIDS may be taking, such as acyclovir, atovaquone (Mepron), or sulfamethoxazole/trimethoprim (SMX/TMP; Bactrim) have no psychotropic drug interactions reported.

The remainder of the chapter examines the metabolism of psychotropics and the ways specific drugs may interact when given to patients receiving HAART. Table 16.3 summarizes the interactions.

ANXIOLYTICS AND SEDATIVE HYPNOTICS

Three benzodiazepines—lorazepam, temazepam, and oxazepam—undergo glucuronidation primarily, have no active metabolites, and are associated with few drug–drug interactions. They have no drug interactions with antiretrovirals. They may also be preferred for patients who have compromised liver function from hepatitis C, a common comorbidity in HIV-infected patients.

The other benzodiazepines are metabolized by CYP3A4. Triazolam, alprazolam, and midazolam are the most sensitive to inhibition of this enzyme and should be used with extreme caution by patients taking medications that are potent or moderate inhibitors. Clonazepam, diazepam, estazolam, and flurazepam may also be affected by CYP3A4 inhibition. The anxiolytic buspirone is also primarily metabolized by CYP3A4, so its serum levels will be affected by 3A4 inhibitors and inducers. Diphenhydramine and hydroxyzine are antihistamines that are sometimes used as anxiolytics; neither of these has reported interactions with antiretrovirals.

There are mixed reports regarding the safety of concurrently prescribing PIs and zolpidem, which is partially metabolized by CYP3A4. Ritonavir inhibits zolpidem metabolism 22% less than it inhibits triazolam metabolism.[5] There were no drug interactions reported between zaleplon or chloral hydrate and antiretroviral medications (Table 16.3).

Among the barbiturates, phenobarbital induces 3A4 as well as other CYP450 enzymes and may decrease serum concentration and antiviral efficacy of the PIs or the NNRTIs. Its use is not recommended for patients receiving HAART. There are no drug interactions reported between other barbiturates and antiretrovirals.

ANTIDEPRESSANTS

Antidepressant side effects and a patient's profile should be considered before medication selection. Decreased side effects lead to improved adherence to medication treatment. Common side effects of PIs and SSRIs include nausea, vomiting, fatigue, and sexual dysfunction; a

TABLE 16.3 Antiretroviral/Psychotropic Drug–Drug Interactions

	Protease Inhibitors						NNRTI		
	Amprenavir	Atazanavir	Indinavir	Nelfinavir	Ritonavir	Saquinavir	Delavirdine	Efavirenz	Nevirapine
Mood Stabilizers									
Lithium	+	+	+	+	+	+	+	+	+
Carbamazepine	++++	++++	++++	++++	++++	++++	++++	++++	+++
Gabapentin	+	+	+	+	+	+	+	+	+
Lamotrigine	+	+	+	+	++	+	+	+	+
Oxcarbazepine	++	++	++	++	++	++	++	+	++
Topiramate	+	+	+	+	+	+	+	+	+
Valproate	+	+	+	+	++	+	+	+	+
Antidepressants									
Tricyclics	++++	++++	+++	+++	++++	+++	++++	+++	++
Duloxetine	+	++	+	++	++	+	++	++	+
Venlafaxine	+	++	++	+	++	+	++	+	+
Citalopram	+	+	+	+	+++	+	++	+	+
Escitalopram	+	+	+	+	+++	+	+++	+	+
Fluoxetine	++	++	++	++	+++	++	+++	+++	++
Fluvoxamine	+++	+++	+++	+++	+++	++	+++	+++	+++
Paroxetine	+	+	+	+	++	+	++	+	+
Sertraline	+	++	++	++	++	+	++	+	+
Bupropion	++	++	++	++	+++	+	++	++	++
Mirtazapine	+	+	+	+	++	+	++	+	+
Nefazodone	++++	++++	++++	++++	++++	++++	++++	++++	++++
Trazodone	++	++	++	++	+++	++	+++	++	++

Antipsychotics								
Haloperidol	+			++		++		++
Thioridazine	++	++		++	++	++		+ ++
Pimozide	+++++	+++	+++++	+++++	+++++	+++++	++	+++
Clozapine	+++	++	+++	+++	+++	+++	+++	++
Olanzapine	++	++	++	++	++	++	++	+
Risperidone	++	++	++	++	++	++	++	+
Aripiprazole	++	++	++	++	++	++	++	+
Quetiapine	++	++	++	++	++	++	++	+
Ziprasidone	++	+	++	++	++	++	++	+
Opioid Agonists								
Methadone	++	++	++	++	++	++	++	+++
Buprenorphine	+	+	+	+ +	+ +	+ +	+ +	+ +
LAAM	+		+	+	+	+		
Erectile Dysfunction Treatment								
Sildenafil	+++	+++	+++	+++	+++	+++	+++	+++
Tadalafil	+++	+++	+++	+++	+++	+++	+++	+++
Vardenafil	+++	+++	+++	+++	+++	+++	+++	+++
Anxiolytics/Hypnotics								
Benzodiazepines								
Lorazepam, oxazepam, temazepam	+	+	+	+	+	+	+	+
Triazolam, alprazolam, midazolam	++++	++++	++++	++++	++++	++++	++++	++++
Zolpidem	++	+++	++	++	++	++	++	+++
Stimulants								
Atomoxetine	+		+	+	+	+	+	+
Dextroamphetamine	+		+	+	+	+	+	+
Modafinil	++	++	++	++	++	++	++	++

(continued)

TABLE 16.3 Antiretroviral/Psychotropic Drug–Drug Interactions (Continued)

Herbals							
Echinacea	+++	+++	+++	+++	+++	+++	+++
Garlic	++	++	++	+++	++	++	++
Ginseng, ginkgo	+++	+++	+++	+++	+++	+++	+++
Kava							
St. John's wort	+++++	+++++	+++++	+++++	+++++	+++++	+++++
Substances of Abuse							
Alcohol	+++	+++	+++	+++	+++	+++	+++
Cannabis	++	++	++	++	+	++	+
Cocaine	+++	+++	+++	++++	++++	+++	++
Crystal methamphetamine	++	++	++	++	++	+++	+
GHB	+++	+++	+++	+++	+++	+++	+++
Ketamine	+++	+++	+++	++	+++	+++	+++
MDMA	++	++	++	+++	+++	+++	+
Phencyclidine (PCP)	+++	+++	+++	+++	+++	+++	+

+ Coadministration is considered safe; no significant interactions have been reported.
++ Use with some caution; interactions of unclear clinical significance have been reported or are theoretically of small risk.
+++ Use with moderate caution; interactions have occasionally been reported or are theoretically possible.
++++ Use with extreme caution; clinically significant interactions have frequently been reported or are theoretically likely, relatively contraindicated.
+++++ Coadministration is absolutely contraindicated.

different antidepressant class may be preferred for patients experiencing these side effects. Although weight gain related to mirtazapine use may be problematic among patients with lipodystrophy and other antiviral-related metabolic abnormalities, the sedating effects of mirtazapine may be helpful in the patient complaining of insomnia. The energizing effects of bupropion may be helpful among patients who experience fatigue from their HIV treatment. The SSRIs undergo extensive oxidative metabolism usually by several CYP450 enzymes, so if one of them is inhibited, others will take over. Thus SSRIs can be given safely along with most antiretrovirals, with the possible exception of ritonavir. Some cases of serotonin syndrome have been reported when fluoxetine was given to patients taking ritonavir.[6] Antiretroviral toxicity should also be monitored among patients taking fluvoxamine because it is a moderate CYP3A4 inhibitor (Tables 16.2 and 16.3).

Three antidepressants thought to be relatively safe to give to patients receiving HAART are venlafaxine, duloxetine, and mirtazapine. Venlafaxine and duloxetine are both metabolized mainly by CYP2D6, with some secondary enzymes also involved. Coadministration with ritonavir could potentially increase serum levels of these drugs, but no clinically significant interactions have been reported. Mirtazapine is metabolized by CYP1A2, 2D6, and 3A4, so there is less potential for drug interactions because if one enzyme is inhibited, the others will take over. However, lower doses of mirtazapine should be considered when given with ritonavir, because this drug can inhibit several enzymes.

Bupropion is metabolized primarily by CYP2B6 and moderately inhibits 2D6. Ritonavir, nelfinavir, and efavirenz may inhibit the metabolism of bupropion and raise its plasma levels, increasing the risk of toxicity; these combinations should be used cautiously.

Ritonavir may inhibit the metabolism of both nefazodone and trazodone via potent CYP3A4 inhibition and thus raise their plasma levels.[7] Adverse effects reported due to nefazodone toxicity include headache, dry mouth, nausea, somnolence, and dizziness, as well as cardiac and neurologic alterations. Adverse effects reported for trazodone toxicity include nausea, hypotension, and syncope. Other potential problems from trazodone toxicity include priapism, respiratory arrest, seizures, and electrocardiographic changes.

Nefazodone itself strongly inhibits CYP3A4 and can lead to inhibition of metabolism of PIs and NNRTIs, increasing the risk of toxicity. Its use demands extreme caution and is relatively contraindicated in patients receiving such medications. In addition, nefazodone should be avoided in HIV-infected patients with compromised liver function, because of the rare but fatal episodes of hepatotoxicity associated with this drug (Tables 16.2 and 16.3).

Tricyclic antidepressants are mainly metabolized by 2D6 with other CYP450 enzymes involved secondarily and may lead to moderate inhibition of 3A4 and 2D6. Again, coadministration of ritonavir, as well as other antiretrovirals, may result in increased levels of tricyclics and the risk of potentially serious toxicity. Serum concentration monitoring is recommended for tricyclic antidepressants when coadministered with PIs and NNRTIs.

There are no published data concerning drug interactions between the monoamine oxidase inhibitors (MAOIs) and antiretrovirals. MAOI use in pharmacotherapy of HIV-infected patients remains very limited because of concerns regarding tolerability, dietary restrictions, and potential for life-threatening hypertensive crises.

MOOD STABILIZERS

With the introduction of several newer anticonvulsant agents, the spectrum of choices for mood stabilization has widened.

Carbamazepine is a potent CYP3A4 inducer (Table 16.2) and has been shown to reduce serum levels of several PIs and NNRTIs. Conversely, carbamazepine levels may be affected by antiretroviral 3A4 inducers and inhibitors. Finally, the potential for overlapping bone marrow toxicity with NRTIs makes carbamazepine a poor choice to give to patients receiving

HAART. Oxcarbazepine is a less potent inhibitor/inducer of CYP3A4 than its parent compound, carbamazepine, so although the potential for interactions with PIs and NNRTIs exist, none have yet been reported.

Valproate, lamotrigine, gabapentin, and topiramate may be the safest mood stabilizers to administer to patients on HAART. Valproic acid may inhibit zidovudine glucuronidation, resulting in higher serum levels; however, the clinical consequences are not clear.[8] Ritonavir and nelfinavir may lead to a decrease in valproate levels by induction of glucuronyl transferase, and monitoring of serum levels would be helpful to ensure efficacy.[9] Lamotrigine is metabolized predominantly by glucuronidation. As with valproic acid, ritonavir and nelfinavir may decrease lamotrigine levels, presumably by enhancing UGT activity, and an increase in dosage may be necessary to avoid loss of lamotrigine efficacy.[9] There is no evidence that lamotrigine either inhibits or induces any CYP450 enzymes. Both gabapentin and topiramate are eliminated essentially unchanged in the urine, and no drug interactions have been reported with either of these medications. Lithium also has no hepatic metabolism, but in practice its use in patients with HIV disease has been limited because of concerns regarding poor tolerability and increased risk of toxicity. Frequently co-prescribed classes of medications, including antibiotics (e.g., tetracyclines, etc.), nonsteroidal anti-inflammatory agents (e.g., ibuprofen, etc.), and cardiovascular drugs (e.g. angiotensin-converting enzyme inhibitors, thiazides, etc.), can lead to serious risks of lithium toxicity (Table 16.3).

NEUROLEPTICS

Most of the typical neuroleptics, with the exception of pimozide, are primarily metabolized by and can lead to moderate inhibition of CYP2D6. Coadministration of ritonavir could potentially lead to neuroleptic toxicity. Although high-potency agents are considered free of clinically significant interactions with antiretrovirals, they should still be given in lower doses to patients in advanced stages of HIV disease because of a higher sensitivity to side effects. Pimozide is primarily metabolized by CYP3A4 and is contraindicated in combination with PIs and NNRTIs because enzyme inhibition can lead to significant prolongation of the QT interval (Table 16.3).

Multiple CYP450 enzymes are usually involved in the metabolism of the atypical neuroleptics, so the potential for drug interactions is most likely with the pan-inhibitors ritonavir and efavirenz. Symptoms of atypical neuroleptic toxicity caused by metabolic inhibition include sedation, hypotension, and extrapyramidal effects. QT interval prolongation would be more problematic and is of particular concern with increased levels of ziprasidone. Clozapine is usually not used in patients with HIV infection because of the risk of agranulocytosis, but further problems could result if its metabolism, mediated by multiple CYP450 enzymes, is inhibited by antiretrovirals.

STIMULANTS

Psychostimulants are used in the management of patients with HIV infection who have depression, anergy, and HIV-associated dementia. Amphetamines are metabolized mainly by deamination and hydroxylation and do not have drug interactions with antiviral medication. However, if a patient has a history of substance abuse, stimulants should be used cautiously. There are also no drug interactions noted between atomoxetine and antiretrovirals. Modafinil is a mild inducer of CYP3A4, and, although no specific drug interactions have been reported, we recommend caution whenever a 3A4 inducer is taken with either a PI or an NNRTI.

OPIOID AGONISTS

Interactions between methadone and efavirenz, nevirapine, or ritonavir leading to an increased rate of methadone metabolism were discussed previously. Although the mechanism is not clear, administration of abacavir may also increase the metabolism of methadone. In addition, methadone may cause a lowered plasma concentration of the NRTIs didanosine and stavudine by causing a decrease in gastrointestinal motility that leads to increased degradation in the gut.[10] In contrast, methadone has been reported to increase zidovudine levels presumably by inhibition of its glucuronidation. Buprenorphine is extensively metabolized by CYP3A4 and should be used cautiously with PIs and NNRTIs.

MEDICATIONS FOR TREATMENT OF ERECTILE DYSFUNCTION

Erectile dysfunction (ED) is not uncommon among men with HIV infection or AIDS, either as a direct complication of the disease or as a medication side effect. Medications currently available for the treatment of ED—sildenafil, vardenafil, and tadalafil—are primarily metabolized by CYP3A4. Elevated serum levels of these drugs due to inhibited metabolism can lead to adverse events, including myocardial infarction, hypotension, visual changes, and priapism. Although sildenafil has been the most studied, potentially serious interactions may occur with any of these medications and the PIs, delavirdine and efavirenz. Current recommendations are for much lower doses of the ED medications when given in the context of HAART.

SUBSTANCES OF ABUSE

A large proportion of patients with HIV infection or AIDS have a current or past substance use disorder, and the clinician should be aware of potential drug interactions with substances of abuse and HIV medications. The literature on this area is speculative, based on known metabolic pathways, or case-report based, and the actual in vivo interaction is often unknown.

Alcohol consumption has been shown to significantly increase the blood serum level of abacavir by competing for alcohol dehydrogenase[11]; however, with chronic use, alcohol can induce CYP3A4 and decrease levels of PIs and NNRTIs.[12] Inhaled marijuana has been shown to decrease the bioavailability of indinavir and nelfinavir, although the precise mechanism is unknown.[13] There is concern that this interaction may occur with other PIs. Cocaine is metabolized to norcocaine by CYP3A4, and inhibitors such as the PIs and some NNRTIs may lead to toxic levels of cocaine.

Methamphetamine and 3,4-methylenedioxymethamphetamine (MDMA, Ecstasy) both are metabolized primarily by CYP2D6. Deaths have been reported among patients who took methamphetamine while being treated with ritonavir.[14] Similarly, a patient being treated with ritonavir and saquinavir died after ingesting MDMA and gamma-hydroxybutyrate (GHB).[15] This patient most likely developed a fatal serotonin syndrome due to inhibited MDMA metabolism, but GHB toxicity was not excluded. Ketamine[16] and phencyclidine (PCP)[17] appear to be primarily metabolized by CYP3A4, and patients should be aware of the potential interaction of these drugs with the inhibitors of this enzyme (Table 16.3).

HERBAL AND ALTERNATIVE TREATMENTS

It is not unusual for patients to take herbal supplements to treat psychiatric and medical conditions. Although they believe that these treatments are safe because they are "natural," these supplements may contain pharmacologically active ingredients that can have drug interactions and/or toxic effects.

Most worrisome is the induction of CYP3A4 by St. John's wort, which can lead to subtherapeutic levels of PIs and NNRTIs. St. John's wort is contraindicated in any patient receiving HAART. Echinacea has been associated with liver damage and should not be combined with other hepatotoxic medications. It also inhibits CYP3A4 and may elevate the serum level of PIs and NNRTIs.[18] Garlic supplements have been shown to decrease the serum levels of saquinavir, although the mechanism is unclear.[19] Kava is a potent CYP3A4 inhibitor that could lead to PI or NNRTI toxicity.[20] In addition, the sale of kava has been banned in many countries because of its potentially fatal hepatotoxicity. Ginseng and ginkgo biloba are capable of inhibiting CYP3A4 and 2C9[21] and should be used with caution among patients receiving HAART (Table 16.3).

REFERENCES

1. Cozza KL, Armstrong SC, Oesterheld JR. *Concise Guide to Drug Interaction Principles for Medical Practice*. 2nd ed. Washington, DC: APPI; 2003.
2. Wynn GH, Zapor MJ, Smith BH, et al. Antiretrovirals, Part 1: Overview, history, and focus on protease inhibitors. *Psychosomatics*. 2004;45:262–270.
3. Zapor MJ, Cozza KL, Wynn GH. Antiretrovirals, Part II: Focus on non-protease inhibitor antiretrovirals (NRTIs, NNRTIs and fusion inhibitors). *Psychosomatics*. 2004;45:524–535.
4. Altice FL, Friedland GH, Cooney EL. Nevirapine induced opiate withdrawal among injection drug users with HIV infection receiving methadone. *AIDS*. 1999;13:957–962.
5. Greenblatt DJ, von Moltke LL, Harmatz JS, et al. Differential impairment of triazolam and zolpidem clearance by ritonavir. *J Acquir Immune Defic Syndr*. 2000;24:129–136.
6. DeSilva K, Le Flore DB, Marston BJ, et al. Serotonin syndrome in HIV-infected individuals receiving antiretroviral therapy and fluoxetine. *AIDS*. 2001;15:1281–1285.
7. Greenblatt DJ, von Moltke LL, Harmatz JS, et al. Short-term exposure to low-dose ritonavir impairs clearance and enhances adverse effects of trazodone. *J Clin Pharmacol*. 2003;43:414–422.
8. Taburet AM, Singlas E. Drug interactions with antiviral drugs. *Clin Pharmacokinet*. 1996;30:385–401.
9. Tseng AL, Foisy MM. Significant interactions with new antiretrovirals and psychotropic drugs. *Ann Pharmacother*. 1999;33:461–473.
10. Rainey PM, Friedland G, McCance-Katz EF, et al. Interaction of methadone with didanosine and stavudine. *J Acquir Immune Defic Syndr*. 2000;24:241–248.
11. McDowell JA, Chittick GE, Stevens CP, et al. Pharmacokinetic interaction of abacavir and ethanol in human immunodeficiency virus-infected adults. *Antimicrob Agents Chemother*. 2000;44:1686–1690.
12. Caballeria J. Current concepts in alcohol metabolism. *Ann Hepatol*. 2003;2:60–68.
13. Kosel BW, Aweeka FT, Benowitz NL, et al. The effects of cannabinoids on the pharmacokinetics of indinavir and nelfinavir. *AIDS*. 2002;16:543–550.
14. Hales G, Roth N, Smith D. Possible fatal interaction between protease inhibitors and methamphetamine. *Antivir Ther*. 2000;5:19.
15. Harrington RD, Woodward JA, Hooton TM, Horn JR. Life-threatening interactions between HIV-1 protease inhibitors and the illicit drugs MDMA and gamma-hydroxybutyrate. *Arch Int Med*. 1999;159:2221–2224.
16. Hijazi Y, Boulieu R. Contribution of CYP3A4, CYP2B6, and CYP2C9 isoforms to N-demethylation of ketamine in human liver microsomes. *Drug Metab Dispos*. 2002;30:853–858.
17. Laurenzana EM, Owens SM: Metabolism of phencyclidine by human liver microsomes. *Drug Metab Dispos*. 1997;25:557–563.
18. Budzinski JW, Foster BC, Vandenhoek S, Arnason JT. An in vitro evaluation of human CYP 3A4 inhibition by selected commercial herbal extracts and tinctures. *Phytomed*. 2000;7:273–282.
19. Piscitelli SC, Burstein AH, Welden N, et al. The effect of garlic supplements on the pharmacokinetics of saquinavir. *Clin Infect Dis*. 2002;34:234–238.
20. Mathews JM, Etheridge AS, Black SR. Inhibition of human CYP activities by kava extract and kavalactones. *Drug Metab Dispos*. 2002;30:1153–1157.
21. Nu H, Timi E. The inhibitory effects of herbal components on CYP2C9 and CYP3A4 catalytic activities in human liver microsomes. *Am J Ther*. 2004;11:206–212.

CHAPTER 17

Pain Syndromes

William Breitbart

Psychiatrists and psychologists are still actively involved in many aspects of the care of patients with acquired immunodeficiency syndrome (AIDS), and so it is necessary for us to be aware of such important quality of care and quality of life issues as pain in AIDS. With the introduction of highly active antiretroviral therapy (HAART) (i.e., combination therapies including protease inhibitors) the face of the AIDS epidemic, particularly for those who can avail themselves of and/or tolerate these new therapies, is indeed changing. Even with advances in AIDS therapies, pain continues to be an important psychiatric and supportive care issue for patients with human immunodeficiency virus (HIV) disease. As the epidemiology of the AIDS epidemic changes in the United States, the challenge of managing pain in patients with AIDS with a history of substance abuse is becoming an ever-growing challenge. Studies have documented that pain in individuals with HIV infection or AIDS is highly prevalent, diverse, and varied in syndromal presentation; associated with significant psychological and functional morbidity; and alarmingly undertreated.[1-12] Pain management needs to be more integrated into the total care of patients with HIV disease. Responses from a self-referred sample of outpatients with AIDS indicate that patients with AIDS experience many distressing physical and psychological symptoms, along with a high level of distress.[13] This chapter describes the prevalence and types of pain syndromes encountered in patients with HIV disease and reviews the psychological and functional impact of pain, as well as the barriers to adequate pain treatment in this population. Finally, principles of pain management, with particular emphasis on the management of pain in HIV-infected patients with a history of substance abuse, are outlined.

PREVALENCE OF PAIN

Estimates of the prevalence of pain in HIV-infected individuals have been reported to range from 30% to over 90%, with the prevalence of pain increasing as disease progresses,[4-8,12,14-16] particularly in the latest stages of illness.

Studies suggest that approximately 30% of ambulatory HIV-infected patients in early stages of HIV disease (pre-AIDS; Category A or B disease) experience clinically significant pain, and as many as 56% have had episodic painful symptoms of less clear clinical significance.[5,7,12]

In a prospective cross-sectional survey of 438 ambulatory patients with AIDS in New York City, 63% reported frequent or persistent pain of at least 2 weeks' duration at the time of assessment.[5] The prevalence of pain in this large sample increased significantly as HIV disease progressed, with 45% of patients with AIDS with Category A3 disease reporting pain, 55% of those with Category B3 disease reporting pain, and 67% of those with Category C1, 2, or 3 disease reporting pain. Individuals in this sample of ambulatory patients with AIDS also were more likely to report pain if they had other concurrent HIV-related symptoms (e.g., fatigue, wasting), had received treatment for an AIDS-related opportunistic infection, or if they had not been receiving antiretroviral medications (e.g., AZT, ddI, ddC,d4t).

In a study of pain in hospitalized patients with AIDS in a public hospital in New York City, over 50% of patients required treatment for pain, with pain being the presenting complaint in 30% and the second most common presenting problem after fever.[8] In a French multicenter study, 62% of hospitalized patients with HIV disease had clinically significant pain.[7] Schofferman and Brody[16] reported that 53% of patients with far-advanced AIDS cared for in a hospice setting had pain; Kimball and McCormick[15] reported that up to 93% of patients with AIDS in their hospice experienced at least one 48-hour period of pain during the last 2 weeks of life.

Larue et al.[17] demonstrated that patients with AIDS being cared for by hospice at home had prevalence rates and intensity ratings for pain that were comparable to, and even exceeded, those of cancer patients. Breitbart et al.[4] reported that ambulatory patients with AIDS in their New York City sample reported a mean pain intensity on average of 5.4 (on the 0 to 10 numerical rating scale of the Brief Pain Inventory) and a mean pain "at its worst" of 7.4. In addition, as with pain prevalence, the intensity of pain experienced by patients with HIV disease increases significantly as disease progresses. Patients with AIDS who are experiencing pain, like their counterparts with cancer pain, typically describe an average of 2.5 to 3 concurrent pains at a time.[4,6]

Frich and Borgbjerg[18] concluded that the incidence of disturbing pain in AIDS is high, specifically in the extremities, gastrointestinal tract, and head. In a study of 95 patients with AIDS, the overall incidence of pain was 88% and 69% of the patients suffered from pain that interfered with daily activity to a degree described as moderate to severe.[18] In patients with AIDS who are approaching end of life, 93% of patients report experiencing pain and discomfort at some time during the last 2 weeks of life.[15] This percentage may be even higher if some pain and discomfort went unrecognized. Most patients experienced at least one 48-hour period of pain and discomfort during the last 2 weeks of life; furthermore, 88% received some sort of opioid analgesia with the majority experiencing some relief afterward.[15]

PAIN SYNDROMES

Pain syndromes encountered in AIDS are diverse in nature and etiology. Pain syndromes seen in HIV disease can be categorized into three types (Table 17.1): (a) those directly related to HIV infection or consequences of immunosuppression, (b) those due to AIDS therapies, and (c) those unrelated to AIDS or AIDS therapies.[2,3,6] In studies to date, approximately 45% of pain syndromes encountered are directly related to HIV infection or consequences of immunosuppression; 15% to 30% are due to therapies for HIV- or AIDS-related conditions, as well as diagnostic procedures; and the remaining 25% to 40% are unrelated to HIV disease or its therapies.[6] The most common pain syndromes reported in studies to date include painful sensory peripheral neuropathy, pain due to extensive Kaposi's sarcoma, headache, oral and pharyngeal pain, abdominal pain, chest pain, arthralgias and myalgias, and painful dermatologic conditions.[5,6,8,10,12,14,16,17,19] In a sample of 151 ambulatory patients with AIDS who underwent a research assessment, which included a clinical interview, neurologic examination, and review of medical records,[6] the most common pain diagnoses included headaches

TABLE 17.1	Pain Syndromes in AIDS Patients

I. Pain related to HIV/AIDS
    HIV neuropathy
    HIV myelopathy
    Kaposi's sarcoma
    Secondary infections (intestines, skin)
    Organomegaly
    Arthritis/vasculitis
    Myopathy/myositis
II. Pain related to HIV/AIDS therapy
    Antiretrovirals, antivirals
    Antimycobacterials, *Pneumocystis jiroveci* (formerly *carinii*) pneumonia (PCP) prophylaxis
    Chemotherapy (vincristine)
    Radiation
    Surgery
    Procedures (bronchoscopy, biopsies)
III. Pain unrelated to AIDS
    Disc disease
    Diabetic neuropathy

(46% of patients, 17% of all pains); joint pains (arthritis, arthralgias, etc., 31% of patients; 12% of pains); painful polyneuropathy (distal symmetric polyneuropathy, 28% of patients; 10% of pains); and muscle pains (myalgia, myositis, 27% of patients; 12% of pains). Other common pain diagnoses included skin pain (Kaposi's sarcoma, infections, 25% of patients; 30% of homosexual males in the sample had pain from extensive Kaposi's sarcoma lesions); bone pain (20% of patients), abdominal pain (17% of patients); chest pain (13%); and painful radiculopathy (12%). Patients in this sample had a total of 405 pains (averaging 3 concurrent pains), with 46% of patients diagnosed with neuropathic pain, 71% with somatic pain, 29% with visceral pain, and 46% with headache (classified separately because of controversy as to pathophysiology). When pain type was classified by pains (as opposed to patients) 25% were neuropathic pains, 44% were nociceptive-somatic, 14% were nociceptive-visceral, and 17% were idiopathic type pains. Patients in this study with lower CD4+ cell counts were significantly more likely to be diagnosed with polyneuropathy and headache. Hewitt et al.[6] demonstrated that although pains of a neuropathic nature (e.g., polyneuropathies, radiculopathies) certainly make up a large proportion of pain syndromes encountered in patients with AIDS (Table 17.2), pains of a somatic and/or visceral nature are also extremely common clinical problems.

WOMEN AND PAIN

The author's group at Memorial Sloan-Kettering Cancer Center has reported on the experience of pain in women with AIDS.[6,20] Although preliminary, our studies suggest that women with HIV disease experience pain more frequently than men with HIV disease and report somewhat higher levels of pain intensity. This may be, in part, a reflection of the fact that women with AIDS-related pain are twice as likely to be undertreated for their pain compared to men.[4] Women with HIV disease have unique gynecologic pain syndromes specifically related to opportunistic infectious processes and cancers of the pelvis and genitourinary tract.[21] Women with AIDS were significantly more likely to be diagnosed with radiculopathy and headache in one survey.[6]

TABLE 17.2 Neuropathies Encountered in HIV/AIDS-Infected Patients

I. Predominantly Sensory Neuropathy (PSN) of AIDS
II. Immune-mediated
    Inflammatory demyelinating polyneuropathies
    Acute (Guillain-Barré syndrome)
    Chronic Inflammatory Demyelinating Neuropathy (CIDP)
III. Infectious
    Cytomegalovirus polyradiculopathy
    Cytomegalovirus multiple mononeuropathy
    Herpes zoster
    Mycobacterial *(Mycobacterium avium intracellulare)*
IV. Toxic/nutritional
    Alcohol, vitamin deficiencies (B_6, B_{12})
    Antiretrovirals
        ddI (didanosine), ddC (zalcitabine), D4T (stavudine)
    Antivirals
    Foscarnet
    PCP prophylaxis
        Dapsone
    Antibacterial
        Metronidazole
    Antimycobacterials
        Isoniazid (INH), rifampin, ethionamide
    Antineoplastics
        Vincristine, vinblastine
V. Other medical conditions
    Diabetic neuropathy
    Postherpetic neuralgia

CHILDREN AND PAIN

Children with HIV infection also experience pain.[22] HIV-related conditions in children that are observed to cause pain include meningitis and sinusitis (headaches); otitis media; shingles; cellulitis and abscesses; severe candida dermatitis; dental caries; intestinal infections, such as *Mycobacterium avium intracellulare* (MAI) and *Cryptosporidium;* hepatosplenomegaly; oral and esophageal candidiasis; and spasticity associated with encephalopathy that causes painful muscle spasms. (The reader is referred to the Chapters 25 and 38 on palliative care in children.)

IMPACT OF PAIN ON QUALITY OF LIFE

Pain, in patients with HIV disease, has a profound negative impact on physical and psychological functioning and overall quality of life.[7,11] In a study of the impact of pain on psychological functioning and quality of life in ambulatory AIDS patients,[11] depression was significantly correlated with the presence of pain. In addition to being significantly more distressed, depressed, and hopeless, those with pain were twice as likely to have suicidal ideation (40%) as those without pain (20%). HIV-infected patients with pain were more functionally impaired.[11] Such functional interference was highly corrlated to levels of pain intensity and depression. Patients with pain were more likely to be unemployed or disabled and reported less social support. Larue et al.[7] reported that HIV-infected patients with pain intensities greater than 5 (on a 0 to 10 NRS) reported significantly poorer quality of life during the week preceding their survey than patients without pain. Pain intensity had an independent negative impact on HIV patients' quality of life, even after adjustment for treatment setting, stage of disease, fatigue, sadness, and depression. Singer et al.[12] also reported an association between the frequency of multiple pains, increased disability, and higher levels of depression. Psychological variables, such as the amount of control people believe they have over pain, emotional associations and memories of pain, fears of death, depression, anxiety, and hopelessness, contribute to the experience of pain in people with AIDS and can increase suffering.[11,23] Our group also reported that negative thoughts related to pain were associated with greater pain intensity, psychological distress, and disability in ambulatory patients with AIDS.[24] Those patients with AIDS who felt that pain represented a progression of their HIV disease reported more intense pain than those who did not see pain as a threat. Vogel et al.[13] assessed 504 ambulatory patients with AIDS to measure symptom distress, physical and psychosocial functioning, and demographic and disease-related factors. As opposed to those who reported sexual contact as a means of transmission, patients who reported intravenous (IV) drug use as route of HIV transmission indicated higher levels of distress and physical symptom distress.[13] Furthermore, Vogel et al.[13] showed that both the number of symptoms and symptom distress were highly associated with psychological distress and poorer quality of life.

MANAGEMENT OF PAIN

ASSESSMENT ISSUES

The initial step in pain management is a comprehensive assessment of pain symptoms. The health professional working in the AIDS setting must have a working knowledge of the etiology and treatment of pain in AIDS. This would include an understanding of the different types of AIDS pain syndromes, as discussed previously, as well as a familiarity with the parameters of appropriate pharmacologic treatment. A close collaboration of the entire health care team is optimal when attempting to adequately manage pain in the patient with AIDS. A careful history and physical examination may disclose an identifiable syndrome (e.g., herpes zoster, bacterial infection, or neuropathy) that can be treated in a standard fashion.[25,26] A standard pain history[27,28] may provide valuable clues to the nature of the underlying process and indeed may disclose other treatable disorders. A description of the qualitative features of the pain, its time course, and any maneuvers that increase or decrease pain intensity should be obtained. Pain intensity (current, average, at best, at worst) should be assessed to determine the need for weak versus potent analgesics and as a means to serially evaluate the effectiveness of ongoing treatment. Pain descriptors (e.g., burning, shooting, dull, or sharp) will help determine the mechanism of pain (somatic, nociceptive, visceral nociceptive, or neuropathic) and may suggest the likelihood of response to various classes of traditional and adjuvant analgesics (nonsteroidal anti-inflammatory drugs [NSAIDs], opioids, antidepressants, anticonvulsants, oral local anesthetics, corticosteroids, etc.).[29–31] Additionally, detailed medical, neurologic, and psychosocial assessments (including a history of substance use or abuse) must be conducted. Where possible, family members or partners should be interviewed and included in the pain management treatment plan. During the assessment phase, pain should be aggressively treated; pain complaints and psychosocial issues are subject to an ongoing process of reevaluation.[27]

PAIN MEASUREMENT/ASSESSMENT TOOLS

An important element in assessment of pain is the concept that assessment is continuous and needs to be repeated over the course of pain treatment. The use of readily available, simple and clinically validated pain self-report measures or tools can make this process simpler and more reliable. There are essentially four aspects of pain experience in AIDS that require ongoing assessment and evaluation, which can be aided by these tools: (a) pain intensity, (b) pain relief, (c) pain-related functional interference (e.g., mood state, general, and specific activities), and (d) monitoring of intervention effects.

Three commonly used self-report pain intensity assessment tools include a simple descriptive pain intensity scale, a 0 to 10 numeric pain intensity scale, and the Visual Analog Scale (VAS) for Pain Intensity. A Pain Faces scale is used in children and in non–English speaking or illiterate populations. The Memorial Pain Assessment Card (MPAC)[32] is a helpful clinical tool that allows patients to report their pain experience. The MPAC consists of visual analog scales that measure pain intensity, pain relief, and mood. The Brief Pain Inventory (BPI) is another pain assessment tool that has been widely used in cancer and AIDS pain research and clinical settings.[33] The BPI has a useful Pain Interference Subscale that assesses pain's interference in seven domains of quality of life and function. There are many other pain assessment tools available for adults and children.

There are four aspects of pain experience in AIDS that require ongoing evaluation: (a) pain intensity, (b) pain relief, (c) pain-related functional interference (e.g., mood state and general and specific activities), and (d) monitoring of intervention effects (analgesic drug side effects and abuse). Several readily available pain assessment tools are easily adapted to the clinical setting. These include the Brief Pain Inventory and the MPAC.

As of January 1, 2001 the Joint Commission on Accreditation of Healthcare Organizations (JCAHO) established new pain management standards for accreditation. These standards include the following statements: (a) individuals served have the right to appropriate assessment and referral for a provision of management of pain and (b) pain must be assessed in all individuals.*

Other sources of help in meeting the pain standards include "Building an Institutional Commitment to Pain Management: The Mayday Resource Manual for Improvement," an excellent compilation of resource material to promote institutional support of pain management; all of the sample resource tools are available on a disc.†

MULTIMODAL APPROACH

Federal guidelines developed by the Agency for Health Care Policy and Research (AHCPR) for the management of cancer pain also address the issue of management of pain in AIDS and state: "The principles of pain assessment and treatment in the patient with HIV positive/AIDS are not fundamentally different from those in the patient with cancer and should be followed for patients with HIV-positive/AIDS."[29] In contrast to pain in cancer, pain in HIV disease may more commonly have an underlying treatable cause.[10] Readers are also directed to an excellent resource for general palliative care in patients with HIV disease and AIDS in the form of Health Resources and Services Administration's *A Clinical Guide to Supportive & Palliative Care for HIV/AIDS*.[34]

---

*The complete standards are available at www.jcaho.org/standard/pm_hap.html.
†Available from Wisconsin Cancer Pain Initiative, 3675 Medical Sciences Center, University of Wisconsin Medical School, 1300 University Avenue, Madison, WI 53706; phone 608-262-0278, fax 608-265-4014; e-mail www.jcaho.org/standard/pm_hap.html, aacpi@aacpi.org, or www.aacpi.org.

Optimal management of pain in AIDS is multimodal and requires pharmacologic, psychotherapeutic, cognitive-behavioral, anesthetic, neurosurgical, and rehabilitative approaches. A multidimensional model of AIDS pain, which recognizes the interaction of cognitive, emotional, socioenvironmental, and nociceptive aspects of pain suggests a model for multimodal intervention.

PHARMACOTHERAPIES FOR PAIN

The World Health Organization (WHO)[30] has devised guidelines for analgesic management of cancer pain that the AHCPR has endorsed for the management of pain related to cancer or AIDS.[29] These guidelines, also known widely as the "WHO Analgesic Ladder," have been well validated.[35] This approach advocates selection of analgesics based on severity of pain, as well as the type of pain (i.e., neuropathic versus non-neuropathic pain). For mild-to-moderate pain, nonopioid analgesics such as NSAIDs and acetaminophen are recommended. For pain that is persistent and moderate to severe in intensity, opioid analgesics of increasing potency (such as morphine) should be utilized. Adjuvant agents, such as laxatives and psychostimulants, are useful in preventing and treating opioid side effects, such as constipation and sedation, respectively. Adjuvant analgesic drugs, such as the antidepressant analgesics, are suggested for use, along with opioids and NSAIDs, in all stages of the analgesic ladder (mild, moderate, or severe pain), but have their most important clinical application in the management of neuropathic pain.

This WHO approach, although not yet validated in AIDS, has been recommended by the AHCPR and clinical authorities in the field of pain management and AIDS.[8,10,12,16,29,36,37] Clinical reports describing the successful application of the principles of the WHO Analgesic Ladder to the management of pain in AIDS, with particular emphasis on the use of opioids, have also appeared in the literature.[9,15,16,38–41]

NONOPIOID ANALGESICS

The nonopioid analgesics (Table 17.3) are prescribed principally for mild-to-moderate pain or to augment the analgesic effects of opioid analgesics in the treatment of severe pain. The use of NSAIDs in patients with AIDS must be accompanied by heightened awareness of toxicity and adverse effects. NSAIDs are highly protein-bound, and the free fraction of available drug is increased in patients with AIDS who are cachectic, wasted, and hypoalbuminic, often resulting in toxicities and adverse effects. Patients with AIDS are frequently hypovolemic, on concurrent nephrotoxic drugs, and experiencing HIV nephropathy and so are at increased risk for renal toxicity related to NSAIDs. The antipyretic effects of the NSAIDs may also interfere with early detection of infection in patients with AIDS.

The major adverse effects associated with NSAIDs include gastric ulceration, renal failure, hepatic dysfunction, and bleeding. The nonacetylated salicylates, such as salsalate, sodium salicylate, and choline magnesium salicylate, theoretically have fewer gastrointestinal side effects and might be considered in cases in which gastrointestinal distress is an issue. Prophylaxis for NSAID-associated gastrointestinal symptoms include histamine H_2-antagonist drugs (cimetidine 300 mg tid to qid or ranitidine 150 mg bid), misoprostol 200 mg qid, omeprazole 20 mg daily, or an antacid). Patients should be informed of these symptoms, issued guaiac cards with reagent, and taught to check their stool weekly. NSAIDs effect kidney function and should be used with caution. NSAIDs can cause a decrease in glomerular filtration, acute and chronic renal failure, interstitial nephritis, papillary necrosis, and hyperkalemia.[42] In patients with renal impairment, NSAIDs should be used with caution, because many (i.e., ketoprofen, feroprofen, naproxen, and carpofen) are highly dependent on renal function for clearance. The risk of renal dysfunction is greatest in patients with advanced age, preexisting

TABLE 17.3	Oral Analgesics for Mild-to-Moderate Pain in AIDS			
Analgesic (by class)	Starting Dose (mg)	Duration (hr)	Plasma Half-life (hr)	Comments
Nonsteroidal				
Aspirin	650	4–6	4–6	The standard for comparison among nonopioid analgesics
Ibuprofen	400–600	—	—	Like aspirin, can inhibit platelet function
Choline magnesium trisalicylate	700–1,500	—	—	Essentially no hematologic or gastrointestinal side effects
Weaker opioids				
Codeine	32–65	3–4	—	Metabolized to morphine; often used to suppress cough in patients at risk of pulmonary bleeding
Oxycodone	5–10	3–4	—	Available as a single agent and in combination with aspirin or acetaminophen
Propoxyphene	65–130	4–6	—	Toxic metabolite norpropoxy accumulates with repeated dosing

renal impairment, hypovolemia, concomitant therapy with nephrotoxic drugs, and heart failure. Prostaglandins modulate vascular tone, and their inhibition by the NSAIDs can cause hypertension and interference with the pharmacologic control of hypertension.[43] Caution should be used in patients receiving β-adrenergic antagonists, diuretics, or angiotensin-converting enzyme inhibitors. Several studies have suggested that there is substantial biliary excretion of several NSAIDs, including indomethacin and sulindac. In patients with hepatic dysfunction, these drugs should be used with caution. NSAIDs, with the exception of the nonacetylated salicylates (e.g., sodium salicylate, choline magnesium trisalicylate), produce inhibition of platelet aggregation (usually reversible, but irreversible with aspirin). NSAIDs should be used with extreme caution, or avoided, in patients who are thrombocytopenic or who have clotting impairment.

OPIOID ANALGESICS

Opioid analgesics are the mainstay of pharmacotherapy of moderate-to-severe intensity pain in the patient with HIV disease (Table 17.4). Several reports describing the safe and effective use of opioid drugs in the management of moderate-to-severe pain in populations of patients with HIV disease (including patients with a history of injection drug use as their HIV transmission factor) have begun to appear in the literature.[15,37–39,40,43] Kaplan et al.[44] conducted a multicenter study in which 44 patients with moderate-to-severe AIDS-related pain were treated with sustained-release oral morphine in an open-label prospective study of

TABLE 17.4 Opioid Analgesics for Moderate-to-Severe Pain in AIDS

Analgesic	Route	Equianalgesic Dose (mg)	Oral Morphine Equivalents (mg)	Analgesic Onset (hr)	Duration (hr)	Plasma Half-life (hr)	Comments
Morphine	PO	30–60*	30–60	1–1½	4–6	2–3	Standard of comparison for the narcotic analgesics; 30 mg for repeat around-the-clock dosing; 60 mg for single dose or intermittent dosing*
	IM, IV, Sub-Q	10	10	½–1	3–6		
Morphine (sustained-release)	PO	90–120	90–120	1–1½	8–12	—	Now available in long-acting, sustained-release forms
Oxycodone	PO	20–30	30–45	1	3–6	2–3	In combination with aspirin or acetaminophen it is considered a weaker opioid; as a single agent it is comparable to the strong opioids, such as morphine. Available in immediate-release and sustained-release preparation.
Oxycodone (sustained-release)	PO	20–40	30–60	1	8–12	2–3	
Hydromorphone	PO	7.5	30–40	½–1	3–4	2–3	Short half-life; ideal for elderly patients. Comes in suppository and injectable forms.
	IM, IV	1.5	15–20	¼–½	3–4	2–3	
Methadone	PO	20	80	½–1	4–8	15–30	Long half-life; tends to accumulate with initial dosing, requires careful titration. Good oral potency.
	IM, IV	10	80	½–1		15–30	
Levorphanol	PO	4	30–60	½–1½	3–6	12–6	Long half-life; requires careful
	IM	2	30–60	½–1		12–16	

(continued)

Analgesic	Route	Equianalgesic Dose (mg)	Oral Morphine Equivalents (mg)	Analgesic Onset (hr)	Duration (hr)	Plasma Half-life (hr)	Comments
Meperidine	PO	300	30–60	1/2–1 1/2	3–6	3–4	dose titration in first week. Note that analgesic duration is only 4 hr. Active toxic metabolite, or meperidine, tends to accumulate (plasma half-life is 12–16 hr), especially with renal impairment and in elderly patients causing delirium, myoclonus, and seizures.
	IM	75	30–60	1/2–1	3–4	3–4	
Fentanyl	TD	0.1	24–30	12–18	48–72	20–22	Transdermal patch is convenient, bypassing GI analgesia until depot is formed. Not suitable for rapid titration.
	IV	0.1	24–30	—	—	—	

GI, Gastrointestinal; IM, intramuscular; IV, intravenous; PO, per oral; Sub-Q, subcutaneous; TD, transdermal.
*Oral morphine equivalents are estimated ranges calculated based on Pereira J, Lawlor P, Vigano A, et al. Equianalgesic dose ratios for opioids: a critical review and proposals for long-term dosing. J Pain Symptom Manage. 2001;22:622–687.

patients treated for up to 18 days. Pain intensity decreased by 65% in the patients who completed treatment, quality of life was good in 80%, acceptability of therapy was 96%, 92% of side effects were resolved, and total morphine dose remained stable through the course of the study. In a pilot study, Newshan and Lefkowitz[45] reported similar findings on the effectiveness and safety of the transdermal fentanyl patch in a small sample of patients with AIDS-related pain. With transdermal fentanyl, pain severity scores decreased, mean pain relief scores increased, and daily functioning measures improved significantly.[45] Furthermore, Newshan and Lefkowitz[45] reported transdermal fentanyl was effective for chronic pain in chemically dependant and nonchemically dependant AIDS patients. In persons with AIDS near the end of life, the use of opioid analgesia remains common practice. The medical records of 185 adult patients with AIDS who receiving hospice care were reviewed by Kimball and McCormick.[15] Most patients (93%) experienced at least one 48-hour period of discomfort during the last 2 weeks of life; the majority (88%) received some form of opioid analgesia.[15] Of these patients, 62% experienced some relief of pain thereafter.[15]

Principles that are useful in guiding the appropriate use of opioid analgesics for pain include the following[31,37,46]:

1. Choose an appropriate drug.
2. Start with lowest dose possible.
3. Titrate dose.
4. Use as-needed doses selectively.
5. Use an appropriate route of administration.
6. Be aware of equivalent analgesic doses.
7. Use a combination of opioid, nonopioid, and adjuvant drugs.
8. Be aware of tolerance.
9. Understand physical and psychological dependence.

In choosing the appropriate opioid analgesic for cancer pain, Portenoy[31] highlights the following important considerations: (a) opioid class, (b) "weak" versus "strong" opioids, (c) pharmacokinetic characteristics, (d) duration of analgesic effect, (e) favorable prior response, and (f) opioid side effects.

Opioid analgesics are divided into two classes, the agonists and the agonist-antagonists, based on their affinity to opioid receptors. Pentazocine, butorphanol, and nalbuphine are examples of opioid analgesics with mixed agonist-antagonist properties. These drugs can reverse opioid effects and precipitate an opioid withdrawal syndrome in patients who are opioid-tolerant or dependent. They are of limited use in the management of chronic pain in AIDS. Oxycodone (in combination with either aspirin or acetaminophen), hydrocodone, and codeine are the so-called weaker opioid analgesics and are indicated for use in Step 2 of the WHO ladder for mild-to-moderate intensity pain. More severe pain is best managed with morphine or another of the stronger opioid analgesics, such as hydromorphone, methadone, levorphanol, or fentanyl. Oxycodone, as a single agent without aspirin or acetaminophen, is available in immediate- and sustained-release forms and is considered a "stronger" opioid in these forms.

The oral route has often been described as the preferred route of administration of opioid analgesics from the perspectives of convenience and cost. However, the transdermal route of administration has gained rapid acceptance amongst clinicians and patients. Patients with HIV infection are burdened with the task of taking 20 to 40 tablets of medication per day and often need to follow complicated regimens in which medication must be taken on an empty stomach, and so on. In a study on patient-related barriers to pain management in AIDS patients, the vast majority of patients with AIDS endorsed a preference to use a pain intervention that required a minimal number of additional pills (e.g., sustained-release preparations of oral opioids) or interventions that did not require taking pills at all (i.e., transdermal opioid system).[4] Immediate-release oral morphine or hydromorphone preparations require that the drug be taken every 3 to 4 hours. Longer-acting, sustained-release oral morphine preparations and oxycodone preparations are available that provide up to 8 to 12 hours or more of analgesia, minimizing the number of daily doses required for the control of persistent pain. Rescue doses of immediate-release, short-acting opioid are often necessary to supplement the use of sustained-release morphine or oxycodone, particularly during periods of titration or pain escalation. The transdermal fentanyl patch system (Duragesic) also has applications in the management of severe pain in AIDS.[40,41] Each transdermal fentanyl patch contains a 48- to 72-hour supply of fentanyl, which is absorbed from a depot in the skin. Levels in the plasma rise slowly over 12 to 18 hours after patch placement, so dosage forms are available. As with sustained-release morphine preparations, all patients should be provided with oral or parenteral rapidly acting, short-duration opioids to manage breakthrough pain. The transdermal system is convenient and can minimize the reminders of pain associated with repeated oral dosing of analgesics. In patients with AIDS, it should be noted that the absorption of transdermal fentanyl could be increased with fever, resulting in increased plasma levels and shorter duration of analgesia from the patch.

It is important to note that opioids can be administered through a variety of routes: oral, rectal, transdermal, intravenous, subcutaneous, intraspinal, and even intraventricularly.[40] There are advantages and disadvantages, as well as indications for use of these various routes. Further discussion of such alternative delivery routes as the intraspinal route are beyond the

TABLE 17.5 | **Medications Commonly Used to Alleviate Opioid Side Effects**

Side Effects	Treatment/Medication Recommendations
Nausea and vomiting	Prochlorperazine (Compazine)
	Thiethylperazine (Torecan)
	Metoclopramide (Reglan)
	Haloperidol (Haldol)
	Droperidol (Inapsine)
	Hydroxyzine (Vistaril)
	Lorazepam (Ativan)
	Granisetron (Kytril)
	Odansetron (Zofran)
Constipation	Increase of fiber consumption
	Mild laxative (Milk of Magnesia)
	Stimulating cathartic drug; bisacodyl, standardized senna concentrate, or hyperosmotic agents
Sedation	Persistent sedation may be helped by reducing the opioid in each dose and increasing the dose frequency. In some patients, switching to another opioid may reduce the sedative effects.
	Caffeine
	Dextroamphetamine
	Methylphenidate
	Pemoline
	Modafinil
Confusion	Lower opioid dose
	Change to a different opioid
	Haloperidol
	Olanzapine
Myoclonus	Clonazepam (Klonopin)
	Diazepam (Valium)
	Baclofen (Lioresal)
Respiratory depression	Preventive: Start opioid analgesics in low doses in opioid-naïve patients, and be cognizant of relative potencies when switching opioid analgesics, routes of administration, or both.
	Opioid antagonists such as naloxone (Narcan), should be used with extreme caution in patients who are opioid tolerant because of the risk of inducing a withdrawal state

scope of this chapter; however, interested readers are directed to the Agency for Health Care Policy and Research *Clinical Practice Guideline: Management of Cancer Pain.*[29*]

Opioid Side Effects

Although the opioids are extremely effective analgesics, their side effects are common and can be minimized if anticipated in advance (Table 17.5). Sedation is a common central nervous system (CNS) side effect, especially during the initiation of treatment. Sedation usually resolves after the patient has been maintained on a steady dosage. Persistent sedation can be alleviated with a psychostimulant, such as dextroamphetamine, pemoline, or methylphenidate. All are prescribed in divided doses in early morning and at noon. Additionally, psychostimulants can improve depressed mood and enhance analgesia.[47–49] Delirium, of an either agitated or somnolent variety, can also occur while on opioid analgesics and is usually accompanied by attentional deficits, disorientation, and perceptual disturbances (visual hallucinations and more commonly illusions). Myoclonus and asterixis are often early signs of neurotoxicity that accompany the course of opioid-induced delirium. Meperidine (Demerol), when administered chronically in patients with renal impairment, can lead to delirium due to accumulation of the neuroexcitatory metabolite normeperidine.[50] Opioid-induced delirium can be alleviated through the implementation of three possible strategies: (a) lowering the dose of the opioid drug presently in use, (b) changing to a different opioid, or (c) treating the delirium with low doses of neuroleptics, such as haloperidol or olanzapine. The third strategy is especially useful for agitation and clears the sensorium.[51] For agitated states, intravenous haloperidol in doses starting at between 1 or 2 mg is useful, with rapid escalation of dose if no effect is noted. Gastrointestinal side effects of opioid analgesics are common. The most prevalent are nausea, vomiting, and constipation.[31] Concomitant therapy with prochlorperazine for nausea is sometimes effective. Because all opioid analgesics are not tolerated in the same manner, switching to another narcotic can be helpful if an antiemetic regimen fails to control nausea. Constipation caused by narcotic effects on gut receptors is a problem frequently encountered, and it tends to be responsive to the regular use of senna derivatives. A careful review of medications is imperative, because anticholinergic drugs such as the tricyclic antidepressants can worsen opioid-induced constipation and can cause bowel obstruction. Respiratory depression is a worrisome but rare side effect of the opioid analgesics. Respiratory difficulties can almost always be avoided if two general principles are adhered to: (a) start opioid analgesics in low doses in opioid-naïve patients, and (b) be cognizant of relative potencies when switching opioid analgesics, routes of administration, or both.

ADJUVANT ANALGESICS

Adjuvant analgesics are the third class of medications frequently prescribed for the treatment of chronic pain and have important applications in the management of pain in AIDS (Table 17.6). Adjuvant analgesic drugs are used to enhance the analgesic efficacy of opioids, treat concurrent symptoms that exacerbate pain, and provide independent analgesia. They may be used in all stages of the analgesic ladder. Commonly used adjuvant drugs include antidepressants, neuroleptics, psychostimulants, anticonvulsants, corticosteroids, and oral and topical local anesthetics.[29,48,49,52]

ANTIDEPRESSANTS

The current literature supports the use of antidepressants as adjuvant analgesic agents in the management of a wide variety of chronic pain syndromes, including cancer pain, postherpetic neuralgia, diabetic neuropathy, fibromyalgia, headache, and low back pain.[53–58] The antidepressants

---

Agency for Health Care Policy and Research's Clinical Practice Guideline: Management of Cancer Pain is available free of charge through 1-800-4-cancer.

TABLE 17.6	Psychotropic Adjuvant Analgesic Drugs for AIDS Pain	
Generic Name	Approximate Daily Dosage Range (mg)	Route
Tricyclic Antidepressants		
Amitriptyline	10–150	PO, IM
Nortriptyline	10–150	PO
Imipramine	15.5–150	PO, IM
Desipramine	10–150	PO
Clomipramine	10–150	PO
Doxepin	12–150	PO, IM
Heterocyclic and Noncyclic Antidepressants		
Trazodone	125–300	PO
Maprotiline	50–300	PO
Selective Serotonin Reuptake Inhibitors		
Fluoxetine	20–80	PO
Paroxetine	10–60	PO
Sertraline	50–200	PO
Newer Agents		
Nefazodone	100–500	PO
Venlafaxine	75–300	PO
Mirtazepine	15–60	PO
Duloxetine	60–120	PO
Psychostimulants		
Methylphenidate	2.5–20 bid	PO
Dextroamphetamine	2.5–20 bid	PO
Pemoline	13.75–75 bid	PO
Modafinil	100–400	PO
Phenothiazines		
Fluphenazine	1–3	PO, IM
Methotrimeprazine	10–20 q6h	IM, IV
Butyrophenones		
Haloperidol	1–3	POA, IV
Pimozide	2–6 bid	PO
Atypical Antipsychotics		
Olanzapine	2.5–20	PO
Antihistamines		
Hydroxyzine	50 q4h–q6h	PO
Anticonvulsants		
Carbamazepine	200 tid–400 tid	PO
Phenytoin	300–400	PO
Valproate	500 tid–1,000 tid	PO
Gabapentin	300 tid–1,000 tid	PO
Pregabalin	150–600	PO
Oral Local Anesthetics		
Mexiletine	600–900	PO

(continued)

TABLE 17.6	Psychotropic Adjuvant Analgesic Drugs for AIDS Pain (Continued)		
Topical Local Anesthetics			
Lidocaine	5%		Patch
Corticosteroids			
Dexamethasone	4–16		PO, IV
Benzodiazepines			
Alprazolam	0.25–2 tid		PO
Clonazepam	0.5–4 bid		PO

bid, twice per day; *IM*, intramuscular; *IV*, intravenous; *PO*, per oral; *q6h*, every 6 hours; *qid*, four times per day; *tid*, three times per day.

are analgesic through a number of mechanisms that include antidepressant activity,[54] potentiation or enhancement of opioid analgesia,[59–61] and direct analgesic effects.[62] The leading hypothesis suggests that both serotonergic and noradrenergic properties of the antidepressants are probably important and that variations amongst individuals in pain (as to the status of their own neurotransmitter systems) is an important variable.[25] Other possible mechanisms of antidepressant analgesic activity that have been proposed include adrenergic and serotonin receptor effects,[63] adenosinergic effects, antihistaminic effects,[63] and direct neuronal effects, such as inhibition of paroxysmal neuronal discharge and decreasing sensitivity of adrenergic receptors on injured nerve sprouts.[64]

There is substantial evidence that the tricyclic antidepressants in particular are analgesic and useful in the management of chronic neuropathic and non-neuropathic pain syndromes. Amitriptyline is the tricyclic antidepressant most studied and has been proved effective as an analgesic in a large number of clinical trials addressing a wide variety of chronic pain syndromes, including neuropathy, cancer pain, fibromyalgia, and others.[25,54,55,65–67] Other tricyclics that have been shown to have efficacy as analgesics include imipramine,[68,69] desipramine,[26,70] nortriptyline,[71] clomipramine,[72,73] and doxepin.[74]

The heterocyclic and noncyclic antidepressant drugs, such as trazodone, mianserin, and maprotiline and the newer selective serotonin reuptake inhibitors (SSRIs) fluoxetine and paroxetine, may also be useful as adjuvant analgesics for chronic pain syndromes.[25,48,49,55,62,69,70,75–79] Fluoxetine, a potent antidepressant with specific serotonin reuptake inhibition activity,[78] has been shown to have analgesic properties in experimental animal pain models,[79] but failed to show analgesic effects in a clinical trial for neuropathy.[70] Several case reports suggest fluoxetine may be a useful adjuvant analgesic in the management of headache and fibrositis.[80] Paroxetine, a newer SSRI, is the first antidepressant of this class shown to be a highly effective analgesic in a controlled trial for the treatment of diabetic neuropathy.[69] Newer antidepressants such as sertraline, nefazodone, venlafaxine, and mirtazapine may also eventually prove to be clinically useful as adjuvant analgesics.

Duloxetine, an antidepressant with potent dual reuptake inhibition of serotonin and norepinephrine has been demonstrated to be a potent analgesic, particularly in such painful syndromes as fibromyalgia and diabetic neuropathy.[81] In a recent double-blind, randomized, placebo controlled trial, duloxetine, at dosages of 60 to 120 mg a day, was shown to be highly effective in reducing pain due to diabetic neuropathy.[81] In clinical practice, the data on duloxetine's efficacy in diabetic neuropathy has led to its widespread use in other painful neuropathies, including those related to AIDS.

Given the diversity of clinical syndromes in which the antidepressants have been demonstrated to be analgesic, trials of these drugs can be justified in the treatment of virtually every type of chronic pain.[52] The established benefit of several of the antidepressants in patients with neuropathic pain,[66,69] however, suggests these drugs may be particularly useful in populations such as patients with cancer and AIDS, where an underlying neuropathic component to the pain(s) often exists.[52] Although studies of the analgesic efficacy of these drugs in HIV-related painful neuropathies have not yet been conducted, they are widely applied clinically using the model of diabetic and postherpetic neuropathies.

Although antidepressant drugs are analgesic in both neuropathic and nonneuropathic pain models, their clinical use is most commonly in combination with opioid drugs, particularly for moderate-to-severe pain. Antidepressant adjuvant analgesics have their most broad application as coanalgesics, potentiating the analgesic effects of opioid drugs.[29] The opioid-sparing effects of antidepressant analgesics have been demonstrated in a number of trials, especially in cancer populations with neuropathic and non-neuropathic pain syndromes.[55,58]

The dose and time course of onset of analgesia for antidepressants when used as analgesics appears to be similar to their use as antidepressants. There is compelling evidence that the therapeutic analgesic effects of amitriptyline are correlated with serum levels, as are the antidepressant effects, and that analgesic treatment failure is due to low serum levels.[66] A high-dose regimen of up to 150 mg of amitriptyline or higher is suggested.[65] The proper analgesic dose for paroxetine is likely in the 40- to 60-mg range, with the major analgesic trial utilizing a fixed dose of 40 mg.[69] There is anecdotal evidence to suggest that the debilitated medically ill (cancer, AIDS) often respond (in regard to depression or pain) to lower doses of antidepressants than are usually required in the physically healthy, probably because of impaired metabolism of these drugs.[48,49] As to the time-course of onset of analgesia, a biphasic process appears to occur. There are immediate or early analgesic effects that occur within hours or days, and these are probably mediated through inhibition of synaptic reuptake of catecholamines. In addition, there are later, longer analgesic effects that peak over a 2- to 4-week period that are probably due to receptor effects of the antidepressants.[65,66]

NEUROLEPTICS AND BENZODIAZEPINES

Neuroleptic drugs, such as methotrimeprazine, fluphenazine, haloperidol, pimozide, and olanzapine, may play a role as adjuvant analgesics[71,82–85] in patients with AIDS who are experiencing pain; however, their use must be weighed against what appears to be an increased sensitivity to the extrapyramidal side effects of these drugs in patients with AIDS who have neurologic complications.[86] Olanzapine, a novel antipsychotic with low potential for extrapyramidal side effects, may be particularly useful in providing adjuvant analgesia in patients with concomitant cognitive impairment and anxiety.[85] Anxiolytics, such as alprazolam and clonazepam, may also be useful as adjuvant analgesics, particularly in the management of neuropathic pains.[87,88]

PSYCHOSTIMULANTS

Psychostimulants, such as dextroamphetamine, methylphenidate, pemoline, and modafinil may be useful antidepressants in patients with HIV infection or AIDS who are cognitively impaired.[47,86] Psychostimulants also enhance the analgesic effects of the opioid drugs.[89] Psychostimulants are also useful in diminishing sedation secondary to narcotic analgesics, and they are potent adjuvant analgesics. Bruera et al.[47] demonstrated that a regimen of 10 mg methylphenidate with breakfast and 5 mg with lunch significantly decreased sedation and potentiated the effect of narcotics in patients with cancer pain. Methylphenidate has also been demonstrated to improve functioning on a number neuropsychological tests, including tests of memory, speed, and concentration, in patients receiving continuous infusions of opioids for cancer pain.[47] Dextroamphetamine has also been reported to have additive analgesic effects when used with morphine in postoperative pain.[90] In relatively low doses, psychostimulants stimulate appetite, promote a sense of well-being, and improve feelings of weakness and fatigue in cancer patients.

Pemoline is a unique alternative psychostimulant that is chemically unrelated to amphetamine but may have similar usefulness as an antidepressant and adjuvant analgesic in patients with AIDS.[49] Advantages of pemoline as a psychostimulant in patients with AIDS who are experiencing pain include the lack of abuse potential, the lack of federal regulation through special triplicate prescriptions, the mild sympathomimetic effects, and the fact that it comes in a chewable tablet form that can be absorbed through the buccal mucosa and thus can be used by AIDS patients who have difficulty swallowing or who have intestinal obstruction. Clinically, pemoline is as effective as methylphenidate or dextroamphetamine in the treatment of depressive symptoms and in countering the sedating effects of opioid analgesics. There are no studies of pemoline's capacity to potentiate the analgesic properties of opioids. Pemoline should be used with caution in patients with liver impairment, and liver function tests should be monitored periodically with longer term treatment. The Food and Drug Administration (FDA) suggests that patients sign an informed consent document, which outlines the potential liver toxicities of pemoline when pemoline is prescribed.

Modafinil, a novel psychostimulant that has shown efficacy in treating excessive daytime sleepiness associated with narcolepsy has recently demonstrated potential for the treatment of depression and fatigue.[91] Modafinil needs further study; however, it appears to be a promising alternative to other psychostimulants in patients who cannot tolerate, or have contraindications to, the use of other stimulants. Modafinil has minimal cardiovascular effects, does not cause tolerance or dependence, has a low abuse potential, and does not require a special triplicate prescription.

ANTICONVULSANT DRUGS

Selected anticonvulsant drugs appear to be analgesic for the lancinating dysesthesias that characterize diverse types of neuropathic pain.[52] Clinical experience also supports the use of these agents in patients with paroxysmal neuropathic pains that may not be lancinating, and to a far lesser extent, in those with neuropathic pains characterized solely by continuous dysesthesias. Although most practitioners prefer to begin with carbamazepine because of the extraordinarily good response rate observed in trigeminal neuralgia, this drug must be used cautiously in patients with AIDS who have thrombocytopenia, those at risk for marrow failure, and those whose blood counts must be monitored to determine disease status. If carbamazepine is used, a complete blood count should be obtained before the start of therapy, after 2 and 4 weeks, and then every 3 to 4 months thereafter. A leukocyte count below 4,000 is usually considered to be a contraindication to treatment, and a decline to less than 3,000 or an absolute neutrophil count of less than 1,500 during therapy should prompt discontinuation of the drug. Other anticonvulsant drugs may be useful for managing neuropathic pain in patients with AIDS, including phenytoin, clonazepam, valproate, and gabapentin.[52]

Several newer anticonvulsants have been used in the treatment of neuropathic pain, particularly in patients with reflex sympathetic dystrophy. These drugs include gabapentin, lamotrigine, and felbamate. Of these newer anticonvulsants, anecdotal experience has been most favorable with gabapentin, which is now being widely used by pain specialists to treat neuropathic pain of various types. Gabapentin has a relatively high degree of safety, including no known drug–drug interactions and a lack of hepatic metabolism.[51] Treatment with gabapentin is usually initiated at a dose of 300 mg/day and then gradually increased to a dose range of 900 to 3,200 mg/day in three divided doses.

Pregabalin, a newly available anticonvulsant, has recently been demonstrated to be an effective analgesic in the management of postherpetic neuropathy and painful diabetic neuropathy.[92] Dosage regimens for pregabalin that have been studied include flexible regimens starting at 150 mg a day, raised weekly by 150 mg to a dose of 600 mg a day, or fixed dosages of 300 mg a day for 1 week then escalated to 600 mg a day.[92]

Baclofen is a gamma-aminobutyric acid (GABA) agonist that has proven efficacy in the treatment of trigeminal neuralgia.[52] On this basis, a trial of this drug is commonly employed in the management of paroxysmal neuropathic pains of any type. Dosing is generally undertaken in a manner similar to the use of the drug for its primary indication, spasticity. A starting dose of 5 mg two to three times per day is gradually escalated to 30 to 90 mg per day and sometimes higher if side effects do not occur. The most common adverse effects are sedation and confusion.

CORTICOSTEROIDS

Corticosteroid drugs have analgesic potential in a variety of chronic pain syndromes, including neuropathic pain and pain syndromes resulting from inflammatory processes.[52] Like other adjuvant analgesics, corticosteroids are usually added to an opioid regimen. In patients with advanced disease, these drugs may also improve appetite, nausea, malaise, and overall quality of life. Adverse effects include neuropsychiatric syndromes, gastrointestinal disturbances, and immunosuppression.

ORAL AND TOPICAL LOCAL ANESTHETICS

Local anesthetic drugs may be useful in the management of neuropathic pains characterized by either continuous or lancinating dysesthesias. Controlled trials have demonstrated the efficacy of oral tocainide[93] and mexiletine, and there is clinical evidence that suggests similar effects from flecainide[94] and subcutaneous lidocaine.[95] It is reasonable to undertake a trial with oral local anesthetic in patients with continuous dysesthesias who fail to respond adequately to, or who cannot tolerate, the tricyclic antidepressants, and with patients with lancinating pain refractory to trials of anticonvulsant drugs and baclofen. Mexiletine is preferred in the United States.[52] Paice et al.[96] studied 26 subjects to test the efficacy of topical capsaicin in the management of HIV-associated pain. Results suggest that capsaicin is ineffective in relieving pain with HIV-associated distal symmetric peripheral neuropathy; however, capsaicin has been shown to be effective in relieving pain associated with other neuropathic pain syndromes.[96] More recently, lidocaine 5% patches used topically have been shown to relieve a variety of neuropathic pain conditions,[97] although no controlled trials have yet been published in HIV-related neuropathies.

DRUG INTERACTIONS: ANALGESICS AND ANTI-HIV DRUG THERAPIES

Many of the available anti-HIV drugs have the potential to interact with other medications prescribed for pain, depression, anxiety, or other medical conditions. These drug interactions can be dangerous, resulting in drug toxicities due to elevated levels of medication, or drug ineffectiveness because of the lowering of drug levels in the serum. Opioid analgesics can interact with certain anti-HIV drug therapies, and these interactions should be kept in mind when prescribing opioids. The protease inhibitor ritonavir (Norvir) can increase the levels of several opioid drugs, including codeine, hydrocodone, oxycodone, methadone, and fentanyl. Patients on ritonavir should not be prescribed meperidine or propoxyphene because of increased risk of serious toxicity. Antidepressant and anticonvulsant analgesics can also interact primarily with ritonavir. Ritonavir can increase the serum levels of bupropion (Wellbutrin, Zyban), fluoxetine, trazodone, and desipramine, resulting in increased drug toxicities (e.g., seizures with bupropion). Both ritonavir and saquinavir (Invirase) may increase levels of anticonvulsants such as phenobarbital, phenytoin, carbamazepine, and clonazepam.

TABLE 17.7	Nonpharmacologic Interventions

Physical Therapies
    Cutaneous stimulation (superficial heat, cold, and massage)
    Transcutaneous electrical nerve stimulation (TENS)
    Acupuncture
    Bed rest

Psychological Therapies
    Relaxation, imagery, biofeedback, distraction, and reframing
    Hypnosis
    Patient education

Neurosurgical Procedures
    Nerve blocks
    Cordotomy

NONPHARMACOLOGIC INTERVENTIONS

A variety of physical and psychological therapies may also prove useful in the management of HIV-related pain (Table 17.7). Physical interventions range from bed rest and simple exercise programs to the application of cold-packs or heat to affected sites. Other nonpharmacologic interventions include whirlpool baths, massage, the application of ultrasound, and transcutaneous electrical nerve stimulation (TENS). Increasing numbers of patients with AIDS have resorted to acupuncture to relieve their pain, with anecdotal reports of efficacy.

Several psychological interventions have demonstrated potential efficacy in alleviating HIV-related pain, including hypnosis, relaxation and distraction techniques such as biofeedback and imagery, and cognitive-behavioral techniques (see Tables 17.7 and 17.8 for sample relaxation and distraction exercises). Where nonpharmacologic and standard pharmacologic treatments fail, anesthetic and even neurosurgical procedures (such as nerve block, cordotomy, and epidural delivery of analgesics) are additional options available to the patient who appreciates the risks and limitations of these procedures.

TABLE 17.8	An Approach to Pain Management in Substance Abusers with HIV Disease

1. Substance abusers with HIV disease deserve pain control; we have an obligation to treat pain and suffering in all of our patients.
2. Accept and respect the report of pain.
3. Be careful about the label "substance abuse"; distinguish between tolerance, physical dependence, and addiction (psychological dependence or drug abuse).
4. Not all substance abusers are the same; distinguish between active users, individuals in methadone maintenance, and those in recovery.
5. Individualize pain treatment.
6. Utilize the principles of pain management outlined for all patients with HIV disease and pain (WHO Ladder).
7. Set clear goals and conditions for opioid therapy: set limits, recognize drug abuse behaviors, make consequences clear, and use written contracts, establish a single prescriber.
8. Use a multidimensional approach: pharmacologic and nonpharmacologic interventions, attention to psychosocial issues, team approach.

UNDERTREATMENT OF PAIN

Reports of dramatic undertreatment of pain in patients with AIDS have appeared in the literature.[8,9] These studies suggest that all classes of analgesics, particularly opioid analgesics, are underutilized in the treatment of pain in AIDS. Our group has reported[5] that less than 8% of individuals in our cohort of ambulatory patients with AIDS reporting pain in the severe range (8 to 10 on a NRS of pain intensity) received a strong opioid, such as morphine, as recommended by published guidelines.[30] In addition, 18% of patients with severe pain were prescribed no analgesics whatsoever, 40% were prescribed a nonopioid analgesic (e.g., an NSAID), and only 22% were prescribed a weak opioid (e.g., acetaminophen in combination with oxycodone). Utilizing the Pain Management Index (PMI),[98] a measure of adequacy of analgesic therapy derived from the BPI's record of pain intensity and strength of analgesia prescribed, our group further examined adequacy of pain treatment. Only 15% of our sample received adequate analgesic therapy based on the PMI. This degree of undermedication of pain in AIDS (85%) far exceeds published reports of undermedication of pain (using the PMI) in cancer populations of 40%. Larue et al.[7] report that in France, 57% of patients with HIV disease reporting moderate-to-severe pain did not receive any analgesic treatment at all and only 22% received a weak opioid.

Opioid analgesics are underutilized; it is also clear that adjuvant analgesic agents, such as the antidepressants, are also dramatically underutilized.[4,7–9] Breitbart et al.[4] report that less than 10% of patients with AIDS reporting pain received an adjuvant analgesic drug (e.g., antidepressants and anticonvulsants), despite the fact that approximately 40% of the sample had neuropathic type pain. This class of analgesic agents is a critical component of the WHO Analgesic Ladder, particularly in managing neuropathic pain and is vastly underutilized in the management of HIV-related pain.

BARRIERS TO PAIN MANAGEMENT

A number of different factors have been proposed as potential influences on the widespread undertreatment of pain in AIDS, including patient, clinician, and health care system–related barriers (Table 17.8).[4,99,100] Sociodemographic factors that have been reported to be associated with undertreatment of pain in AIDS include gender, education, and substance abuse history.[5] Women, less educated patients, and patients who reported injection drug use as their HIV risk transmission factor are significantly more likely to receive inadequate analgesic therapy for HIV-related pain.

Breitbart et al.[99] surveyed 200 ambulatory AIDS patients utilizing a modified version of the Barriers Questionnaire (BQ),[101] which assesses a variety of patient-related barriers to pain management (resulting in patient reluctance to report pain or take opioid analgesics). Results of this study demonstrated that patient-related barriers (as measured by BQ scores) were significantly correlated with undertreatment of pain (as measured by the PMI) in AIDS patients with pain. Additionally, BQ scores were significantly correlated with higher levels of psychological distress and depression, indicating that patient-related barriers contributed to undertreatment for pain and poorer quality of life. The most frequently endorsed BQ items were those concerning the addiction potential of opioids, side effects and discomfort related to opioid administration, and misconceptions about tolerance. Although there were no age, gender, or HIV risk transmission factor associations with BQ scores, non-White and less educated patients scored higher on the BQ. Several additional AIDS specific patient-related barriers examined[99] reveal that 66% of patients are trying to limit their overall intake of medications (i.e., pills) or utilize nonpharmacologic interventions for pain, 50% of patients cannot afford to fill a prescription for analgesics or have no access to pain specialists, and about 50% are reluctant to take opioids for pain out of a concern that family, friends, physicians will assume they are misusing or abusing these drugs.

TABLE 17.9	Barriers to Pain Management in AIDS

Clinician-Related Factors
Focus on treating life-threatening opportunistic infections
Inability to properly assess pain
Limited knowledge of current pharmacotherapeutic approaches
Fears of causing addiction or contributing to drug abuse
Concern about regulation of controlled substances

Patient-Related Factors
Limited expectation regarding pain relief
Reluctance to bring up pain as a focus of care
Limited capacity to communicate as AIDS dementia increases
Fears of addition or readdiction

Social and Economic Factors
Restrictive regulation of controlled substances
Access to health care; availability of treatments
Inadequate reimbursement, financial concerns

In a survey of approximately 500 AIDS care providers[100] clinicians (primarily physicians and nurses) rated the barriers to AIDS pain management they perceived to be the most important in the care of AIDS patients. The most frequently endorsed barriers were those regarding lack of knowledge about pain management or access to pain specialists and concerns regarding the use and addiction potential of opioid drugs in the AIDS population. The top five barriers endorsed by AIDS clinicians included the following: Lack of knowledge regarding pain management (51.8%); Reluctance to prescribe opioids (51.5%); Lack of access to pain specialists (50.9%); Concern regarding drug addiction and/or abuse (50.5%); and Lack of psychological support/drug treatment services (43%). Patient reluctance to report pain and patient reluctance to take opioids were less commonly endorsed barriers, with about 24% of respondents endorsing those barriers. In contrast, past surveys of oncologists rated patient reluctance to report pain or take opioids as two of the top four barriers. Like AIDS care providers, oncologists also endorsed highly a reluctance to prescribe opioids, even to a population of cancer patients with a significantly lower prevalence of past or present substance abuse disorders. Both oncologists and AIDS care providers report they have inadequate knowledge of pain management and pain assessment skills.

PAIN MANAGEMENT AND SUBSTANCE ABUSE

Individuals who inject drugs are amongst the AIDS exposure categories with the highest rate of increase over the past 5 years, especially in large urban centers. Pain management in the substance-abusing patient with AIDS is perhaps the most challenging of clinical goals. Fears of addiction and concerns regarding drug abuse affect both patient compliance and physician management of pain and use of narcotic analgesics, often leading to the undermedication of HIV-infected patients with pain.

Studies of patterns of chronic narcotic analgesic use in patients with cancer, burns, and postoperative pain, however, have demonstrated that, although tolerance and physical dependence commonly occur, addiction, that is, psychological dependence and drug abuse, are rare and almost never occur in individuals who do not have histories of drug abuse.[102–104] More relevant to the clinical problem of pain management in AIDS patients, however, is the issue of managing pain in the growing segment of HIV infected patients who have a history of substance abuse or who are actively abusing drugs. The use, specifically of opioids for pain control in patients with HIV infection and a history of substance abuse, raises several difficult pain treatment questions, including how to treat pain in people who have a high tolerance to narcotic analgesics; how to mitigate this population's drug-seeking and potentially manipulative behavior; how to deal with patients who may offer unreliable medical histories or who may not comply with treatment recommendations; and how to counter the risk of patients spreading HIV while high and disinhibited.

Perhaps of greatest concern to clinicians is the possibility that they are being lied to by a substance-abusing patient with AIDS who is complaining of pain. Clinicians must rely on a patient's subjective report, which is often the best or only indication of the presence and intensity of pain, as well as the degree of pain relief achieved by an intervention. Physicians who believe they are being manipulated by drug-seeking patients often hesitate to use appropriately high doses of narcotic analgesics to control pain. The fear is that the clinician is being "duped" into prescribing narcotic analgesics, which will then be abused or sold. Clinicians do not want to contribute to or help sustain addiction. This leads to an immediate defensiveness on the part of the clinician and an impulse to avoid prescribing opioids and even to avoid full assessment of a pain complaint. Because concerns are often raised regarding the credibility of patients with AIDS' report of pain, particularly where there is a history of injection drug use, Breitbart et al.[2,3] conducted a study of 516 ambulatory patients with AIDS, in which they compared the report of pain experience and the adequacy of pain management among patients with and without a history of substance abuse. This study found that there were no significant differences in the report of pain experience (i.e., pain prevalence, pain intensity, and pain-related functional interference) among patients who reported injection drug use as their HIV transmission risk factor and those who reported other transmission factors (non–injection drug use). Furthermore, there were no differences in the report of pain experience among patients who acknowledged current substance abuse, those in methadone maintenance, and those who were in drug-free recovery. The description of HIV-related pain was comparable among intravenous drug users (IDUs) and non-IDU groups. What was different was the treatment received by these two groups. Patients in the IDU group were significantly more under-medicated for pain compared to the non-IDU group. A survey of 211 HIV-infected patients was conducted to assess pain reporting in HIV-infected patients with and without intravenous drug use.[105] Martin et al.[105] demonstrated that non-IDUs showed a strong correlation between pain and disease stage, CD4 levels, and mortality rates. However, IDUs did not display the same correlation between pain and disease parameters. Finally, Martin et al.[105] concluded that pain was more prominent in IDUs compared to non-IDUs, suggesting the need to differentiate risk groups in pain-related studies.

Unfortunately, the existence or severity of pain cannot be objectively proven. The clinician must accept and respect the report of pain in spite of the possibility of being duped and proceed in the evaluation, assessment, and management of pain.

Experience from the cancer pain literature suggests that it is possible to adequately manage pain in substance abusers with life-threatening illness and to do so safely and responsibly utilizing opioid analgesics and several sound principles of pain management (Table 17.9).[106–108] Most clinicians experienced in working with this population of patients recommend that practitioners set clear and direct limits. Although this is an important aspect of the care of IDUs with HIV disease, it is by no means the whole answer. As much as possible, clinicians should attempt to eliminate the issue of drug abuse as an obstacle to pain management by dealing directly with the problems of opiate withdrawal and drug treatment. Clinicians should err on the side of believing patients when they complain of pain and should utilize knowledge of specific HIV-related pain syndromes to corroborate the report of a patient perceived as being unreliable. Messiah et al.[109] sought to demonstrate whether physicians were able to accurately identify IDUs and treat them appropriately. The results suggest that identification of active intravenous drug use may be partially based on incorrect interpretations of subjective cues.[109]

The clinician must be familiar with, and understand the current terminology relevant to, substance abuse and addiction. It is important to distinguish between the terms *tolerance*, *physical dependence*, and *addiction* or *abuse* (psychological dependence). Tolerance is a pharmacologic property of opioid drugs defined by the need for increasing doses to maintain an (analgesic) effect. Physical dependence is characterized by the onset of signs and symptoms of withdrawal if narcotic analgesics are abruptly stopped or a narcotic antagonist is administered. Tolerance usually occurs in association with physical dependence. Addiction or abuse (also often termed psychological dependence) is a psychological and behavioral syndrome in which there is drug craving, compulsive use (despite physical, psychological, or social harm to user), other aberrant drug-related behaviors, and relapse after abstinence.[36] The term "pseudo-addiction" has been coined to describe the patient who exhibits behavior that clinicians associate with addiction, such as requests for higher doses of opioid, but in fact is due to uncontrolled pain and inadequate pain management.[110]

The clinician must also distinguish between the "former" addict who has been drug free for years, the addict in a methadone maintenance program, and the addict who is actively abusing illicit and/or prescription drugs. Actively using addicts and those on methadone maintenance who are experiencing pain must be assumed to have some tolerance to opioids and may require higher starting and maintenance doses of opioids. Preventing withdrawal is an essential first step in managing pain in this population. In addition, "active" addicts with AIDS will understandably require more in the way of psychosocial support and services to adequately deal with the distress of their pain and illness. Former addicts may pose the challenge of refusing opioids for pain because of fears of relapse. Such patients can be assured that opioids, when prescribed and monitored responsibly, may be an essential part of pain management, and the use of the drug for pain is quite different from its use when they were abusing similar drugs. Some authorities emphasize the importance of conducting a comprehensive pain assessment to define the pain syndrome. Specific pain syndromes often respond best to specific interventions (e.g., neuropathic pains respond well to antidepressants or anticonvulsants). Adequate assessment of the cause of pain is essential in all patients with AIDS and particularly in the substance abuser. It is critical that adequate analgesia be provided while diagnostic studies are underway. Often treatments directed at the underlying disorder causing pain are very effective as well. For example, headache from CNS toxoplasmosis responds well to primary treatments and steroids.

When deciding on an appropriate pharmacologic intervention in the substance abuser, it is advisable to follow the WHO Analgesic Ladder. This approach advocates selection of analgesics based on severity of pain; however, clinicians also often take into account the nature of the pain syndrome in selecting analgesics. For mild-to-moderate pain, NSAIDs are indicated. The NSAIDs are continued with adjuvant analgesics (antidepressants, anticonvulsants, neuroleptics, steroids) if a specific indication exists. Patients with moderate-to-severe pain or those who do not achieve relief from NSAIDs are treated with a weak opioid, often in combination with NSAIDs and adjuvant drugs, if indicated.

It has been pointed out that it is critical to apply appropriate pharmacologic principles for opioid use. Data by Kaplan et al.[111] suggest that patients with AIDS with prior drug use history benefited by opioid analgesia but required substantially more morphine than nonusers. One should avoid using agonist-antagonist opioid drugs. The use of as-needed dosing often leads to excessive drug-centered interactions with staff that are not productive. Although patients should not necessarily be given the specific drug or route they want, every effort should be made to give patients more of a sense of control and a sense of collaboration with the clinician. Often a patient's report of beneficial or adverse effects of a specific agent are useful to the clinician.

The management of pain in substance-abusing AIDS patients requires a team approach. Early involvement of pain specialists, psychiatric clinicians, and substance abuse specialists is critical. Nonpharmacologic pain interventions should be appropriately applied, not as a substitute for opioids but as an important adjunct. Realistic goals for treatment must be set, and problems related to inappropriate behavior around the handling of prescriptions and interactions with staff should be anticipated.

Hospital staff must be educated and made aware that such difficult patients evoke feelings that if acted on could interfere with providing good care. Clear limit setting is helpful for both the patient and treating staff. Sometimes, written rules about what behaviors are expected and what behaviors are not tolerated and the consequence should be provided. The use of urine toxicology monitoring, restrictions of visitors, and strict limits on amount of drug per prescription can all be very useful. It is important to also remember that rehabilitation or detoxification from opioids is not appropriate during an acute medical crisis and should not be attempted at that time. Once more stable medical conditions exist, referral to a drug rehabilitation program may be very useful. Constant assessment and reevaluation of the effects of pain interventions must also take place to optimize care. Special attention should be given to points in treatment where routes of administration are changed or where opioids are being tapered. It must be made clear to patients what drugs and/or regimen would be introduced to control pain when opioids are tapered or withdrawn and what options are available if that nonopioid regimen is ineffective.

Finally, it is important to recognize that substance abusers with AIDS are quite likely to have comorbid psychiatric symptoms, as well as multiple other physical symptoms, which can all contribute to increased pain and suffering. Adequate attention must be paid to these physical and psychological symptoms for pain management to be optimized.

SUMMARY

Pain in AIDS, even in this era of protease inhibitors and decreased AIDS death rates, is a clinically significant problem contributing greatly to psychological and functional morbidity. Pain can be adequately treated and so must be a focus of psychiatric and supportive care in the patient with AIDS. Substance abusers and women are particularly undertreated segments of the population with AIDS pain and need special attention. Managing pain in patients with AIDS who have a history of substance abuse is a particularly challenging problem, which mental health professionals who provide care to patients with AIDS will be facing with increasing frequency.

REFERENCES

1. Breitbart W. Pharmacotherapy of pain in AIDS. In: Wormser G, ed. *A Clinical Guide to AIDS and HIV*. Philadelphia: Lippincott-Raven; 1996;359–378.
2. Breitbart W, Rosenfeld B, Passik S, et al. A comparison of pain report and adequacy of analgesic therapy in ambulatory AIDS patients with and without a history of substance abuse. *Pain*. 1997;72:235–243.
3. Breitbart W. Pain in AIDS. In: Jensen J, Turner J, Wiesenfeld-Hallin Z, eds. *Proceedings of the 8th World Congress on Pain: Progress in Pain Research and Management*. Vol 8. Seattle: IASP Press; 1997:63–100.
4. Breitbart W, Rosenfeld B, Passik S, et al. The undertreatment of pain in ambulatory AIDS patients. *Pain*. 1996;65:239–245.
5. Breitbart W, McDonald MV, Rosenfeld B, et al. Pain in ambulatory AIDS patients, I: Pain characteristics and medical correlates. *Pain*. 1996;68:315–321.
6. Hewitt D, McDonald M, Portenoy R, et al. Pain syndromes and etiologies in ambulatory AIDS patients. *Pain*. 1997;70:117–123.
7. Larue F, Fontaine A, Colleau S. Underestimation and undertreatment of pain in HIV disease: multicentre study. *Br Med J*. 1997;314:23–28.
8. Lebovits AK, Lefkowitz M, McCarthy D, et al. The prevalence and management of pain in patients with AIDS: a review of 134 cases. *Clin J Pain*. 1989;5:245–248.
9. McCormack JP, Li R, Zarowny D, et al. Inadequate treatment of pain in ambulatory HIV patients. *Clin J Pain*. 1993;9:247–283.

10. O'Neill WM, Sherrard JS. Pain in human immunodeficiency virus disease: a review. *Pain*. 1993;54:3–14.
11. Rosenfeld B, Breitbart W, McDonald MV, et al. Pain in ambulatory AIDS patients, II: Impact of pain on psychological functioning and quality of life. *Pain*. 1996;68:323–328.
12. Singer EJ, Zorilla C, Fahy-Chandon B, et al. Painful symptoms reported for ambulatory HIV-infected men in a longitudinal study. *Pain*. 1993;54:15–19.
13. Vogel D, Rosenfeld B, Breitbart W, et al. Symptom prevalence, characteristics, and distress in AIDS outpatients. *J Pain Symptom Manage*. 1999;18:253–262.
14. Breitbart W, Passik S, Bronaugh T, et al. Pain in the ambulatory AIDS patient: prevalence and psychosocial correlates [abstract]. 38th Annual Meeting, Academy of Psychosomatic Medicine, Atlanta, Georgia, October 17–20, 1991.
15. Kimball LR, McCormick WC. The pharmacologic management of pain and discomfort in persons with AIDS near the end of life: use of opioid analgesia in the hospice setting. *J Pain Symptom Manage*. 1996;11:88–94.
16. Schofferman J, Brody R. Pain in far advanced AIDS. In: Foley KM, et al., eds. *Advances in Pain Research and Therapy*. Vol 16. New York: Raven Press; 1990:379–386.
17. Larue F, Brasseur L, Musseault P, et al. Pain and HIV infection: a French national survey [abstract]. *J Palliat Care*. 1994;10:95.
18. Frich LM, Borgbjerg FM. Pain and pain treatment in AIDS patients: a longitudinal study. *J Pain Symptom Manage*. 2000;19:339–347.
19. Penfold R, Clark AJM. Pain syndromes in HIV infection. *Can J Anaesth*. 1992;39:724–730.
20. Breitbart W, McDonald M, Rosenfeld B, et al. Pain in women with AIDS [abstract]. Proceeding of the 14th Annual Meeting, American Pain Society, Los Angeles, Calif, 1995.
21. Marte C, Allen M. HIV-related gynecologic conditions: overlooked complications. *Focus Guide AIDS Res Counsel*. 1991;7:1–3.
22. Strafford M, Cahill C, Schwartz T, et al. Recognition and treatment of pain in pediatric patients with AIDS [abstract]. *J of Pain and Symp Manage*. 1991;6:146.
23. Breitbart W. Suicide risk and pain in cancer and AIDS patients. In: Chapman R, Foley KM, eds. *Current Emerging Issues in Cancer Pain: Research and Practice*. New York: Raven Press; 1993:49–65.
24. Payne D, Jacobsen P, Breitbart W, et al. Negative thoughts related to pain are associated with greater pain, distress and disability in AIDS pain [abstract]. 13th annual Scientific Meeting, American Pain Society, Miami, Fla, November 1994.
25. Watson CP, Chipman M, Reed K, et al. Amitriptyline versus maprotiline in post herpetic neuralgia: a randomized double-blind, cross-over trial. *Pain*. 1992;48:29–36.
26. Kishore-Kumar R, Max MB, Scafer SC, et al. Desipramine relieves post-herpetic neuralgia. *Clin Pharmacol Ther*. 1990;47:305–312.
27. Portenoy R, Foley KM. Management of cancer pain. In: Holland JC, Rowland JH, eds. *Handbook of Psychooncology*. New York: Oxford University Press; 1989:369–382.
28. Foley KM. The treatment of cancer pain. *N Engl J Med* 1985:313:84–95.
29. Jacox A, Carr D, Payne R, et al. *Management of Cancer Pain*. Clinical Practice Guideline No. 9. Washington, DC: U.S. Department of Health and Human Services, Public Health Service, Agency for Health Care Policy and Research, Publication 94-0592:139–41; 1994.
30. World Health Organization. *Cancer Pain Relief*. Geneva: World Health Organization; 1986.
31. Portenoy RK. Pharmacologic approaches to the control of cancer pain. *J Psychosocial Oncol*. 1990;8:75–107.
32. Fishman B, Pasternak S, Wallenstein SL, et al. The Memorial Pain Assessment Card: a valid instrument for the evaluation of cancer pain. *Cancer*. 1987;60:1151–1158.
33. Daut RL, Cleeland CS, Flanery RC. Development of the Wisconsin Brief Pain Questionnaire to assess pain in cancer and other diseases. *Pain* 1983;117:197–210.
34. O'Neill JF, Selwyn P, Schietinger H, eds. *A Clinical Guide to Supportive & Palliative Care for HIV/AIDS*. Washington, DC: Health Resources and Services Administration; 2003.
35. Ventrafridda V, Caraceni A, Gamba A. Field testing of the WHO guidelines for cancer pain relief: summary report of demonstration projects. In: Foley KM, Bonica JJ, Ventrafridda V, eds. *Proceedings of the Second International Congress on Pain*. Vol 16. *Advances in Pain Research and Therapy*. New York: Raven Press; 1990:155–165.
36. Lefkowitz M, Breitbart W. Chronic pain and AIDS. *Innovat Pain Med*. 1992;36:2–3, 18.
37. American Pain Society. *Principles of Analgesic Use in the Treatment of Acute Pain and Cancer Pain*. 3rd ed. Skokie, Ill: American Pain Society; 1992.
38. Newshan G, Wainapel S. Pain characteristics and their management in persons with AIDS. *J Assoc Nurs AIDS Care*. 1993;4:53–59.
39. Anand A, Carmosino L, Glatt AE. Evaluation of recalcitrant pain in HIV-infected hospitalized patients. *J Acquir Immune Defic Syndr*. 1994;7:52–56.
40. Patt RB, Reddy SR. Pain and the opioid analgesics: alternate routes of administration. *PAACNOTES*. November 1993:453–458.
41. Lefkowitz M, Newshan G. An evaluation of the use of Duragesic for chronic pain in patients with AIDS [abstract]. 16th Annual Meeting, American Pain Society, New Orleans, La, 23–26, November 1997.
42. Murray MD, Brater DC. Adverse effects of nonsteroidal anti-inflammatory drugs on renal function. *Ann Intern Med*. 1990;112:559–560.
43. Radeck K, Deck C. Do nonsteroidal anti-inflammatory drugs interfere with blood pressure control in hypertensive patients? *J Gen Int Med*. 1987;2:108–112.

44. Kaplan R, Conant M, Cundiff D, et al. Sustained-release morphine sulfate in the management of pain associated with acquired immune deficiency syndrome. *J Pain Symptom Manage.* 1996;12:150–160.
45. Newshan G, Lefkowitz M. Transdermal fentanyl for chronic pain in AIDS: a pilot study. *J Pain Symptom Manage.* 2001;21:69–77.
46. Foley KM, Inturrisi CE. Analgesic drug therapy in cancer pain: Principles and practice. In: Payne R, Foley KM, eds. *Cancer Pain Medical Clinics of North America.* Philadelphia: WB Saunders; 1987:207–232.
47. Bruera E, Chadwick S, Brennels C, et al. Methylphenidate associated with narcotics for the treatment of cancer pain. *Cancer Treat Rep.* 1987;71:67–70.
48. Breitbart W. Psychotropic adjuvant analgesics for cancer pain. *Psycho-Oncology.* 1992;7:133–145.
49. Breitbart W, Mermelstein H. Pemoline: an alternative psychostimulant in the management of depressive disorder in cancer patients. *Psychosomatics.* 1992;33:352–356.
50. Kaiko R, Foley K, Grabinski P, et al. Central nervous system excitation effects of meperidine in cancer patients. *Ann Neurol.* 1983;13:180–183.
51. Breitbart W. Psychiatric management of cancer pain. *Cancer.* 1989;63:2336–2342.
52. Portenoy RK. Adjuvant analgesics in pain management. In: Doyle D, Hanks GWC, MacDonald N, eds. *Oxford Textbook of Palliative Medicine.* 2nd ed. New York: Oxford University Press; 1998:361–390.
53. Butler S. Present status of tricyclic antidepressants in chronic pain therapy. In: Benedetti C, et al, eds. *Advances in Pain Research and Therapy.* Vol 7. New York: Raven Press; 1986:173–196.
54. France RD. The future for antidepressants: treatment of pain. *Psychopathology.* 1987;20:99–113.
55. Ventafridda V, Bonezzi C, Caraceni A, et al. Antidepressants for cancer pain and other painful syndromes with deafferentation component: comparison of amitriptyline and trazodone. *Ital J Neurol Sci.* 1987;8:579–587.
56. Getto CJ, Sorkness CA, Howell T. Antidepressant and chronic malignant pain: a review. *J Pain Symptom Control.* 1987;2:9–18.
57. Magni G, Arsie D, Deleo D. Antidepressants in the treatment of cancer pain: a survey in Italy. *Pain.* 1987;29:347–353.
58. Walsh TD. Controlled study of imipramine and morphine in chronic pain due to advanced cancer. In Foley KM, et al., eds. *Advances in Pain Research and Therapy.* Vol 16. New York: Raven Press; 1986;155–165.
59. Botney M, Fields HC. Amitriptyline potentiates morphine analgesia by direct action on the central nervous system. *Ann Neurol.* 1983;13:160–164.
60. Malseed RT, Goldstein FJ. Enhancement of morphine analgesics by tricyclic antidepressants. *Neuropharmacology.* 1979;18:827–829.
61. Ventafridda V, Branchi M, Ripamonti C, et al. Studies on the effects of antidepressant drugs on the antinociceptive action of morphine and on plasma morphine in rat and man. *Pain.* 1990;43:155–162.
62. Spiegel K, Kalb R, Pasternak GW. Analgesic activity of tricyclic antidepressants. *Ann Neurol.* 1993;13:462–465.
63. Gram LF. Receptors, pharmacokinetics and clinical effects. In: Burrows GD, et al., eds. *Antidepressants.* Amsterdam: Elsevier; 1983:81–95.
64. Devor M. Nerve pathophysiology and mechanisms of pain in causalgia. *J Autonom Nerv Syst.* 1983;7:371–384.
65. Pilowsky I, Hallet EC, Bassett EL, et al. A controlled study of amitriptyline in the treatment of chronic pain. *Pain.* 1982;14:169–179.
66. Max MB, Culnane M, Schafer SC, et al. Amitriptyline relieves diabetic neuropathy pain in patients with normal and depressed mood. *Neurology.* 1987;37:589–596.
67. Sharav Y, Singer E, Dione RA, et al. The analgesic effect of amitriptyline on chronic facial pain. *Pain.* 1987;31:199–209.
68. Young RJ, Clarke BF. Pain relief in diabetic neuropathy: the effectiveness of imipramine and related drugs. *Diabet Med.* 1985;2:363–366.
69. Sindrup SH, Gram LF, Brosen K, et al. The selective serotonin reuptake inhibitor paroxetine is effective in the treatment of diabetic neuropathy symptoms. *Pain.* 1990;42:135–144.
70. Max MB. Effects of desipramine, amitriptyline, and fluoxetine on pain and diabetic neuropathy. *N Engl J Med.* 1992;326:1250–1256.
71. Gomez-Perez FJ, Rull JA, Dies H, et al. Nortriptyline and fluphenazine in the symptomatic treatment of diabetic neuropathy: a double-blind cross-over study. *Pain.* 1985;23:395–400.
72. Langohr HD, Stohr M, Petruch F. An open and double-blind crossover study on the efficacy of clomipramine (Anafranil) in patients with painful mono- and polyneuropathies. *Eur Neurol.* 1982;21:309–315.
73. Tiegno M, Pagnoni B, Calmi A, et al. Chlorimipramine compared to pentazocine as a unique treatment in post-operative pain. *Int J Clin Pharmacol Res.* 1987;7:141–143.
74. Hammeroff SR, Cork RC, Scherer K, et al. Doxepin effects on chronic pain, depression and plasma opioids. *J Clin Psychiatr.* 1982;2:22–26.
75. Davidoff G, Guarracini M, Roth E, et al. Trazodone hydrochloride in the treatment of dysesthetic pain in traumatic myelopathy: a randomized, double-blind. placebo-controlled study. *Pain.* 1987;29:151–161.
76. Costa D, Mogos I, Toma T. Efficacy and safety of mianserin in the treatment of depression of woman with cancer. *Acta Psychiatr Scand.* 1985;72:85–92.
77. Eberhard G, von Khorring L, Nilsson HL, et al. A double-blind randomized study of clomipramine versus maprotiline in patients with idiopathic pain syndromes. *Neuropsychobiology.* 1988;19:25–32.
78. Feighner JP. A comparative trial of fluoxetine and amitriptyline in patients with major depressive disorder. *J Clin Psychiatr.* 1985;46:369–372.
79. Hynes MD, Lochner MA, Bemis K, et al. Fluoxetine, a selective inhibitor of serotonin uptake, potentiates morphine analgesia without altering its discriminative stimulus properties or affinity for opioid receptors. *Life Sci.* 1985;36:2317–2323.

80. Geller SA. Treatment of fibrositis with fluoxetine hydrochloride (Prozac). *Am J Med.* 1989;87:594–595.
81. Goldstein DJ, Lu Y, Detke MJ, et al. Duloxetine vs. placebo in patients with diabetic neuropathy. *Pain.* 2005;116:109–118.
82. Beaver WT, Wallerstein SL, Houde RW, et al. A comparison of the analgesic effect methotrimeprazine and morphine in patients with cancer. *Clin Pharmacol Ther.* 1966;7:436–466.
83. Maltbie AA, Cavenar SO, Sullivan JL, et al. Analgesia and haloperidol: a hypothesis. *J Can Psychiatry.* 1979;40:323–326.
84. Lechin F, Vander Dijs B, Lechin ME, et al. Pimozide therapy for trigeminal neuralgia. *Arch Neurol.* 1989;9:960–964.
85. Khojainova N, Santiago-Palma J, Kornick C, et al. Olanzapine in the management of cancer pain. *J Pain Symptom Manage.* 2002;23:346–350.
86. Breitbart W, Marotta RF, Call P. AIDS and neuroleptic malignant syndrome. *Lancet.* 1988;2:1488.
87. Swerdlow M, Cundhill JG. Anticonvulsant drugs used in the treatment of lacerating pains: a comparison. *Anesthesia.* 1981;36:1129–1134.
88. Caccia MR. Clonazepam in facial neuralgia and cluster headache: clinical and electrophysiological study. *Eur Neurol.* 1975;13:560–563.
89. Bruera E, Breuneis C, Patterson AH, et al. Use of methylphenidate as an adjuvant to narcotic analgesics in patients with advanced cancer. *J Pain Symptom Manage.* 1989;4:3–6.
90. Forrest H. Dextroamphetamine with morphine for the treatment of post-operative pain. *N Engl J Med.* 1977;296:712–715.
91. Menza MA, Kaufman KR, Castellanos AM. Modafinil augmentation of antidepressant treatment in depression. *J Clin Psychiatry.* 2000;61:378–381.
92. Freynhagen R, Strojek K, Griesing T, et al. Efficacy of pregabalin in neuropathic pain evaluated in a 12 week, randomized, double-blind, multicentre, placebo-controlled trial of flexible- and fixed-dose regimens. *Pain.* 1995;115:254–263.
93. Lyndstrom P, Lindbloom T. The analgesic tocainide for trigeminal neuralgia. *Pain.* 1987;28:45–50.
94. Dunlop R, Davies RJ, Hockley J, et al. Letter to the editor. *Lancet.* 1989;1:420–421.
95. Brose WG, Cousins MJ. Subcutaneous lidocaine for treatment of neuropathic cancer pain. *Pain.* 1991;45:145–148.
96. Paice J, Ferrans CE, Lahley FR, et al. Topical capsaicin in the management of HIV-associated peripheral neuropathy. *J Pain Symptom Manage.* 2000;19:45–52.
97. Devers A, Galer B. Topical lidocaine patch relieves a variety of neuropathic pain conditions: an open label study. *Clin J Pain.* 2000;16:205–208.
98. Zelman D, Cleeland C, Howland E. Factors in appropriate pharmacological management of cancer pain: a cross-institutional investigation. *Pain Suppl.* 1987;S136.
99. Breitbart W, Passik S, McDonald M, et al. Patient-related barriers to pain management in ambulatory AIDS patients. *Pain.* 1998;76:9–16.
100. Breitbart W, Kaim M, Rosenfeld B. Clinician's perceptions of barriers to pain management in AIDS. *J Pain Symptom Manage.* 1999;18:203–212.
101. Ward SE, Goldberg N, Miller-McCauley C, et al. Patient-related barriers to management of cancer pain. *Pain.* 1993;52:319–324.
102. Kanner RM, Foley KM. Patterns of narcotic use in a cancer pain clinic. *Ann N Y Acad Sci.* 1981;362:161–172.
103. Porter J, Jick H. Addiction rare in patients treated with narcotics. *N Engl J Med.* 1980;302:123.
104. Perry S, Heidrich G. Management of pain during debridement: a survey of US burn units. *Pain.* 1982;13:267–278.
105. Martin C, Pehrsson P, Osterberg A, et al. Pain in ambulatory HIV-infected patients with and without intravenous drug use. *Eur J Pain.* 1999;3:157–164.
106. Macaluso C, Weinberg D, Foley KM. Opioid abuse and misuse in a cancer pain population. *J Pain Symptom Manage.* 1988;3:54.
107. McCaffery M, Vourakis C. Assessment and relief of pain in chemically dependent patients. *Orthop Nurs.* 1992;11:13–27.
108. Portenoy RK, Payne R. Acute and chronic pain. In: Lowinson JH, Ruiz P, Millman RB, eds. *Comprehensive Textbook of Substance Abuse.* Baltimore: Williams and Wilkins; 1992:691–721.
109. Messiah A, Loundou A, Maslin V, et al. Physician recognition of active injection drug use in HIV-infected patients is lower than validity of patient's self-reported drug use. *J Pain Symptom Manage.* 2001;21:103–112.
110. Weissman DE, Haddox JD. Opioid pseudoaddiction and iatrogenic syndrome. *Pain.* 1989;36:363–366.
111. Kaplan R, Slywka J, Slagle S, et al. A titrated morphine analgesic regimen comparing substance users and non-users with AIDS-related pain. *J Pain Symptom Manage.* 2000;19:265–273.

CHAPTER 18

Sexually Transmitted Infections

Angela L. Stotts, Mark Evans, Shelly L. Sayre, Katherine A. McQueen

Exchange of body fluids through sexual contact is the primary mechanism for transmission of the human immunodeficiency virus (HIV).[1] High-risk sexual activity that exposes individuals to HIV similarly exposes an individual to comorbid infection with other sexually transmitted infections (STIs). Among HIV-infected persons, data indicate that STI rates are no longer declining as they did in the late 1980s and 1990s and are, in fact, increasing in certain subpopulations (i.e., men who have sex with men [MSM]).[2] Due to compromised immune systems, persons living with HIV infection or acquired immunodeficiency syndrome (AIDS) must be concerned with prevention of infections that could lead to disease progression or interfere with receiving appropriate treatments such as highly active antiretroviral therapy (HAART).

STIs and HIV are believed to have a synergistic relationship. Although biologic mechanisms have not been fully elucidated, STIs increase acquisition and transmission of HIV by increasing viral load and HIV virulence.[1,3] Disruptions to the usual mucosal barriers promote HIV infection by luring HIV-susceptible inflammatory cells to the genital tract. In turn, STIs promote shedding of HIV in the genital tract, thereby increasing transmission to noninfected partners. This enhanced transmissibility occurs with both ulcerative and nonulcerative STIs. HIV-positive individuals with comorbid STIs experience an accelerated progression toward developing AIDS.[4] Given this relationship, early identification and successful treatment of STIs is important for reducing both HIV transmission and progression to AIDS.

The common STIs can be categorized as bacterial, viral, and protozoan (Table 18.1). Gonorrhea, chlamydia, and syphilis are the most common bacterial infections; herpes simplex virus 2 (HSV-2), human papillomavirus (HPV), hepatitis B and C (HBV; HCV), and cytomegalovirus (CMV) the most important sexually transmitted viral infection; trichomoniasis the most common sexually transmitted protozoan infection. Although much work has been done to study the effects of these infections on HIV disease, less is known about the impact of HIV on STIs. Findings from prospective studies, though, suggest that HIV may increase rates of acquiring genital ulcerative disease (e.g., HSV-2, CMV), chlamydia, and gonorrhea.[5]

BACTERIAL INFECTIONS

Gonorrhea, chlamydia, and syphilis are all included on the Centers for Disease Control and Prevention's (CDC's) list of nationally reportable infectious diseases.[6] Gonorrhea (commonly referred to as "the clap") infects the penis, vagina, or anus and causes pain, burning,

TABLE 18.1 Common Sexually Transmitted Infections, Transmission Modalities, and Implications for Those with HIV Infection

STI	Type of Transmission	Number of U.S. Cases (2003)[a]	Potential Concerns for Those with HIV
Gonorrhea	Bacterial	335,104	Increases progression toward AIDS
Chlamydia	Bacterial	877,478	
Syphilis (primary and secondary)	Bacterial	7,177	
Herpes simplex 2 (HSV-2)	Viral	203,000	Promotes HIV shedding and infectiousness; more severe infections, including encephalitis
Human papillomavirus (HPV)	Viral	6.2 million	Increased likelihood of anogenital cancers[b] and CIN
Cytomegalovirus (CMV)	Viral	Annual is unknown, 50% to 80% of adults seropositive	May cause blindness
Hepatitis B (HBV)	Viral	Over 300,000	May result in poorer response to some HIV treatments
Hepatitis C (HCV)	Viral	~25,000	Causes more rapid progression of liver disease; poorer response to both HIV and HCV treatment
Trichomoniasis	Protozoan	7.4 million	Early treatment reduces vaginal shedding of HIV RNA

[a]Figures are according to the Centers for Disease Control and Prevention.[6]
[b]From Klausner JD, Kent CK. HIV and sexually transmitted diseases: latest views on synergy, treatment, and screening. *Postgrad Med.* 2004;115:79–84.
AIDS, Acquired immunodeficiency syndrome; *CIN*, cervical intraepithelial neoplasia; *HIV*, human immunodeficiency virus; *RNA*, ribonucleic acid.

and discharge. Although the 2003 infection rate may appear high—116.2 cases per 100,000—it actually represents a declining trend and is the lowest U.S. rate ever reported for this infection. There are no significant differences in rates between women and men.[7]

In contrast, chlamydia is a nonulcerative infection with few symptoms, especially in women. Rates of this infection rose 5.1% to 304.3 cases per 100,000 people between 2002 and 2003. Rates of chlamydia are three times higher in women than in men. Infection with gonorrhea or chlamydia can lead to pelvic inflammatory disease (PID), an infection of the womb, fallopian tubes, and reproductive organs leading to infertility, ectopic pregnancies, abscesses, and pelvic pain.[7]

Syphilis, which had been on the decline in the United States, has been increasing since 2001. Most of the increased incidence appears to be in men, and incidence rates are five times higher in African Americans than in Whites. Although the 2003 rate of 2.5 per 100,000 seems low compared to that of other bacterial STIs, close monitoring is warranted. Syphilis is readily treated in its early stages, but has the capability to spread throughout the body, affecting the heart, brain, and nerves and, as a result, may present clinically with more debilitating features.[7] HIV can lead to reactivation of latent syphilis. In particular, HIV-positive individuals have earlier neurologic involvement and higher risk of developing neurosyphilis, an infection of the brain or spinal cord, than their HIV-negative counterparts.[8]

VIRAL INFECTIONS

Viral STIs are frequently asymptomatic, and most are difficult to treat or incurable. The lack of effective treatments for viral STIs necessitates that individuals at risk be tested frequently to ensure that they are not unwittingly transmitting infections to others. The most common viral infections include HSV-2, HPV, CMV, HBV, and HCV. With the exception of HBV, none of these infections is included on the CDC's list of nationally reportable infectious diseases; therefore infection rates are typically estimated from initial visits to doctors' offices. HSV-2 produces ulcers in many of the mucosal regions and is readily transmitted through exchange of body fluids during, and in the days surrounding, an outbreak. Between outbreaks, the virus lies dormant in the nerves surrounding the genital area. During outbreaks, viral shedding is more active and risk of infection of both HSV-2 and HIV is greater. Sexual contacts should be avoided when HSV-2 is symptomatic, particularly for coinfected persons. Individuals with AIDS have more severe outbreaks, and ulceration can occur on other body surfaces (e.g., skin, eye, mouth, ear). The virus can also disseminate to the central nervous system (CNS), leading to encephalitis and resultant permanent neurologic damage or death. In the United States, HSV-2 is prevalent and in high-risk subpopulations seropositivity rates are as high as 50%.[7]

HPV, also known as genital warts, presents as wartlike growths or abnormal cell changes in the genital area and cervix. At any given time in the United States, 20 million people have HPV and approximately 6.2 million are newly diagnosed each year. Although HPV cannot be cured, the infection usually subsides on its own. HPV is more prevalent in women, and approximately 80% of the female population acquiring HPV will do so by the age of 50. Women are usually diagnosed by a Pap test, which screens for cervical cancer.[7] The rate of coinfection of HPV with HIV is 60% to 77% in women. HIV-positive women have been shown to have a higher rate of persistent types of HPV often associated with cervical intraepithelial neoplasia (CIN) and cervical cancer.[9]

CMV is a member of the herpesvirus family and can remain dormant for long periods. CMV is transmitted via body fluids (including semen, urine, blood, saliva, tears, and breast milk) of infected individuals. The infection is not highly contagious and often can be prevented by simple hand washing. However, CMV antibody can be detected in 50% to 85% of U.S. adults by the time they are 40 years of age. Signs of infection include mononucleosis-like syndrome, prolonged fever, and mild hepatitis. Once infected, the virus can lie dormant for years unless the immune system is suppressed. CMV is of particular concern for HIV-infected individuals. As immune function decreases (i.e., CD4 count reduction), this infection can cause pneumonia, retinitis (eye infections, which can lead to blindness), mucosal ulcers, and gastrointestinal disease. Approximately 5% of HIV-positive individuals have active CMV infection.[10]

HBV and HCV, blood-borne infections that affect the liver, can be transmitted via body fluids (most commonly blood and semen). The coinfection rate of HBV is 70% to 90%, with higher rates representing those with a history of intravenous drug use. Although conflicting data exist on the effect of HBV on HIV infection, it does not appear that HBV significantly affects HIV progression. However, HBV carriage rates in HIV-positive individuals are 25% compared to 5% in HIV-negative individuals, indicating HIV affects HBV replication and clearance.[11]

Approximately 4 million people in the United States have been infected with HCV. At highest risk of contracting HCV are individuals who inject drugs and share needles, those who body pierce or tattoo with unsterilized needles, and health care workers who come into direct contact with blood. Although blood-borne transmission through injection behaviors are the primary source of infection, the CDC now estimates that 15% to 20% of HCV infections are contracted through sexual transmission.[7] Although most infected individuals are asymptomatic, HCV can develop as a chronic condition characterized by flulike symptoms, fatigue, jaundice, and liver pain 15 to 20 years postinfection. Because of the potentially long asymptomatic period of HCV, estimating the incidence of new infections is difficult and under-reporting is a problem.[12] Approximately one fourth of HIV-positive individuals are coinfected with HCV. In coinfected individuals, HCV infection progresses at a faster rate than in those with HCV alone and response to HCV treatment is decreased. HCV, however, does not increase the rate of HIV multiplication, though damage caused to the liver can make it difficult for some HIV medications to be absorbed. Consequently, medications may be less effective and medication side effects may be more pronounced.[13] Similarly, coinfection increases the risk of hepatotoxicity of HAART, making treatment of HIV problematic. Because of this stress on the liver, coinfected individuals must be mindful of risk factors that could result in an additional hepatitis infection. As a precaution, coinfected individuals are advised to be vaccinated against HBV.

PROTOZOAN INFECTION

Trichomoniasis is a protozoan infection most often affecting the vagina and urethra of women. It is transmitted through penis-to-vagina or vulva-to-vulva contact. Thus women can contract it from infected male or female partners, but men typically contract it from infected female partners. Symptoms, more common in women, include discolored vaginal discharge with a strong odor and genital irritation and itching. One of the most common STIs in women, trichomoniasis is treatable and can typically be cured with a single dose of an antiprotozoal medication. Women with trichomoniasis are more susceptible to contracting HIV due to inflammation of their genitals. Conversely, women who are coinfected with HIV and trichomoniasis have an increased likelihood of passing HIV on to their partners.[7]

ASSESSMENT AND SCREENING FOR STIS

Recent prevalence data suggest a halt in the decline of STI rates among the HIV-infected population.[2] Possible explanations for the increase in high-risk behaviors associated with STI and HIV transmission include changes in community norms, alcohol and other drug use, and a decrease in fear of AIDS resulting from more effective treatments (e.g., HAART). Attempting to combat these unfortunate trends in risky behaviors and to prevent a resurgence in newly acquired HIV infections, public health officials are increasingly emphasizing STI screening, diagnosis, and treatment. The CDC's Advisory Committee for HIV and STI Prevention (ACHSP) specifically recommends early detection and treatment of curable STIs suspected of facilitating HIV transmission.[14]

BEHAVIORAL RISK AND SEXUALLY TRANSMITTED INFECTION HISTORY ASSESSMENT

A thorough behavioral and medical evaluation is necessary to determine the extent to which an individual is at risk for acquiring an STI, which in turn determines frequency of routine STI testing.[8] A complete evaluation includes performing a sexual and substance use risk assessment, gathering STI history information, and eliciting current signs or symptoms consistent with the presence of an STI. Specific sexual and substance use behaviors increase acquisition risk, and individuals who have been diagnosed previously with an STI are at higher risk of reinfection. The full evaluation should be conducted at any initial medical contact and repeated every 3 months.

Specific sexual and substance use risk indicators include the following:

- Being of adolescent age
- Having a sex partner with a known STI diagnosis

- Having more than one recent sex partner (past 1 to 4 months)
- Having a sex partner who has had other recent sex partners (past 1 to 4 months)
- Inconsistently using barrier methods
- Acquiring a new partner within the last 2 or 3 months
- Reporting a history of sexual assault or abuse
- Trading sex for money or drugs
- Currently using substances, particularly injection drugs (self or partner)

Collecting accurate sexual and substance use history information requires skill and rapport. Establishing rapport may start by explaining and reinforcing confidentiality, along with any limits to confidentiality, and inquiring about and addressing concerns of the patient. Once a relationship has been established the patient should be asked directly and nonjudgmentally about specific STI risk behaviors. Sexual activity should be defined using a range of specific anatomic and behavioral terms to enhance accuracy and prevent omission of important information. For example, sex partners are defined as anyone with whom the patient has had intimate sexual contact at oral, genital, or rectal sites. This includes sex with men, women, or both. After obtaining a detailed sexual history, the provider should ask about condom use, including pattern of use (i.e., never, sometimes, always), use with different sites of exposure (i.e., vaginal, oral, rectal), use with steady versus new partners, and circumstances of nonuse (e.g., substance use). It is also important to obtain a prior history of STIs and genitourinary infections (e.g., number of episodes, date of last treatment), including associated signs and symptoms. Finally, a thorough substance use history should also be obtained targeting all drugs of abuse and routes of administration, but in particular crack cocaine, amphetamine, and injection drug administration. Use of safety practices should be determined, such as rinsing needles with bleach or never using shared needles. Sexual activity related to acquisition or use of drugs should also be explored in detail.

SEXUALLY TRANSMITTED INFECTION SCREENING AND DETECTION

Most STI infections are asymptomatic (especially in the initial stages), making routine screening and comprehensive physical examination (including skin, mouth, and anogenital regions) critical aspects of medical care for those with and without HIV. Individuals at risk for STIs often present to health care settings for reasons other than STI testing or treatment. STI screening should be a standard part of medical care for high-risk individuals in all health care settings.[14] Thorough physical examinations are particularly important for hospitalized patients. Regular screening resulting in early STI detection and treatment in the HIV-infected population may be particularly effective and cost-beneficial in reducing HIV transmission for several reasons: (a) most STIs promote increased shedding of HIV, (b) the number of HIV-infected persons is smaller than the number of persons at risk for becoming infected, and (c) HIV-infected persons often are receiving regular medical care.

General ACHSP guidelines recommend the following[14]:

- All sexually active males and females younger than 25 years of age who visit a health care provider for any reason should be screened for chlamydia, gonorrhea, HPV, and, among women, trichomoniasis at least once per year. More selective screening criteria can be used in settings or geographic areas in which prevalence rates have been determined to be low. Adolescents and young MSM populations are particularly at high risk for HIV and other STIs and are critically important to reach for STI screening. Health care settings such as family planning clinics, prenatal clinics, emergency rooms, walk-in clinics, community health centers, school-based and adolescent clinics, correctional facilities, mental health facilities, and primary care provider offices should have active screening procedures in place.

- Older, high-risk males and females who visit a health care provider for any reason should also be routinely screened for chlamydia and gonorrhea once per year. In general, as mentioned previously, higher risk individuals include those who use and/or misuse substances, have a history of STIs, have more than one sex partner per year, trade sex for money or drugs, are in correctional facilities, or live in communities with high rates of STI or HIV infection.
- Serologic syphilis screening should be conducted in high-risk persons at least yearly. Syphilis rates vary considerably by region and among subpopulations, and therefore local epidemiologic and/or pilot data should be used to guide local screening efforts.
- For high-risk individuals, testing for HBV and HCV is recommended every 6 months. Detectable antibodies may not be present for up to 6 to 8 weeks, and therefore initial testing may yield false negative results. A person with two negative antibody tests conducted over a 6-month period (with no high-risk activity during that time) can be considered truly negative for hepatitis; at which time vaccinations are recommended for high-risk patients.

Screening guidelines are generally the same for individuals infected with HIV; however, it is even more important that routine screening occur.[14] All HIV-infected persons who may be at risk for contracting STIs should be screened at least yearly for curable STIs, including gonorrhea, chlamydia, syphilis, and, among women, trichomoniasis. In addition, persons with HIV disease or AIDS should be evaluated for genital herpes and HPV infection. For women in particular the CDC recommends two pelvic examinations with Pap smear screening during the first year after HIV diagnosis, with yearly Pap smears and pelvic examinations thereafter if initial results are normal. Screening frequency should be modified based on an individual's risk behaviors, potential risk behavior of the individual's partner(s), and the incidence of STIs in the local population. Screening should be performed more frequently if any STIs are detected.

PREVENTION AND TREATMENT OF SEXUALLY TRANSMITTED INFECTIONS

The prevention and treatment of STIs in the HIV-infected population require a multifaceted approach with attention to the STI–HIV synergistic relationship. The approach involves three primary components: medical management, behavior management, and partner management.[8] Although each component is distinct, integrating them into a comprehensive case management plan for patients with HIV is highly recommended. Ideally, patients should receive all relevant services within one provider practice.

MEDICAL MANAGEMENT

Complex interactions exist between HIV infection and other STIs. As noted, HIV has been found to alter the manifestation and course of various STIs, and certain STIs may alter the transmission of HIV infection. Standard treatment regimens recommended for particular STIs may require modification for HIV-infected patients.[1] HIV status may influence the choice of medications, duration of treatment, and follow-up care in managing STIs. Although it is beyond the scope of this chapter to detail specific pharmacologic treatments for each STI, those for which there are specific prevention or treatment considerations due to positive HIV status are presented.[8] For STIs not listed, first-line treatments are generally the same for both HIV-infected and noninfected patients.

Hepatitis B Virus and Hepatitis A Virus

Preexposure vaccination is available and recommended to prevent both HBV and HAV in HIV-infected patients. The HBV vaccine is recommended for all patients who do not have serologic evidence of immunity to HBV infection. The HAV vaccine is recommended for illegal drug users, MSM, persons with chronic liver disease, and those who engage in anal-oral sexual contact or anal intercourse without condoms.

Syphilis

Penicillin is the drug of choice for HIV-infected patients. However, treatment failures with currently recommended oral regimens for syphilis have been reported, and therefore longer duration intramuscular regimens may be the preferred treatment. HIV may increase the progression of neurosyphilis, and no effective alternative treatment regimen to prevent this has been identified.[8]

Human Papillomavirus

Increased rates of HPV infection have been found for HIV-infected persons.[9] Multiple treatments exist that are chosen based on the extent of the disease (e.g., wart size and number). Persons who are immunosuppressed due to HIV or other reasons may not respond as well as immunocompetent persons to genital wart treatment. They also may have more frequent recurrences after treatment. Treatment is recommended only if the individual is symptomatic. Lesions that fail to resolve after treatment with multiple modalities deserve biopsy for detection of neoplastic features. Women with coinfection are more likely to develop neoplasia, and initial colposcopy followed by annual Pap tests are recommended.

Pelvic Inflammatory Disease

Treatment recommendations for HIV-infected women with PID are similar to those for noninfected women; more aggressive management is not indicated.[8] However, some experts do recommend initial hospitalization and parenteral antimicrobial regimens in HIV-infected women, particularly those with low CD4 lymphocyte counts.

Trichomoniasis

HIV-infected women (and men) should receive the same treatment as HIV-negative persons. Interestingly, though, Wang et al.[15] found that treatment of trichomoniasis in HIV-infected women reduced the vaginal shedding of HIV ribonucleic acid (RNA) but not deoxyribonucleic acid (DNA).

BEHAVIORAL MANAGEMENT

Because STIs facilitate both the acquisition and transmission of HIV, an integrated behavioral approach to HIV infection and STI primary and secondary prevention is ideal. The CDC recommends the following counseling components be covered for HIV-positive individuals with a newly diagnosed STI[14]:

- Assessment of frequency and type of sexual behaviors
- Determining the number and HIV status of recent sexual contacts
- Counseling and educating HIV-positive individuals with a new STI on the synergistic relationship between the infections and the need to eliminate unprotected sexual behavior, especially with persons of HIV-negative or unknown HIV status
- Counseling as to proper and effective treatment interventions for the newly diagnosed STI and referral for HIV-infection or AIDS treatment if the individual does not have a provider
- Partner notification issues as mandated by state/federal regulatory agencies

Traditionally, patient education was the only counseling strategy used to elicit behavior change in patients with HIV disease or STIs. Although this is an important component, education alone is not sufficient for sustained behavior change.[16] The CDC now recommends HIV science-based counseling that is: (a) interactive, (b) focused on personal risks and circumstances, and (c) directed toward helping clients set and reach specific goals.[16]

Counseling interventions should also be tailored specifically to both HIV and STIs and for specific populations (e.g., drug using, non–drug using; heterosexual, homosexual). Sexual behaviors that transmit HIV are also involved in the transmission of certain STIs, including chlamydia, gonorrhea, and syphilis. Thus it is often assumed that preventive methods effective against HIV infection will be equally effective against other STIs. Unfortunately this is not the case. Traditional barrier methods advocated for HIV prevention do not necessarily eliminate risk for other STIs.[17] For example, condoms are more likely to be effective in reducing cumulative HIV risk, but STI risk is more likely to be diminished by reducing number of partners.[17] Traditional HIV counseling has also been found less effective than expected in reducing HCV risk.[18] Thus, traditional HIV risk reduction counseling strategies and interventions may not be sufficient to stop the recent increase in STI infections; specific STI risk reduction strategies must be integrated into HIV counseling protocols.

A recent example of an integrated counseling program is reported by Evans et al.,[18] in which HCV education and counseling were integrated into an established HIV program within a substance abuse research treatment facility. HIV counseling and testing were initiated for all participants using the CDC model of client-centered HIV prevention counseling.[16] HCV counseling was incorporated into this model by the clinic, with all counselors undergoing in-house training on HCV transmission, risk identification, and risk reduction. Training in HIV counseling had been conducted previously. Measures assessing HIV and HCV knowledge and risk exposure served as data collection instruments as well as diagnostic tools used to assist in developing an individualized risk reduction counseling intervention. Counseling and testing, including the HIV and HCV knowledge and risk exposure measures, were conducted during the intake assessment and again at a follow-up appointment 10 weeks later.

In addition to the provision of quality HIV and HCV counseling services, data collected yielded interesting results. In the first study, a positive relationship was found between HIV and HCV knowledge scores ($r = .52$; $N = 110$; $p < .01$), indicating that higher levels of HIV knowledge were associated with higher levels of HCV knowledge.[18] However, clients tended to score proportionally better on the HIV knowledge scale (73.7% correct) than on the HCV scale (45.3% correct), indicating that specific knowledge of HCV transmission and acquisition was lacking. In fact, the majority of HCV items were answered either incorrectly or "Don't know." The substance-abusing sample was also divided into two subgroups: individuals who reported past or present intravenous (IV) drug use and those who did not. IV drug users answered more items correctly on both the HIV and HCV risk factors and prevention strategies. Finally, a second, follow-up study demonstrated significant improvement in both HIV and HCV transmission and risk behavior knowledge at 10 weeks postcounseling.[19]

These data highlight: (a) the need for STI-specific education and counseling, (b) the feasibility of integrating STI counseling into existing HIV prevention programs, (c) the importance of attending to individual differences (e.g., IV drug use) in developing personalized HIV infection and STI programs, and (d) the effectiveness of STI-specific counseling and testing delivered within a specialty clinic setting for improving knowledge about specific STIs.

PARTNER MANAGEMENT

For health care providers, partner management involves two primary components: (a) notification and referral and (b) medical evaluation and treatment.

Notification and Referral

Partner notification was established in 1937 by Thomas Parran, Surgeon General, as a public health practice and has been implemented with success since the 1940s for STI control and prevention.[8] For patients with HIV and an additional STI, partner management involves confidential procedures to inform the sexual and/or needle-sharing partners of disease exposure and to encourage them to seek medical evaluation. Partner management is especially important in order for partners to have the opportunity for early diagnosis and treatment of STI or HIV infection. On a larger scale, partner notification assists in interrupting disease transmission and preventing complications by referring exposed people for medical evaluation. It is also an opportunity to address high-risk behaviors and provide education and counseling to many individuals who may not be otherwise identified as being at-risk.

CDC Guidelines[20] recommend that HIV-infected patients should be asked to notify their partner(s) about their disease and to refer them to counseling and testing. Health care providers are important in facilitating this process either directly or by referral to health department partner notification programs. If patients are unwilling or deemed unlikely to notify partners, physicians or health department personnel should use confidential procedures to do so. State laws vary and should be consulted to determine when (and if) confidential notification may be undertaken. Similar procedures should be in place for other STIs, as well, particularly for the diseases that require reporting in all states (i.e., syphilis, gonorrhea, chlamydia, AIDS).

Medical Evaluation and Treatment

Beyond notification, specific partner evaluation and treatment recommendations exist for each sexually transmitted infection, based on incubation or latency periods, times of highest transmission risk, and other particular characteristics of the disease.[8] For example, sexual transmission of *Treponema pallidum*, which causes syphilis, occurs only when mucocutaneous syphilitic lesions are present, and such manifestations are uncommon after the first year of infection. Persons exposed within 90 days preceding the diagnosis of syphilis in a sex partner might be infected even if seronegative and therefore should be treated presumptively. In the case of gonorrhea, partner management recommendations include evaluating and treating all partners with whom sexual contact has been made within 60 days before the onset of symptoms or diagnosis. If a patient's last sexual contact was prior to 60 days, then the most recent sex partner should be treated. Specific partner management strategies for the majority of STIs have been identified by the CDC.[20]

SUMMARY

STIs and HIV infection are inextricably linked. Risk factors for acquisition are similar, if not identical, and, although varied, short- and long-term consequences are potentially life altering, if not life threatening. It is incumbent upon primary care and mental health practitioners who work with patients with HIV disease or AIDS to have a clear understanding of the various types of STIs, as well as the synergistic relationships that exist between HIV and STIs. As high-risk behaviors continue to increase in certain populations, health care professionals must be able to assess and identify individual risk, counsel, and provide proper referrals as needed (including referrals for medical treatment, vaccination, additional counseling or behavioral interventions, and partner notification, as needed). It is feasible to integrate STI and HIV counseling into a joint counseling and educational unit, and such programs must be specifically tailored to address issues related to both HIV infection and STIs, as well as different at-risk populations. Successful treatment of STIs may not only increase life expectancy and quality of life for HIV-infected individuals, but reduce the burden on the health care system and, through education and intervention with these clients, may serve to prevent the spread of disease.

REFERENCES

1. Cohen MS. HIV and sexually transmitted diseases: lethal synergy. *Top HIV Med.* 2004;12:104–107.
2. Bachmann LH, Grimley DM, Waithaka Y, et al. Sexually transmitted disease/HIV transmission risk behaviors and sexually transmitted disease prevalence among HIV-positive men receiving continuing care. *Sex Transm Dis.* 2005;32:20–26.
3. Klausner JD, Kent CK. HIV and sexually transmitted diseases: latest views on synergy, treatment, and screening. *Postgrad Med.* 2004;115:79–84.
4. Rottingen JA, Cameron DW, Garnett GP. A systematic review of the epidemiologic interactions between classic sexually transmitted diseases and HIV: how much really is known? *Sex Transm Dis.* 2001;28:579–597.
5. McClelland RS, Lavreys L, Katingima C, et al. Contribution of HIV-1 infection to acquisition of sexually transmitted disease: a 10-year prospective study. *J Infect Dis.* 2005;191:333–338.
6. Centers for Disease Control and Prevention. *2003 STD Surveillance Report*. Atlanta: Centers for Disease Control and Prevention; 2004.
7. Centers for Disease Control and Prevention. *2005 STD Fact Sheets*. Atlanta: Centers for Disease Control and Prevention.
8. Ratelle S, Brzankalski G, Cherneskie T, et al. *Prevention and Management of Sexually Transmitted Diseases in Persons Living with HIV/AIDS*. Boston, MA: Eastern Quadrant STD/HIV Prevention Training Centers; 2003.
9. Sun XW, Kuhn L, Ellerbrock TV, et al. Human papillomavirus infection in women infected with the human immunodeficiency virus. *N Engl J Med.* 1997;337:1343–1349.
10. Centers for Disease Control and Prevention. *Cytomegalovirus (CMV) Infection*. Atlanta: Centers for Disease Control and Prevention; 2002.
11. Khalili M. Coinfection with hepatitis viruses and HIV. In: HIVInSite, ed. *Knowledge Base Chapters*. San Francisco: University of California San Francisco; 2004.
12. Kim WR. The burden of hepatitis C in the United States. *Hepatology.* 2002;36(5 suppl 1):S30–S34.
13. Thiemann L, Lalazeri J. *Double Jeopardy: The HIV/HCV Co-Infection Handbook*. New York: Community Prescription Service; 1999.
14. Centers for Disease Control and Prevention: HIV prevention through early detection and treatment of other sexually transmitted diseases: United States. *MMWR Morbid Mortal Wkly Rep.* 1998;47:1–25.
15. Wang CC, McClelland RS, Reilly M, et al. The effect of treatment of vaginal infections on shedding of HIV type1. *J Infect Dis.* 2001;183:1017–1022.
16. Centers for Disease Control and Prevention: Revised guidelines for HIV counseling, testing, and referral. *MMWR Morbid Mortal Wkly Rep.* 2001;50:1–62.
17. Pinkerton SD, Layde PM, DiFranceisco W, Chesson HW. All STDs are not created equal: an analysis of the differential effects of sexual behaviour changes on different STDs. *Int J STD AIDS.* 2003;14:320–328.
18. Evans M, Stotts AL, Graham S, Schmitz J, Grabowski J: Hepatitis C knowledge assessment and counseling within the context of substance use treatment. *Addict Disord Treat.* 2004;3:18–26.
19. Evans M, Hokanson P, Augsburger J, et al. Increasing knowledge of HIV and hepatitis C during substance abuse treatment. *Addict Disord Treat.* 2005;4:71–76.
20. Centers for Disease Control and Prevention: Sexually transmitted diseases treatment guidelines 2002. *MMWR Morbid Mortal Wkly Rep.* 2002;50:1–82.

CHAPTER 19

Psychiatric Comorbidities in Medically Ill Patients with HIV/AIDS

Stephen J. Ferrando, Constantine G. Lyketsos

The psychiatric care of medically hospitalized patients with human immunodeficiency virus (HIV) disease or acquired immunodeficiency syndrome (AIDS) is complex, requiring a thorough understanding of the epidemiology of psychiatric disorders in HIV disease and AIDS, the neuropsychiatric manifestations of HIV itself, and multiple differential diagnostic considerations. Although some of these issues have been covered elsewhere in this volume, this chapter focuses on those issues most critical to the psychiatric diagnosis and treatment of the medically hospitalized patient with HIV disease or AIDS.

The following case illustrates the complex differential diagnostic issues encountered in the hospitalized HIV/AIDS patient:

A 34-year-old Hispanic woman is escorted by her mother to the medical emergency room with complaints of fever, weight loss, severe vaginal yeast infections, and increasingly erratic behavior in the context of a recent positive HIV-1 antibody test. Physical examination is remarkable for gaunt appearance; pressured, disorganized speech; disorientation; temperature of 101° F; mild abdominal tenderness; and severe vaginal and oral candidiasis. Chest x-ray film and electrocardiogram are normal. Laboratory examination is significant for anemia, normal white blood cell count with concurrent lymphopenia, elevated liver enzymes, normal rapid toxicology screen, and negative blood alcohol level. Tests for lymphocyte subsets, HIV-1 antibody and viral load, and hepatitis B and C (HBV, HCV) serologies are performed.

The patient is admitted to the inpatient HIV/AIDS specialty care unit, where she has a 24-hour companion to prevent elopement. A psychiatric consultant obtains history from the patient's mother suggesting no prior psychiatric or substance use history. Over the past 4 weeks the patient has become increasingly irritable, has not been sleeping at night, and has become "very religious," stating that she can see God and defeat the devil. On mental status examination, the patient is found to be disheveled, wearing several crucifixes around her neck, and praying. She repeats to herself "I and God are one" and, when questioned, begins yelling "leave God's house at once!" The patient was given an emergency dose of intramuscular ziprasidone with good results. A magnetic resonance imaging (MRI) scan and lumbar puncture are performed.

Test results reveal repeat positive HIV-1 antibody test, HIV ribonucleic acid (RNA) viral load of 346,000 copies/ml, CD4+ lymphocyte count of 57 cells/mm^3, and positive HCV antibody findings. MRI scan reveals no focal lesions, generalized cortical atrophy inappropriate for age, and multifocal increased signal intensity in the basal ganglia and periventricular white matter. Lumbar puncture is significant for white blood cell pleocytosis and increased β2-microglobulin; cerebrospinal fluid (CSF) HIV-1 RNA is 732,000 copies/ml.

A diagnosis of HIV-associated mania, with possible HIV-associated cognitive motor disorder is made. Cognitive impairment related to HCV coinfection is also considered. The patient is started on a standing regimen of olanzapine 10 mg twice daily, which she takes at the constant urging of her mother. Intermittent doses of lorazepam given for acute agitation appear to make her more confused, so this is discontinued. After 6 days, she becomes calmer, more conversant, and less delusional, but remains somewhat pressured and cognitively impaired. Cognitive examination using the HIV Dementia Scale reveals a score of 6 (<10 is suggestive of HIV-associated dementia [HAD]), with impairment in orientation, psychomotor processing speed, and short-term memory.

In conjunction with the medical team, discussion is initiated regarding the necessity of initiating highly active antiretroviral therapy (HAART) to address both systemic and central nervous system (CNS) HIV infection, in addition to the institution of a mood stabilizer and possible psychiatric hospitalization. More extensive neuropsychological testing is suggested both before and 3 to 6 months after the initiation of antiretroviral therapy, in addition to follow-up MRI.

MEDICAL HOSPITALIZATION AND THE CHANGING SCOPE OF THE HIV EPIDEMIC

With the widespread availability of HAART for HIV infection in developed countries occurring in the mid-1990s, rates and reasons for medical hospitalization of HIV-infected patients have changed. Multiple studies conducted after the dissemination of HAART documented dramatic declines in inpatient censuses, ranging from 33% to 75%, occurring primarily between 1995 and 1997.[1–4] In the late 1990s and early 2000s, rates stabilized or rebounded slightly.

Data on the changing reasons for medical hospital admissions reflect the impact of HAART on AIDS-related opportunistic infections and cancers. In two urban hospital studies, a uniform drop in hospital admissions due to opportunistic infections and cancers was observed, contrasting with a rise in nonopportunistic complications.[3,4] Mean CD4 counts of HIV-infected inpatients were seen to increase by over 100 cells/mm^3 from 1995 to 2001.[3]

Factors that appear to confer risk for medical hospitalization in the HAART era include low CD4 count, female gender, lack of antiretroviral treatment, and injection drug use.[3,4] The sociodemographic characteristics of those at risk reflect the shifting demographics of the HIV epidemic, limited access to care, and adherence to antiretroviral treatment.

EPIDEMIOLOGY OF PSYCHIATRIC DISORDERS IN MEDICAL INPATIENTS

In contrast to the extensive epidemiologic data for psychiatric disorders in ambulatory patients with HIV infection or AIDS, there are relatively few data on rates of psychiatric disorders among medical inpatients. Nearly all published studies describing outcomes of psychiatric consultations in inpatients with HIV disease or AIDS in the pre-HAART era include small samples and do not employ standardized psychiatric diagnostic instruments. Despite these limitations, available data reflect those clinical problems that the consulting psychiatrist is most likely to encounter.

Table 19.1 summarizes the literature to date.[5–9] Across studies, the most frequently diagnosed disorders are in the depressive spectrum (range 27% to 83%), including depression secondary to medical condition (or organic mood disorder), major depressive disorder, or dysthymic disorder. Delirium is diagnosed in 8% to 29% of patients, regardless of HIV stage, and

TABLE 19.1 Frequency of Psychiatric Disorders Reported in the Inpatient Medical Setting

Reference	N	Male (%)	HIV Risk (%)	Medical Illnesses (%)	Depressive Disorders (%)	Dementia (%)	Delirium (%)	Substance Use Disorder (%)	Other Psychiatric Disorders (%)
Perry, Tross, 1984[5]	52 AIDS	98	Homosexual, 79 Homosexual + IVDU, 12 Other, 9	OI, 71 KS, 17 OI + KS, 12	Any, 83	11	29	11	Schizophrenia, 2
Dilley et al, 1985[6]	13 AIDS	100	Homosexual, 100	OI, 70 OI + KS, 15 Other, 15	Adjustment disorder, 54 MDD, 15	8	8	31	Panic, 8
O'Dowd, McKegney, 1990[7]	67 AIDS	69	Not reported	Not reported	Adjustment disorder, 42 MDD, 3	22	27	20	Axis II, 6
Bialer et al, 1996[8]	433 AIDS 116 HIV+	79	Not reported	Not reported	Organic mood disorder, 13 Adjustment disorder, 13 MDD, 1	22	29	36	Axis II, 9
Ferrando SJ et al, 1998[9]	36 AIDS 4 HIV+	60	Homosexual, 34 IVDU, 31 Heterosexual, 31	OI, 89	MDD or dysthymic disorder, 31	19	19	19	Mania/hypomania, 11 Anxiety, 8

AIDS, Acquired immunodeficiency syndrome; *HIV*, human immunodeficiency syndrome; *IVDU*, intravenous drug users; *KS*, Kaposi's sarcoma; *MDD*, Major depressive disorder; *OI*, opportunistic infections.

is often reported to be concurrent with HIV-associated dementia, diagnosed in 8% to 22% of cases. Substance use disorders are diagnosed in 11% to 36% of inpatients with AIDS and up to 63% in HIV-positive patients who do not have AIDS. Only one study explicitly addressed bipolar spectrum disorders, including primary bipolar disorder and HIV-associated mania, which occurred in 11% of patients.[10]

DIFFERENTIAL DIAGNOSIS

Differential diagnosis is paramount in evaluating psychiatric disorders and symptoms in medical inpatients with HIV disease or AIDS, especially when investigating for medical and neuropsychiatric etiologic factors related to HIV illness and its treatment. Table 19.2 lists the major differential diagnostic considerations.

Of patients with HIV infection, 60% to 70% have one or more psychiatric disorders before contracting HIV illness.[10,11] Medical hospitalization can serve as a triggering stressor for relapse of primary psychiatric disorders once HIV infection is diagnosed. Thus, in assessing the hospitalized patient, it is important to query for personal and family psychiatric history in order to assess for vulnerability to relapse. However, even in the presence of a prior psychiatric history, it is most important to rule out potentially exacerbating, if not etiologic, medical factors. As discussed in Chapter 12, HIV-associated neurocognitive disorders are associated with a range of cognitive and behavioral symptoms, including apathy, depression, sleep disturbances, mania, and psychosis. CNS opportunistic illnesses and cancers can also present with a wide range of behavioral symptoms, most often in the context of delirium, as a result of both focal and generalized neuropathologic processes. Table 19.3 lists the major CNS opportunistic infections, their symptom presentations, and their diagnostic workup.

Substance intoxication and withdrawal are also common in the medical inpatient setting (see Chapter 14). Most notable in this context is that HIV-infected substance users have high rates of preexisting comorbid psychopathology that may be exacerbated by ongoing substance use. Further, these individuals often abuse multiple substances concurrently, which compounds the complexity of assessing behavioral symptoms and presents the challenge of treating mixed withdrawal states.

HCV infection, independent of HIV coinfection and interferon/ribavirin therapy, is associated with multiple neuropsychiatric complaints, most frequently fatigue, depression, and cognitive dysfunction. The pattern of cognitive impairment is similar to that in HIV disease, with impairment in attention, concentration, psychomotor processing speed, verbal memory, and executive dysfunction. Patients with end-stage liver disease and cirrhosis experience superimposed delirium (hepatic encephalopathy). Combination pegylated interferon alfa-2a

TABLE 19.2	Differential Diagnosis of Psychiatric Disorders and Symptoms in Medical Inpatients with HIV Disease and AIDS

- Primary psychiatric disorder
- Central nervous system (CNS) HIV infection (minor cognitive motor disorder and HIV-associated dementia)
- CNS opportunistic illnesses and cancers
- Substance intoxication and withdrawal
- Neuropsychiatric complications of hepatitis C and its treatments
- Neuropsychiatric side effects of HIV medications
- Drug interactions
- Endocrine abnormalities (e.g., hypogonadism, adrenal insufficiency)

TABLE 19.3 Opportunistic Illnesses (OI) of the Central Nervous System in AIDS

OI	CD4	Signs	Focal	CT/MRI	Lumbar Puncture
Toxoplasmosis	<100	Delirium Fever Headache Seizures	Y	Ring enhancing lesions • Basal ganglia • Gray-white junction	*Toxoplasma gondii* antibody or PCR High specificity/low sensitivity
Cytomegalovirus	<50	Delirium Infections found at diagnosis • Retina • Blood • Adrenal gland • GI tract	N (Y)	Ventricular enlargement Increased periventricular signal (T2 image)	CMV PCR Variable specificity and sensitivity Elevated protein level, pleocytosis, hypoglycorrhachia
Cryptococcal meningitis	<100	Fever Delirium Not universally seen Increased ICP (50%) • Seizures	N [Y 10%]	Nonspecific	*Crytococcus neoformans*, India ink, latex agglutination, or PCR High specificity/high sensitivity

Condition	CD4	Clinical features	Focal	Imaging	Diagnostics
Progressive multifocal leukoencephalopathy	<100	Monoparesis/hemiparesis Dysarthria Gait disturbance Sensory deficit Progressive dementia Occasional • Visual loss • Seizures	Y	Attenuated signal/ (T2 images) Periventricular white matter Other areas • Gray matter • Brainstem • Cerebellum • Spinal cord	JCV PCR High specificity/high sensitivity Other routine CSF studies not generally diagnostic
Central nervous system neoplasms/ lymphoma	<100	Afebrile Delirium Seizures 10% Increased ICP	Y	Lesions • Hypodense/patchy • Nodular enhancing SPECT thallium: differentiates from toxoplasmosis	EBV PCR High specificity/high sensitivity Other routine CSF evaluation not useful.

CMV, Cytomegalovirus; CSF, cerebrospinal fluid; EBV, Epstein-Barr virus; GI, gastrointestinal; ICP, intracranial pressure; JCV, JC Virus; PCR, polymerase chain reaction; SPECT, single photon emission computed tomography.

treatment for HCV infection has been extensively documented to cause neuropsychiatric side effects, including depression, suicidal ideation, anxiety, sleep disturbance, fatigue, mania, psychosis, confusion, and cognitive dysfunction.[12]

Multiple antiretroviral and other medications used in the context of HIV have been reported to have neuropsychiatric side effects. These include zidovudine,[13] didanosine,[14] abacavir,[15] nevirapine,[16] efavirenz, and interferon alfa-2a. Most of these are uncommon or rare, and causal relationships are often difficult to determine. The most widespread clinical concern has been generated by reports of sudden-onset depression and suicidal ideation associated with interferon alfa-2a and efavirenz. Early reports suggested that efavirenz may be associated with at least transient neuropsychiatric side effects in more than 50% of patients.[17] Reported effects are protean and include depression, suicidal ideation, vivid nightmares, anxiety, insomnia, psychosis, cognitive dysfunction, and antisocial behavior.

Drug interactions between antiretroviral and psychotropic medications, covered extensively in Chapter 16, are an important aspect of differential diagnosis and treatment planning in the inpatient medical setting. Clinically significant drug interactions are more likely to be seen in this setting because of medical illness severity, prior substance abuse, the likelihood of multiple medications being initiated simultaneously, changes in volume of distribution and protein binding, and hepatic and renal impairment. In one study, medical inpatients with HIV disease or AIDS were prescribed an average of seven medications during their admission.[9]

Inpatients with HIV disease or AIDS often experience endocrinologic derangements that may produce behavioral symptoms. These include clinical and subclinical hypothyroidism,[18] hypogonadism,[19] and adrenal insufficiency,[20] as well as Graves' disease (autoimmune thyroiditis).[18] Thyroid deficiency, including its subclinical forms, is present in approximately 16% of HIV-infected patients.[18] Testosterone deficiency, with clinical symptoms of hypogonadism is present in up to 50% of men with symptomatic HIV infection or AIDS and is likely to be present with concurrent acute medical illness.[19] Deficiency of adrenal glucocorticoid production is present in up to 50% of severely ill HIV-infected patients.[20] These endocrine deficiency states have been associated with fatigue, low mood, low libido, and loss of lean body mass and may be ameliorated by correction of the deficiency. Graves' disease presents in the acute stages with activation symptoms including anxiety, irritability, insomnia, weight loss, mania, and agitation.

DIAGNOSTIC EVALUATION

The psychiatric evaluation of the inpatient with HIV disease or AIDS is consistent with the broad differential diagnosis and is initially focused on identifying potentially reversible underlying etiologies. A thorough psychiatric evaluation, including presenting symptoms, personal and family history of psychiatric illness and substance abuse, as well as a cognitive functioning examination are essential. Although a complete medical evaluation is implicit, the psychiatric consultant may suggest additional diagnostic testing based on the clinical situation. Table 19.4 contains a listing of such diagnostic tests.

In general, the diagnostic workup should include complete blood count with differential, serum chemistries (including liver and renal function tests, fasting blood glucose, and creatine phosphokinase), chest x-ray, electrocardiogram, blood and urine cultures (if indicated), toxicology screen, and psychotropic medication serum levels (when available). Depending on the clinical presentation, assays of thyroid function, vitamins B_6 and B_{12}, *Treponema pallidum* IgG, serum total, free and/or bioavailable testosterone, adrenocorticotropic hormone (ACTH) stimulation, and 24-hour urinary cortisol may be obtained. If brain imaging is required, MRI of the brain with gadolinium contrast is preferred over computed tomographic scanning because it produces better visualization of brain tissue, subcortical and posterior fossa structures, and focal lesions. A lumbar puncture may be obtained, if necessary, under

TABLE 19.4	Diagnostic Evaluation of the Medical Inpatient with HIV/AIDS and Psychiatric Symptoms

- Medical evaluation with screening laboratories: complete blood count, chemistry screen (including liver and renal function tests), urinalysis, chest x-ray, electrocardiogram, blood and urine cultures (when applicable)
- Psychiatric diagnostic interview, including personal and family history
- Cognitive screen (HIV Dementia Scale)
- Additional laboratory studies when applicable: illicit drug toxicology screen, serum psychotropic drug levels, thyroid function tests, antithyroid antibodies, vitamin B_6 and B_{12} levels, total or bioavailable testosterone, dehydroepiandrosterone sulfate, adrenocorticotropic hormone stimulation test, 24-hour urine cortisol
- Evaluation for hepatitis C (including viral load)
- Review of antiretroviral regimen for neuropsychiatric side effects
- Review of psychotropic mediations for efficacy, neuropsychiatric side effects, drug interactions
- Neuroimaging (magnetic resonance imaging, magnetic resonance spectroscopy)
- Lumbar puncture

sedation with fluoroscopic guidance. Results are often nonspecific, but important studies include opening pressure, culture (viral, fungal, mycobacterial), cell count, protein, neopterin, β2-microglobulin, and polymerase chain reaction (PCR) testing for CMV, Epstein-Barr virus, JC Virus, herpes simplex virus, and HIV-1.

PSYCHIATRIC DISORDERS AND THEIR TREATMENT

Readers are referred to other chapters in this volume that address the outpatient diagnosis and treatment of psychiatric and substance use disorders, neurocognitive disorders, pain, fatigue, and sleep; most of these issues will apply in the inpatient medical setting. Depression, delirium, HIV-associated mania, and psychosis are discussed later in more detail because there is an increased likelihood they will be encountered in the inpatient setting.

DEPRESSION

Depression is the most common psychiatric symptom and diagnosis among medical inpatients with HIV disease or AIDS. Symptoms are often attributed to adjustment disorder or to medically related ("organic") factors that may be transient, related to onset and then improvement in physical symptoms. However, in one prospective study assessing depressive symptoms at admission and discharge, 28% of medical inpatients with HIV disease or AIDS had severe depressive symptoms that persisted at discharge.[21] In another study, 76% of patients who had a depressive disorder during their admission continued to have significant depressive symptoms 3 to 6 weeks after discharge, with significant predictors of depression during and after medical hospitalization being female gender, AIDS diagnosis, and poor social support.[9]

In the medical inpatient setting in particular, the diagnosis of depressive disorder in HIV-infected patients may be confounded by somatic symptoms common to depression and HIV illness and its complications, including fatigue, appetite loss, sleep disturbance, and difficulty with attention or concentration. The preponderance of evidence in the HIV literature suggests that in the presence of persistent depressed mood or loss of interest, an inclusive approach toward somatic symptoms is preferred. This is based on the fact that affective and somatic subscales of depression screening instruments (e.g., the Beck Depression Inventory) are highly intercorrelated, that these symptoms are more closely linked to measures of depression than to measures of HIV disease severity, and that both affective and somatic symptoms improve with antidepressant treatment.[22,23]

The treatment of depression in HIV disease is discussed in Chapter 10. In the medical inpatient setting, when antidepressant medication treatment is considered, particular attention must be paid to the side effect profile, hepatic and renal function, and potential for drug interactions. In addition to standard antidepressants such as serotonin and serotonin/norepinephrine reuptake inhibitors (see Chapter 10), the initiation of psychostimulants and anabolic steroids, particularly testosterone, may be more frequent in the inpatient setting and will be given more attention here.

Psychostimulants have been studied for the treatment of depressed mood, fatigue, and cognitive impairment in the context of HIV infection, particularly in advanced illness and where rapid onset of action is desirable. Agents studied include methylphenidate (5 to 90 mg/day), dextroamphetamine (5 to 20 mg/day), pemoline (35 to 150 mg/day), and the wakefulness agent modafinil (50 to 200 mg/day).[24–27] These agents are efficacious in treating depressive symptoms in patients with advanced HIV disease. The primary side effect is overstimulation.

Testosterone deficiency, with clinical symptoms of hypogonadism (depressed mood, fatigue, diminished libido, decreased appetite, and loss of lean body mass) is present in up to 50% of men and women with symptomatic HIV disease or AIDS.[19] The most common screening test for testosterone deficiency is total serum testosterone (deficiency is defined as less than 300 to 400 ng/dl in men); however, serum-free (deficiency: less than 5 to 7 pg/ml in men; <3 pg/ml in women) and bioavailable testosterone may be more accurate measures. For testosterone replacement in men, commonly used testosterone preparations include esterified depot testosterone (propionate, enanthate, cypionate, initiated at 100 to 200 mg intramuscularly [IM] every 2 weeks, maximum 400 mg IM weekly), transdermal skin patches (1 to 2 patches, 5 to 10 mg, to clean, dry skin daily), and transdermal testosterone gel (1 to 4 packets, 25 to 100 mg, to clean, dry skin daily), with the depot preparations being the least expensive and most studied. Patch and gel formulations may produce less variability in serum testosterone levels and, therefore, in target symptoms. In women, transdermal testosterone 150 mcg per day or equivalent may be used.[28] Reported side effects include irritability, tension, reduced energy, hair loss, testicular atrophy, reduced ejaculate volume, and acne.

DELIRIUM

In contrast to ambulatory patients with HIV disease or AIDS, delirium is common among hospitalized patients with HIV disease or AIDS, diagnosed in 11% to 29% of patients. There are no data regarding specific or distinguishing symptom characteristics for the delirium seen in HIV-infected patients. Both the hypoactive and hyperactive variants of delirium are seen, and in addition to cognitive disturbance, symptom manifestations include apathy, dysphoria, agitation, fearfulness, delusions, and hallucinations.

Delirium in the HIV/AIDS patient is often superimposed on HIV-associated neurocognitive disorders, particularly dementia, and patients with these disorders are at increased risk for the development of delirium when medically hospitalized. The etiology of delirium in HIV/AIDS patients is generally multifactorial. Breitbart et al.[28] reported a mean of 12.6 medical complications in 30 patients with AIDS who were experiencing delirium, with the most common being hematologic (anemia, leukopenia, thrombocytopenia, hypoalbuminemia) and infectious diseases (e.g., septicemia, systemic fungal infections, *Pneumocystis jiroveci* (formerly *carinii*) [PCP] pneumonia, tuberculosis, and disseminated viral infections). Other potential etiologies are discussed in the previous section on differential diagnosis.

Central to the treatment of delirium is treatment of its underlying medical cause(s). Symptomatic treatment includes educational, environmental, and psychopharmacologic interventions. Education regarding the risk and nature of delirium delivered to patients, their family, and the treatment team can be preventive and can result in earlier treatment and improved outcomes. Environmental interventions include titrating the level of stimulation, having the patient assume the sitting position, placing the patient next to a window, frequently checking the patient's orientation to surroundings, stabilizing sleep–wake cycles, and placing familiar people and orienting objects in the room.

In terms of pharmacologic treatment, most practitioners treat delirium with atypical antipsychotics, including olanzapine (available with dissolving oral preparation and for intramuscular injection), risperidone, quetiapine, and ziprasidone (available for intramuscular injection). However, the only double blind clinical trial of delirium treatment compared haloperidol, chlorpromazine, and lorazepam.[28] In that study, Breitbart et al.[28] screened medical inpatients with HIV disease for delirium. Thus, treatment was initiated early, when symptoms were mild to moderate in degree. Patients were severely medically ill; 9 (30%) of the 30 patients died within 1 week after completing the protocol. There were three important findings. First, haloperidol (mean dose 2.8 mg/day acutely and 1.4 mg/day maintenance) and chlorpromazine (mean dose 50 mg/day acutely and 36 mg/day maintenance) were equally efficacious. Second, the lorazepam arm (mean dose 3 mg acutely) was stopped early because of worsening delirium symptoms, including oversedation, disinhibition, ataxia, and increased confusion. Thus benzodiazepines should be used with extreme caution, if at all, and adjunctively with neuroleptics. Third, adverse effects in the antipsychotic arms were limited and included mild parkinsonian symptoms of decreased expressiveness, increased rigidity and tremor, and mild akathisia.

In sum, delirium is common in hospitalized patients with HIV disease or AIDS; these patients should be assessed frequently for early detection and treatment. A combination of psychoeducational, environmental, and pharmacologic interventions, primarily with neuroleptic medications, will provide the best outcomes.

MANIA

Manic symptomatology has been reported in 11% of all medically hospitalized patients with HIV disease or AIDS[9] and may be seen in conjunction with primary bipolar illness or with CNS HIV infection (HIV-associated mania). Descriptively, HIV-associated mania is found to be a late-onset, secondary affective illness associated with HIV infection of the brain, being less associated with a personal or family history of mood disorder. In addition, the symptomatology of HIV-associated mania may include more irritability, less hyper-talkativeness, and more psychomotor slowing and cognitive impairment compared to primary bipolar mania. Given that HIV-associated mania is directly related to HIV brain infection, antiretroviral agents that penetrate the blood–brain barrier may offer some protection from incident mania.[29]

Practice guidelines recommend lithium, valproic acid, or carbamazepine as standard therapy for a manic episode of bipolar affective illness. However, in the context of HIV infection, there are particular considerations regarding their use, especially in later stage illness.

There is relatively little research on the psychopharmacologic treatment of HIV-associated mania. A case report on the use of lithium for HIV-associated mania in a patient with AIDS showed control of symptoms at a dosage of 1,200 mg daily; however, significant neurotoxicity (cognitive slowing, fine tremor) occurred, leading to discontinuation.[30] The most commonly used mood stabilizer in the treatment of HIV-associated mania is valproic acid. Valproic acid, up to 1,750 mg daily, led to significant improvement in acute manic symptoms, at serum levels more than 50 mcg/L, with few adverse effects.[31] There have been reports of valproic acid increasing HIV replication in vitro in a dose-dependent manner, and one report of increased cytomegalovirus (CMV) replication, perhaps mediated by alterations in intracellular glutathione, which is an important mediator of HIV replication. The clinical relevance of these findings remains controversial, and, to date, there are no reports of valproic acid causing elevations in viral load in vivo. Most recently, the anticonvulsant lamotrigine has received

Food and Drug Administration (FDA) approval for maintenance therapy in bipolar illness, has been tested for HIV-associated peripheral neuropathy, and may be useful for treating mania in HIV infection. This anticonvulsant requires careful upward dose titration because of risk for severe hypersensitivity.

Given the limitations of mood stabilizers, there is widespread clinical use of atypical antipsychotics for acute and maintenance treatment of HIV-associated mania. Effective agents in this regard include olanzapine, risperidone, and quetiapine, but data are limited. Benzodiazepines may be useful for adjunctive therapy, but acute and maintenance treatment may be complicated by tolerance, dependence, and cognitive impairment.

PSYCHOSIS

HIV infection may be directly linked to the onset of psychosis, which is defined by the presence of thought disorder, hallucinations, or delusions. Psychosis in HIV is most often a manifestation of substance intoxication or withdrawal, delirium, HIV-associated neurocognitve disorders, mood disorders with psychotic features, or schizophrenia. Estimates of the prevalence of new-onset psychosis in patients with HIV infection range from 0.5% to 15%.[32] One study compared 20 HIV-infected patients with new-onset psychosis (and no prior psychotic episodes or current substance abuse) with 20 demographic and HIV illness–matched, nonpsychotic patients. The former group tended to have worse global neuropsychological impairment, was more likely to have a prior history of substance abuse, and had significantly higher mortality at follow-up, suggesting that psychotic patients with HIV disease or AIDS had an increased CNS vulnerability.[33]

HIV-infected patients with primary psychotic disorders such as schizophrenia and schizoaffective disorder may have poor access to HIV care, may present to the emergency and medical inpatient setting with untreated illness, and may be at risk for poor adherence to care, unless provided with comprehensive supportive services including psychiatric treatment, housing, and community case management.

In general, treatment with antipsychotic medication requires awareness of HIV-infected patients' susceptibility to neuroleptic-induced extrapyramidal symptoms (EPS) as a result of HIV-induced neuronal damage to the basal ganglia. In fact, movement disorders (acute dystonia, parkinsonism, ataxia) can be seen in advanced HIV disease in the absence of antipsychotic exposure. General recommendations include avoidance of high-potency D2 blocking agents, avoidance of depot neuroleptics, and the consideration that maintenance antipsychotic medication may not be necessary for the complete remission of new-onset or transient psychotic symptoms. Most clinicians prefer the use of atypical antipsychotics in this population.

A literature search on the use of antipsychotic medication in HIV disease and AIDS revealed six studies published since 1993; these studies described treatment of psychosis occurring in delirious, schizophrenic, and manic patients. Agents reported in the literature include haloperidol (mean dose, 3 mg)[34]; thioridazine (mean dose, 145 mg/day)[35]; molindone (20 to 180 mg/day)[36]; clozapine (mean dose, 27 mg/day)[35]; risperidone (mean dose, 3.3 mg/day),[37] and olanzapine (10 to 15 mg/day).[38] Haloperidol was reported to have a high incidence of EPS,[36] and caution is encouraged with clozapine because of the risk for agranulocytosis and interaction with ritonavir.

SYSTEM OF CARE ISSUES

The delivery of inpatient care for individuals with HIV disease or AIDS varies greatly. In nonepicenter cities, patients with HIV disease or AIDS are most often integrated into the general hospital population. In major urban hospitals there are more likely to be HIV/AIDS specialty care units. Such units provide patients with access to dedicated nursing, physician, mental health, and other clinical expertise with HIV/AIDS care, a high standard of cooperative interaction, and continuity with ongoing outpatient care. Such units have generally had more success hiring and retaining staff than those of other medical specialties. Further, they have been found to offer important benefits to patients with HIV disease or AIDS, including lower odds of dying within 30 days of admission, higher patient satisfaction, and care meeting professional standards. In general, this multidisciplinary specialty model of care is most effective for patients with HIV disease or AIDS who have comorbid psychiatric and substance use disorders. Concerns have been raised regarding the wisdom of centralizing the care of these patients because of issues of confidentiality and segregation; however, most centers provide patients with the choice of occupying specialty or nonspecialty unit beds, with the vast majority choosing the former.

PROVIDER ISSUES

Working with patients with HIV disease or AIDS can be extremely rewarding, and staff burnout may actually be lower than in other specialties of medicine.[39] This is most likely to be true in integrated specialty units because of an enhanced sense of community and centrality of purpose. Nonetheless, staff stress inevitably results from working in the acute setting, especially where acting out behavioral disorders occur as a result of treating patients with the triple diagnosis of HIV-related medical problems, psychiatric disorders, and substance use disorders. Staff members often comment (jokingly or not) that the inpatient HIV medical unit seems like a psychiatric unit. Medical nursing and other staff may not feel adequately equipped to manage such issues. Thus it is vital to have readily available psychiatric staff to educate and support other clinicians, to assist in diagnosis and behavioral management, and to facilitate transfer to psychiatric or substance abuse treatment as indicated.

A further issue of heightened concern for staff in the medical inpatient setting is occupational exposure to HIV, HBV, and HCV. Although fear of contagion may be an absolute deterrent to work with patients with HIV disease or AIDS for some individuals, all staff, including mental health professionals, working with these patients must assess their own underlying degree of concern and take appropriate precautions. The widespread application of Universal Precautions was largely spurred by the HIV epidemic. As of 2001, there were 56 definite and 138 probable cases of HIV infection from occupational exposure to HIV.[40] The risk of infection from a single percutaneous needlestick injury with blood from a known HIV-positive patient is approximately 1 in 300 (0.3%) and from a single mucocutaneous exposure is 1 in 1,000 (0.09%). In the case of occupational exposure to HIV, the Centers for Disease Control and Prevention guidelines recommend postexposure prophylaxis (PEP) with two or three antiretroviral drugs, depending on the route and volume of exposure, commencing immediately and continued for 4 weeks. Distress in the affected individual and colleagues may inevitably occur because of high-risk exposure. Although affected staff members are told that a low risk exists for HIV infection, a 4-week regimen of PEP might be recommended, and they are asked to commit to behavioral measures (e.g., sexual abstinence or condom use) to prevent secondary transmission, all of which influence their lives for several weeks to months. Mental health staff members should be available for general emotional support and referral for the individual at risk and should be aware of the ripple of concern among other staff, providing individual or group intervention where indicated.

SUMMARY

Although the overall frequency and reasons for inpatient medical admission of patients with HIV disease or AIDS have changed over the past decade, comorbid psychiatric and substance use disorders continue to be common. In the medical inpatient setting, these comorbid disorders will often present in the acute stages in patients with poor access and adherence to HIV care. In contrast to the outpatient setting, in the inpatient medical setting, delirium, substance-induced disorders and withdrawal states, psychosis, and mania are more likely to be seen. In this context, differential diagnosis can be complex and requires a thorough consideration of the neuropsychiatric manifestations of HIV, associated illnesses such as HCV infection, substance intoxication and withdrawal states, and the possible neuropsychiatric side effects of medical treatments. Thus, readily available and informed psychiatric consultation and liaison services are an essential component of the comprehensive evaluation and management of these patients.

REFERENCES

1. Fleishman JA, Hellinger FJ. Trends in HIV-related inpatient admissions from 1993–1997: a seven-state study. *J Acquir Immune Defic Syndr.* 2001;28:73–80.
2. Fleishman JA, Hellinger FH. Recent trends in HIV-related inpatient admissions 1996–2000: a seven-state study. *J Acquir Immune Defic Syndr.* 2003;34:102–110.
3. Paul S, Gilbert HM, Lande L, et al. Impact of antiretroviral therapy on decreasing hospitalization rates of HIV-infected patients in 2001. *AIDS Res Hum Retroviruses.* 2002;18:501–506.
4. Cebo KA, Diener-West M, Moore RD. Hospitalization rates in an urban cohort after the introduction of highly active antiretroviral therapy. *J Acquir Immune Defic Syndr.* 2003;27:143–152.
5. Perry S, Tross S. Psychiatric problems of AIDS inpatients at the New York Hospital: preliminary report. *Public Health Rep.* 1984;99:200–205.
6. Dilley JW, Ochitill HN, Perl M, Volberding PA. Findings in psychiatric consultations with patients with acquired immune deficiency syndrome. *Am J Psychiatry.* 1985;142:82–86.
7. O'Dowd MA, McKegney FP. AIDS patients compared with others seen in psychiatric consultation. *Gen Hosp Psychiatry.* 1990;12:50–55.
8. Bialer P, Wallack J, Prenzlauer S, Bogdonoff L, Wilets I. Psychiatric comorbidity among hospitalized AIDS patients vs. non-AIDS patients referred for psychiatric consultation. *Psychosomatics.* 1996;37:469–475.
9. Ferrando SJ, Rabkin J, Rothenberg J. Psychiatric disorders and adjustment of HIV and AIDS patients during and after medical hospitalization. *Psychosomatics.* 1998;39:214–215.
10. Perry S, Jacobsberg LB, Fishman B, et al. Psychiatric diagnosis before serological testing for the human immunodeficiency virus. *Am J Psychiatry.* 1990;147:89–93.
11. Williams JBW, Rabkin JG, Remien RH, Gorman JM, Ehrhardt AA. Multidisciplinary baseline assessment of homosexual men with and without human immunodeficiency virus infection. II. Standardized clinical assessment of current and lifetime psychopathology. *Arch Gen Psychiatry.* 1991;48:124–130.
12. Crone C, Gabriel GM. Comprehensive review of hepatitis C for psychiatrists: risks, screening, diagnosis, treatment and interferon-based therapy complications. *J Psychiatr Pract* 2003;9:93–110.
13. Maxwell S, Scheftner WA, Kessler HA, Busch K. Manic syndrome associated with zidovudine treatment. *JAMA.* 1988;259:3406–407.
14. Brouillette MJ, Chouinard G, Laloonde R. Didanosine-induced mania in HIV infection. *Am J Psychiatry.* 1994;151:1839–1840.
15. Foster R, Taylor C, Everall IP. More on abacavir-induced neuropsychiatric reactions. *AIDS.* 2004;18:2449.
16. Morlese JF, Qazi NA, Gazzard BG, Nelson MR. Nevirapine-induced neuropsychiatric complications, a class effect of non-nucleoside reverse transcriptase inhibitors? *AIDS.* 2002;16:1840–1841.
17. Staszewski S, Morales-Ramirez J, Tashima KT, et al. Efavirenz plus zidovudine and lamivudine, efavirenz plus indinavir, and indinavir plus zidovudine and lamivudine in treatment of HIV-1 infection in adults. Study 006 team. *N Engl J Med.* 1999;341:1865–1873.
18. Chen F, Day SL, Metcalfe RA, et al. Characteristics of autoimmune thyroid disease occurring as a late complication of immune reconstitution in patients with advanced human immunodeficiency virus (HIV) disease. *Medicine (Baltimore).* 2005;84;98–106.
19. Mylonakis E, Koutkia P, Grinspoon S. Diagnosis and treatment of androgen deficiency in human immunodeficiency virus-infected men and women. *Clin Infect Dis.* 2001;33:857–864.
20. Mayo J, Callazos J, Martinez E, Ibarra S. Adrenal function in the human immunodeficiency virus-infected patient. *Arch Intern Med.* 2002;162:1095–1098.
21. Mierlak D, Leon A, Perry S. Does physical improvement reduce depressive symptoms in HIV-infected medical inpatients? *Gen Hosp Psychiatry.* 1995;17:380–384.
22. Rabkin JG, Williams JB, Remien RH, et al. Depression, distress, lymphocyte subsets and human immunodeficiency virus symptoms on two occasions in HIV-positive homosexual men. *Arch Gen Psychiatry.* 1992;48:111–119.
23. Ferrando SJ, Goldman JG, Charness W. SSRI treatment of depression in symptomatic HIV infection and AIDS: improvements in affective and somatic symptoms. *Gen Hosp Psychiatry.* 1997;19:89–97.
24. Holmes VF, Fernandez F, Levy JK. Psychostimulant response in AIDS-related complex patients. *J Clin Psychiatry.* 1989;50:5–8.

25. Wagner GJ, Rabkin R. Effects of dextroamphetamine on depression and fatigue in men with HIV: a double-blind, placebo-controlled trial. *J Clin Psychiatry.* 2000;61:436–440.
26. Breitbart W, Rosenfeld B, Kaim M, Funesti-Esch J. A randomized, double-blind, placebo-controlled trial of psychostimulants for the treatment of fatigue in ambulatory patients with human immunodeficiency virus disease. *Arch Intern Med.* 2001;161:411–420.
27. Rabkin JG, McElhiney M, Rabkin R, Ferrando SJ: Modafinil treatment of fatigue in HIV+ patients. *J Clin Psychiatry.* 2004;65:1688–1695.
28. Breitbart W, Marotta R, Platt MM, et al. A double-blind trial of haloperidol, chlorpromazine, and lorazepam in the treatment of delirium in hospitalized AIDS patients. *Am J Psychiatry.* 1996;153:231–237.
29. Mijch AM, Judd FK, Lyketsos CG, Ellen S, Cockram A. Secondary mania in patients with HIV infection: are antiretrovirals protective? *J Neuropsychiatry Clin Neurosci.* 1999;11:475–480.
30. Tanquary J. Lithium neurotoxicity at therapeutic levels in an AIDS patient. *J Nerv Ment Dis.* 1993;181:518–519.
31. Halman MH, Worth JL, Sanders KM, Renshaw PF, Murray GB. Anticonvulsant use in the treatment of manic syndromes in patients with HIV-1 infection. *J Neuropsychiatry Clin Neurosci.* 1993;5:430–434.
32. McDaniel JS, for the Working Group on HIV/AIDS. Practice guideline for the treatment of patients with HIV/AIDS. *Am J Psychiatr.* 2000;157:1–62.
33. Sewell DD, Jeste DV, Atkinson JH, et al. HIV-associated psychosis: a study of 20 cases. San Diego HIV Neurobehavioral Research Center Group. *Am J Psychiatry.* 1994;151:237–242.
34. Sewell DD, Jeste DV, McAdams LA, et al. Neuroleptic treatment of HIV-associated psychosis: HNRC group. *Neuropsychopharmacology.* 1994;10:223–229.
35. Lera G, Zirulnik J. Pilot study with clozapine in patients with HIV-associated psychosis and drug-induced parkinsonism. *Mov Disord.* 1999;14:128–131.
36. Fernandez F, Levy JK. The use of molindone in the treatment of psychotic and delirious patients infected with the human immunodeficiency virus: case reports. *Gen Hosp Psychiatry.* 1993;15:31–35.
37. Singh AN, Golledge H, Catalan J. Treatment of HIV-related psychotic disorders with risperidone: a series of 21 cases. *J Psychosom Res.* 1997;42:489–493.
38. Meyer JM, Marsh J, Simpson G. Differential sensitivities to risperidone and olanzapine in a human immunodeficiency virus patient. *Biol Psychiatry.* 1998;44:791–794.
39. Lopez-Castillo J, Gurpegui M, Ayuso-Mateos JL, Luna JD, Catalan J. Emotional distress and occupational burnout in health care professionals serving HIV-infected patients: a comparison with oncology and internal medicine services. *Psychother Psychosom.* 1999;68:348–356.
40. Centers for Disease Control and Prevention. Updated U.S. Public Health Service guidelines for the management of occupational exposures to HBV, HCV, and HIV and recommendations for postexposure prophylaxis. *MMWR Morbid Mortal Wkly Rep.* 2001;50(RRII):1–42.

SECTION V

Special Populations

CHAPTER 20

HIV/AIDS Among Hispanic Americans

Pedro Ruiz, Francisco Fernandez

During the last several decades, the United States has become a multiethnic, pluralistic society. The Hispanic population in the United States has grown and represents the largest ethnic minority group in this country. Currently, the Hispanic population is 35.3 million or about 12.5% of the total U.S. population.[1] The 11 million undocumented Hispanic immigrants are not included in this number. The current growth rate of Hispanics in the United States is 58%, compared to 50% for the Asian/Pacific Islander population, 17% for the Alaskan Native population, 16% for the African-American population, and 3% for the White population.[1] Hispanics tend to marry young and have the highest number of offspring compared to other ethnic minority groups in the United States. Thus Hispanics and the Hispanic culture pose special challenges to the understanding and containment of the human immunodeficiency virus (HIV) and acquired immunodeficiency syndrome (AIDS) epidemic in this significant portion of the population.

Culture, race, and ethnicity have always been a consideration in the identification of risk factors involved in acquiring and transmitting HIV infection and AIDS. For example, AIDS-defining conditions are more common among certain racial or ethnic groups.[2] For example, the prevalence of extrapulmonary tuberculosis is found to be higher among Hispanics, Blacks, Asians/Pacific Islanders, and Native Americans/Alaskan Natives suffering from HIV disease or AIDS than among Whites. Likewise, the prevalence of isosporiasis and toxoplasmosis is higher among Hispanics than among African-American or non-Hispanic Whites.[2]

This chapter defines the Hispanic population of patients with HIV disease and AIDS, addresses the most important risk factors pertaining to HIV disease and AIDS among Hispanics, and reviews the most relevant clinical considerations related to this diverse ethnic group.

HIV/AIDS EPIDEMIOLOGY AMONG HISPANICS

The current HIV/AIDS epidemic represents a very serious threat to the U.S. Hispanic community. Although Hispanics comprise 12.5% of the population in the United States, they account for nearly 20% of people with AIDS.[3] In addition to being a population disproportionately affected by HIV disease and AIDS, Hispanics in the United States continue to face major challenges in accessing health care, in securing health-related prevention services, and in receiving effective antiretroviral treatment. In 2001, HIV disease/AIDS was the third leading cause of death among Hispanic men aged 35 to 44 and the fourth leading cause of death among Hispanic women in the same age-group.[3] Survival rates in Hispanics with AIDS are significantly lower (61%) than in Whites (64%) and Asians/Pacific Islanders (69%). Only Native Americans/Alaskan Natives (58%) and African Americans (55%) had lower survival rates.[4] Hispanics also have the second highest rate of new AIDS cases in the United States compared to other racial and ethnic groups, with the African-American community being the highest. Table 20.1 denotes the estimated number of cases with HIV disease or AIDS diagnosed in 2002 according to race.[4]

As depicted in Table 20.1, Hispanics accounted for 13% of new HIV infection or AIDS cases diagnosed in 2002. Among Hispanics, from 1999 to 2002, the number of new HIV infection or AIDS cases diagnosed increased 26%.[4] Table 20.2 shows the rate of AIDS cases in the United States in 2003.[5]

Table 20.3 depicts the percentage of AIDS cases in Hispanics from the 859,000 AIDS cases reported to the Centers for Disease Control and Prevention (CDC) through 2002.[5]

In 2003, an estimated 11,498 women had a diagnosis of AIDS; this number represented 27% of the 43,171 AIDS cases diagnosed in that year.[6] The rate of AIDS diagnosis for Hispanic women in 2003 was 12.4/100,000; this rate was higher than the rate for White women (2/100,000) and second only to that of African-American women (50.2/100,000).[6] African-American and Hispanic women make up 83% of all AIDS cases diagnosed in 2003, with African-American women having a risk that is 16 times that of White women.[6] Thus, HIV infection and AIDS among U.S. Hispanics present a major health/mental health challenge.

RISK FACTORS FOR HIV/AIDS AMONG HISPANICS

The primary risk factor for exposure to HIV in U.S. Hispanics varies for different groups. It is therefore imperative to be fully aware of these risk factors in order to attempt to deal with the diversity pertaining to age, gender, nationality, migratory experience, and acculturation as it relates to medical, psychiatric, and public health perspectives. For example, the Hispanic migration to the United States originates from many countries and varying regions therein. Thus the Hispanic community in the United States is not a culturally homogeneous group. This fact needs to be taken into consideration when discussing these risk factors related to HIV disease and AIDS.

Research and investigational efforts have demonstrated that Hispanics born in different countries and regions may depict different behavioral risk factors for HIV disease and AIDS. For example, it has been documented that Hispanics born in Puerto Rico or who are of Puerto Rican descent are more likely to become HIV infected as a result of injection drug use than any other subgroup of Hispanics. By contrast, men who have sex with men (MSM) are

TABLE 20.1	2002 Estimated HIV Cases in the United States (N = 26,464)
	(%)
African American	53
White	32
Hispanic	13
Asian/Pacific Islander	1
American Indian/Alaska Native	1

TABLE 20.2	2003 Estimated AIDS Cases			
Ethnicity	Male		Female	
	Cases	Rate per 100,000	Cases	Rate per 100,000
White, not Hispanic	10,450	12.8	1,725	2.0
Black, not Hispanic	13,624	103.8	7,551	50.2
Hispanic	6,087	40.3	1,744	12.4
Asian/Pacific Islander	408	8.3	8.6	1.6
American Indian/ Alaska Native	150	16.2	46	4.8
Total	30,851	26.6	11,211	9.2

considered the primary route of HIV transmission among men born in Mexico or who are of Mexican descent.[7] Table 20.4 denotes the 2002 exposure category for Hispanic countries and regions compared with that of the United States.[5]

CLINICALLY RELEVANT CULTURAL FACTORS

LANGUAGE

Culturally competent health care starts with common and shared understanding and communication. From the perspective of a monolingual Hispanic patient, this requires either a linguistically competent provider or the use of a translator. In HIV/AIDS care, the use of a translator is fraught with problems. For example, assessing sexual risk factors and injection drug use may be complicated by an inadequate or erroneous translation due to the nuance variations between the two languages. At other times, the nonprofessional translator, out of *respeto* (respect) or *verguenza* (shame), may not directly inquire about specific sexual practices, which may result in misinformation. For similar reasons, one should avoid the use of the patient's family or friends. Moreover, the identified patient may not be truthful or may have difficulty disclosing such intimate information through friends or family. Ideally, professional medical translators should be used. However, even with such individuals, one should, whenever possible, obtain a translator of the same gender and ideally of the same cultural subgroup or background as the patient.

LA FAMILIA (THE FAMILY)

Familiarismo (familism) is another common cultural norm within the Hispanic community.[7] This cultural value and norm is characterized by a strong sense of loyalty and reciprocity to the

TABLE 20.3	AIDS in Hispanics Through 2003 (Total = 902,223)
• 19% of total cases	
• 19% of women cases	
• 22% of heterosexual cases	
• 23% of children cases	

20% of AIDS cases reported in 2003 were among Hispanic adults and adolescents.

TABLE 20.4	2004 AIDS Cases by Exposure Category				
Exposure Category	United States (%)	Mexico (%)	Puerto Rico (%)	Cuba (%)	Central and South America (%)
Male-male sexual contact	43	60	20	59	52
Injection drug use	25	11	39	13	13
Male-male sexual contact and injection drug use	5	3	4	5	2
Heterosexual contact	25	25	37	23	32
Other	1	1	1	0	1

nuclear family, as well as members of the extended family (*compadres/comadres* [godparents], *primos/primas* [cousins], and *tios/tias* [uncles/aunts]). Familiar participation by these groups is as significant as the true sociobiologic equivalents.

Although usually a source of strength and support, such relationships may present significant challenges when dealing with issues such as disclosure of HIV status, sexual orientation, and drug use. *Falta de armonia* (lack of harmony) is a common complaint reflecting lack of tangible support and interpersonal struggles over these issues, as well as socioeconomic functioning. Clinicians must consider these factors in treatment planning, including the possible need to rely on alternative support systems for the patient.

MACHISMO

A cultural factor such as *machismo* (exaggerated sense of manliness or hypermanliness) is another contributing factor to increasing risk and promoting transmission of HIV infection in the Hispanic community. Hispanic men may be reluctant to acknowledge and accept high-risk behaviors such as having sex with other men. This may lead Hispanic MSM to inaccurately portray their sexual drives and behaviors in favor of identifying themselves as heterosexuals.[5] This further limits access to education, prevention, and treatment efforts.

In some households where *machismo* is prevalent, Hispanic women are likely to feel powerless regarding their individual risks for HIV infection and AIDS.[8] For example, it may be rather difficult to impose or advise them to use safe-sex practices such as condom use because of a culture that might also impose on them social and physical sanctions against such assertive behaviors. In these households, *machismo* can often lead to family violence and physical abuse if women attempt to become assertive in their homes. Moreover, use of condoms in these cases might also be culturally unacceptable because it implies lack of trust among both partners and violation of religious practices and is thus considered sinful.[8]

Other potentially negative effects of *machismo* may involve lack of knowledge about HIV infection and AIDS and modes of transmission and prevention strategies.[8] These may negatively affect psychoeducational or community involvement regarding HIV/AIDS in Hispanics.

MARIANISMO (VIRGIN MARY IN LIKENESS)

Being virginous is another potential cultural confound in Hispanic women. Women's virginity still is highly valued in many Hispanic households based on cultural norms.[9] Single Hispanic women are most likely infected with HIV as a result of heterosexual contacts. Sexual contacts of any kind before marriage are not sanctioned in most Hispanic communities. This may in part account for why the use of condoms by Hispanic women is very low.[5]

In marriage, Hispanic women, in many instances, are expected to play a submissive, obedient, and subservient role to their husbands. Because of this cultural value, many Hispanic women center their life around their husband and children and are expected to avoid self-indulgence and sensuality, as well as be always available to the sexual desires of their men/husbands.[9]

HOMOSEXUALITY

In most Hispanic communities, homosexuality is morally rejected, scorned, and often considered a character flaw.[10] Gay, bisexual, and lesbian Hispanics often have difficulty integrating their sexuality and often live in isolation from their families. The clinician may face great difficulty in diagnosing and treating medical conditions that are sexually related in this population (see Chapters 28 and 29).

Machismo presents an added attitudinal barrier influencing acceptance of sexual preferences and other lifestyle issues. Many Hispanic MSM do not regard themselves as homosexuals or even bisexual. Assuming the dominant sexual role (insertive as opposed to receptive) and/or continuing to engage in heterosexual sex practices gives sanction to this sexual practice as long as the male fulfills his "masculine" (dominant, heterosexual) role.[9] Again, this has major implications for prevention efforts in HIV infection and AIDS.

POVERTY

Poverty is a major factor that needs to be recognized and dealt with when addressing the needs of U.S. Hispanics. According to the 2000 census, about 22% of Hispanic families live below the poverty level; also, Hispanic families have an annual income of about $30,735, compared to $44,366 for White families; additionally, 39.4% of Puerto Rican families are led by women.[1,11] A variety of socioeconomic problems associated with poverty, including substance use and abuse, prostitution, and limited access to high-quality health and mental health care, directly and indirectly increase the risk for HIV infection and AIDS.[12]

SUBSTANCE USE AND ABUSE

Substance use and abuse is another major risk factor for HIV infection among Hispanics. The role of drug use and abuse in HIV infection among Hispanics is steadily increasing. Comorbid factors related to drug use and abuse greatly complicate the diagnosis and treatment of Hispanics with HIV infection or AIDS, including compliance, thereby increasing morbidity and mortality across all disease states.[13] Injection drug use alone accounts for an increasing proportion of HIV infection among Hispanics and other ethnic minorities. Hispanic intravenous drug users and abusers, particularly those using opioids or cocaine, often share dirty needles and engage in unsafe sexual practices because of drug-induced hypersexuality or exchanges of sex for drugs.[13] Hispanic drug users or abusers who are homosexual or bisexual and who frequently use alcohol or noninjecting drugs of abuse also tend to engage in high-risk sexual activities and thus are at increased risk of becoming infected with HIV.[14]

The co-occurrence of some psychiatric disorders and drug use or abuse also represents a significant risk for becoming infected with HIV. This type of comorbidity leads to clinical considerations such as impaired judgment, poor impulse control, lack of insight, and promiscuity. All of these negatively affect adherence to more positive health behaviors and increase the risks for acquiring infection with HIV or transmission of HIV.[13] Among these disorders are schizophrenia, schizoaffective disorder, antisocial personality disorder, borderline personality disorder, and impulse-control disorder.[13] Additionally, substance users and abusers who become infected with HIV may develop higher and sustained levels of stress. This might lead to further use or abuse of drugs and high-risk sexual activity.

CULTURALLY SANCTIONED SEXUAL BEHAVIORS

High-risk sexual behaviors are known vectors for HIV in the Hispanic community. For example, both Hispanic men and women engage in anal sexual practices as a way of protecting the women's virginity and avoiding pregnancies. Other sexual practices have also been sanctioned by culture among Hispanic communities. For example, homosexual extramarital relations for both men and women might be considered preferable if they lead to ongoing family stability; that is, they are less threatening to the family. Ongoing sexual relations with prostitutes, particularly for men, is also sanctioned. Unfortunately, prostitutes often avoid the use of condoms for fear that they might give a message to their male partners that they might be considered infected with a sexually transmitted disease.[9]

Other studies on HIV infection and AIDS focusing on high-risk sexual practices among Hispanics who live in high-risk cities have shown that Hispanic males with multiple sexual partners tend to be unmarried (31%), Cuban (28%), aged 18 to 29 years (25%), better educated (21%), of lower income status (23%), and highly acculturated (20%).[15] Similarly, Hispanic women with multiple sex partners tend to be highly acculturated (87%). It should also be noted that among Hispanic men with multiple sex partners, only 20% used condoms regularly with their primary partner and only 29% used condoms regularly with their secondary partner. Among Hispanic men, condom use tends to decrease as the number of sex partners increases.[15]

SEXUALLY TRANSMITTED INFECTIONS

Young Hispanic women between 15 and 24 years of age are vulnerable in that their sexual behaviors also increase their propensity to contract sexually transmitted infections (STIs), including HIV infection. For example, Hispanics are twice as likely to suffer from gonorrhea and syphilis as Whites.[16] Women are twice as likely as men to contract an STI or HIV during vaginal intercourse. Undoubtedly, these cultural norms regarding sex practices have major implications in prevention and treatment of HIV infection and AIDS.

Table 20.5 denotes the sexual risks for HIV infection and AIDS among Hispanic adults and adolescents during 2002.[5]

RELIGION

In the Hispanic community, religion is a core element of life. It often takes on a life of its own and is very public. Catholicism in Central and Latin America and the Caribbean is over 500 years old. Its teachings provide the framework to living a good life and therefore are hard to modify or let go. American Catholics for many years have made a distinction between what they believe and how they behave—not so for Hispanic Catholics.

Growing rates of HIV infection among Hispanics are distinctly influenced by questions of choice in complex decisions concerning premarital and extramarital relationships, contraception,

TABLE 20.5 2004 Risk Factors for HIV/AIDS Among Hispanic Adults and Adolescents

	Male (%)	Female (%)
Male-male sexual contact	54	N/A
Injection drug use	26	30
Male-male sexual contact and injection drug use	6	N/A
Heterosexual contact	14	68
Other	1	2

pregnancy, and abortions.[17] All too often, the solutions to these concerns are influenced by religious teachings that directly affect individual and family influences and social pressures. Trust in religious teachings creates almost an adversarial reaction in some Hispanic groups (whether Catholic, Pentecostal, Baptist, or Protestant) in which HIV education and prevention efforts appear to subvert the religious rules and family values.

Although essential changes are occurring, they are slow.[18] Hispanic AIDS initiatives showing *respeto* for spiritual beliefs and how they affect prevention of infection and its devastating effects on families are beginning to take hold.[19]

SUMMARY

We have attempted to define the Hispanic population of the United States and addressed the risk factors that make Hispanics vulnerable to HIV infection and AIDS. Major sociocultural characteristics of Hispanics that pose clinical challenges have been reviewed in the context of the HIV/AIDS epidemic. This information is essential for mental health practitioners who assess and treat HIV disease and AIDS among Hispanic populations, as well as in preparing the design of successful preventive strategies to control the current HIV infection and AIDS epidemic among Hispanic populations in this country and abroad.

REFERENCES

1. Ruiz P. La Psiquiatria en las Minorias Etnicas: El Ejemplo de Estados Unidos. In: Vallejo Ruiloba J, Leal Cercos C, eds. *Tratado de Psiquiatria*. Vol. II. Barcelona: Ars Medica; 2005:2273–2280.
2. Hu DJ, Fleming PL, Castro KG, et al. How important is race/ethnicity as an indicator of risk for specific AIDS-defining conditions? *J Acquir Immune Defic Syndr Hum Retrovirol*. 1995;10:374–380.
3. Anderson RN, Smith BL. Deaths: leading causes for 2001. *Natl Vital Stat Rep*. 2003;52:51–53.
4. National Center for HIV, STD and TB Prevention, Division of HIV/AIDS Prevention. *HIV/AIDS Among Hispanics in the United States*. Fact Sheet. November 16, 2004:1–6.
5. Centers for Disease Control and Prevention. *HIV/AIDS Among Hispanics*. Atlanta: Centers for Disease Control and Prevention; November 2004:1–4.
6. National Center for HIV, STD and TB Prevention, Division of HIV/AIDS Prevention. *HIV/AIDS Among Women*. Fact Sheet, December 2, 2004:1–7.
7. Gaines SO, Rios DI, Buriel R. Familism and personal relationship process among Latina/Latino couples. In: Gaines SO, Buriel R, Liu JH, Rios DI, eds. *Culture, Ethnicity, and Personal Relationship Processes*. New York: Rutledge; 1977:41–46.
8. Fernandez F, Ruiz P, Bing EG. The mental health impact of aids on ethnic minorities. In: Gaw AC, ed. *Culture, Ethnicity, and Mental Illness*. Washington, DC: American Psychiatric Press; 1993:573–586.
9. Peragallo N. Latino women and AIDS risk. *Public Health Nurs*. 1996;13:217–222.
10. Bing EG, Nichols SE, Goldfinger SM, et al. The many faces of AIDS: Opportunities for intervention. In Goldfinger SM, ed. *Psychiatric Aspects of AIDS and HIV Infection*. San Francisco: Jossey-Bass; 1990:69–81.
11. Diaz T, Chu S, Buehler J, et al. Socioeconomic differences among people with AIDS: results from a multi-state surveillance project. *Am J Prev Med*. 1994;10:217–222.
12. Ruiz P, Guynn RW, Matorin AA. Psychiatric considerations in the diagnosis, treatment, and prevention of HIV/AIDS. *J Psychiatr Pract*. 2000;6:129–139.

13. Ruiz P. Living and dying with HIV/AIDS: a psychosocial perspective. *Am J Psychiatry*. 2000;157:110–113.
14. Ruiz P, Lile B, Matorin AA. Treatment of a dually diagnosed gay male patient: a psychotherapy perspective. *Am J Psychiatry*. 2002;159:209–215.
15. Sabogal F, Faigeles B, Catania JA. Multiple sexual partners among Hispanics in high risk cities. *Fam Plann Perspect* 1993;25:257–262.
16. Fleming DT, Wasserheit JN. From epidemiological synergy to public health policy and practice: the contribution of other sexually transmitted diseases to sexual transmission of HIV infection. *Sex Transm Infect*. 1999;75:3–17.
17. Amaro H. Love, sex, and power: considering women's realities in HIV prevention. *Am Psychol*. 1995;50:437–447.
18. Gomez CA, Hernandez M, Faigeles B: Sex in the New World: an empowerment model for HIV prevention in Latina immigrant women. *Health Educ Behav*. 1999;26:200–212.
19. Marin G. AIDS prevention among Hispanic needs, risk behaviors and cultural values. *Public Health Rep*. 1989;104:411–415.

CHAPTER 21

HIV/AIDS Among African Americans

William B. Lawson, Janice G. Hutchinson, Dianne L. Reynolds

HIV/AIDS AND THE AFRICAN AMERICAN COMMUNITY

Human immunodeficiency virus (HIV) and acquired immunodeficiency syndrome (AIDS) together are a worldwide pandemic that continues to be a major health problem despite treatments that bring lengthy periods of remission. It does not affect all segments of the U.S. population equally. AIDS is now the number one cause of death for African Americans between the ages of 25 and 44.[1] African-Americans represent only 12% of the total U.S. population, yet almost half of all new AIDS cases reported in 2003 were African Americans. Over three quarters of all women with AIDS were Black or Hispanic, and 81% of all children with AIDS were Black or Hispanic.[1] Thus African-American women are 23 times more likely to be infected with AIDS than White women.[2] African-American men are almost 9 times more likely to be infected with AIDS than White men. Moreover, from 1999 to 2003 the numbers of HIV infection and AIDS diagnoses were consistently higher among non-Hispanic Blacks than among other races and ethnicities. In the 32 states with HIV infection reporting, the HIV infection and AIDS diagnosis rate in 2003 was 74 per 100,000 for Blacks, 25 per 100,000 for Hispanics, 11 per 100,000 for American Indians/Alaska Natives, 9 per 100,000 for Whites, and 7 per 100,000 for Asians/Pacific Islanders. The rates for persons living with HIV disease or AIDS at the end of 2003 were highest for Blacks (765 per 100,000) and Hispanics (220 per 100,000).[3]

The pattern of how the disease is acquired appears to differ by ethnicity. African Americans appear to be at greater risk of heterosexual and substance abuse spread rather than men with men. The majority of Black women with HIV contracted it from heterosexual sex.[2] However, a disproportionate number of their partners also had male partners, were substance abusers, or both. A survey of low-income women found that AIDS was ranked as the most important health concern.[4] There continues to be a steady rate of increase of new cases, especially among teenagers and those in their twenties. This suggests that current efforts in HIV prevention strategies have failed in the African-American communities.

We will present a case report that shows the complexity of these issues.

George is a 35-year-old African-American male who recently tested positive for HIV. He presented to a mental health clinic seeking advice on how to disclose his HIV status to his family. He also complained of having "anxiety attacks" since learning of his HIV status 1 week previously. George had never received mental health services before, nor had he sought treatment for what he referred to as a "moody personality." He stated that his current visit to the clinic is the result of a referral he received from the testing center. George reports having had many visits to the emergency room for "bad nerves," for which he received treatment. George also reported having a past alcohol and cocaine problem, which he managed on his own. The current HIV problem was too much for George to manage on his own. George is a father of two children, ages 7 and 11. He has been married for 11 years to a woman he met in college. He is not aware of how he contracted HIV, but figures that it must have been through sexual contacts.

At first glance, the major risk factor seems to be a history of substance abuse. Injectable agents such as opioids contribute to spread because of their risk for intravenous transmission. Cocaine and even alcohol or marijuana can increase the risk of contracting AIDS because they can increase the likelihood of high-risk sexual behavior. However, there is another factor that George admitted almost as an afterthought, and which contributed to his anxiety. He had had male sexual encounters. He fervently denied being gay.

George is one of many African-American men living "on the down low," which along with having addicted partners, probably contributes to significant heterosexual spread of AIDS and the increased risk of infection for African-American women.[5,6] The down low represents a secret sexual lifestyle for Black men who are married or have girlfriends, but are also secretly sleeping with men. Down low men distinguish themselves from gay men by not embracing the gay culture, and not being in "relationships." Down low refers to "gratification not orientation"; that is, the desire to have male-to-male sex. There are perhaps several reasons for the secrecy. One is the taboo of homosexuality in the African-American community; a taboo that visits shame on the family and implies weakness of character for the homosexual member. Also, many African-American women see men who choose a gay lifestyle as reducing the pool of available African-American men at a time when there is a shortage of potential male sex partners.[7] This openly discriminatory attitude, pervasively practiced within the African-American community, invokes fear of disclosure of one's sexual orientation.

In addition, many African-American men who see themselves as heterosexual may participate in homosexual behavior for opportunistic reasons, which may be a factor in the development of the down low culture. Men in settings where there are no women available, such as the correctional system, may participate in such sex and continue the behavior once they are released.

African-American men make up 50% of correctional system inmates and are far more likely to be incarcerated than their White counterparts.[8] Some of the highest rates of HIV infection are found among jails and prisons because of the high frequency of drug-related sentences and high-risk behaviors that occur within these institutions. When former felons are released to the community, they may continue this high-risk sexual behavior and become infected or they may already be infected. The result is a public health concern and an important contributor to the heterosexual spread and risk for women and their children.

HIV/AIDS AND MENTAL ILLNESS

HIV is neuropathic, invading the central nervous system (CNS) early during the initial period of infection. Although HIV does not infect neurons in the CNS, it causes neuronal death by other mechanisms. HIV infection of microglial cells in the CNS causes the elaboration of neurotoxins that, in turn, cause neuronal damage.[9] Consequently, HIV infection can lead to neuropsychiatric syndromes that can occur at various stages of infection.[10] AIDS has been proposed as a direct contributor to mental disorders because the AIDS virus infects neurons early in the course of the illness. Anxiety disorders are the most common, but other neuropsychiatric disorders may also be seen, including depression, dementia, and psychosis.[11,12]

Awareness of AIDS is also a risk factor for depression and anxiety, as the case report discussed illustrates. AIDS awareness has also been associated with post-traumatic disorder.[13]

Patients with mental disorders can be at greater risk for AIDS because substance abuse is often a comorbid condition with mental illness.[14] Moreover, mental disorders and substance abuse illnesses may lead to high-risk behavior associated with HIV spread.[15]

Mental disorders may affect the course of AIDS.[16,17] Depression may occur in as many as a third of AIDS patients and may be associated with increased morbidity and mortality.[18] It may also contribute to the higher suicide rate associated in gays with AIDS.[16]

Mental illnesses can decrease medication compliance and treatment plan adherence. Multiple and timed pill taking are still necessary in AIDS treatment, although highly active antiretroviral therapy (HAART) has reduced many neuropsychiatric complications. However, studies of antiretroviral treatment continue to indicate that near-perfect adherence is needed to adequately repress viral replication. About 95% adherence is necessary to prevent the emergence of resistant strains.[19] The importance of mental health treatment is shown by the finding that depression is associated with poor adherence and the finding that ongoing high-risk sexual behavior is predicted by higher levels of depression and recreational drug use.[15] Moreover, 10% of men with severe mental disorders, such as schizophrenia, reported same-sex sexual encounters, despite denying that they were bisexual or gay, thus suggesting that the mental disorder may affect judgment of high-risk behavior.[20]

MENTAL ILLNESS IN AFRICAN AMERICANS

Disparities in the burden of mental illness for African Americans have been well documented. African Americans are more likely to be diagnosed with a severe mental illness, such as schizophrenia, when they have a mood disorder.[21] As noted above, psychiatric disorders affect many aspects of HIV infection. For example, failure to recognize a psychiatric disorder could result in the missing of a key determinant of morbidity and the course of illness. Mood disorders are often not diagnosed or misdiagnosed in African Americans.[22] Yet, as noted, depression has been associated with both a shortened survival and poor adherence.

African Americans are less likely to be treated for mental disorders. The Surgeon General commissioned a study of ethnicity and mental illness, which concluded that ethnic differences in prevalence of mental disorders were relatively small.[23] However, African Americans experienced more illness burden. A subsequent Surgeon General report and a nationwide survey of diagnosis and treatment services found that, for a variety of reasons, treatment is less accessible, especially state-of-the-art treatment.[24,25] Psychotherapy is often not provided. Medication or emergency care is more likely to be provided as treatment when services are provided. Antipsychotic medication, in particular, is more likely to be provided in higher doses, which increases the risk for side effects.[25] Patient issues are also important because African Americans are less likely to seek mental health treatment because of stigma. Medication is also more likely to be refused, and noncompliance is more common.[26] However, provider variables are also important because many ethnic differences disappear when the provider is willing to engage with the patient.[27]

The number of HIV-positive, mentally ill African Americans has not been reported. Nevertheless, one recent study estimated that 13% of people with HIV disease receiving care in the United States in 1996 had co-occurring psychiatric symptoms and either or both drug dependence symptoms or heavy drinking.[28] Sixty-nine percent of those with a substance-related condition also had psychiatric symptoms; 27% of those with psychiatric symptoms also had a substance-related condition. Comorbidity was also more common in heterosexual African-American men. The convergence of these disorders has clearly contributed to the devastation that this virus causes in the African-American community. The combination of stigma associated with AIDS and mental illness, the lack of services for both conditions, and the under-recognition of both conditions, early in their courses, certainly contribute to the spread and poorer prognosis of HIV infection in the African-American community.

Affective disorders are the most common psychiatric diagnosis among HIV-positive men. Although HIV may have a direct effect on the brain, leading to depression, psychosocial factors certainly play a role, including the loss of loved ones and friends who might have been infected. Moreover, in a well-controlled study, depression was found to contribute both to nonadherence to AIDS pharmacotherapy and to a faster disease progression.[29] Mania or frank bipolar disorder has been associated with AIDS and may be directly related to the infection of key areas of the brain.[30,31] Mania has also been associated with AIDS pharmacotherapy.[32] As noted above, anxiety is also common, which is produced either from the virus directly or from the chronic worry associated with having this disease and the resulting disruption in the usual activities of daily living.[11]

Mood and anxiety disorders are frequently underdiagnosed in the African-American community.[26] As a consequence of this, African Americans run the risk of being nonadherent to treatment because of unrecognized and untreated depression. Moreover, the course of the disease may be worsened, and the patient may suffer from both the burden of AIDS and undiagnosed depression. African Americans with mood disorders are often misdiagnosed as having schizophrenia.[22] They may have their psychiatric problems inappropriately treated and their AIDS undertreated because many providers assume that the severely mentally ill should not be aggressively treated. Anxiety disorders are also underdiagnosed in African Americans or misdiagnosed. As a consequence, these individuals are also at risk for inappropriate treatment with the wrong psychotropic agents and undertreatment of AIDS.[33]

Depression and anxiety are common in gays and bisexuals with AIDS, the result to a large extent of the bias against their lifestyle in American culture and other social factors related to their often unaccepted lifestyle.[34] African-American gays face the stigma of race that may exclude them from support available to their White counterparts. In addition, the greater stigmatization by the African-American community toward gays further contributes to alienation and despair.[3,6,17,18]

As noted above, under-recognition, especially of depression, is common among African Americans. Two of us (JH and DR) administered the Hamilton Depression Scale and the Brief Symptom Inventory to AIDS patients. All suffered from low self-esteem. Most of these patients were found to have met diagnostic criteria over a period of years; however, they were never diagnosed or treated. Many met criteria for serious mental illnesses (Bipolar Disorder, Psychosis, and Major Depressive Disorder). They had unrecognized suicidal attempts, but did not recognize them as possible symptoms to treatable conditions. Nor were they aware of where services were available, given that they had little or no medical insurance.

HIV infection is over-represented in the African-American population, especially among women and children. Moreover, mentally ill African Americans are over-represented among the homeless and in the prison population.[8,23] Many of these individuals are at great risk of becoming HIV-positive related to victimization and risky sexual behavior. They often do not have access to routine reliable mental heath services. Problems of adherence and accessibility are magnified by their lifestyle and undertreated mental disorders.

PSYCHIATRIC ASPECTS OF HIV/AIDS IN CHILDREN AND ADOLESCENTS

One of the first known cases of HIV infection and AIDS occurred in 1988. The patient presented to the emergency room of a St. Louis, Missouri, public hospital complaining of fever, weakness, rash, and malaise. He was thin and walked with difficulty. Doctors admitted the patient because of his debilitated state and conducted a complete and thorough evaluation of all organ systems. There was extensive lymphedema of the genitalia and lower extremities. Chlamydial organisms were widely disseminated. The patient's history was positive for sexual activity with females. Doctors were baffled but provided supportive palliative care for this unknown illness. After 16 months with an unknown generalized illness, the patient died. At autopsy, there was evidence of widespread dissemination, including the perianal region, of an aggressive form of Kaposi's sarcoma. Years later, subsequent evaluation of stored blood samples were found positive for HIV infection. The patient was a 15-year-old African-American male teen.[35] This case heralded an epidemic that has been devastating to African-American youth.

Children who are HIV-negative but whose parents are HIV-positive represent the largest group affected by AIDS. They have disabled and deceased parents. They feel shame, anger, and sadness. Family members may reluctantly and angrily assume primary care, or foster care systems may provide guardianship and homes, but they often will not. In the African-American community, informal adoption is common but an infected parent may be alienated from the rest of the community. The children themselves have questions but few answers. Young children want to know who will take care of them, preparing meals, providing safety, giving baths. African-Americans youth are far more likely to be living in poverty even when parents are present, so these issues are often more immediate.[22] Older children want to know how they will get to school and who will buy their clothes. Living with and through the prospect of loss of ones' parents embraces issues of death and dying, grief, and bereavement. Effective emotional management should include visits and time with disabled parents, who often do not have the economic resources. The psychiatrist can facilitate communication and help the children understand their parent's illness. Ongoing planning is another goal of treatment. Collaboration with social services agencies and other programs to address psychosocial issues and access to treatment is essential.

A growing number of children will lose one or both parents to HIV disease. The consequence is unsupported grieving. Psychiatrists need to explore the capacity of families to communicate about HIV disease and the children's understanding of their parent's illness. Disclosure is difficult for many parents who worry about revealing stigmatized behaviors that are often unacceptable in the African-American church, a primary support provider in the African-American community, or overwhelming a child with information.[36] It is also confounded by the reluctance of African Americans to utilize mental health services to deal with distress.[37] Permanency planning is an essential step in communication and collaboration with social agencies and mental health providers. For African-American children in particular, bereavement is complicated by the psychosocial and economic problems that existed before HIV disease that are then compounded by disintegration of the immediate family. Family-based, multidisciplinary team approaches may be effective in providing access to care, and needed follow-up services are often essential in the African-American community. Many ethnic minorities find the religious community or body of the church to be the network that most effectively addresses their need for support in crises. It becomes important then to include the church in an AIDS comprehensive support program, despite the African-American's church difficulty in reconciling the AIDS crisis with its value orientation.

Suicide is an unrecognized but serious problem in the African-American community. A study of suicide among 15- to 25-year-old men who have sex with men (MSM) found that African Americans had higher rates of suicide.[38] The discomfort and suspicion with which people of color view mental health practitioners remains a deterrent to timely, effective consultation. The myth that African Americans do not commit suicide further complicates intervention.[39]

Pressures of intracultural expectations can make young men be what they are not. Families and communities of color are more likely to regard young males with a same-sex identification or interest as "acting White, being punks or sissies, and not being real men." The demasculinization of African-American males historically creates pressure in young males to be "real men." For many, this translates to engaging in behaviors that may be covertly same-sex, but overtly opposite-sex. It is not unusual to find that African-American male teenagers have a girlfriend(s) and boyfriend(s). In this scenario, same-sex contraction of HIV infection then lends itself to heterosexual spread to females. This scenario as well as the opportunistic sex and down low lifestyle may explain why 50% of infected adolescents are female but 29% of infected individuals older than 25 years old are female.[1] Synchrony with peer attitudes and behaviors is an important part of normal adolescent development. Dissonance is disquieting and often leads to poor, desperate choices.

Adolescent females tend to have notions of masculinity that are stereotypical and naïve. They identify heterosexual boys as the ones who are athletes, who behave aggressively, and who express or demonstrate a sexual interest in females. They identify the same-sex interested male as someone with a limp wrist, a female gait, and flashy, tight clothing. Younger teen girls also have cervical and vaginal histology that allows easier passage of the virus.

A history of sexual victimization also appears to contribute to the spread of HIV among teens, including African-Americans teens. All but one HIV-positive teen in the mental health system in Washington, D.C. from 1990 to 1995 had been a victim of sexual assault (unpublished data; JH). None had received a mental health intervention. All were African American. These teens subsequently contracted HIV directly from the assault or from the impulsive, risky, depressed, angry behaviors that resulted. Girls who are molested tend to eventually engage in sexual activity with multiple sexual partners, tend to associate themselves with abusive men, and are not able to protect their own children. Boys who are molested will sometimes molest smaller children, often irrespective of gender. Psychiatrists must always include sexual abuse histories in their evaluation of adolescents. Early and frequent abuse has been related to the development of post-traumatic stress, borderline, bipolar, and substance abuse disorders that may make the teens more susceptible to the risky, unprotected behaviors associated with HIV transmission.

There is also a new generation of HIV-positive teens who are primarily African American and who were born HIV-positive. They represent the longest living cohort of in utero infected youth to date. The life span had not been more than 5 to 6 years. With the advent of new, improved treatments, these children are living into at least early adolescence. This is a time of sexual interest and activity, impulsivity, explorations, and expressions of independence. Psychiatrists have to help this group cope with feelings of peer dissonance. They feel different because their choices and options are different. These teens often suffer from low self-esteem and depression because they do not feel as free as peers to be the teens they are. They also feel restricted and compromised in every aspect of adolescent development.

Even before adolescence, caretakers have difficult decisions. When do you tell children that they are HIV-positive and how do you explain the medications that are multiple and taken several times a day? Early in their short lives there are multiple doctor visits, needlesticks, x-ray films, and other examinations, some of which are invasive. There are treatments with medications that bring side effects and medication schedules that other children are not facing. Do you tell the teacher and school officials? Frequent illnesses may compromise physical health, preventing full participation in childhood activities. HIV infection is also associated with CNS compromise, so that school can also be a challenge for learning.

There may be an episode of bleeding resulting from not uncommon nose bleeding or injury during a sporting event. How do you help this child monitor self-disclosure to others, given the possibility of rejection and cruel responses from both other children, as well as adults.

Helping the child and adolescent cope with these issues is a critical focus of treatment planning. Individual, family, and group therapy are valuable interventions. Individual therapy can help the child address angers and fears; family therapy can facilitate communication between caretakers by uncovering the family secret; and group therapy can help youth know they are not alone and can survive. Unsupported and rejected youth can end up homeless, facing the vulnerabilities and dangers of life on the streets.

TREATMENT

Modern antiviral therapy has greatly changed the prognosis of AIDS. HAART in particular has contributed to AIDS becoming primarily a chronic and not immediately lethal disorder. Adherence to antiretroviral therapy regimens is critical because 95% adherence to treatment was associated with complete viral suppression; failure rates increased sharply with less than 95% adherence.[19]

As depression and other neuropsychiatric disorders worsen compliance and greatly affect treatment outcomes, medication treatment of the mental disorder can be an important intervention. Although traditional antidepressants are effective, they are not tolerated as well as newer antidepressants. Consequently, selective serotonin reuptake inhibitors (SSRIs) and selective norepinephrine reuptake inhibitors (SNRIs) are recommended over tricyclic antidepressants.[40,41] Unfortunately, African Americans are much less likely to choose psychotropic medications than other ethnic groups.[42] African Americans are more likely to have negative feelings and less likely to be adherent to AIDS medication.[43] Culturally based education can change these attitudes.[44] Unfortunately, African Americans are less likely to be prescribed antidepressant medication.[45,46] When African Americans are prescribed antidepressants, they are less likely to be prescribed SSRIs.[47] Although there are no data on HIV-positive African Americans, there is no reason to assume that similar prescribing patterns will not be seen. Consequently, education of prescribers is necessary as well.

Sometimes, antipsychotic medications are necessary to treat psychotic symptoms resulting from AIDS, the medications used to treat AIDS, or a preexisting psychiatric disorder. First-generation antipsychotic medications when given to patients with advanced HIV infection are associated with an increased incidence of extrapyramidal side effects. High-potency first-generation antipsychotics can be associated with severe dystonia, rigidity, akathisia, and parkinsonism.[48] Even low-potency first-generation neuroleptics can result in severe extrapyramidal side effects, but overall they appear to be less problematic than high-potency neuroleptics. Onset of tardive dyskinesia has been reported within a period as short as 6 weeks or within months. These agents would be especially problematic for African Americans. Tardive dyskinesia and other movement disorder side effects may be twice as common among African Americans.[49] There are so far no published reports on these agents in HIV-infected African Americans. Second-generation or atypical antipsychotic agents appear to be better tolerated, with fewer serious side effects. However, as with newer antidepressants, African Americans are less likely to be prescribed these agents.[50]

Depakote thus far has been well tolerated. Lithium must be used with great caution in patients who develop HIV-related nephropathy. Lithium has been associated with toxicity in some AIDS patients, even without renal disease.[51] Lithium should be used with great caution in patients who develop HIV-related nephropathy, a generally irreversible complication that can lead to decreased lithium clearance and possible lithium toxicity. When given at doses necessary to maintain serum lithium concentrations, between 0.5 and 1.5 mEq/L, lithium has been associated with signs of toxicity in some HIV-positive patients, even among patients without renal disease. African Americans seem to be at greater risk for lithium side effects because of a higher red blood cell to plasma ratio.[52] Thus lithium should be avoided in African-American patients with probable AIDS mania or advanced HIV disease.

Since the beginning of the AIDS epidemic, psychosocial support has emerged as a cornerstone of the comprehensive treatment for many persons infected and affected by HIV disease or AIDS. African Americans, however, often choose such support from individuals outside of the mental health system or are unable to access such support at all. More needs to be done with these organizations, such as the church, to make such support available. For many HIV-infected patients, psychotherapy and psychosocial interventions have been invaluable in the search for meaning during the course of living with HIV disease.[53]

The ideal intervention is prevention. Intervention, even early intervention, although clearly cost effective in addressing this expensive disorder, still leaves the individual with an illness that is either highly lethal even with treatment or chronic and requiring lifelong expensive treatment. Ethic minorities, in particular, often have limited individual and community resources to address this epidemic. To reduce rates of HIV infection and AIDS, effective and culturally appropriate prevention interventions must be developed and implemented.[54,55]

Those programs that are culturally based are clearly more effective. Programs can vary from AIDS awareness to substance abuse prevention. Unfortunately, there are no published studies on prevention programs in mentally ill African Americans. Given the increased burden of being mentally ill, disparities in services, and the heavy burden of AIDS, more must be done to address the needs of African Americans with HIV disease and AIDS and mental illness.

REFERENCES

1. Centers for Disease Control and Prevention. *HIV/AIDS Surveillance Report*. Atlanta: Centers for Disease Control and Prevention; 2003.
2. Whitmore SK, Satcher AJ, Hu S. Epidemiology of HIV/AIDS among non-Hispanic black women in the United States. *J Natl Med Assoc*. 2005;97(suppl 7):19S-24S.
3. Dean HD, Steele CB, Satcher AJ, Nakashima AK. HIV/AIDS among minority races and ethnicities in the United States, 1999–2003. *J Natl Med Assoc*. 2005;97(suppl 7):5S–12S.
4. Carey MP. HIV and AIDS relative to other health, social, and relationship concerns among low-income urban women: a brief report. *J Womens Health Gend Based Med*. 1999;8:657–661.
5. Miller M, Serner M, Wagner M. Sexual diversity among black men who have sex with men in an inner-city community. *J Urban Health*. 2005;82:26–34.
6. King JL. *On the Down Low: A Journey into the Lives of "Straight" Black Men Who Sleep with Men*. Broadway Books; 2004.
7. Lemelle AJ Jr, Battle J. Black masculinity matters in attitudes toward gay males. *J Homosex*. 2004;47:39–51.
8. Primm AB, Osher FC, Gomez MB. Race and ethnicity, mental health services and cultural competence in the criminal justice system: are we ready to change? *Community Ment Health J*. 2005;41:557–569.
9. Kolson DL, Lavi E, Gonzalez-Scarano F. The effects of human immunodeficiency virus in the central nervous system. *Adv Virus Res*. 1998;50:1–47.
10. McDaniel JS, Campos PE, Purcell DW, et al. A national, randomized survey of HIV/AIDS attitudes and knowledge among psychiatrists-in-training. *Acad Psychiatry*. 1998;22:107–116.
11. Lyketsos CG, Hutton H, Fishman M, Schwartz J, Treisman GJ. Psychiatric morbidity on entry to an HIV primary care clinic. *AIDS*. 1996;10:1033–1039.
12. Rabkin JG, Ferrando SJ, Jacobsberg LB, Fishman B. Prevalence of Axis I disorders in an AIDS cohort: a cross-sectional, controlled study. *Compr Psychiatry*. 1997;38:146–154.
13. Olley BO, Zeier MD, Seedat S, Stein DJ. Post-traumatic stress disorder among recently diagnosed patients with HIV/AIDS in South Africa. *AIDS Care*. 2005;17:550–557.
14. Kessler RC, McGonagle KA, Zhao S, et al. Lifetime and 12 month prevalence of DSM III-R psychiatric disorders in the United States. *Arch Gen Psychiatry*. 1994;51:8–19.
15. Kelly JA, Murphy DA, Bahr GR, et al. Factors associated with severity of depression and high-risk sexual behavior among persons diagnosed with human immunodeficiency virus (HIV) infection. *Health Psychol*. 1993;12:215–219.
16. Marzuk PM, Tardiff K, Leon AC, et al. HIV seroprevalence among suicide victims in New York City, 1991–1993. *Am J Psychiatry*. 1997;154:1720–1725.
17. Judd F, Komiti A, Chua P, et al. Nature of depression in patients with HIV/AIDS. *Aust N Z J Psychiatry*. 2005;39:826–832.
18. Mayne TJ, Vittinghoff E, Chesney MA, Barrett DC, Coates TJ. Depressive affect and survival among gay and bisexual men infected with HIV. *Arch Intern Med*. 1996;156:2233–2238.
19. Paterson DL, Swindells S, Mohr J, et al. Adherence to protease inhibitor therapy and outcomes in patients with HIV infection. *Ann Intern Med*. 2000;133:21–30.
20. Cournos F, Guido JR, Coomaraswamy S, Meyer-Bahlburg H, Sugden R, Horwath E. Sexual activity and risk of HIV infection among patients with schizophrenia. *Am J Psychiatry*. 1994;151:228–232.
21. Lawson WB, Hepler N, Holladay J, Cuffel B. Race as a factor in inpatient and outpatient admissions and diagnosis. *Hosp Community Psychiatry*. 1994;45:72–74.
22. Strakowski SM, Keck PE Jr, Arnold LM, et al. Ethnicity and diagnosis in patients with affective disorders. *J Clin Psychiatry*. 2003;64:747–754.
23. U.S. Department of Health and Human Services. *Mental Health: A Report of the Surgeon General*, Rockville, Md: U.S. Department of Health and Human Services, Public Health Service, Office of the Surgeon General; 1999.
24. U.S. Department of Health and Human Services. *Mental Health: Culture, Race, and Ethnicity—A Supplement to Mental Health: A Report of the Surgeon General*, Rockville, Md: U.S. Department of Health and Human Services, Public Health Service, Office of the Surgeon General; 2001.

25. Wang PS, Lane M, Olfson M, Pincus HA, Wells KB, Kessler RC. Twelve-month use of mental health services in the United States: results from the National Comorbidity Survey Replication. *Arch Gen Psychiatry*. 2005;62:629–640.
26. Lawson WB. Issues in the pharmacotherapy of African Americans. In: Ruiz P, ed. *Ethnicity and Psychopharmacology, Review of Psychiatry*, Vol. 19. Washington, DC: American Association Press; 2000.
27. Segal SP, Bola J, Watson M. Race, quality of care, and antipsychotic prescribing practices in psychiatric emergency services. *Psychiatr Serv*. 1996;47:282–286.
28. Galvan FH, Burnam MA, Bing EG. Co-occurring psychiatric symptoms and drug dependence or heavy drinking among HIV-positive people. *J Psychoactive Drugs*. 2003;35(suppl 1):153–160.
29. Bouhnik AD, Preau M, Vincent E, et al; MANIF 2000 Study Group. Depression and clinical progression in HIV-infected drug users treated with highly active antiretroviral therapy. *Antivir Ther*. 2005;10:53–61.
30. Ellen SR, Judd FK, Mijch AM, Cochram A. Secondary mania in patients with HIV infection. *Aust N Z J Psychiatry*. 1999;33:353–360.
31. Lyketsos CG, Schwartz J, Fishman M, Treisman G: AIDS mania. *J Neuropsychiatry Clin Neurosci*. 1997;9:277–279.
32. Brouillette MJ, Chouinard G, Lalonde R. Didanosine-induced mania in HIV infection [letter]. *Am J Psychiatry*. 1994;151:1839–1840.
33. Paradis CM, Hatch M, Friedman S. Anxiety disorders in African Americans: an update. *J Natl Med Assoc*. 1994;86:609–612.
34. Mayne TJ, Vittinghoff E, Chesney MA, Barrett DC, Coates TJ. Depressive affect and survival among gay and bisexual men infected with HIV. *Arch Intern Med*. 1996;156:2233–2238.
35. Garry RF, Witte MH, Gottlieb AA, et al. Documentation of an AIDS virus infection in the United States in 1988. *JAMA*. 1988;260:2085–2087.
36. Rotheram-Borus MJ, Draimin BH, Reid HM, Murphy DA: The impact of illness disclosure and custody plans on adolescents whose parents live with AIDS. *AIDS*. 1997;11:1159–1164.
37. Neighbors HW. The distribution of psychiatric morbidity in black Americans: a review and suggestion for research. *Community Ment Health J*. 1984;20:169–181.
38. Remafedi G. Suicidality in a venue-based sample of young men who have sex with men. *J Adolesc Health*. 2002;31:305–310.
39. Dula A, Williams S. When race matters. *Clin Geriatr Med*. 2005;21:239–253.
40. Klesmer J, Badescu R. Pharmacologic treatment of mood disorders in acquired immune deficiency syndrome (AIDS). *Curr Psychiatry Rep*. 2002;4:222–227.
41. Elliott AJ, Uldall KK, Bergam K, Russo J, Claypoole K, Roy-Byrne PP. Randomized, placebo-controlled trial of paroxetine versus imipramine in depressed HIV-positive outpatients. *Am J Psychiatry*. 1998;155:367–372.
42. Cooper LA, Gonzales JJ, Gallo JJ, et al. The acceptability of treatment for depression among African-American, Hispanic, and white primary care patients. *Med Care*. 2003;41:479–489.
43. Siegel K, Karus D, Schrimshaw EW. Racial differences in attitudes toward protease inhibitors among older HIV-infected men. *AIDS Care*. 2000;12:423–434.
44. Primm AB, Cabot D, Pettis J, Vu HT, Cooper LA. The acceptability of a culturally-tailored depression education videotape to African Americans. *J Natl Med Assoc*. 2002;94:1007–1016.
45. Blazer DG, Hybels CF, Simonsick EM, Hanlon JT. Marked differences in antidepressant use by race in an elderly community sample: 1986–1996. *Am J Psychiatry*. 2000;157:1089–1094.
46. Blazer DG, Hybels CF, Fillenbaum GG, Pieper CF. Predictors of antidepressant use among older adults: have they changed over time? *Am J Psychiatry*. 2005;162:705–710.
47. Melfi CA, Croghan TW, Hanna MP, Robinson RL. Racial variation in antidepressant treatment in a Medicaid population. *J Clin Psychiatry*. 2000;61:16–21.
48. Sewell DD, Jeste DV, McAdams LA, et al.; HNRC Group. Neuroleptic treatment of HIV-associated psychosis. *Neuropsychopharmacology*. 1994;10:223–229.
49. Glazer WM, Morgenstern H, Doucette J. Race and tardive dyskinesia among outpatients at a CMHC. *Hosp Community Psychiatry*. 1994;45:38–42.
50. Herbeck DM, West JC, Ruditis I, et al. Variations in use of second-generation antipsychotic medication by race among adult psychiatric patients. *Psychiatr Serv*. 2004;55:677–684.
51. Parenti DM, Simon GL, Scheib RG, et al. Effect of lithium carbonate in HIV-infected patients with immune dysfunction. *J Acquir Immune Defic Syndr*. 1988;1:119–124.
52. Strickland TL, Lin K-M, Fu P, Anderson D, Zheng Y. Comparison of lithium ratio between African-American and Caucasian bipolar patients. *Biol Psychiatry*. 1995;37:325–330.
53. Dean HD, Steele CB, Satcher AJ, Nakashima AK. HIV/AIDS among minority races and ethnicities in the United States, 1999–2003. *J Natl Med Assoc*. 2005;97(suppl 7):5S–12S.
54. Marcus MT, Walker T, Swint JM, et al. Community-based participatory research to prevent substance abuse and HIV/AIDS in African-American adolescents. *J Interprof Care*. 2004;18:347–359.
55. Baptiste DR, Paikoff RL, McKay MM, Madison-Boyd S, Coleman D, Bell C. Collaborating with an urban community to develop an HIV and AIDS prevention program for black youth and families. *Behav Modif*. 2005;29:370–416.

CHAPTER 22

HIV/AIDS Among Asian and Pacific Islander Americans

Lynette J. Menezes, Todd S. Wills, Karina D'Souza

Human immunodeficiency virus (HIV) infection and acquired immunodeficiency syndrome (AIDS) are fast emerging as a significant public health problem in one of the fastest growing ethnic groups in the United States—Asian and Pacific Islanders (APIs). With over 929,985 cumulative AIDS cases nationwide, there are 7,166 reported cases of AIDS among APIs.[1] The relatively low AIDS rate may falsely suggest that the epidemic has spared this group. However, recent trends indicate otherwise. Compared to the national population, APIs have experienced a 35% increase—the largest—in the number of AIDS diagnoses in the past 5 years.[1] Yet the published literature on HIV disease and AIDS among APIs is limited, and research is mainly confined to small samples, specific subgroups, and the English-speaking segments of this population. This lack of attention in part is because traditionally APIs were considered a model minority group and sensitive health issues such as HIV disease and AIDS were thought to afflict high-risk groups among other minority populations. This chapter examines the extent of the HIV and AIDS problem among APIs, discusses the psychosocial and cultural factors—protective and risk—that influence epidemiologic trends, describes the impact of the disease on mental health, discusses the role of clinicians, provides an overview of current prevention and intervention programs, and concludes with a discussion on need for research and culturally competent risk reduction strategies.

EPIDEMIOLOGY

At 12.5 million and comprising 4.4% of the U.S. population, the term Asian/Pacific Islanders refers to individuals having origins in the Far East, Southeast Asia, the Indian subcontinent, Hawaii, Guam, Samoa, or other Pacific Islands.[2] Though classified for surveillance purposes as one group, the term is used for a wide variety of subgroups that differ both culturally and linguistically. Additionally, the majority of this population is concentrated in the West and Northeast, with over half of individuals that identify themselves as Asian living in the West.[2]

According to reports from the Centers for Disease Control and Prevention (CDC), as of December 2002, men account for 87% and women 13% of cumulative AIDS cases among APIs.[3] Individuals aged 25 to 34 years had the highest number of diagnoses.[3] For API men living with HIV disease or AIDS, the most significant risk factor was male–male sexual contact. Sixty-seven percent of men diagnosed with HIV infection or AIDS were men who had sex with men (MSM).[1] This statistic is among the highest compared to MSM in other ethnic groups. Examining temporal trends, McFarland et al.[4] found that from 1999 to 2002, sexually transmitted infection (STI) incidence and sexual risk behavior such as unprotected anal intercourse among API MSM had exceeded that of White MSM. Other risk factors have also been documented among API men. For example, CDC data from 33 areas revealed other forms of exposure, including heterosexual contact (16%), injection drug use (12%), and male–male sexual contact in conjunction with injection drug use (4%).[1] However, for API women, heterosexual contact was the most important risk factor (81%), followed by injection drug use (14%).

The number of reported AIDS cases in APIs varies proportionately by geographic location. Most cases of AIDS are concentrated in the metropolitan areas of Los Angeles, New York City, and San Francisco.[5] This finding could also be related to the failure of reporting APIs as a separate racial/ethnic group in the majority of the United States. Currently, only Hawaii, California, New Mexico, and the Pacific Island jurisdictions report HIV disease and AIDS cases in APIs as a separate racial/ethnic group.[5] Other obstacles facing researchers in collection of HIV and AIDS surveillance data, namely lack of reporting, underreporting, and misclassification, hinder the reliability of data on APIs. All of these factors suggest that the number of HIV infection and AIDS cases are probably higher than reported. Additionally, rates of HIV infection in Asia have been drastically rising. This factor, in relation to high rates of immigration to the United States underscores the fact that rates of HIV infection among APIs will rise in the future.[5,6]

PSYCHOSOCIAL FACTORS

KNOWLEDGE AND PERCEPTIONS RELATED TO HIV/AIDS

There is substantial evidence in the published literature on HIV disease and AIDS that both inadequate and inaccurate knowledge related to HIV acquisition and transmission increases the risk of HIV infection. In a study of junior high school students, API adolescents had the lowest levels of knowledge compared to African-American, Latino, and White students,[7] suggesting that API adolescents might be at increased risk for HIV infection. Among Asian Indian adolescents, although 86% answered correctly regarding modes of transmission, a substantial number retained myths and misconceptions about the role of blood donation, blood testing, use of public toilets, and being gay in HIV transmission.[8] Likewise, Gellert et al.[9] found high levels of knowledge regarding actual modes of transmission among Vietnamese adults, but misconceptions related to HIV acquisition through casual contact, shared utensils, and public toilets persisted in a significant proportion. In terms of gender, the authors noted that women had lower levels of knowledge than men; however, acculturated younger women (younger than 35 years) had higher levels of knowledge than less acculturated men and women and comparable levels to acculturated young men.

The risk of HIV infection is further compounded when individuals at high risk perceive themselves at low risk for contracting HIV. For instance, API MSM who perceived themselves to be at low risk for acquiring and transmitting HIV were more likely to engage in unprotected anal intercourse.[10] Additionally, stereotypes in the gay community that APIs are at low risk may result in increasingly unsafe sex behavior among APIs and their partners. Choi et al.[11] found that API MSM were less likely to use protection during anal intercourse with API partners compared to non-API partners. The authors argue that these perceptions, in part, persist because of the low rates of HIV prevalence in the API MSM community and that earlier studies showed lower rates of unsafe sexual practices in this population. In the heterosexual API community, perceptions of AIDS as a disease of the gay and White communities continue to persist.[6] API's perceptions of low risk were also influenced by their HIV-negative status after unprotected sex with multiple sex partners.[6]

CULTURAL ATTITUDES, BELIEFS, AND VALUES

Compared to Western society, which values individualism, Asians strongly believe in collectivism. Typically, Asian communities believe in group harmony and therefore individuals must conform to the happiness of the group and the community. Engaging in premarital and extramarital sex is generally disapproved of in the API community, and communication on sexual matters is rarely encouraged in API families. For example, Vietnamese women (55%) were more likely than men (22%) to disapprove of premarital sex, whereas 87% of the participants, both men and women disapproved of extramarital sex.[9] There have been reports of late initiation and low rates of sexual activity among API adolescents compared to those in adolescents from other ethnic communities.[12] Although disapproval of premarital sex might be a culturally protective factor reducing risk of exposure to HIV, it might negatively influence self-reports of sexual activity, resulting in an inaccurate picture of the extent of risk behaviors among API youth. Further, because of familial disapproval of sensitive sexual topics, API youth might seek information regarding HIV from sources that might not be helpful. The majority of Asian Indian youth in one study reported using media such as television, movies, talk shows, and magazines as information sources, but only a minority found them useful.[8]

Homophobia is widely prevalent in API communities. API gay or bisexual men are less inclined to disclose their sexual orientation to maintain family honor. In Kanuha's study in Hawaii,[13] API gay and bisexual men reported a constant pressure between concealing and publicly disclosing their gay identities to protect relationships with family members. API MSM may be stigmatized and ostracized in their communities, leading to social isolation. One can surmise that API MSM with HIV infection will be most affected. Stigma due to HIV can marginalize both API MSM and heterosexual APIs because of widely prevalent cultural beliefs that HIV is acquired through socially unaccepted behaviors such as homosexuality, substance use, sexual promiscuity, and commercial sex work.

API women are particularly vulnerable to HIV infection and its impact because of sociocultural norms regarding women's subservient roles and status in the family. Cultural beliefs regarding condom use pose a substantial risk for women. Negotiating condom use is rarely a choice for API women because of traditional male privilege in their community. Women are afraid to ask their partners to use condoms because the partner might suspect they are having an affair or label them as promiscuous or because it might imply that the partner is promiscuous. Another popular belief that sex with condoms is less pleasurable compounds the risk for API women. In the API community, female massage parlor workers are receiving some attention as a high-risk group for spreading HIV. Nemoto et al.[14] found that API masseuses reported inconsistent condom use, despite knowing about the risks of contracting HIV and other STIs. Reasons mentioned by API masseuses were financial considerations, competition for customers, and demanding clients who refuse to use condoms. Besides, some masseuses believed that regular customers are safe. These women were also at risk for abuse from customers and API gangs, and several women reported instances of physical and psychological abuse. Traditionally, violence against API women was condoned and used to discipline wives and maintain prescribed roles. Research studies on violence against immigrant API women in the past decade[15] attest to the persistence of these attitudes. Not surprisingly, threats of physical abuse are likely deterrents to the use of condoms in a sexual encounter.

IMMIGRANT STATUS

The immigration experience for APIs is often characterized by exploitation, financial hardship, unemployment, loss of status, and social and geographic isolation. Linguistic difficulties combined with adjusting to a new culture leads to a great deal of psychosocial stress for many immigrants. Yoshikawa et al.[6] suggest that experiences of racism, poverty, and homophobia are likely to increase the risk for HIV infection among APIs through decreased levels of self-esteem and higher levels of social isolation. The authors further argue that cultures of origin may have differential norms related to HIV risk and protective behaviors from the United States. As API immigrants begin to adjust to the diverse communities with which they have contact, they may assimilate new beliefs and behaviors from already existing API communities, mainstream U.S. communities, and mainstream gay communities. These communities may have differential rates of HIV prevalence, beliefs related to substance use, sexual practices, condom use, and perceptions regarding HIV risk, all important predictors of unsafe sex behaviors.[6]

SUBSTANCE USE

The published literature on AIDS is replete with studies demonstrating an association between drug use and unsafe sexual behaviors. There is growing evidence of the relationship between substance use and sexual risk behaviors among APIs.[10,16] Substance use was the strongest predictor of unprotected anal intercourse in a study of 241 API MSM in San Francisco.[10] An emerging concern is the use of methamphetamine as a sex-enhancing drug, especially in the gay population. The review by Reback et al.[17] of recent research indicates that methamphetamine use is strongly associated with HIV-related risk behaviors such as infrequent condom use, exchanging sex for money, and multiple sexual partners. Among APIs, a recent study of Filipino methamphetamine users revealed that the frequency of methamphetamine use was highly associated with unprotected sex and commercial sex activity.[16] In general, the emerging effect of methamphetamine, its lowering of inhibitions, and use among APIs portend a grim epidemic.

SOCIAL SUPPORT

A pervasive theme within the HIV API community is the absence of social support from family, friends, and the local community. Reduced social and sexual networks due to HIV-related stigma, internalized fears of being ostracized, and geographic isolation add to the already existing psychological distress. Undocumented immigrants living with HIV disease or AIDS tend to be more socially isolated and seek minimal support from family and friends.[18] Not only self-imposed isolation, but feelings of alienation from the API community due to sexual stigma and from the mainstream gay community due to racism[19] add to the overall sense of loss. API MSM in this study expressed an intense desire for intimacy and positive reinforcement from people other than APIs and gay members. As a result, API MSM reported engaging in high-risk sex to satisfy these pressing emotional desires.[19]

HELP-SEEKING PATTERNS AND ACCESS TO SERVICES

There is a scarcity of prevention and intervention programs targeted specifically to the API community. The stereotype of a "model minority" has led to APIs with HIV infection or AIDS not only being overlooked in local, state, and national HIV prevention programs and care services, but also APIs underutilizing existing services.[20] The API community has one of the lowest rates of knowledge about HIV status and access to treatment once diagnosed. In a study conducted in New York City among MSM, APIs had the highest rate of persons who had never been tested for the HIV virus (18%) and whose HIV serostatus was unknown (18%).[19] Findings from an ongoing CDC-sponsored behavioral surveillance project revealed that 46% of APIs were tested because of illness compared to 38% of Whites, and 16% of APIs did not know their CD4 count compared to 8% of Whites.[21]

PSYCHIATRIC ISSUES

Many of the psychosocial barriers that impede access to care and treatment for HIV infection in Asian and Pacific Islanders are magnified when managing mental heath disorders. Any practitioner caring for APIs must be aware of the specific cultural and personal characteristics that may affect both the clinical presentation of disease as well as success of therapy.

PSYCHIATRIC DISORDERS IN ASIANS AND PACIFIC ISLANDERS

The incidence of mood disorders among APIs in the United States is poorly quantified. Reasons for the paucity of data in this population may include the limited population size (4.4% of the population), diversity of subgroups, and difficulty in applying *Diagnostic and Statistical Manual of Mental Disorders (DSM-IV)* criteria in a culturally relevant way. Recent immigrants may be susceptible to mood and anxiety disorders including post-traumatic stress disorder, especially recent refugees. Although some studies have suggested that APIs may have a higher rate of mental illness than the general population, they are less likely to seek treatment than Whites, African Americans, or Hispanic Americans. As discussed previously, reasons for this lack of treatment-seeking behavior may include language barriers, stigma within the API community, and cultural explanations for symptoms that exclude the consideration of mental illness.[22] Suicide rates among Asian Americans are generally less than those in other racial groups; however, surprising variation exists. For example, API women have the highest suicide rate among all women older than 65 in the U.S.[22]

The incidence of mood disorders in APIs with HIV infection is even less defined. Some specific characteristics of APIs with HIV infection may have implications on the frequency of mental illness in this population. As noted earlier, the majority of men diagnosed with AIDS identified male–male sexual contact as the mode of transmission. Although fewer APIs with HIV infection have concomitant substance abuse problems, Asian and Pacific Islander MSM with HIV bear the significant burden of stigma associated with HIV and with being gay. Despite the well-known effects of HIV-stigma in other communities, little attention has been directed to the physical and psychological impact of HIV-related stigma in APIs. In assessing psychological sequelae to HIV-related stigma among 53 documented and undocumented immigrants, Kang et al.[18] found that HIV-related stigma was associated with psychological distress. HIV-related stigma was assessed using five dimensions: social rejection, negative self-worth, perceived interpersonal insecurity, financial security, and discretionary disclosure. Nonspecific psychological distress included hopelessness, sense of dread, confused thinking, sadness, and anxiety. Social rejection, negative self-worth, and perceived interpersonal insecurity were significantly associated with psychological distress. Undocumented immigrants experienced greater distress than legal immigrants and had higher scores on the above three components.

PATIENT ENCOUNTERS

Health care providers must be aware of the specific cultural traits that may affect encounters with API and hinder diagnostic accuracy. Michael Menaster[23] describes an interesting factor that may affect encounters between APIs and health care providers. Menaster describes a "Model Minority Myth," which is especially important in interactions with API. The primary components of this myth are the common perceptions of Asian Americans as productive workers with significant family support for education, low rates of substance abuse, and low rates of alcohol consumption compared to other racial groups.

Providers unaware of their own assumptions about APIs may pursue a diagnosis of mood disorders, including major depression, less frequently because of countertransference related to the model minority myth. This lack of awareness may contribute to the lower rates of reported mental illness in APIs than in other ethnic groups. Equally, the model minority myth creates a perception of decreased vulnerability to diseases such as HIV infection where behavior pays a significant role in transmission. Health care providers must identify any biases or assumptions they hold toward APIs in order to pursue an objective diagnostic workup. An important tool in encounters with APIs is the use of permissive language regarding both mental health complaints and sexual behavior. Permissive language places a wide spectrum of behavior within an expected "normal" range and may allow API patients to speak about mental illness or sexual behavior with less concern about straying outside the expectations of the model minority myth.

The accurate diagnosis of mental illness in APIs is hampered by several factors. Most significant among these factors is a shortage of health care providers with language fluency and cultural competency in the many cultures that make up this heterogeneous ethnic group. Without such cultural competency, both underdiagnosis and overdiagnosis of mental illness is possible. A significant difference between models of health between East and West may confound health care providers. Many APIs believe in a unity of mind and body. This belief secondarily may lead to increased somatization in the presence of psychiatric disease and the possibility of underdiagnosis of mental illness.

Conversely, overdiagnosis of mental illness also occurs in a setting of limited cultural competency. In many Asian cultures, the physician is held as an authority figure. Limited eye contact and spontaneous conversation by an API may reflect deference to an authority figure rather than blunting of affect. Deference to an authority figure may also be manifest as frequent "yes" answers on screening questionnaires because of a lack of understanding of the questions posed. In the case of screening instruments for depression, a false positive diagnosis may result.[24]

Many of these limitations may be overcome with the use of well-trained translators. In many situations, health care providers rely on family members or close friends of a patient to act as a translator. This should be avoided if at all possible in most encounters, especially when dealing with potentially stigmatizing issues such as mental illness, HIV infection, or other sexually transmitted diseases. Well-trained translators can provide additional insight into fluency of speech and patient affect that may otherwise be imperceptible to the health care provider. Unfortunately, such translation services are unavailable in most clinic settings.

THERAPY CONSIDERATIONS

Limited data exist on the specific effect of pharmacotherapy and psychotherapy for mental illness in APIs and even less for the subgroups of APIs with HIV. Further study is necessary to determine the most effective drug regimens for the treatment of mood disorders, anxiety states, and psychosis. The most effective use of psychotherapy is yet to be determined. The limitations previously discussed regarding cultural and language fluency are even more significant for any practitioner lacking a shared culture with the patient.

Many scientists have postulated that APIs may be more sensitive to medications than other racial groups. It is well known that many APIs have low levels of alcohol dehydrogenase, leading to slow metabolism of alcohol and intoxication at lower levels of consumption.[25,26] Further research into pharmacogenomics may reveal other unique variations in metabolism among APIs. Possible results of impaired drug metabolism in APIs may include effective therapy at lower doses than required for other racial groups but an increased risk for medication sensitivity and toxicity. Practitioners treating mental illness in APIs must be especially vigilant to avoid drug interaction that may impair patient tolerance to both antiretroviral and psychiatric medications.

FUTURE RESEARCH

Many avenues for future research on mental illness and neurocognitive disorders in APIs with HIV disease or AIDS remain open. The validity of standard neuropsychiatric screening and testing tools on the multiple cultures that make up APIs in the United States must be assessed further. The role of psychotherapy in APIs with HIV disease is an important question, especially whether differences exist in the success of such therapy based on the culture and language of both patient and physician. Finally, further characterization of the clinical manifestations of neurocognitive disorders in APIs with HIV disease and AIDS is needed, including the presentation of neurologic opportunistic infections in APIs with AIDS. Such investigations will improve the quality of health care to this growing segment of the U.S. population.

HIV PREVENTION AND INTERVENTION PROGRAMS

Prevention is the cornerstone of risk reduction in HIV disease. The growing numbers of patients with HIV infection in this population suggests an urgent need to develop prevention programs targeting the API community. Although prevention programs for other ethnic groups abound, there are few culturally specific programs that have been evaluated for their effectiveness in the API community. Any culturally sensitive program must recognize the linguistic and cultural differences and variability in immigration experiences across subgroups of APIs. And therefore understanding the role of factors such as stigma, attitudes and health beliefs, geographic and social isolation, social support, and access to care in influencing how APIs seek education, treatment, and other care-related services is critical. However, HIV researchers have focused primarily on the API MSM community, neglecting emerging risk groups in the heterosexual community, in particular women, adolescents, and transgender individuals.

A second notable issue is the theoretical basis of many of these prevention programs. For too long HIV prevention programs in the United States have relied on models that draw from individual-based theories of change. More specifically, the health belief model, stages of change, AIDS risk reduction, and self-efficacy theories have been traditionally used in informing prevention programs.[6] Although these models have been widely applied across diverse ethnic groups, the focus has been on individuals, dissociated from their context. By focusing on individuals' ability to change their behavior and ignoring contextual factors such as the social environment, including stigma, social support, cultural norms and beliefs, and access to care, these prevention programs have failed to resonate within the API community and participation has been marginal. Instead, prevention and intervention programs that draw from an ecologic framework are more likely to succeed.

Research has shown that an effective method of reaching the API community is through peer educators, who engage most often in direct client contact.[6] In a study by Yoshikawa et al.,[6] peer educators participated in a focus group to discuss their experiences within API community-based organizations. They identified several factors that were most effective and successful in encouraging health-protective behaviors in the API community. Working within social networks, rather than individual-based prevention efforts, was the most effective method, according to the participants. For example, distributing condoms and HIV information through a network of grocery store owners, a setting that is frequented by Bangladeshi immigrants, has been a useful method of communicating safer sex practices.[6]

These strategies highlight a few examples of successful efforts in education and prevention programs directed toward APIs in the United States. However, continuing research on this issue must be conducted in order to raise awareness in this community. Incorporating network-level strategies that begin with social groups and community-based organizations, rather than with the individuals, will be less threatening and more effective for APIs. For example, promoting safe sex and other protective health behaviors within churches and schools may be more appealing to individuals because information will be presented to them in a familiar and comfortable environment. Additionally, because of the shared value of collectivism within the API community, inclusion of family, friends, and other members of the community in prevention efforts is essential. The Internet could be a novel vehicle for presenting preventive programs. Computers have become an integral part of daily life both in work and school for the API community. Providing information and education on prevention, treatment, and other care-related services on easily accessible websites would greatly benefit individuals who might want to access services anonymously or prefer information in this format.

Not only cultural barriers, but also language barriers in this community must be overcome. With over 100 dialects within the API community, language is one of the most pressing issues for prevention programs. Distributing information in brochure format in different languages will be helpful, as would public service announcements, a project that has already begun in California.[20] Community-based organizations staffed by ethnically and culturally diverse personnel are more likely to elicit the participation of APIs in prevention activities.

SUMMARY AND IMPLICATIONS FOR RESEARCH AND PRACTICE

The foregoing discussion on the different factors that influence risk reduction and prevention in the API population underscores the need to examine the problem of HIV infection and AIDS among APIs through a cultural lens. Whether APIs with HIV disease access help depends on their perception of the problem, their knowledge about services and resources that exist, and whether they perceive the services as beneficial. Cultural variability in immigration experiences, traditional values of collectivism and family sanctity, dysfunctional social networks, and lack of culturally competent services clearly play a role in increasing risk for HIV infection. Despite the increasing numbers of APIs with HIV, the inherent diversity within and across subgroups makes researching this population a difficult task. Research studies have been limited by small sample sizes, nonrandom samples, qualitative studies, and single group studies, reducing generalizability. In addition, standardized measures to assess stigma, psychological stress, attitudes and perceptions, access to care, and social support are based on the mainstream population and may not be appropriate with an ethnically diverse population. Investigating cultural variability in risk and protective behaviors, acculturation, social support, stigma, and access to care across diverse groups by utilizing indigenously developed standardized measures is a daunting task but one that needs to be addressed by HIV/AIDS researchers and social scientists. Clearly, we need to better understand whether there is variability within and across specific subgroups to initiate and continue safe sex behaviors.

Finally, although HIV infection rates in the API community have been steadily increasing, the API community has been bypassed in terms of education and prevention programs compared to other ethnic groups in the United States. Understandably, the diverse needs of APIs with HIV disease makes it difficult for organizations to provide services to this multiethnic population. Additionally, inadequate funding initiatives for HIV prevention and treatment programs deter organizations from providing much needed preventive and treatment services. Involving the API community through outreach and collaboration with local minority community organizations can be effective in providing improved services to this population. Although policy has been slow to recognize the needs of APIs, the creation of the Asian American Pacific Islander Initiative (AAPI) in 1997 is a significant step in the right direction. The current AAPI action agenda clearly states the need to increase access to health, mental health, and social services to the Asian-American population.[27] Ultimately, prevention, early identification, and intervention with this group can significantly reduce HIV acquisition and transmission, leading to better health outcomes in this unique population.

REFERENCES

1. Centers for Disease Control and Prevention. HIV/AIDS surveillance report: cases of HIV infection and AIDS in the United States, 2003. 2004;15. Available: http://www.cdc.gov/hiv/stats/2003SurveillanceReport.htm. Accessed August 1, 2005.
2. Reeves T, Bennett C. *The Asian and Pacific Islander Population in the United States: March 2002. Current Population Reports, P20–540.* Washington, DC: U.S. Bureau of the Census; 2003.
3. Centers for Disease Control and Prevention. HIV/AIDS surveillance supplemental report: cases of HIV infection and AIDS in the United States, by race/ethnicity, 1998-2002. 2004;10. Available: http://www.cdc.gov/hiv/stats/hasrsuppVol10No1.htm. Accessed August 1, 2005.
4. McFarland W, Chen S, Weide D, Kohn R, Klausner J. Gay Asian men in San Francisco follow the international trend: increases in rates of unprotected anal intercourse and sexually transmitted diseases, 1999-2002. *AIDS Educ Prev.* 2004;16:13–18.
5. Sy FS, Chng CL, Choi ST, Wong FY. Epidemiology of HIV and AIDS among Asian and Pacific Islander Americans. *AIDS Educ Prev.* 1998;10(suppl A):4–18.
6. Yoshikawa H, Wilson PA, Hsueh JA, Rosman EA, Chin J, Kim JH. What front-line CBO staff can tell us about culturally anchored theories of behavior change in HIV prevention for Asian/Pacific Islanders. *Am J Community Psychol.* 2003;32:143–158.
7. Siegel DLN. AIDS knowledge, attitudes, and behavior among inner city, junior high school students. *J School Health.* 1991;61:160–165.
8. Bhattacharya G, Cleland C, Holland S. Knowledge about HIV/AIDS, the perceived risks of infection and sources of information of Asian-Indian adolescents born in the USA. *AIDS Care.* 2000;12:203–209.
9. Gellert GA, Maxwell RM, Higgins KV, Mai KK, Lowery R, Doll L. HIV/AIDS knowledge and high risk sexual practices among southern California Vietnamese. *Genitourin Med.* 1995;71:216–223.
10. Choi KH, Coates TJ, Catania JA, et al. High HIV risk among gay and Asian and Pacific Islander men in San Francisco. *AIDS.* 1995;9:306–308.
11. Choi K-H, Operario D, Gregorich SE, Han L. Age and race mixing patterns of sexual partnerships among Asian men who have sex with men: implications for HIV transmission and prevention. *AIDS Educ Prev.* 2003;15(suppl 1):53–65.
12. Faryna EL, Morales E. Self-efficacy and HIV-related risk behaviors among multiethnic adolescents. *Cult Divers Ethnic Minor Psychol.* 2000;6:42–56.
13. Kanuha VK. The impact of sexuality and race/ethnicity on HIV/AIDS risk among Asian and Pacific Island American (A/PIA) gay and bisexual men in Hawai'i. *AIDS Educ Prev.* 2000;12:505–518.
14. Nemoto T, Iwamoto M, Wong S, Le MN, Operario D. Social factors related to risk for violence and sexually transmitted infections/HIV among Asian massage parlor workers in San Francisco. *AIDS Behav.* 2004;8:475–483.
15. Raj A, Silverman J. The roles of culture, context, and legal immigrant status on intimate partner violence. *Viol Against Immigr Women.* 2002;8:367–398.
16. Nemoto T, Operario D, Soma T. Risk behaviors of Filipino methamphetamine users in San Francisco: implications for prevention and treatment of drug use and HIV. *Public Health Rep.* 2002;117(suppl 1):S30–S38.
17. Reback CJ, Larkins S, Shoptaw S. Changes in the meaning of sexual risk behaviors among gay and bisexual male methamphetamine abusers before and after drug treatment. *AIDS Behav.* 2004;8:87–98.
18. Kang E, Rapkin BD, Remien RH, Mellins CA, Oh A. Multiple dimensions of HIV stigma and psychological distress among Asians and Pacific Islanders living with HIV illness. *AIDS Behav.* 2005;9:145–154.
19. Nemoto T, Operario D, Soma T, Bao D, Vajrabukka A, Crisostomo V. HIV risk and prevention among Asian/Pacific islander men who have sex with men: listen to our stories. *AIDS Educ Prev.* 2003;15(suppl 1):7–20.
20. National Alliance of State and Territorial AIDS Directors (NASTAD). Focus on Asian and Pacific Islander (A&PI) issues. Available: http://www.nastad.org/DOCUMENTS/PUBLIC/PUB_PREVENTION/200251MAY2002HVPREVENTIONBULLETIN.PDF. Accessed August 1, 2005.
21. Wong FY, Campsmith ML, Nakamura GV, Crepaz N, Begley E. HIV testing and awareness of care-related services among a group of HIV-positive Asian Americans and Pacific Islanders in the United States: findings from a supplemental HIV/AIDS surveillance project. *AIDS Educ Prev.* 2004;16:440–447.
22. Department of Health and Human Services. *Mental Health: Culture, Race, and Ethnicity: A Supplement to Mental Health—A Report of the Surgeon General.* Washington, DC: U.S. Department of Health and Human Services Substance Abuse and Mental Health Services Administration, Center for Mental Health Services; 2001:105–122.
23. Menaster M. Asian American mental health issues. Asia Pacific: perspectives 2003. 2003;3:31–34. Available: http://www.pacificrim.usfca.edu/research/perspectives. Accessed August 1, 2005.
24. Estin P. Spotting depression in Asian patients. *RN.* 1999;62:39–40.
25. Frackiewicz E, Sramek J, Herrera J. Ethnicity and antipsychotic response. *Ann Pharmacother.* 1997;31:1360–1369.
26. Lin K, Cheung F. Mental health issues for Asian Americans. *Psychiatr Serv.* 1999;50:774–780.
27. Office of Minority Health. AAPI: action agenda, 1998. May 1, 2000. Available: http://www.omhrc.gov/omh/Asian%20Americans/3rdpgasian/agenda.htm. Accessed August 1, 2005.

CHAPTER 23

HIV/AIDS Among American Indians and Alaska Natives

Carol E. Kaufman, Janette Beals, Sara Jumping Eagle, Christina M. Mitchell

American Indians and Alaska Natives (AI/ANs)* made up less than 1% of the total number of AIDS cases diagnosed in the United States in 2003 (n = 3,026),[1] yet that number represents more than a 10-fold increase in the number of AIDS cases among AI/ANs since 1990 (n = 233).[2] Indeed, according to the Centers for Disease Control and Prevention (CDC), the rate of AIDS cases for AI/ANs (8.1 per 100,000) is higher than for the White, non-Hispanic population (6.1 per 100,000).[1] At the same time, recent psychiatric epidemiologic studies have found that disorders such as alcohol use disorders (AUD) and post-traumatic stress disorder (PTSD), are found at elevated levels in this population.[3] Rates of major depressive episode, as assessed by common structured interviews, have been shown to be lower than the general U.S. population for some tribes.[4,*] Each of these disorders has been linked to various points in the transmission or progression of HIV infection and AIDS in other populations. Yet, little research exists to understand the connections between psychiatric problems and HIV infection and AIDS among AI/ANs. Even less exists that examines the cultural framing of those connections and the critical ties to family, community, and religious or spiritual beliefs.

In this chapter, we begin to examine the psychiatric aspects of HIV disease and AIDS among AI/ANs, with specific reference to cultural underpinnings. First, we begin with a brief overview of the demographic characteristics of AI/ANs and then review the statistics of HIV infection and AIDS and predominant risk factors for this population. We then assess the psychiatric epidemiology of AI/ANs and delineate the cultural parameters of those disorders as they relate to HIV infection and AIDS. Finally, we review the role of families, communities, and prevention and intervention programs.

---

*In March 1977, the National Congress of American Indians and the National Tribal Chairmen's Association issued a joint resolution that the people and their descendants who were originally indigenous to the U.S. portion of North America before colonization should be referred to as American Indians. In keeping with the resolution, we also use the term American Indians, together with Alaska Natives, and abbreviate to AI/AN solely for space considerations.

BACKGROUND AND CONTEXT

According to the 2000 census, the AI/AN population represents less than 2% of the total population. Their small numbers mean that they are often not well represented in most national surveys; thus we know surprisingly little about this population. Their diversity contributes additional complexity to understanding their communities and characteristics. AI/ANs comprise 562 federally recognized tribes and Alaska Native Villages. Estimates derived from national surveys regarding AI/ANs can be misleading because this diversity is rarely accounted for within sample design or analyses. With this inherent weakness in most national or sample surveys, census data provide one of the main sources of information on this group. The statistics are striking. About 12% of the national population lives below the poverty line, compared to 28% of all AI/ANs and 36% of AI/AN children living on reservations. Unemployment rates are above 10% for most tribes;[4,**] households are usually very crowded; and educational achievement lags behind that of other Americans, with only 10% of all reservation-resident AIs holding a bachelor's degree or higher, compared with 24% in the U.S. general population.[5]

AI/ANs also endure elevated levels of mortality and morbidity. Age-adjusted mortality rates, for example, show that AI/ANs are over 7 times more likely to die from alcoholism compared to the U.S. general population, 1.5 times as likely to die from firearm wounds, almost twice as likely to experience a homicidal death, and over 3 times as likely to die in a car accident. AI/ANs are also at increased risk of suicide, with age-adjusted suicide rates for AI/ANs estimated to be 72% higher than for the general population.[6] As yet, we know little about how this challenging environment may shape the relationship between HIV and AIDS status and psychiatric disorder. These statistics also do not reveal the strengths of family and community life. AI/ANs, on and off the reservation, often have strong ties to extended family, tribal communities, and cultural traditions, ceremonies, and beliefs. Distant relatives or friends may be referred to as "aunties" or "grandfathers"; cousins may be referred to as "brothers" or "sisters." Honoring ceremonies, powwows, and funerals bring even the most urbanized AI/ANs together. Such ties and community strength may act as protective factors in risk behavior associated with HIV transmission and in mental illness.

HIV/AIDS TRENDS AND PATTERNS

The number of AIDS cases among AI/ANs have undergone over a 1,000% increase from 1990 (223 cases) to 2003 (3,026 cases). AI/ANs experience a faster progression, from HIV infection to AIDS than any other racial group in the United States. In 2001, 48% of AI/ANs diagnosed with HIV infection were subsequently diagnosed with AIDS within 12 months, compared to 40% for the general population. They also experience one of the lowest survival rates after an AIDS diagnosis is made. Among those with AIDS, AI/ANs are slightly younger than the national population on average. Among AI/ANs diagnosed with AIDS, youth aged 13 to 24 years make up 6% of all cases, cumulatively, compared to 4% in the general population.[2] The percent of AI/ANs diagnosed with AIDS who were women or girls ranged between 22% and 31% from 1999 to 2002, with no discernible trend. The current level, 26% in 2002, is second only to that in Blacks, in which women and girls comprise 34% of all diagnosed cases.[2]

These HIV infection and AIDS statistics for AI/ANs are even more concerning because they are likely to be underestimated due to racial or ethnic misclassification.[7] Further, national

---

**The unemployment rate as calculated by the census does not include persons who are not actively looking for work. In many reservation settings, where jobs are scarce, many have simply given up looking. The unemployment rate as calculated thus substantially deflates the level of real unemployment.*

trends tend to dilute local experiences of HIV disease and AIDS. AI/ANs are residentially concentrated in a relatively limited geographic area—about 60% of the total AI/AN population resides in about 11 states.[5,***] Finally, many of those states, such as Alaska, California, and New York, do not require confidential name-based HIV infection reporting; thus, we know very little about HIV status for substantial sectors of the AI/AN population. Indeed, we did not reference HIV trends because of the likely biases they contain because reporting policies are not uniform across states.[5,†]

The predominant mode of transmission has been men having sex with men (MSM) sexual contact, comprising 60% of transmission cumulatively, slightly more than 54% of the national general population. Although many tribes traditionally accepted and even revered those people who were "two spirited" or *winkte*, the influence of mainstream American culture has resulted in the stigmatization of those members of an AI/AN community who are gay, lesbian, bisexual, or transgender (GLBT); this also puts them at increased risk because they are more likely to engage in clandestine activities. Little research exists on the complexity of GLBT issues in AI/AN communities, but anecdotal evidence suggests that such persons may engage in homosexual behavior only when under the influence of drugs or alcohol, because their disinhibiting influence may allow them, first, to pursue such activities and, second, because they may not be held accountable, socially, for such actions if intoxicated. Additionally, GLBT AI/ANs may pursue differential identity strategies, depending on where they are. That is, in reservation communities, they may present themselves as heterosexual and engage in heterosexual activities there. When they travel to (or live in) urban communities, they may see themselves as GLBT individuals and engage in different sexual activity. This shifting identification likely increases stress and anxiety, which in turn may be linked to increases in risk taking. It is also likely to increase risk exposure to HIV for persons residing in reservations and who are sexually active with persons who do not disclose their own sexual identity or possible risk of HIV infection.

Although AIDS incidence reports had indicated a shift in proportion from transmission via MSM to transmission via heterosexual contact and injection drug use (IDU), data for 2001 and 2002 show that concrete trends are not yet established. From 1999 to 2002, MSM transmission levels have begun to increase again since reaching a low of 47% in 2000, rising to a high of 55% in 2002 (which includes MSM and IDU as dual mode of transmission category); levels of IDU transmission rates similarly have varied over that same period, ranging between 33% and 43%; and rates for heterosexual transmission have remained roughly unchanged at about 20%, a level similar to that for Blacks and Hispanics. Of importance, IDU as a mode of transmission is the highest among AI women and girls (43%) compared to women and girls of any other race groups (Whites, 38%; Blacks, 28%; Hispanics, 26%; Asian and Pacific Islanders, 18%).[2]

Sexual risk taking and substance use are among the main risk factors for AI/AN populations. The prevalence of sexually transmitted infections (STIs), a marker of sexual risk taking, is 2 to 6 times higher among AI/ANs than in the general U.S. population.[8] According to the National Study of Drug Use and Health (NSDUH),[††] in 2002, about 60% of AI/ANs reported illicit drug use at some point in their lives, compared to 46% nationally.[9] Related to AI/AN drug use, the elevated levels of diabetes among AI/ANs, and the commensurate

---

***Sixty-two percent of AI/ANs live in Alaska, Arizona, California, Florida, Michigan, New Mexico, New York, North Carolina, Oklahoma, Texas, and Washington, compared to only 44 percent of the U.S. population.[5]

†Bertolli et al.[7] list a number of data sources for HIV-related information. However, as those authors point out, each of these is limited in its own way and of minimal use in a broad overview such as this.

††Caveats about the AI/AN sample size in the NSDUH apply. Specifically, the survey includes a nationally representative sample of 67,784 persons aged 12 years and older. AI/AN categories are based on those respondents marking AI/AN as their only race, or just over 600 persons.

increase in insulin injections, have resulted in a greater availability of discarded needles, which are then used for illicit injection drugs. According to the NSDUH of 2001,[9] although AI/ANs reported less lifetime alcohol use (by 10 points) than the general population, about 30% reported binge or heavy drinking, compared to 26% nationally. Thus, alcohol, like drug use, may be a factor for some AI/ANs, but will likely vary considerably in whether it plays a role in risk taking for or coping with HIV disease or AIDS.

Location may also be a factor in risk. AI/ANs are more likely to reside in rural areas, often remote reservation areas or villages, compared to other race groups. Although the relative isolation of many of these communities may appear to afford some protection, in fact, in most cases, these communities are not so isolated. AI/ANs travel back and forth between urban areas and reservations to attend school or work or to participate in cultural and family events. This pattern of urban–rural circulation, coupled with high levels of STIs and substance use, places even remote rural communities at risk. Further, persons living in remote areas are less likely to have access to appropriate testing, counseling, and treatment services. A number of other additional factors may also foster HIV and AIDS transmission for this population. The small and often tightly knit communities in which AI/ANs live mean that stigma, fear of a breach of confidentiality in medical services, and wide-ranging taboos and proscriptions on sexual behavior, including same-sex sexual behavior may increase risk. Sexual networks also can be extensive in AI/AN communities, as evidenced by a recent well-publicized incident of HIV exposure. The often long distances to health care facilities may also make prevention, testing, and care challenging. As we note later in the chapter, many facilities of the Indian Health Service (IHS), estimated to serve approximately 60% of the eligible AI/AN population, are inadequately staffed and trained and they often lack appropriate medications, especially for HIV disease and AIDS, providing further disincentive to seek testing or treatment. In urban areas, while HIV/AIDS-related services may be more available, IHS services are not. About 60% of AI/ANs live in urban areas, but only three urban IHS-funded clinics exist, and only 1% of the total IHS budget is designated for urban services. Many AI/ANs speak languages other than English, and even when English is spoken, terms and phrasing may differ between local use and medical provider use. Moreover, some AI/AN groups adhere to forms of communication that may increase social distance to providers, such as avoiding eye contact, prolonged periods of silence, or a soft handshake. Finally, it is worth noting that some traditions and ceremonies involve skin piercing or tattooing. Absent sterile implements, these practices may also elevate risk of HIV transmission.

PSYCHIATRIC EPIDEMIOLOGY OF AMERICAN INDIANS AND ALASKA NATIVES

Our understanding of the complex pattern of associations between psychiatric disorders and HIV/AIDS is woefully inadequate. For the AI/AN population, understanding this association presents even a greater challenge, because little is known about psychiatric disorders in this group. National efforts, such as the National Comorbidity Survey (NCS), do not include sufficient numbers of AIs for independent estimates. Indeed, the 2001 Surgeon General's report, *Mental Health: Culture, Race, and Ethnicity*,[10] concluded that the most basic data about the relative mental health burdens borne by AI/ANs were lacking, thus precluding accurate assessments of treatment need. We present in the following section an emerging picture of mental health among AI/ANs, as a background with which to understand connections to HIV/AIDS.

Evidence for psychiatric disorders among AI/ANs is thin and tends to focus on AI tribes, rather than AN villages or communities or urban populations. However, several targeted studies of AI mental health do exist. In an early effort, Shore et al.[11] found that 69% of a small tribal village (n = 100) in the Northwest had definite or probable psychiatric impairment (using *Diagnostic and Statistical Manual of Mental Disorders* (*DSM-I* and *DSM-II*). The most common disorder was alcoholism. A second interview 19 years later in the same village (n = 98) using the *DSM-III-R* version of the Schedule for Affective Disorders and Schizophrenia–Lifetime Version found elevated rates of lifetime alcohol use disorders (AUDs; 57%) and major depressive episode (MDE; 21%) and somewhat elevated rates of lifetime PTSD (5%) compared to the large catchment area samples of that time.[12]

The American Indian Service Utilization, Psychiatric Epidemiology, Risk and Protective Factors Project (AI-SUPERPFP), conducted from 1996 to 1999, was a large-scale project designed to directly address gaps in AI/AN psychiatric epidemiology. The study included representative samples from two major tribes of the United States, one from the Southwest and one from the Northern Plains. Using a computerized diagnostic interview, results of this study showed that *DSM*-defined lifetime drug abuse or dependence rates ranged from 5.2% for Southwest women to 15.4% among Northern Plains men—levels that were about equivalent to the those found in the NCS.[13] Lifetime rates of alcohol dependence for men in both tribes were 50% higher than those found in the NCS. For Northern Plains women, however, rates of lifetime alcohol dependence were twice those of women in the NCS, but Southwestern women had rates similar to those of the national sample.[14] Major anxiety and depression levels ranged between 6.8% and 13.0%, levels slightly lower than for those estimated for the national population (16.2%).[4] Beals et al.[3] warn, however, that questions that are used in the calculus of a depression diagnosis may be interpreted and answered with specific cultural lenses (see later discussion). In contrast, lifetime *DSM-IV-R* PTSD rates for AI/ANs in this sample were substantially higher than those for the general population. Overall, AUD and PTSD were the most common disorders in these two tribal populations, with substantial comorbidity between substance use and depressive/anxiety disorders.[3]

CULTURAL PERSPECTIVES ON PSYCHIATRIC CONDITIONS

Individuals at high risk for HIV infection may also be at high risk for psychiatric disorders. Causality may work in both directions. Disorders may occur before infection, or they may come about as a consequence of learning of the diagnosis. However, even in cases in which a psychiatric diagnosis occurs before infection, the diagnosis does not necessarily precede the *behaviors* that put a person at risk for HIV infection. A variety of mechanisms may link psychiatric disorders with HIV-risk behaviors. Important here, cultural influences may shape those mechanisms. Yet the role of culture in the connection between psychiatric disorders and the initiation and maintenance of risk behaviors has had little research attention. Understanding the cultural foreground of those associations, especially for AI/ANs, will provide for more effective care by clinicians or service providers. As suggested in the 2001 Surgeon General's Report, cultural beliefs, family processes, and community conditions are key components of mental illness and subsequent service use,[10] particularly in AI populations in which kinship and community are integral to daily life. The focus of this section, then, is to highlight the specific cultural underpinnings of psychiatric disorders and their relationship to HIV disease among AIs.

Three main disorders are addressed in the following section—substance use (including both alcohol and drug), depression, and PTSD. Each diagnosis is discussed with its sociocultural validity; that is, with an informed consideration of culture and meaning for each disorder. The disorder is considered from both emic (from inside the culture) and etic (from outside the culture) perspectives, underscoring the importance of local idioms and local explanations of distress.

SUBSTANCE USE

Alcohol and drug use has been shown to be closely involved with HIV disease and AIDS, both in transmission (e.g., through disinhibition and increased sexual risk behavior or through IDU), and in disease progression (e.g., in cognitive function or viral load). For AI/ANs, links with

HIV infection and AIDS risk or progression are important to consider within cultural context. Cultural beliefs, practices, and values assigned to alcohol and drug use vary dramatically across tribes. As Heath et al.[15] argue, depending on cultural context, alcohol can be viewed as medicine or poison, as sacramental or sacrilegious, or as a stimulant or relaxant. Similar arguments can be made for drug use, especially because many tribes use substances in spiritual traditions or healing ceremonies. The meanings of symptoms of disorder also are likely influenced by cultural context, as evidenced by the changing interpretations of the seriousness of driving under the influence in recent years or medical use of marijuana.[15] Thresholds for "illness" likely vary cross-culturally. Certain alcohol- or drug-related behaviors may be considered normative in some contexts but not in others. Ethnographic studies within AI communities, for example, show that drinking, even at levels qualifying for diagnosis, and sometimes using drugs may be valued as a demonstration of kinship and sharing, even at the same time that harmful consequences are also noted.[16]

For assessing substance use in relation to HIV disease and AIDS, the clinician or service provider must remember that excessive drug or alcohol use by AI/ANs is a stereotype. Many in this group do not use substances at all. For those who do, some drug or alcohol use may include important ceremonial or social links. It is use tied with risk behavior, such as shared needles or increased likelihood of sexually unsafe practices, that is most critical to identify. Understanding the social context and expected behavior in situations that include substance use will provide starting points for treatment.

DEPRESSION

An extensive literature has emerged on the relationship of depression and depressive symptoms and HIV disease and AIDS, including effect on progression and HIV-risk behavior. An extensive literature also exists on the cultural phenomenology of depression.[17] Ethnographic research has identified several critical factors in the cross-cultural experience of depression. First, the Euro-American construct of "depression" refers to a mood or emotional state, a symptom, and an illness, with these typically considered as denoting increased levels of severity. Other cultures may not have this hierarchy and also may adopt different norms for normal versus pathologic.[18,19] Also, in depression, cultures vary in the degree to which the emotion associated with MDE is sociocentric (rather than egocentric) and thus best understood in terms of the person's relationships with others.[19] Among some AIs, for example, "loneliness" is a common metaphor for depression, clearly invoking considerations of an individual's social network.[20] Further, the suffering commonly labeled as depressed affect may be constructed differently across cultures. Another theme in ethnographic studies of depression is the role of somatic symptoms; many non–Euro-American populations may not differentiate between mind and body symptoms. Further, not all of those who otherwise meet criteria for MDE may acknowledge depressed mood or dysphoria (at least one of which is necessary for a diagnosis of MDE). Finally, other social factors, such as gender or social class, likely condition or mediate the expression or recognition of depression within a particular culture.[17–19]

Depression and its links with HIV disease and AIDS may be at first obscure to service providers. A perfunctory review of statistics of depression among AI/ANs may simply reinforce a lack of connection between depression and HIV, because depression as measured by *DSM* algorithms from data collected by lay interviewers reveals low levels in this group. The lessons of psychiatric epidemiology and ethnography, however, indicate that this would be a simplistic and possibly harmful view. Depression appears to manifest itself, or be described, in different ways among AI/ANs. Establishing expected behavior of patients' community, their own description of the degree of similarity or divergence from that, and their level of comfort with that distance may be useful in establishing depressive or anxiety symptoms.

For example, a gay AI may have little difficulty when living in a large urban area. Yet, returning to his reservation community, he may be unable to disclose his gay identity because of taboos or stigma. The disjuncture in identity may bring about both depressive symptoms and increased risk behavior. However, without asking about the two different worlds, and understanding his response, no apparent sign of depression or risk may be forthcoming.

POST-TRAUMATIC STRESS DISORDER

Although PTSD was introduced only recently (*DSM-III* in 1980), it has been the focus of a substantial ethnographic literature. Diagnosis is dependent on a traumatic etiologic event, defined in *DSM-IV*[21] as "an event or events that involved actual or threatened death or serious harm, or a threat to the physical integrity of self or others and the person's response involved intense fear, helplessness, or horror." This wording represents a marked improvement, from a sociocultural stance, on the *DSM-III-R* definition that defined trauma as "outside the range of usual human experience"; yet ethnographers have shown that cultural factors continue to be important. Manson et al.[22] provide the example of how a broken leg, while normally not seen as a trauma, might qualify when the cause is culturally attributed to witchcraft. He suggests that PTSD has been adopted as a metaphor for the social and psychological burdens AIs experience, using the cultural idiom of "wounded spirit." Manson[23] concluded that the *DSM* definitions of PTSD function similarly in AI Vietnam veterans as in others, with the war experience as a major influence on phenomenology; however he also anticipated that the presentation of symptoms may differ among nonveterans, suggesting, for example, that the value on stoicism may make the identification of avoidance symptoms difficult.

For AI/ANs, the examination of a possible association of trauma (if not PTSD) with HIV risk or infection is key. As noted above, these populations experience elevated risks of trauma compared to the national population; clinicians who may not investigate this link extensively with their other clients should take time to explore this link with AI/AN patients.

SERVICE PROVISION

AI/AN communities have a unique services ecology, including the IHS, tribally funded health programs, private clinics, federally administered services, not-for-profit agencies, and traditional healers whose roles vary dramatically by tribe and by illness. The IHS is the primary source of biomedical services in many communities, estimated to have served about 60% or 1.6 million AI/ANs in the United States.[24] Yet this agency is dramatically underfunded, particularly with respect to mental health services. As a result, such services are scarce, with many provided by paraprofessionals; typically, psychiatric medications are provided either by primary care physicians or by traveling psychiatrists, who provide medication management on a monthly basis. The majority of IHS facilities are on or near AI/AN reservations and communities, and many persons who live in urban areas do not have access to these facilities. More than a quarter of AI/ANs do not have any health insurance at all.[24] Moreover, there is considerable misinformation about Medicaid eligibility; many believe that AI/ANs are not eligible for this state-administered program because federally recognized tribes are sovereign nations and are not generally subject to state laws (or rights). Although the law requires states to provide Medicaid assistance to eligible AI/ANs regardless of tribal affiliation or residence on or off the reservation, this frequently does not happen. HIV disease and AIDS, in particular, is a challenging disease for this patchwork of clinics or hospitals that serve AI/ANs. Many IHS facilities simply do not have staff that are adequately trained, the money to purchase the necessary medications for treatment, or a commitment to providing HIV/AIDS services.[25]

Although federal programs have provided funds to AI/AN-focused HIV/AIDS services, many of these programs are competitive 3- to 5-year awards, which dampen continuity and may weaken stability of services. Thus many AI/ANs do not have access to adequate care for HIV/AIDS. Although a recent study of the Ryan White Comprehensive AIDS Resource Emergency (CARE) Act show no differences between AI/ANs and persons of other racial groups receiving services provided through this funding mechanism,[26] the study included only grantees of CARE funds and thus only a small number of AI/AN clients (314 AI/ANs out of over 41,700 patient records). Of importance, the lack of continuity also likely means that many AI/ANs do not receive the comprehensive care of physical, emotional, mental, and spiritual needs they may require over the course of the disease.

A few HIV/AIDS programs, or models for programs, in AI/AN communities are important to mention.[25,27,28] Vernon and Jumper-Thurman[25] advance the community readiness model, a community-based approach that assesses, and then builds upon, the level of acceptance and support for prevention activities. Duran and Walters[27] present a postcolonial perspective on HIV/AIDS programs for AI/ANs, one that uses indigenous ways of healing with Western medicines and therapies, based on community self-assessment of need, support, and involvement. Tafoya[28] elaborates the power of story-telling for prevention in AI/AN communities. Finally, many tribes have rite-of-passage ceremonies that may provide opportunity for HIV/AIDS prevention.

To our knowledge, none of these approaches or practices has been rigorously evaluated. However, they all have in common the foregrounding of cultural experience—whether through culturally based participation, traditional healing, storytelling, or treatment links to medical and nonmedical practitioners—in the prevention, treatment, and care of HIV disease and AIDS. In short, AI/ANs often have a broad view and experience of health and illness, such as HIV disease and AIDS. The link to mental health is only one part of the whole. Many AI/ANs do not make distinctions among mental, emotional, spiritual, and physical health. Both prevention and treatment are likely to be most effective if presented within a holistic framework. Any psychiatric evaluation of HIV disease or AIDS with an AI/AN client should include a broad view of health and links with community and family life.

SUMMARY

This chapter presents an overview of the links between HIV disease and AIDS and psychiatric disorders among AI/ANs, with special attention to a few of the cultural factors that may underpin those links. Indeed, mostly we have stressed the lack of information, especially for ANs. We know little about psychiatric disorders, HIV disease and AIDS, or the cultural context that may influence transmission or disease progression among AI/ANs. For clinicians and service providers, this may be particularly frustrating, because little empirical guidance exists. As outlined above, a few models of care or approaches to treatment have been proposed as being particularly useful with AI/AN persons. Whatever approach or model is selected, any psychiatric evaluation of AI/ANs with respect to HIV disease and AIDS should account for cultural understanding or interpretation of symptoms and consequences. Also, treatment plans should include specific address of cultural challenges, along with a systematic review of services options or benefits so that the multiple needs of a client can be as comprehensively addressed as is possible.§

---

§*A number of important AI/AN-specific resources are listed within the references for this chapter. The following websites may also be useful: http://www.ihs.gov/MedicalPrograms/aids/ hiv-coe-native-american-aids-specific-resources.asp; www.nnaapc.org; http://www.ac.wwu.edu/ ~culture/medicine.htm.*

ACKNOWLEDGMENTS

Support for this project came from the National Institute of Mental Health grant R01 MH69086 (Kaufman, PI) and R01 DAD17803 (Beals, PI).

REFERENCES

1. Centers for Disease Control and Prevention. Cases of HIV infection and AIDS in the United States, 2003. In: *HIV/AIDS Surveillance Report*. Atlanta: Centers for Disease Control and Prevention; 2004.
2. Centers for Disease Control and Prevention. Cases of HIV infection and AIDS in the United States, by race/ethnicity, 1998–2002. In: *HIV/AIDS Surveillance Supplemental Report*. Atlanta: Centers for Disease Control and Prevention; 2003.
3. Beals J, Manson SM, Whitesell NR, et al. Prevalence of DSM-IV disorders and attendant help-seeking in two American Indian reservation populations. *Arch Gen Psychiatry*. 2005;62:99–108.
4. Beals J, Manson SM, Whitesell NR, et al., and the AI–SUPERPFP team (2005). Prevalence of major depressive episode in two Amercian Indian reservation populations: unexpected findings with a structured interview. *Am J Psychiatry*. 2006;162:1713–1722.
5. U.S. Bureau of the Census Bureau. Census 2000 summary files 1, 2, 3 (SF1, SF2, SF3). 2002. American Factfinder. Available: http://www.census.gov. Accessed April 10, 2005.
6. U.S. Department of Health and Human Services. *Trends in Indian Health 1998–1999*. Rockville, Md: U.S. Department of Health and Human Services; 2001.
7. Bertolli J, McNaghten AD, Campsmith M, et al. Surveillance systems monitoring HIV/AIDS and HIV risk behaviors among American Indians and Alaska Natives. *AIDS Educ Prev*. 2004;16:218–237.
8. Centers for Disease Control and Prevention. *Sexually Transmitted Disease Surveillance 2002*. Atlanta: U.S. Department of Health and Human Services, Centers for Disease Control and Prevention, Division of STD Prevention; 2003.
9. Substance Abuse and Mental Health Services Administration. *Results from the 2002 National Survey on Drug Use and Health: National Findings. 2003*. Rockville, Md: Office of Applied Studies; 2003.
10. U.S. Department of Health and Human Services. *Mental Health: Culture, Race, and Ethnicity—A Supplement to Mental Health: A Report of the Surgeon General*. Rockville, Md: U.S. Department of Health and Human Services, Substance Abuse and Mental Health Services Administration, Center for Mental Health Services; 2001.
11. Shore JH, Kinzie JD, Hampson JL, & Pattison EM. Psychiatric epidemiology of an Indian village. *Psychiatry*. 1973;36:70–81.
12. Kinzie JD, Leung PK, Boehnlein J, et al. Psychiatry epidemiology of an Indian village: a 19-year replication study. *J Nerv Ment Dis*. 1992;180:33–39.
13. Mitchell CM, Beals J, Novins DK, et al. Drug use among two American Indian populations: prevalence of lifetime use and DSM-IV substance disorders. *Drug Alcohol Depend*. 2003;69:29–41.
14. Spicer P, Beals J, Mitchell CM, et al. The prevalence of alcohol dependence in two American Indian reservation populations. *Alcohol Clin Exp Res*. 2003;27:1785–1797.
15. Heath AC, Whitfield JB, Madden PA, et al. Towards a molecular epidemiology of alcohol dependence: analysing the interplay of genetic and environmental risk factors. *Br J Psychiatry Suppl*. 2001;40:S33–S40.
16. Spicer P. Toward a (dys)functional anthropology of drinking: ambivalence and the American Indian experience with alcohol. *Med Anthropol Q* 1997;11:306–323.
17. Kirmayer LJ, Groleua D. Affective disorders in cultural context. *Psychiatr Clin North Am*. 2001;24:465–487.
18. Kleinman A. *Rethinking Psychiatry: From Cultural Category to Personal Experience*. New York: Free Press; 1988.
19. Manson SM. Culture and DSM-IV: Implications for the diagnosis of mood and anxiety disorders. In: Mezzich J, Kleinman A, Fabrega H, et al., eds. *Culture and Psychiatric Diagnosis*. Washington, DC: American Psychiatric Association Press; 1996.
20. O'Nell TD. Cultural formulation of psychiatric diagnosis: psychotic depression and alcoholism in an American Indian man. *Culture Med Psychiatry*. 1998;22:123–136.
21. American Psychiatric Association. *Diagnostic and Statistical Manual of Mental Disorders*. 4th ed. Washington, DC: American Psychiatric Association; 1994.
22. Manson S, Beals J, O'Nell T, et al. Wounded spirits, ailing hearts: PTSD and related disorders among American Indians. In: Marsella AJ, Friedman MJ, Gerrity ET, et al., eds. *Ethnocultural Aspects of Posttraumatic Stress Disorder: Issues, Research, and Clinical Applications*. Washington, DC: American Psychological Association; 1996:255–284.
23. Manson SM. The wounded spirit: a cultural formulation of post-traumatic stress disorder. *Culture Med Psychiatry*. 1996;20:489–498.
24. U.S. Commission on Civil Rights. *Broken Promises: Evaluating the Native American Health Care System*. Washington, DC: U.S. Commission on Civil Rights, Office of the General Counsel; 2004.
25. Vernon IS, Jumper-Thurman P. Prevention of HIV/AIDS in Native American communities: promising interventions. *Public Health Rep*. 2002;117(suppl 1):S96–S103.
26. Ashman JJ, Perez-Jimenez D, Marconi K. Health and support service utilization patterns of American Indians and Alaska Native diagnosed with HIV/AIDS. *AIDS Educ Prev*. 2004;16:238–249.
27. Duran B, Walters KL. HIV/AIDS prevention in "Indian Country": current practice, indigenist etiology models and postcolonial approaches to change. *AIDS Educ Prev*. 2004;16:187–201.
28. Tafoya T. Unmasking Dashkayah: Storytelling and HIV prevention. *Am Indian Alsk Native Ment Health Res*. 2000;9:53–65.

CHAPTER 24

HIV/AIDS Among Neonates and Infants

Andrea Stolar, Johanna Goldfarb

EPIDEMIOLOGY OF HIV INFECTION IN CHILDREN

Since its recognition as a new disease in the United States in 1981, acquired immunodeficiency syndrome (AIDS) has spread throughout the world. Although the epidemic in the United States began in homosexual men, it quickly spread into heterosexual populations, and with infection in young women, infection in children followed. Most infection in childhood is the result of vertical transmission from mother to infant during the perinatal period.

Estimated rates of human immunodeficiency (HIV) infection in children in the United States range widely (see Chapter 25 for details). However, the epidemiology of HIV among children reflects the demographic trends of their infected mothers. In 2004, among reported cases of vertically infected children in the United States, 89% were non Caucasian, of these, 71% were African American and 18% were Hispanic.[1]

VERTICAL TRANSMISSION

Women are increasingly at the forefront of the pandemic, with 17.5 million women of childbearing age estimated to be living with HIV worldwide.[2] In sub-Saharan Africa, 60% of adults living with HIV are women. Young women are particularly vulnerable to infection, not only because male-to-female transmission is twice as likely as female-to-male, but also as an effect of poverty, with sex as a commodity to secure basic necessities. Where the pandemic is firmly entrenched among women, pregnancy and the potential for vertical transmission follow. In Sub-Saharan Africa, up to a third of pregnant women are HIV-infected. Globally, the changing face of HIV disease and AIDS has been recognized and initiatives are aimed toward empowering women in order to stem the course of the pandemic. In the meantime, vertical transmission remains a critical focus in an increasingly young and female disease.

Without prophylaxis, there is a 30% risk for vertical HIV transmission, ranging from 24% to 65% depending on virologic, host, and placental factors.[3] Infection can occur at conception, via vaginal or seminal virus, or through placental transfer, although 50% of infection occurs around the time of birth. Advanced maternal age, recent infection or more progressed disease state, increased viral load, and multiply infected or an otherwise medically compromised host increases the risk. Disruption of mucosal or placental integrity eases the passage of the virus, implicating nutritional (vitamin deficiency) and behavioral (smoking) factors. Obstetric procedures that increase the exposure of the neonate to maternal blood and cervical and vaginal secretions increase the risk of perinatal infection. Genetic determinants of the developing infant may also play a role in the risk of transmission and disease progression. Infants with immune environments genetically similar to those of their mothers inherit a system that has failed to control maternal virus; thus immunologic maternal–fetal concordance is associated with an increased risk of vertical transmission.[4] A small percentage of infection occurs postnatally due to breast feeding, with variables at this stage including the duration of breast feeding, maternal disease, and the antibody content of breast milk.[5]

PREVENTION OF VERTICAL TRANSMISSION

A decade ago the AIDS Clinical Trial Group 076 demonstrated that antiretroviral therapy with AZT begun during the third trimester of pregnancy, continued through labor, and given to the newborn during the first weeks of life could markedly decrease the risk of HIV transmission from mother to newborn.[6] By the mid-1990s, pregnant women in the United States were voluntarily screened for HIV and offered AZT prophylaxis. Other studies identified that birthing method,[7] vigorous antiretroviral therapies in pregnant women (to keep maternal viral loads low), and bottle feeding in lieu of breast feeding, could further reduce HIV transmission from mother to child. These strategies resulted in a striking reduction in the number of cases of perinatal HIV infections and led to the Centers for Disease Control and Prevention's (CDC's) 2003 recommendation of the "opt-out" approach to HIV testing of pregnant women. The CDC's goal is the universal testing of HIV in pregnancy, with the aim to institute as early as possible the strategies that had been found to reduce HIV transmission. The "opt-out" recommendations include making HIV education a part of routine prenatal care and the addition of HIV testing to the battery of routine prenatal laboratory tests, unless the woman "opts-out." This approach has helped to identify the majority of pregnant HIV-infected women.[8] The dramatic decline in the number of newly diagnosed pediatric AIDS cases in the United States reflects the success of these public health initiatives. Intrapartum transmission can now be less than 2% in women with good prenatal and intrapartum care.

IMPLICATIONS FOR PRENATAL CARE

As it became clear that HIV transmission could be interrupted from mother to infant, identification of HIV-infected pregnant women has become a priority. Access and acceptance of medical care may be compromised in the population at highest risk for HIV infection. Poor women and women of color are less likely than other women to receive optimal HIV care. Women whose risk for HIV includes substance abuse (either directly or in her sexual partner) are often less likely to receive good prenatal care or any prenatal care at all. A pregnant woman with a substance use disorder may be fearful of accessing medical care (assuming appropriate care is available) and entering a system that may criminalize her substance use during pregnancy. Some municipalities have interpreted legislation regarding the delivery of drugs to minors to include prenatal and perinatal transmission, indicting women for drug use and child endangerment on the basis of their substance use[9] and in at least one case for the murder of her stillborn child.[10] This political environment may deter high-risk women from seeking prenatal care. Adolescents and unregistered aliens similarly may be reticent to access medical care, fearing vulnerability to legal repercussions. Inadequate insurance, a lack of transportation or daycare, cultural issues, language, and education all may serve as additional barriers to the crucial early identification and treatment of the HIV-infected mother.

Once a pregnant woman has accessed prenatal care and has been identified for HIV screening (see Chapter 27 for testing guidelines in pregnant women), whether she agrees to the testing is largely a function of her ability to make an informed decision. Education is crucial. Among those offered HIV testing, a significant factor weighing toward compliance is the belief that such testing will benefit the infant.[11] Although the message has spread that treatment for HIV can lengthen survival for those infected, there are still many who are unaware of the potential for prevention of perinatal transmission.[12] Further, despite great educational efforts and popular awareness of HIV and AIDS early in the epidemic, recent years have found a growing complacency about the disease among Americans. With breakthroughs in treatment has come reduced concern about the severity of HIV.[13]

For those who are engaged in prenatal care and offered HIV testing, there may be rational deterrents to acceptance. Pregnancy is a time of increased vulnerability to domestic violence, and disclosure of HIV infection may increase that risk. Women may also fear rejection, discrimination, or abandonment by family, support networks, or even by their health care providers with the discovery of their HIV status. There is no universal agreement among state laws regarding the confidentiality of HIV-related information, nor regarding discrimination on the basis of HIV status.[14] A woman may rightly be concerned that her HIV status, or her decisions with regard to testing and treatment, may be used against her.[15]

The long-term effect of retroviral therapy during pregnancy to prevent HIV transmission to her fetus can have an effect on the mother's own personal long-term therapeutic needs. Even brief exposures to an antiretroviral may induce resistance, perhaps limiting a woman's options for treatment in the future. Informed consent for HIV testing during pregnancy, therefore, must include not only the rationale for testing and the potential benefits to mother and child, but also the risks. Each woman must be educated about what rights she maintains with regard to the confidentiality of her test results. She must be assured that her testing decision will not adversely affect her right to prenatal care, and a plan to address the repercussions of a positive result must be in place.[16] As any effective treatment and transmission prophylaxis depend on the cooperation and compliance of the mother, her informed decision-making at the start of this process increases the likelihood of a successful outcome.

IMPLICATIONS FOR TREATMENT AT LABOR AND DELIVERY

According to the CDC, approximately 40% of the mothers of HIV-infected infants born in 2000 were not known to be HIV-positive before delivery.[17] Women with no or limited prenatal care are more likely to be infected than women who have received care. Consideration should be given to the empiric treatment of women arriving in labor with no prenatal care, but can be better directed if a rapid test is available to help guide therapy.[18] Though not as effective as therapy begun during gestation, beginning therapy at delivery does significantly decrease transmission rates.[19] Infants can be treated until the mother's HIV status can be clarified, and, if negative, the therapy is then discontinued.[20] The availability of rapid HIV testing makes last-minute prevention strategies possible, and some states have adopted policies of universal screening of newborns. Less intrusive than the mandatory screening of pregnant women, obligatory screening of newborns allows for the immediate treatment of those infants found antibody-positive. Beginning therapy after delivery, though not as effective as starting therapy during pregnancy, does reduce the risk of transmission and may reduce the rate of maternal–child transmission by 50%.[21]

At times the discovery of an HIV-infected infant is the first indication of infection in the mother. In the context of the availability of prenatal testing through the opt-out approach, when an HIV-infected infant is the first indication of disease in the mother, it is likely that her treatment will be confounded by the psychosocial obstacles that led to her unrecognized serostatus before delivery. Sensitivity to such issues is perhaps even more critical when identification is delayed until delivery, and supportive intervention for the mother increases the likelihood of instituting appropriate preventive intervention and medical care for the neonate and mother.

Medical Treatment Guidelines to Prevent Vertical Transmission

Guidelines for management of HIV infection in pregnancy have been reviewed in detail[22] (see Chapter 27 for details). Important concepts for therapy include reducing maternal HIV ribonucleic acid (RNA) levels, usually with multiple drugs, even if the woman does not otherwise meet criteria for treatment. The goal is to keep viral levels below 1,000 copies of virus/ml and to avoid development of resistance. This requires maintaining regimens with excellent suppression, maintaining adherence to medications, and starting and stopping all drugs together, never separately. Zidovudine should be one of the antiretrovirals used for therapy in pregnancy unless there is a contraindication (Table 24.1).

Cesarean delivery should be considered in women with high viral levels (>1,000 copies/ml) because this may additionally decrease transmission risk. To be effective, cesarean delivery must occur before the rupture of membranes. The role of cesarean delivery in women with HIV RNA levels below 1,000 copies/ml is unclear, and presently should be discussed, but cannot be definitively recommended without considering the risks and benefits of surgical delivery for each woman individually. Intravenous zidovudine is recommended 2 hours before surgical delivery or during labor for vaginal delivery. The infant is started immediately on oral zidovudine, and oral therapy is then continued for the first 6 weeks of life.[23] Shorter courses of therapy are less effective.[24] Using parts of the planned treatment, such as starting zidovudine only at labor or after delivery in the newborn (within 48 hours) each add some benefit, but are less effective than the complete protocol.[25]

Studies from the developing world have demonstrated that oral nevirapine given to the pregnant woman at onset of labor is effective at decreasing transmission.[26] This regimen is much less expensive, but not as effective, as the standard described previously. The role for nevirapine in women presenting without prenatal care needs to be clarified, but should be considered for women presenting with known HIV infection and no prenatal care, with oral AZT and/or a dose of nevirapine for the newborn. The rare occurrence of acute liver failure associated with nevirapine has raised concern about the use of this drug in prevention. A CDC website keeps an update on recommended therapy for prevention of perinatal transmission (www.cdc.gov/hiv/projects/perinatal). Other recommendations to avoid exposing the newborn

TABLE 24.1 Zidovudine (AZT) Regimen for Decreasing Perinatal Transmission of the Human Immunodeficiency Virus

During pregnancy	Begin AZT after week 14 (200 mg three times/day or 300 mg twice/day). Continue maternal therapy to keep viral levels as low as possible, optimally undetectable.
Labor and delivery	2 mg/kg AZT intravenously during the first hour and then 1 mg/kg/hour until infant is delivered.
Newborn	2 mg/kg AZT given four times/day orally for the first 6 weeks of life.

Centers for Disease Control and Prevention. U.S. Public Health Service Task Force recommendations for use of antiretroviral drugs in pregnant HIV infected women for maternal health and for interventions to reduce perinatal HIV-1 transmission in the United States. *MMWR Morb Mortal Wkly Rep.* 2002;51:1–38.

to maternal blood include avoiding episiotomies and scalp electrodes whenever possible and bathing the infant before giving intramuscular injections such as vitamin K.

THE HIV-POSITIVE INFANT

The diagnosis of HIV infection is most difficult to make in the first months of life. The presence or absence of HIV antibody in the newborn is a reflection only of maternal serostatus. Immunoglobulin G (IgG) is actively transported across the placenta to the unborn fetus, and thus a positive HIV antibody test at birth is not diagnostic of infection, but does reflect the presence of IgG antibody in the mother. Uninfected children will serorevert by 8 months and certainly by 15 months of age. Children who are infected will begin to produce their own immunoglobulin in the first months of life, and that antibody persists as maternal antibody fades. A small number of very ill children with active disease and malnutrition do not produce antibody and remain seronegative despite infection. A positive serologic test after the age of 15 months can be assumed to be true evidence of infection in the infant. However, a negative test in an ill and especially in a malnourished infant can be falsely negative. Better diagnostic tests in infancy are viral culture or an antigen test—PCR assay by deoxyribonucleic acid (DNA) or RNA. Currently it is recommended that screening of infants at birth should be by HIV PCR assay by DNA at birth, and by PCR assay by RNA serially over time. PCR tests are cheaper and faster than viral culture. Infection should be diagnosed only if two separate tests of two different specimens are positive.

Infants born to HIV-infected mothers should also be started on trimethoprim/sulfamethoxazole (TMP/SMX) prophylaxis at about 4 to 6 weeks of age. This recommendation is based on the observation that some infected infants present with *Pneumocystis* pneumonia before the accurate diagnosis of HIV infection. If the infant is determined to be uninfected, the medication is discontinued. The HIV-positive infant should be continued on TMP/SMX until 1 year of age. Continuation of treatment after 1 year of therapy is determined by the immune status of the infected child.

Other pediatric care should be routine. Children should receive all standard vaccines in the first year of life, regardless of serostatus, including inactivated poliomyelitis vaccine (IPV), diphtheria-pertussis-tetanus (DPT), hepatitis B, pneumococcal, *Haemophilus influenzae* type B (HIB), and mumps-measles-rubella (MMR) at the appropriate ages. The only vaccine to avoid in the infected infant and young child is the chickenpox vaccine, because it is a live viral vaccine. However, in children with adequate immune function, consideration should be given to including this vaccine. The MMR is given despite being a live viral vaccine and appears safe. Exposure of the HIV-infected child without vaccine immunity to active cases of chickenpox or measles is an indication for passive protection by giving varicella-zoster immune globulin (chickenpox) or immune globulin (measles), because these infections can be life threatening in a child with serious immune deficiency. Children should receive the influenza vaccine each year. Uninfected children living in a home with infected adults should receive the same vaccines, avoiding the oral polio vaccine, which is no longer standard in this country.

With the development of highly active antiretroviral therapy (HAART) against HIV, long-term survival of both adults and children with HIV infection has improved and fewer children have a rapidly progressive course of disease. Untreated HIV infection in children infected during the perinatal period usually presents in the first years of life. The clinical diagnosis of HIV infection can be suggested by finding typical manifestations of an immunodeficiency, such as failure to thrive and diarrhea, or opportunistic infections such as severe persisting thrush. Recurrent bacterial infections, such as otitis media, may be the first manifestation of the progressive immunodeficiency associated with HIV infection. Untreated children occasionally present with HIV encephalopathy, others with parotitis and diffuse lymphadenopathy with hepatosplenomegaly. Some children remain well and undiagnosed until much later, maintaining steady HIV serum levels and stable T cell function for years. (For the manifestations and the CDC system of describing the severity of pediatric HIV infection, refer to Chapter 25) The decision to start treatment in children is based on viral levels and the clinical status of the child. Children with high viral loads that persist beyond the first months of life are at highest risk for rapid progression and death if untreated. Recommendations for treatment, with frequent updates available based on the latest data, can be found at www.aidsinfo.nih.gov.

The survival of children, like that of adults with HIV, is dependent on complex regimens of antiretroviral medications, usually involving multiple medications with significant side effects. Resistance occurs quickly if medications are not taken reliably and as directed. The issue of adherence to medication is perhaps the most serious psychosocial issue facing children with HIV.[27] Children born into poverty and into difficult social situations are those most likely to experience difficulty with medication adherence. In one series, the social stigma of HIV infection, especially in African-American women with children, appeared to intensify the chronic sorrow, social isolation, poverty, and social pain of being infected with HIV.[28]

DEVELOPMENTAL AND NEUROBIOLOGIC ISSUES

Most HIV-infected newborns appear normal at birth and begin to develop normally. However, infant neurodevelopmental delay and impairment does occur in some HIV-infected infants and may be directly related to infection. However, other factors frequently complicate the evaluation of young children with HIV infection. These include prenatal or perinatal distress, other disease processes, including opportunistic infections, as well as the many psychosocial stressors found among HIV-infected mothers. Recent studies that have included seroreverted HIV-negative siblings as controls have provided a greater appreciation of the complexity of factors contributing to infant and childhood neurobehavioral development in the context of HIV infection. For example, a longitudinal study of perinatally infected children found that the high rate of emotional and behavioral problems previously associated with pediatric HIV infection was found to be similar to that of their noninfected siblings.[29] In fact, neither HIV status nor prenatal drug use predicted the behavioral problems that were highly prevalent in this cohort. Other factors, such as the disruption of primary caregiver or residence, impoverished developmental environment, and maternal illness or loss may provide as significant a contribution to the long-term neurobehavioral development of HIV-positive children as does their HIV serostatus. More than once, a child with severe failure to thrive, at first attributed to HIV infection, has grown normally when removed from a difficult social situation and placed in a stable home.

As a neurotropic virus, HIV displays a predilection for the central nervous system (CNS), and it is therefore the CNS that appears to be the primary pathway by which the virus can affect the mental and physical development of the child. In the developing infant, delayed neurodevelopmental milestones or the failure to acquire these milestones may be the presenting symptom of HIV infection. This is a nonspecific finding, occurring with any serious illness or infection in the young infant. For example, an infant with untreated miliary tuberculosis will also fail to make milestones and may lose those already acquired.

In a study comparing HIV-positive infants and their seroreverting counterparts, HIV infection predicted lower scores on individually administered psychometric assessments of developmental function in infants less than 30 months of age,[30] and baseline scores on the Bayley Scales of Infant Development independently predicted mortality in a cohort of vertically infected HIV-positive infants.[31]

Progressive encephalopathy may be a manifestation of HIV infection due to direct CNS involvement. A child who has been developing normally gradually begins to lose milestones despite adequate nutrition, in contrast to the nonspecific loss of milestones in a very sick child. The child who was walking well begins to toe walk, then has trouble walking at all, difficulty sitting alone, and eventually is unable to roll over. The first manifestation of progressive encephalopathy is increased tone and brisk reflexes in the lower extremities which, if sought, will be present before the loss of function. The child is initially alert and appears oriented to person and place despite the progressive loss of motor function. Ultimately, the untreated child becomes quiet and poorly responsive and death will follow. Before standard screening and treatment was available, progressive HIV encephalopathy occurred in up to 35% of children infected with HIV; since the implementation of HAART the rate has declined to less than 2%.[32]

The diagnosis of HIV-related encephalopathy can be confirmed by demonstrating HIV in cerebrospinal fluid (CSF). Often there is a mild pleocytosis and perhaps a mildly elevated CSF protein. Glucose is usually normal. Brain scans such as magnetic resonance imaging or computed tomography may show nonspecific findings associated with sick infants such as calcifications in the basal ganglia. Atrophy will be present in late stages. Encephalopathy may result from other pathogens that may occur with AIDS, such as cytomegalovirus. However, the slowly progressive loss of milestones and hyper-reflexia in a child with HIV infection is very characteristic of HIV disease and should suggest this diagnosis in an infant, even without known HIV infection. HIV testing is indicated, and if HIV infection is found, treatment should be started immediately.

The encephalopathy is responsive to treatment of the HIV infection with antiretrovirals. Even in the first studies that used a single agent, AZT, the encephalopathy was noted to be responsive to therapy, although viral resistance is more likely with monotherapy. The response can be impressive; the infant begins to become more interested in the world and to relearn recently lost skills, correlating with a fall in viral titers. There is no specific drug to be used; the goal is to control the systemic infection, and therapy should be guided by such factors as likely resistance patterns in the infant. The aim is to control the viral load in the serum and, with this, the CSF. With the availability of HAART, progressive HIV encephalopathy can be arrested, although relapse remains a risk should viral control be lost and residual cognitive and neurologic impairments may persist.

In end-stage AIDS, when disease has become unresponsive to treatment, there is progressive infection. Death is often related to encephalopathy or a severe wasting syndrome. In a prospective longitudinal study, the immediate cause of death in infants who died from AIDS was most often infection; in older children, wasting and HIV-related cardiac disease became more common.[33]

THE ROLE OF THE PSYCHIATRY LIAISON

The identification of the HIV-infected infant calls for the education and support of the family. Basic family and environmental needs must be identified, supported, and/or met before optimal long-term benefit can be achieved through medical and pharmacotherapy. The psychiatry liaison can play a vital role in assessing and supporting adherence with recommendations. The caregiver of the newborn must be educated regarding the need for confirmatory testing, the regimen for HIV prophylaxis, and the importance of medication adherence to increase the likelihood of viral inhibition and reduce the risk of developing drug resistance. The HIV-positive mother must be informed about the possibility of HIV transmission with breast feeding and encouraged to choose the safer alternative of bottle feeding. The caregiver must be educated regarding the signs and symptoms that may indicate HIV-associated complications, such as fever, respiratory symptoms, persistent thrush or diaper rashes, changes in mental status, and slowed growth or failure to achieve, or loss of, developmental milestones. Siblings may require testing and evaluation. Finally, the maintenance of mental and physical well-being of mother is crucial to the well-being of her infant. It has been noted that women are less likely than men to receive optimal HIV and AIDS therapy,[34] and mothers burdened by caregiving responsibilities have been found to have very low rates of antiviral adherence.[35]

These considerations assume the availability of family and willingness of caregivers to follow medical recommendations. Conflict may arise when parental choice differs from what is felt to be in the best interest of the child. During pregnancy, overriding parental choice intrudes on the privacy rights of the mother. After birth, however, parental nonadherence with the medical care of an infant may constitute neglect. Investigating the basis of the noncompliance may identify misconceptions regarding treatment or barriers to care that can be addressed. For example, cultural issues may factor into infant feeding decisions and be amenable to additional education and support. However, neglect may also arise from the incapacity of the parent to make informed decisions regarding her child, due to her own psychiatric illness or substance use. There may be instances in which a competency evaluation of the parent and involvement of the legal system become necessary for the appropriate care of the infant. Cooperative involvement with the caregiver is always preferable to forced care, which invariably strains the doctor–patient relationship. A team approach from the outset, whenever possible, increases the likelihood of optimally engaging the infant and caregiver.

SUMMARY

Medical breakthroughs in the treatment and prevention of HIV infection and AIDS have offered the hope of the elimination of perinatal infection in the United States, while highlighting the disparity between the United States and the Third World. In sub-Saharan Africa, children made up almost 8% of those living with HIV disease in 2004, with the overwhelming majority infected through vertical transmission. Three quarters of HIV-infected sub-Saharan African young people between the ages of 15 and 24 are female, and fewer than 10% of pregnant women are offered services proven to prevent vertical HIV transmission; thus there is a reasonable expectation that this 8% will rise.[36] Even in the United States, the changing epidemiology of HIV disease and AIDS underscores the increasing divide between those who have access to care and those who do not. As the infection takes hold among women and children globally, and among women of color locally, it is found increasingly among the poor and disenfranchised. Our scientific progress will be of limited value if it does not reach those in need. Integrated treatment and prevention efforts with appropriate funding hold the greatest hope for controlling HIV infection and AIDS.[37] Such integrated treatment and prevention is best exemplified in the management of the at-risk pregnant woman in which optimal care includes education and support, efforts toward prevention of transmission, and comprehensive prenatal and HIV disease care for the mother.

REFERENCES

1. www.cdc.gov/hiv/topics/surveillance/resources/reports/2004report/table23.htm.
2. Available at: www.unaids.org/epi/2005/doc/EPIupdate2005_pdf_en/epi-update2005_en.pdf. Accessed February 5, 2006.
3. Ahmad N. The vertical transmission of human immunodeficiency virus type 1: molecular and biological properties of the virus. *Crit Rev Clin Lab Sci*. 2005;42:1–34.
4. Kuhn L, Abrams EJ, Palumbo P, et al. Maternal versus paternal inheritance of HLA class I alleles among HIV-infected children: consequences for clinical disease progression. *AIDS*. 2004;18:1281–1289.
5. Goldfarb J: Breastfeeding: AIDS and other infectious diseases. *Clin Perinatol*. 1993;20:225–243.
6. Sperling RS, Shapiro DE, Coombs RW, et al. Maternal viral load, zidovudine treatment and the risk of transmission of human immunodeficiency virus type 1 from mother to infant. *N Engl J Med*. 1996;335:1621–1629.
7. The International Perinatal HIV Group. The mode of delivery and the risk of vertical transmission of human immunodeficiency virus type 1. *N Engl J Med*. 1999;340:977–987.
8. Schuman P, Jones TB, Ohmit S, Marbury C, Laken MP. Voluntary HIV counseling and testing of pregnant women: an assessment of compliance with Michigan public health statutes. *Med Gen Med*. 2004;6:52.

9. Paltrow LM, Cohen DS, Carey CA. Women's Law Project & National Advocates for Pregnant Women: year 2000 overview—governmental responses to pregnant women who use alcohol and other drugs. October 2000. Available at: http://www.advocatesforpregnantwomen.org/articles/gov_response_review.pdf. Accessed February 5, 2006.
10. *The State, Respondent v. Regina McKnight*, Supreme Court of South Carolina, 352 S.C. 635; 576 S.E. 2d 168; 2004 S.C. Lexis 23. TX and OK legislation.
11. Fernandez MI, Wilson TE, Ethier KA, Walter EB, Gay CL, Moore J. Acceptance of HIV testing during prenatal care. *Public Health Rep*. 2000;115:460–468.
12. Anderson JE, Ebrahinm SH, Sansom S. Women's knowledge about treatment to prevent mother-to-child human immunodeficiency virus transmission. *Obstet Gynecol*. 2004;103:165–168.
13. Demmer C. Quality of life and risk perception among predominantly heterosexual, minority individuals with HIV/AIDS. *AIDS Patient Care STDs*. 2001;15:481–489.
14. Wolf LE, Lo B, Gostin LO. Legal barriers to implementing recommendations for universal, routine prenatal HIV testing. *J Law Med Ethics*. 2004;32:137–147.
15. Mutcherson KM. No way to treat a woman: creating an appropriate standard for resolving medical treatment disputes involving HIV-positive children. *Harv Womens Law J*. 2002;25:221–279.
16. Wolf LE, Lo B, Gostin LO. Legal barriers to implementing recommendations for universal, routine prenatal HIV testing. *J Law Med Ethics*. 2004 Spring;32:137–147.
17. Office of the Inspector General. Reducing obstetrician barriers to offering HIV testing. 2002. Available: http://oig.hhs.gov/oei/reports/oei-05-01-00260.pdf. Accessed February 5, 2006.
18. Lampe M, Branson B, Paul S, Burr C, et al. Rapid HIV antibody testing during labor and delivery for women of unknown HIV status. Atlanta: Centers for Disease Control and Prevention; 2004. Available at: www.cdc.gov/hiv/projects/perinatal.Accessed February 5, 2006.
19. Aynalem G, Mendoza P, Frederick T, Mascola L. Who and why? HIV-testing refusal during pregnancy: implication for pediatric HIV epidemic disparity. *AIDS Behav*. 2004;8:25–31.
20. American Academy of Pediatrics. *Redbook of the American Academy of Pediatrics*. Elk Grove Village, Ill; 2004.
21. Minkoff H. HIV infection in pregnancy. *Obstet Gynecol*. 2003;101:797–810.
22. Watts DH. Management of human immunodeficiency virus infection in pregnancy. *N Engl J Med*. 2002;346:1879–1891.
23. Centers for Disease Control and Prevention. Guidelines for national human immunodeficiency virus case surveillance, including monitoring for human immunodeficiency virus infection and acquired immunodeficiency syndrome. *MMWR Morb Mortal Wkly Rep*. 1999;48:1–28.
24. Lallemant M, Jourdain G, Le Coeur S, et al. A trial of shortened zidovudine regimens to prevent mother-to-child transmission of human immunodeficiency virus type 1: perinatal HIV trial (Thailand) investigators. *N Engl J Med*. 2000;343:982–991.
25. Wade NA, Birhead GS, Warren BL, et al. Abbreviated regimens of zidovudine prophylaxis and perinatal transmission of the human immunodeficiency virus. *N Engl J Med*. 1998;339:1409–1414.
26. Guay LA, Musoke P, Fleming T, et al. Intrapartum and neonatal single-does nevirapine compared with zidovudine for prevention of mother-to-child transmission of HIV in Kampala, Uganda. *Lancet*. 1999;354:795–802.
27. Mellins CA, Brackis-Cott E, Dolezal C, Abrams EJ. The role of psychosocial and family factors in adherence to antiretroviral treatment in human immunodeficiency virus-infected children. *Pediatr Infect Dis J*. 2004;23:1035–1041.
28. Lichtenstein B, Laska MD, Clair JM. Chronic sorrow in the HIV-positive patient: issues of race, gender and social support. *AIDS Patient Care STDs*. 2002;16:27–38.
29. Mellins CA, Smith R, O'Driscoll P, et al. High rates of behavioral problems in perinatally HIV-infected children are not linked to HIV disease. *Pediatrics*. 2003;111:384–393.
30. Knight WG, Mellins CA, Levinson RL, Arpadi SM, Kairam R. Brief report: effects of pediatric HIV infection on mental and psychomotor development. *J Pediatr Psychol*. 2000;25:583–587.
31. Llorente A, Brouwers P, Charurat M, et al. Women and Infant Transmission Study Group: Early neurodevelopmental markers predictive of mortality in infants infected with HIV-1. *Def Med Child Neurol*. 2003;45:76–84.
32. Chiriboga CA, Fleishman S, Champion S, Gaye-Robinson L, Abrams EJ. Incidence and prevalence of HIV encephalopathy in children with HIV infection receiving highly active anti-retroviral therapy (HAART). *J Pediatr*. 2005:146:402–407.
33. Langston C, Cooper ER, Goldfarb J, et al. Human immunodeficiency virus-related mortality in infants and children: data from the pediatric pulmonary and cardiovascular complications of vertically transmitted HIV (P2C2) study. *Pediatrics*. 2001;107:328–338.
34. Shapiro MF, Morton SC, McCaffrey DF, et al. Variations in the care of HIV-infected adults in the United States: results from the HIV cost and utilization study. *JAMA*. 1999;281:2305–2315.
35. Murphy DA, Greenwell L, Hoffman D. Factors associated with antiretroviral adherence among HIV- infected women with children. *Women Health*. 2002;36:97–111.
36. Joint United Nations Programme on HIV/AIDS (UNAIDS) World Health Organization (WHO), AIDS Epidemic Update 2004. Available at: http://www.unaids.org/wad2004/EPIupdate2004_html_en/epi04_00_en.htm. Accessed February 2005.
37. Farmer P. AIDS as a global emergency. *Bull World Health Org*. 2003;81:699.

CHAPTER 25

HIV/AIDS Among Children and Adolescents

Andres J. Pumariega, Margaret A. Shugart, JoAnne B. Pumariega

EPIDEMIOLOGY, RISK FACTORS, AND CONSEQUENCES

Worldwide, 1 million of the 7 million people with acquired immunodeficiency syndrome (AIDS) are children and adolescents and 2 million children and adolescents have died from AIDS, with 90% of those infected living in developing nations. Half of the approximately 6 million infections diagnosed worldwide annually occur among people 15 to 24 years of age; approximately 25% of the 40,000 new infections per year in the United States occur in people 13 to 21 years of age. In the United States, mortality from human immunodeficiency virus (HIV) infection and AIDS has decreased in people under 24 years of age, but the hopes presented by new treatments and preventive efforts have been darkened by the continuous increase in risk reported among American youth.[1-3]

Pediatric AIDS is seen disproportionately among children of color. Of the 3,788 children under the age of 13 living with AIDS in 2003, 570 were non-Hispanic White, 2,461 were African American, 853 were Hispanic/Latino, 17 were Asian-American, and 10 were American Indian. The children that run the highest risk of infection from HIV-infected mothers are infants born to mothers who are prostitutes or intravenous drug users (IDUs); mothers whose sexual partners are bisexual, have hemophilia, or abuse drugs; infants with a history of blood transfusions; and infants who have hemophilia. Children can also become infected with HIV through exposure to nonsterilized needles, or by breast feeding from an infected mother. Most cases among children and youth in the United States occur in the coastal states and large urban areas. Socioeconomic and cultural factors among Latino and African-American populations, such as poverty, high drug use, and sexual lifestyles are also factors in the prevalence of AIDS among their descendants.[1-3]

Based on current trends, a young person aged 13 to 21 years is infected with the HIV virus in the United States every hour of every day. HIV spreads sexually among the adolescent population more than in any other group. Adolescents who are homosexual or use drugs, youthful offenders who drop out of school or run away from home, and immigrant youth are especially vulnerable to HIV infection. These youth are frequently difficult to reach through prevention and education efforts and have limited access to medical insurance. The African-American and Latino populations are disproportionately represented amongst adolescents contracting HIV infection, accounting for over 85% of AIDS cases in 2002. Adolescent females also represent a higher proportion of new HIV and AIDS cases, with 50% of new cases between ages 13 and 19, compared in 2002, and 66% of adolescent females infected in heterosexual encounters. School dropouts constitute approximately 3 million adolescents in the United States (12.7%) and are primarily youth of color. This group of youth has a high frequency of behaviors (particularly unprotected sexual activity and intravenous drug use) that place them at risk for contracting HIV or some other sexually transmitted disease and have the least accessibility to prevention programs.[1-3]

AIDS is the seventh leading cause of death among children from 1 to 4 years of age and the sixth main cause of death between ages 15 and 24 years in the United States. The first children infected with HIV were described in 1983. From that beginning, the global epidemic of HIV has had a deep impact on the health of children and their survival. At least all the infections of HIV among young children are due to vertical transmission, which can occur in utero, intrapartum (through exposure to maternal blood products or transfusions), or postpartum through breast feeding. Detection during the interpartum period with more sophisticated screening and diagnostic tests provides a crucial opportunity for prevention. Transmission after childbirth through the mother contributes about a third to half of the world's vertical transmission, which can be prevented with timely maternal treatment with retrovirals. In the absence of maternal antiretroviral treatment, the risk of HIV infection among infants is approximately 25% (ranging from 10% in European studies to 45% in African studies), but can go down to 4% to 8% with maternal and infant antiretroviral treatment. Carefully designed studies of the epidemic are clarifying immunologic, virologic, genetic, and behavioral factors that affect the risk of transmission of HIV from the mother to the infant, as well as response to antiretrovirals, and the natural history of the HIV infection in prenatally infected children.[1] Major advances in pediatric AIDS, however, have been the dramatic decrease in the number of new cases under the age of 13 (from 952 in 1992 to 50 in 2003), as well as the decrease in mortality from HIV disease and AIDS in both the under-13 and 14- to 24-year age-groups in the United States. This has been the result of perinatal maternal testing and of more effective antiretroviral therapies.[3]

A major remaining challenge is the translation of these advances to poorer, underserved populations and Third World regions of the world. One geographic area that has not received much attention related to the HIV/AIDS epidemic is Latin America. Given its proximity to the United States and its contribution to immigration, particularly of young immigrants, it merits much closer attention. The Pan American Health Organization reports that today there is probably a higher rate of HIV infection in Latin America than in the United States. As of 1997, approximately 470,000 people have died of AIDS in the hemisphere, with 90,000 orphans resulting in Latin America alone, but these figures are considered underestimates. Among the 812,000 cases reported in the hemisphere, all but 14,000 are pediatric cases. Among the 22.6 million people worldwide that are considered living with HIV disease or AIDS, 1.6 millions live in the Latin American and Caribbean region. Unless prevention programs are refocused on these affected groups, the HIV virus could become the main cause of death among youth in Latin America and the Caribbean.[4]

Providing care to these populations, to patients and their families in these countries, is an enormous task given the limited resources of developing nations. Additionally, the lower socioeconomic status of women and children substantially limits the effectiveness of programs for care and prevention in developing nations.[4]

NEUROCOGNITIVE ASPECTS OF HIV/AIDS IN CHILDREN

Among children, HIV penetrates early into the central nervous system (CNS) during the course of the illness. Abnormalities of the CNS are significant and frequent complications of AIDS in infants and children. Although their causes can be related to HIV infection, malnutrition and poor prenatal and postnatal care can also contribute significantly to such problems. Other factors that affect the neuropsychological function of seropositive children include prenatal insults and other diseases, such as other infections, strokes, and neoplasms.[1]

Neurocognitive deterioration appears to be associated with the increased replication of the HIV virus, resulting in HIV-associated progressive encephalopathy (HIV-PE). HIV-PE is associated with a triad of symptoms: impaired brain growth, progressive motor dysfunction, and loss or plateauing of developmental milestones. HIV-PE has an estimated prevalence of 13% to 23% among infected children. The course of HIV-PE in infants or young children is determined by its timing in the child's brain development, the strain of HIV, and genetic vulnerabilities. Three patterns of abnormal neurocognitive development have been described with HIV-PE: rapid HIV-PE with loss of attained milestones, subacute progression of encephalopathy with relatively stable periods, and static encephalopathy with failure to achieve new milestones. Longitudinal assessments allow the differentiation between HIV-PE and mental retardation resulting from other factors, such as maternal drug addiction and poor prenatal care. There is no obvious correlation between immunologic status and the development of HIV-PE.[5,6]

Autopsy studies on patients with HIV-PE reveal decreased brain weight, inflammatory changes, calcifications of basal ganglia vessels, white matter deterioration, and astrocytosis.[6] Proposed mechanisms for the pathogenesis of HIV disease in the CNS include direct neuronal injury, macrophage destruction resulting in neurotoxicity, dysfunction caused by viral products, neuroreceptor blockade, coinfection with other agents, autoimmune reactions, antibody-mediated cellular toxicity, integration of the provirus in CNS cell lines, alteration of the blood–brain barrier, and brain vascular changes.[5,6] High frequencies of vascular lesions, ranging from aneurysms to infarctions, have been found using neuroimaging studies.[7] The overall computed tomography (CT) brain scan severity rating and the level of the neurotoxin quinolinic acid in the cerebrospinal fluid have been found to be highly predictive of the level of cognitive functioning and impairment in children.[8]

Among children, the deterioration of language skills commonly occurs with HIV infections, particularly expressive more than receptive language. The periodic evaluation of language development should be part of the regular monitoring of infants and children with HIV infection as a method of evaluating the progression of the illness and the effectiveness of prescribed treatment. Visual-spatial and visual-motor skills are cognitive functions sensitive to the stage of the illness, method of transmission, and the environment in which the child lives.[5] In one recent study, HIV-infected patients and control children had similar performance on a panel of neuropsychological tests except for spatial learning and memory using the Children's Memory Scale total score. Choline levels in the hippocampus correlated positively with the delayed spatial memory tests in the patients, but not in the controls.[9] Learning disabilities associated with cognitive impairment can be seen in elementary school–age children infected with HIV, which can be associated with gradual diminution in their mental function because of the disruption of cortical or subcortical structures.[10]

The use of the retroviral medications can moderate some of the functional difficulties faced by these children and improve cognitive deficits, at least for a period of time. There is greater efficacy of retroviral treatment associated with greater brain impairment before treatment and better CNS penetration of the antiretroviral agent. However, the effect of retroviral treatment has not been sustained in many children beyond 6 months of treatment, with cognitive decline in the face of virologic and immunologic improvement, though recent advances have been made in this area. Specific neuropathologic and neuropsychological deficits are probably permanent, and there are limitations posed by the mechanisms of action of retroviral treatment (resulting in mutations and viral resistance), as well as interactions amongst multiple drugs.[1,11]

PSYCHOLOGICAL IMPACT OF PEDIATRIC AIDS

HIV infection and AIDS have a very significant psychosocial impact on patients, their families, and society in general, including psychological, cognitive, emotional, and social effects. This illness in children has important and durable effects on their families. Additionally, most families affected by HIV disease are of minority and disadvantaged backgrounds and are already discriminated against and stigmatized in the society. AIDS affects many children and adolescents with parents who are also victims of the disease themselves. There are thousands of children with fathers who are close to death or already dead, and thousands with mothers who have died from AIDS or are too ill to serve their role of primary parent or caregiver. Even when the parents live, psychological pressures on the parents, the use of drugs, and their sexual lifestyles are parts of the conflicts between parents infected with HIV and their adolescents.[1,12,13]

In the year 2000, approximately 100,000 children younger than 18 years of age lost their mothers to AIDS. Approximately one third of these children live with a father who is HIV-positive, one third with a grandmother, and one third in an orphanage or adoptive care. Most of the caretakers for children with HIV disease are single mothers who face the biggest challenges in their lives alone, and are overextended with the responsibility of caregiving. Those families are primarily African American and Latino of low socioeconomic levels and of limited economic resources. The children have been sensitized to loss and anticipated separation, and their caretakers feel a great burden of anguish and anticipatory grief. The caretakers of these children need to be aware of the problems of children infected with HIV. The physical and psychological care of these children and infected adolescents are a major challenge, and it affects the whole family system.[12] At the other end of the spectrum, the transition from adolescence to adulthood and greater self-sufficiency also present significant challenges to HIV-infected youth. Youth need to address a number of adaptations, ranging from greater demands for self-management of their health care, the impact of their illness on their emerging sexuality and independence, and the often difficult transition from familiar pediatric health care settings to unfamiliar adult providers.[2]

There is great psychological impact on the increasing numbers of adolescents and children acquiring the HIV infection and developing AIDS from the medical and psychosocial consequences of the illness. Many of them have lost parents, other relatives, and friends to AIDS, leading to a double psychological impact. These children are beneficiaries of the greater openness around the diagnosis of HIV infection and AIDS, but there are many other cultural and social conditions that complicate their future adaptation. The stigmatizing public response, with fear of contagion, association with drugs and homosexuality, and anxiety about the threat of contracting the disease, lead to feelings of isolation and rejection.[1]

Children and adolescents with HIV disease or AIDS experience more subjective distress than their uninfected peers, including dysphoria from the physiologic effects of the illness, hopelessness, preoccupation with their illness, and poor body image. Facing and understanding their own possible death are major challenges faced by children and youth with HIV infection. The cognitive and emotional maturity of the child often determines their level of awareness about their own mortality, as well as their coping skills and defenses to deal with this realization. Children's reactions can range from unawareness of the finality of death in very young children, to increasing awareness and anxiety in the elementary age period, to major existential conflicts in teenagers. Negative and traumatic life events such as forced disclosure about their illness, a history of abuse (physical or sexual), and loss of a parent or sibling contribute to heightened distress. Coping with HIV infection may trigger many emotional responses, including social withdrawal, loneliness, anger, confusion, fear, numbness, and guilt. Various adaptive cognitive approaches and coping styles are used by HIV-infected children and youth, including denial, reaction formation, resignation, self-calming, and distraction.

Some adolescents with HIV infection or AIDS report more sexual risk-taking behaviors and conduct and hyperactivity disorders, at times driven by their underlying distress. Also contributing to the level of experienced distress is the cultural context within which HIV disease or AIDS is experienced by the child or adolescent. People of different racial/ethnic and socioeconomic backgrounds cope with HIV/AIDS in different ways, according to their social mores and cultural traditions, thus experiencing varying levels of stigma, shame, or social support. The success or failure of these coping reactions or strategies not only influence the level of emotional distress experienced by children with HIV disease or AIDS, but also the distress they experience from pain and their demands for pain relief.[1,14,15]

Children with HIV disease suffer of a wide spectrum of psychiatric manifestations that extend from depression to anxiety to behavioral disturbances. Among adults with HIV disease or AIDS, lifetime rates of depression range from 32% to 56%, and suicidality is common among homosexual and bisexual men. In one study of 34 HIV-positive adolescents using structured diagnostic interviews, 44% presented with current major depression, 85% had at least one *Diagnostic and Statistical Manual of Mental Disorders (DSM)* diagnosis, and 53% had a history of psychiatric disorders before HIV infection. Another study comparing children with HIV infection with children with asthma showed that anxiety disorders were more common in the HIV-infected group than in the asthma group. Children who have depression are isolated and fear an early and unavoidable death. They also suffer anxiety accompanied by the fear of transmission and feel guilty to be a burden to their family.[1,15,16]

The brothers and sisters of children suffering with HIV disease experience numerous emotional difficulties. Frequently, those not affected by the illness report anger because they have to assist their sibling with the illness. Many of the siblings feel guilty to not be the one affected, and they feel isolated and fearful of contracting the illness. The fear of contracting the illness by the nonaffected sibling is influenced by numerous factors such as their age, level of education, knowledge of and understanding about the illness, and attitudes about the illness.[1]

INTERVENTION AND PSYCHOLOGICAL AND PSYCHIATRIC TREATMENT

The family with children with HIV disease is generally a family dealing with crisis, illness, lack of resources, and social isolation and in need of support and medical, psychological, and social services. There is also a high frequency of comorbid drug abuse and mental disorders in HIV-infected parents. It is important to assist these children and their families through interdisciplinary interventions oriented to improving the child's and family's quality of life. Family-centered approaches have been advocated that address family stresses, adaptation, and cultural factors affecting the whole family. They also provide developmentally appropriate supports for the infected child and siblings and connect families to services and community resources and supports (including medical, mental health, social welfare services, and such critical services as respite care) through case management.[1,17,18]

Comprehensive psychiatric, psychological, and neurologic assessments are critical components in the overall care for children and youth with HIV disease. Psychiatric evaluation is important in assessing the presence of depressive, anxiety, and psychotic symptoms (such as hallucinations) related to the psychological impact of the illness on the child and/or the effects of retroviral treatment. Mental status evaluation is important in determining the presence of any symptoms of attention deficits, memory impairment, or even full-blown dementia in advanced cases. Neurologic examination is important to detect the presence of such signs as abnormal reflexes, bradykinesis, and spasticity. Neuroimaging tests are also important in such comprehensive evaluations when more advanced neuropsychiatric complications are suspected. Electroencephalography (EEG) is important whenever there is any suspicion of seizure activity or focal neurologic findings.[1,2,11]

Psychological and neuropsychological testing and neuroimaging tests are important in providing objective baseline assessment of cognitive and developmental progress and whenever there is suspicion of developmental delay or cognitive dysfunction. These include the Weschler Intellectual Scales for Children (4th edition), the Children's Memory Scale (CMS, a spatial memory test), and the CMS Long Delay (spatial memory after long delay) in older children and youth and the Bailey Scales of Development and the Vineland scales in younger children.[5,8–10] Computed tomography (CT) of the head can be used to evaluate structural changes associated with neuropsychiatric complications, such as microcalcifications (especially in the basal ganglia) and brain atrophy with increased ventricular size and increased cerebral sulci. Magnetic resonance imaging (MRI) of the head can be used to evaluate cerebrovascular findings, such as signs of ischemic strokes and cerebral artery aneurysms and the presence of mass lesions from toxoplasmosis or CNS lymphoma.[2,6–8]

Therapeutic support has the greatest role in the care of the children with HIV disease. Supportive and cognitive therapy for these children and their parents and families is essential because they are most vulnerable to separation and loss. Support groups and structured programs for HIV-infected youth have demonstrated effectiveness. The use of active strategies within these groups, such as problem-solving and help-seeking, have been shown to be helpful, though these are more consistent with Western cultural orientations. Two important areas of focus in support groups are those of disclosure of HIV infection and adherence with treatment, with failure of disclosure out of fear of social stigma often leading to poor treatment adherence. Improving adherence with HIV treatment regimens and approaches to disclosure of HIV status can also be the target of psychosocial and support group interventions, with youth sharing effective strategies for addressing both challenges.[1,2,19]

Safe-sex practice interventions have been developed for HIV-infected youth to enhance the use of condoms, build social skills, improve self-efficacy, and create supportive peer norms. These interventions target the cognitive immaturity and exploratory learning behaviors commonly seen in adolescents, as well as other factors such as impulsivity, distress, and adverse life experiences. Both psychotherapeutic and psychoeducational approaches have been shown to be effective in reducing risky sexual behaviors. For example, a study by Brown et al.[1] reported a 12-month motivational skills intervention with 111 adolescents living with hemophilia and HIV disease and demonstrated significant increases in condom use, safer sexual practices, and increased self-efficacy.

The care of children infected with HIV is very difficult and affects the whole family system. Psychological supportive therapy for the family and caregivers of infected children is an area of mental health services in very high demand and need. These services help reduce isolation, promote family function, and teach coping skills and abilities.[12]

The most frequent psychodynamic themes for children infected with HIV involve guilt, self-esteem, and matters related to death. Mental health professionals can help the child face guilt feelings, feelings of being punished, depression, and fears of death. Both individual and group therapies are effective. Individual therapy could be brief or long-term and could be supportive, cognitive, behavioral, or psychodynamic in focus. It is very important to form a strong alliance with the family in the treatment of children with HIV disease. The parents and family of children with HIV disease feel extremely guilty about the transmission of the illness.[15]

Psychopharmacologic treatment of seropositive children and adolescents with HIV is the subject of a lot of debate. A balance of risks versus benefits in the use of pharmacotherapy needs to be determined for each individual case. The hyperactivity associated with HIV encephalopathy in children has been treated with methylphenidate and clonidine, with good results. Although psychotherapy should be used in the treatment of anxiety in patients with HIV disease or AIDS, the use of anxiolytics could be necessary. It is preferred to use an anxiolytic with short-acting rather than longer-acting pharmacokinetics. Many experts believe that depression in patients with AIDS should be treated aggressively with antidepressant medications. Selected serotonin reuptake inhibitor (SSRI) antidepressants have been used with very good results in older patients with AIDS; tricyclic antidepressants can worsen the confusion associated with HIV encephalopathy.[20,21] With children, it is especially important to begin with a small dose and then increase it slowly until the therapeutic effect and dose are reached. It is also important to be aware of drug interactions between psychiatric and neurologic medications (such as sedative hypnotics, amphetamines, anticonvulsants, and some antidepressants) and some retrovirals, either through direct interactions or the inhibition of hepatic metabolism. These may result in the child or adolescent with HIV disease or AIDS not being able to use some psychiatric medications (such as sedative hypnotics and amphetamines) or requiring lower doses (such as with carbamazepine and bupriopion[1]).

Changes in antiretroviral therapy may be indicated when there is toxicity or intolerance of the current regimen, failure of the current regimen, or evidence that another regimen offers superior results. In the case of failure of highly active antiretroviral therapy (HAART), a careful evaluation to exclude nonadherence is indicated. Poor adherence to antiretroviral agents results in subtherapeutic levels that lead to emergence of viral drug resistance that may affect all other members of that class of drug, thus reducing treatment options. A comprehensive assessment of adherence issues must be undertaken. Factors involved include the type of drug preparation acceptable to younger children (liquid and palatable), caretaker function, challenges presented by disclosure, and denial of the severity of illness. When adherence cannot be ensured, treatment should be discontinued. Emergence of life-threatening toxicity also requires discontinuation of antiretroviral therapy. In these cases, only follow-up is advised.[21]

SUMMARY

The scientific advances in medical treatment of HIV disease and AIDS have been highly significant over the past 10 years, and these promise to improve the longevity and quality of life for children and youth infected with HIV. Additionally, prenatal testing and community preventive approaches targeting safe-sex practices and intravenous drug abuse should also contribute to stemming and reduction in this dreaded disease among children and youth. However, the context of HIV disease and AIDS within poverty, minority status, and disenfranchised and underserved populations (not only in the United States, but also worldwide) presents significant barriers to the application of these scientific advances. Effective approaches and models that address the psychosocial, cultural, and systemic context of this epidemic will prove to be as important, if not more important, than the biologic advances in diagnosis and treatment.[20]

Pediatric HIV disease and AIDS affect the child, family, and community on many levels; there is a significant parallel with the multilevel impact of serious emotional disturbances on children and families. There may be significant value in the adaptation of systems of care approaches developed in the child mental health arena for serious emotional disturbances. These approaches have promoted interdisciplinary and interagency collaboration, services that are culturally competent and delivered within the child's own community, individualized care that is driven by and empowers children/youth and families, use of community supports, and the reduction of stigma. These approaches have been demonstrated to be particularly successful in delivering mental health services for disenfranchised, underserved populations, similar to those among whom HIV infection and AIDS is most rapidly increasing.[22]

REFERENCES

1. Brown L, Lourie K, Pao M. Children and adolescents living with HIV and AIDS: a review. *J Child Psychol Psychiatry*. 2000;41:81–96.
2. Futterman D, Chabon B, Hoffman N. HIV and AIDS in adolescents. *Pediatr Clin North Am*. 2000;47:171–188.

3. Centers for Disease Control and Prevention. *HIV/AIDS Surveillance Report: Cases of HIV Infection and AIDS in the United States, 2003*. Vol. 15. Atlanta: Centers for Disease Control and Prevention; 2004.
4. Pan American Health Organization. *AIDS Surveillance in the Americas*. Washington, DC: Pan American Health Organization; 1997.
5. Coplan J, Contello KA, Cunning CK, et al. Early language development in children exposed to or infected with human immunodeficiency virus. *Pediatrics*. 1998;102:e8.
6. Stolar A, Fernandez F. Psychiatric perspective of pediatric human immunodeficiency virus infection. *South Med J*. 1997;90:1007–1016.
7. Patsalides A, Wood L, Atac G, Sandifer E, Butman J, Patronas N. Cerebrovascular disease in HIV-infected pediatric patients: neuroimaging findings. *Am J Roentgenol*. 2002;179:999–1003.
8. Brouwers P, De Carli C, Civitello L, Moss H, Wolters P, Pizzo P. Correlation between computerized tomographic brain scan abnormalities and neuropsychological function in children with symptomatic human immunodeficiency virus disease. *Arch Neurol*. 1995;52:39–44.
9. Keller MA, Venkatraman TN, Thomas A, et al. Altered neurometabolite development in HIV-infected children: correlation with neuropsychological tests. *Neurology*. 2004;62:1810–1817.
10. Frank EG, Foley GM, Kuchuka A. Cognitive functioning in school-age children with human immunodeficiency virus. *Percept Motor Skills*. 1997;85:267–272.
11. Civitello L. Neurologic aspects of HIV infection in infants and children: therapeutic approaches and outcome. *Curr Neurol Neurosci Rep*. 2003;3:120–128.
12. Joslin D, Harrison R. The hidden patient: older relatives raising children orphaned by AIDS. *J Am Med Womens Assoc*. 1998;53:65–71, 76.
13. Rotheram-Borus MJ, Robin L, Reid HM, Draimin BH. Parent-adolescent conflict and stress when parents are living with AIDS. *Fam Process*. 1996;37:422–435.
14. Martin S, Wolters P, Klaas P, Perez L, Wood L. Coping styles among families of children with HIV infection. *AIDS Care*. 2004;16:283–292.
15. Aronson S. The bereavement process in children of parents with AIDS. *Psychoanalyt Study Child*. 1996;51:422–435.
16. Moss H, Base S, Wolters P, Brouwners P. A preliminary study of factors associated with psychological adjustment and disease course in school-age children infected with the human immunodeficiency virus. *J Dev Behav Pediatr*. 1998;19:18–25.
17. Boland M. Caring for the child and family with HIV disease. *Pediatr Clin North Am*. 2000;47:189–202.
18. Wight R, Aneshensel C, Le Blanc A. Stress buffering effects of family support in AIDS caregiving. *AIDS Care*. 2003;15:595–613.
19. Blasini I, Chantry C, Cruz C, et al. Disclosure model for pediatric patients living with HIV in Puerto Rico: design, implementation, and evaluation. *J Dev Behav Pediatr*. 2004;25:181–189.
20. Forsyth B. Psychological aspects of HIV infection in children. *Child Adolesc Psychiatr Clin North Am*. 2003;12:423–437.
21. Anabwani GM, Woldetsadik EA, Kline MW. Treatment of human immunodeficiency virus (HIV) in children using antiretroviral drugs. *Semin Pediatr Infect Dis*. 2005;16:116–124.
22. Pumariega AJ, Winters NC, eds. *Handbook of Community Systems of Care: The New Child & Adolescent Community Psychiatry*. San Francisco: Jossey Bass; 2003.

CHAPTER 26

HIV/AIDS Among Older Adults

Maria D. Llorente, Julie E. Malphurs

There is a growing evidence base regarding human immunodeficiency virus (HIV) and older adults, although at times the available information consists of anecdotal case reports, small case series, and extrapolations from the general HIV-negative geriatric or younger HIV-positive adult fields. Within the context of HIV infection, the Centers for Disease Control and Prevention (CDC) defined "older adults" as persons aged 50 and older. Although these individuals share features in common with younger HIV-positive persons and the HIV-negative geriatric population, they also exhibit unique characteristics.

RISK, DIAGNOSIS, COURSE, TREATMENT, AND AGING

EPIDEMIOLOGY

Older adults account for 10% to 18% of those estimated to be infected with HIV. More than half of this older HIV-positive group are of African-American and Hispanic origin, indicating greater risk for ethnic and racial minority older adults. Currently, approximately 17% of people in the United States living with AIDS are 50 years old or older, but there are geographic variations.[1] In addition to primary infection in later life, with the wide use of highly active antiretroviral therapy (HAART), adults who were infected in earlier life are living longer. As a result, the proportion of older people living with HIV disease quintupled between 1988 and 2000.

HIV RISK AND AGING

HIV has traditionally been thought of as a disease of young persons. However, the primary routes of transmission, sexual activity and drug use, usually associated with young adulthood and middle age, are also the most common routes for infection for older adults. Many health care providers do not know this and thus do not discuss issues of sexuality or substance use with seniors. Older adults themselves are often unaware of the risk factors for HIV infections or do not see themselves as being at risk for infection. Compounding this issue is that older adults are not typically targeted for prevention or safe-sex education.

For older men in the United States, the most frequent exposure category is men having sex with men, but heterosexual and intravenous drug use exposures are increasing. Certain factors increase the risk for older men. First, unlike younger men, older men are less likely to reveal their sexual orientation to health care workers, limiting the opportunities for prevention education. Second, drugs such as sildenafil (Viagra) have contributed to increased rates of heterosexual, homosexual, and bisexual activity, but many seniors do not use condoms consistently. Third, reports from Florida reveal an added risk for older men. Prostitutes who are HIV-positive have used older men's insulin needles to inject drugs and then returned the syringes to their packaging to avoid detection. The unsuspecting older men then used the dirty needles.

Older women are more commonly exposed through heterosexual transmission, but intravenous drug use is also a route of exposure. Older women are more vulnerable to HIV infection than their younger counterparts because of age-related changes in vaginal mucosa after menopause. The vaginal wall is thinner and lubrication is reduced, leading to a greater likelihood of vaginal trauma during intercourse. Older women associate condom use with prevention of pregnancy and, because this is no longer a concern after menopause, are less likely than younger women to use condoms. A recent source of intravenous drug use exposure among older adults with diabetes is the sharing of insulin needles, syringes, and glucose monitoring needles to save money.

HIV DIAGNOSIS, COURSE, AND AGING

There are unique characteristics that distinguish the presenting symptoms, diagnosis, and course of HIV disease in older adults. Seniors are less likely to be tested for HIV than younger persons, because HIV infection symptoms are attributed to other diseases common among the elderly. Thus HIV infection often is first diagnosed at later stages of infection. Older HIV-positive adults are more likely than younger adults to have comorbid medical conditions commonly seen in the aging population and to require concomitant medications, complicating symptom assessment and treatment choices. Age-related declines in immune function leave older adults more vulnerable to opportunistic infections, with increased rates of HIV-related complications, more rapid progression to AIDS, and lower survival rates than in younger adults with HIV disease.[2]

TREATMENT

Although HIV treatment guidelines have been developed for other patient populations, no specific treatment recommendations exist for older adults. Nevertheless, administration of HAART to HIV-positive older adults is effective and produces greater reductions in mortality rates compared to those in younger HIV-positive adults. Little is known about age-specific HAART drug actions, drug–drug interactions, drug–disease interactions, or adverse events. For example, recent studies have found that older adults are more likely to experience toxicities from HAART, including dyslipidemia, insulin resistance, and pancreatitis. A person's age does not interfere with HAART's ability to reduce viral load, but CD4 recovery was lower in older people compared to younger ones, likely due to age-related decreased activity of the thymus gland, where CD4 cells are made.

NORMAL AGING AND HIV INFECTION

Normal aging is associated with declines in physical functioning, receptor number and affinities, and metabolism so that an older adult may be unable to respond to increased demands for cellular repair or activity. Age-related changes in immune function and pharmacokinetics are of particular importance in HIV disease.[3]

IMMUNE SYSTEM FUNCTIONING AND AGING

With aging, the total numbers of immune cells and concentration of immunoglobulins do not change, but a redistribution does occur.[4] Increases in immunoglobulin (Ig)A and IgG and decreases in IgM are seen. The main age-related cellular changes, however, occur in the ratios of subpopulations of T lymphocytes. There are increases in immature cell forms and reductions in cytotoxic and natural killer cells. The delayed-sensitivity reaction is less vigorous, and immunity to virus infections is reduced. T cells have been shown to have fewer surface receptors and B cells fewer immunoglobulin markers. As a result of these changes, at time of HIV diagnosis, older adults have lower CD4 counts than younger patients.

PHARMACOKINETIC CHANGES AND AGING

Hepatic metabolic functioning declines with age, in part reflecting reduced hepatic perfusion and reductions in liver size. The oxidative pathways, especially cytochrome isoenzymes 2D6 and 1A2, are those most affected, particularly in men, with relative sparing of conjugation. These functional changes result in increases in the bioavailability of drugs (through half-life prolongation) and metabolites that are normally inactivated through phase I of hepatic enzyme biotransformation. Ritonavir itself can inhibit the activity of cytochrome P 2D6, so that in an older adult, use of this antiretroviral can increase both beneficial and adverse effects of many psychotropic medications.

Renal function normally declines with aging as a result of a decrease in glomerular filtration rate and renal blood flow, leading to reductions in creatinine clearance. This has important implications for drugs excreted through the kidneys, such as lithium and buspirone. Older adults are more susceptible to develop the syndrome of inappropriate antidiuretic hormone secretion (SIADH) from medications, such as the selective serotonin reuptake inhibitors (SSRIs) and carbamazepine.

Plasma concentrations are reduced with aging and malnutrition, and hepatic disease causes further declines. The consequence of this reduction is that free plasma concentrations of protein-bound medications (i.e., the pharmacologically active component) remain the same, but the bound portion is reduced. Thus the therapeutic and toxic effects occur at lower total drug plasma concentrations. This is particularly relevant for anticonvulsants used to treat mood disorders.

PSYCHIATRIC DISORDERS, HIV, AND AGING

There is some early evidence suggesting that older HIV-positive adults are at risk for elevated rates of psychiatric disorders. This group generally has fewer social and institutional supports, lack caregivers, have often lost peers to HIV disease, and perceive less acceptance of HIV status among family and friends.[5] When a social network is present, they report more conflict, particularly gay older men.[6] Fear of rejection from grown children and loss of interaction with grandchildren furthers the sense of isolation. Additionally, a complex relationship exists between greater medical comorbidity and an increased incidence of certain psychiatric disorders, including depression and dementia. Serious and chronic mental illnesses (including substance use disorders, schizophrenia, and mania) are themselves risk factors for HIV infection and often precede the infection, and are associated with poorer compliance and poorer outcomes physically and mentally.

PSYCHOTIC DISORDERS

SCHIZOPHRENIA

The prevalence of schizophrenia in older HIV-positive adults (3%) is higher than in the general population, but similar to the prevalence in younger HIV-positive adults. Mortality in persons with schizophrenia is 2 to 4 times greater than in the general population, and nonadherence to nonpsychiatric medications is a major contributing factor.[7,8] Successful treatment of HIV infection requires consistent adherence to 90% of prescribed antiretrovirals; thus patients with schizophrenia have poorer treatment success. This partly explains the high prevalence of schizophrenia (12.8%) among HIV-positive nursing home residents with dementia.[6]

HIV-RELATED PSYCHOSIS

HIV infection may be associated with new-onset psychotic symptoms, typically occurring in later stages of HIV or AIDS. Persecutory, grandiose, or somatic delusions are common, with prominent auditory hallucinations and occasional affective symptoms. A prior history of methamphetamine use disorders, untreated HIV infection, and dementia are associated with psychosis and increase vulnerability.

Treatment

The treatment of psychotic disorders is very similar whether the symptoms are due to an existing disorder or of new onset. Adults with AIDS are reported to have twice the risk of developing extrapyramidal symptoms (EPS) or tardive dyskinesia with conventional antipsychotics compared to patients who do not have AIDS because of the loss of dopaminergic neurons from HIV-related injury to the basal ganglia. Loss of dopaminergic neurons and decreased dopamine levels normally occur with aging, so that older HIV-positive adults are at particularly high risk for developing EPS and tardive dyskinesia. Atypical antipsychotics are therefore the treatment of choice for psychosis. Clozapine, which can cause bone marrow suppression, is highly anticholinergic and causes orthostatic hypotension; it should be used very cautiously in this population. Response to antipsychotics typically occurs in doses one fourth to one half of those required for treating comparable HIV-negative and younger populations.

Drug–drug interactions should also be considered. Ritonavir and lopinavir/ritonavir may increase serum levels of clozapine and risperidone and decrease serum levels of olanzapine. Doses of these antipsychotics would need to be adjusted accordingly. Fluconazole can prolong the QT interval, and there should be concern in coadministration with risperidone, quetiapine, and especially ziprasidone, which can all prolong QT intervals, particularly in older adults with comorbid cardiac disease.

Increasing age, HIV seropositivity, and schizophrenia are all independent risk factors for the development of metabolic syndrome and diabetes mellitus, so that older HIV-positive persons with schizophrenia are at particularly high risk. The use of HAART further increases this risk, as do some atypical antipsychotics. Metabolic disruptions occur more commonly with clozapine and olanzapine than with other available agents. HIV-positive older adults with psychotic disorders should be screened for risk factors for metabolic syndrome (Table 26.1), and the American Diabetes Association Consensus Guidelines[9] for ongoing monitoring of diabetes risk should be followed (Table 26.2).

MOOD DISORDERS

DEPRESSIVE SPECTRUM

Depressive disorders among HIV-positive older adults are highly prevalent, ranging from 15% to 61% for the spectrum of depressive disorders from dysthymia to major depression[10–12] and typically precede the infection. HIV-positive persons are 2 to 7 times more likely than age-matched adults to meet criteria for major depression, and older adults are at particularly high risk.[12] Depressive symptoms in older adults with HIV infection are associated with poorer

TABLE 26.1	Metabolic Syndrome: Any 3 of these 5 Criteria	
Criteria	Men	Women
Obesity: waist size	>40 inches	>35 inches
HDL cholesterol	<40 mg/dl	<50 mg/dl
Triglycerides	≥150 mg/dl	
Blood pressure	≥130 mm Hg systolic or 85 mm Hg diastolic	
Fasting blood glucose	≥100 mg/dl	

TABLE 26.2	American Diabetes Association Consensus Guidelines on Antipsychotic Drugs, Obesity, and Diabetes: Monitoring Protocol					
Risk Factor	Baseline Screen	4 Weeks	8 Weeks	3 Months	6 Months	12 Months
Family history	X					
Personal history (includes gestational diabetes)	X					X
Weight (BMI)	X	X	X	X	X	X
Waist circumference	X					X
Blood pressure	X			X		X
Fasting glucose	X			X		X
Fasting lipids	X			X		X

More frequent assessments may be clinically indicated.

adherence and physical or mental functioning and are a significant predictor of HIV disease progression and survival.

PRESENTING SYMPTOMS

Similar to HIV-negative older persons, HIV-positive seniors have symptoms that fail to meet diagnostic criteria for major depression, but are associated with significant functional disability. These subsyndromal disorders co-occur with chronic medical conditions and present with prominent somatic and anxiety components. Older adults, specifically older White men, have the highest rates of completed suicide, and these rates are especially high among older men with chronic medical illnesses. HIV-positive individuals additionally have other risk factors for suicide, including psychiatric disorders, substance use disorders, and, for older adults, lack of social supports.[13]

DIFFERENTIAL DIAGNOSIS

It can be difficult to diagnose major depression in this population due to subsyndromal conditions, confusion with physical symptoms of HIV infection or other comorbid diseases, or medication side effects, especially HAART. Recently, the Patient Health Questionnaire depression scale (PHQ-9)[14] has become a commonly used, self-administered instrument to assist primary care providers in making an initial diagnosis of depression, determining its severity, and tracking the outcomes of treatment. This instrument, although not specifically tested in an HIV-infected population, is likely to be beneficial, because it is sensitive and specific in medically ill populations. The Geriatric Depression Scale (GDS),[15] a self-administered instrument, has several versions that are sensitive and specific for screening (4- and 10-item versions) and measure depression severity (15- and 30-item versions). In patients with dementia, determination of depressive symptoms often requires input from a caregiver. The Cornell Scale for Depression in Dementia[16] was specifically designed to assess severity of depression in dementia, although not specifically tested in older adults with HIV-associated dementia.

TREATMENT

Several general principles guide the pharmacologic management of depression. First, doses of antidepressants are started at half of the dose used in younger adults and titrated gradually to clinical efficacy. Second, because HIV-positive patients are typically taking multiple medications, choosing medications with minimal drug–drug interactions and simplifying the dosing regimen to once or twice daily dosing is preferred. Sertraline, citalopram, venlafaxine, and, more recently, duloxetine, are often chosen because of the lower frequency of drug–drug interactions.[12] Patients receiving both HAART and SSRIs may be at increased risk for hyperserotonergic syndrome due to increased serum levels of SSRIs. Further, indinavir, saquinavir, and efavirenz may interfere with the metabolism of bupropion.[17]

HIV-positive older adults reportedly have poorer response rates to antidepressant treatment than younger adults.[17] In older HIV-negative adults, the rate of chronicity for depression, particularly for late-onset depression, approaches 40% and is associated with cerebrovascular disease, executive dysfunction or dementia, less frequent family history of mood disorders, and high severity of depression. This may also hold true for HIV-positive older adults with late-onset depressive disorders. Electroconvulsive therapy is effective for depression in HIV-positive older adults, even if complicated by dementia. Psychostimulants, as mono- or combination therapy can treat depressive symptoms, including fatigue, in HIV-positive patients.

The Stressor-Support-Coping Model for Psychosocial Intervention is an effective psychotherapy to improve mood and anxiety in HIV-positive older adults.[18] Social support group therapy facilitates the building of networks of mutual support and can improve coping skills. The impact of supportive therapy on decreasing distress and increasing well-being is more pronounced among older HIV-positive men. In the primary care setting, collaborative care models of therapy, using mental health case managers, have consistently been found to be more effective than usual care for depressed older adults, regardless of their ethnicity.[19] Exercise may benefit mood in older persons with HIV who are able to participate in an exercise regimen, including walking.

MANIA

In a sample of 795 older HIV-positive patients, the prevalence of bipolar disorder was 2%, significantly higher than previously reported in a community sample, in which no mania cases were identified among 923 elderly persons. The manic symptoms of hypersexuality, impulsivity and grandiosity, and participation in higher risk sex acts increase the risk for contracting and transmitting HIV. In those HIV-positive individuals in whom onset of manic symptoms occurs after the age of 40, HIV neurotoxicity should be considered. The related mood symptom of irritability has been shown to be a sequela of neurologic injury to the prefrontal or subcortical structures and fronto-subcortical projections as occurs in HIV-associated dementia (HAD).

Treatment

CNS-penetrating antiretroviral medications have been found to offer some protection against mania; however, manic episodes, whether from primary or secondary etiologies, respond well to guideline-based treatments with mood stabilizers. The use of lithium, however, is potentially problematic in older adults who may have cognitive impairment or HIV-associated nephropathy or who are more susceptible to developing a fine tremor and myoclonus, even with therapeutic levels. In addition, age-associated reductions in renal clearance may cause older adults to have high plasma levels at relatively low oral doses. Usually half to two thirds of the dose required for younger patients is effective for older adults.

Anticonvulsants are likely to be effective. Many older HIV-positive individuals have chronic infections with hepatitis B and/or C, chronically abuse alcohol, and are thus more susceptible to liver damage,[2] so liver function tests must be monitored. Thrombocytopenia occurs as a side effect of valproic acid among older adults and is associated with high trough serum levels, and carbamazepine is associated with leukopenia in 2% of treated patients, so complete blood counts should be monitored frequently. Carbamazepine is problematic in older adults, who are more sensitive to the side effects of sedation, ataxia, and confusion. For older patients in a depressive phase of bipolar disorder, lamotrigine, in conjunction with lithium and valproate, has shown effectiveness in a small sample of geriatric patients.

SUBSTANCE USE DISORDERS

CLINICAL FEATURES

Older age is generally considered to result in a maturation effect with decline in drug use. The diagnosis of substance use disorders can be difficult in older adults, however. Current *Diagnostic and Statistical Manual of Mental Disorders (DSM-IV)* for substance abuse requires assessment of the impact of drug abuse on work, school, and family life, areas that are less affected by drug abuse in older adults who may be retired or living alone. Physiologic age-related changes in responses to drugs may lead to lower consumption with continued adverse consequences, including a greater likelihood of developing hepatitis, heart problems, diabetes, cancer, and arthritis.

In studies comparing older and younger samples of substance abuse in HIV-positive subjects, the older cohort was more likely to have a history of arrests; be disabled, retired, or unemployed; live alone; be uninsured; and have lower incomes.[10] Sexually active older drug users engaged in similar rates of risky sexual behavior as did younger users, with those who smoked crack cocaine at highest risk of infection. Some adults do begin to smoke crack cocaine in later life. Women who are late-onset crack users reported more lifetime partners, higher levels of sexual activity, and lower levels of condom use than women who began crack use earlier in life. Men who start crack in later life are introduced to crack through younger female users.

TREATMENT

For men, treatment is often initiated as a result of an acute and at times life-threatening medical illness, such as a myocardial infarction. Among women, treatment of drug use is often initiated as an alternative to a jail sentence. Very little is known about the efficacy of treatment of substance use disorders in an older HIV-positive population. The goals of treatment are similar to those for younger adults, that is, abstinence from consumption, treatment for comorbid psychiatric and medical conditions, and development of alternative coping strategies to reduce relapse risk. Because older HIV-positive adults have a high prevalence of comorbidity, however, collaborative models that integrate mental health and primary care are more likely to be successful.

HIV-ASSOCIATED DEMENTIA

The growing use of HAART has improved survival of patients with AIDS and decreased the incidence of HAD from a cumulative prevalence of 17% to 25% during the course of AIDS, to current prevalence rates of 7% to 10%. HAART, unfortunately, does not provide full protection against neurologic damage, partly because some of the antiretrovirals have poor penetration into the CNS.

PATHOGENESIS

The principal causative factor is thought to be the activation of macrophages and microglia, with subsequent release of chemical intermediaries that lead to neuronal injury, dysfunction, and death. As a response to microglial activation, neuroprotective astrocyte up-regulation should occur. With aging, however, astrocytic activation occurs more slowly, is less pronounced, and persists for shorter periods than in younger brains. Thus the aging brain's environment favors the harmful effects of microglial activation and limits compensatory responses. These pathologic pathways are seen in other dementias, such as Alzheimer's disease, dementia of Parkinson's disease, and cerebrovascular injuries.

RISK FACTORS

Jannssen et al.[20] found a linear increase in the incidence of HAD with increasing age, as follows: 15 to 34 years (6%), 35 to 54 (8%), 55 to 74 years (12%), and 75 and older (19%). Age is thus a very significant risk factor for HAD for a variety of reasons. First, age is an important risk factor for other dementias, most notably Alzheimer's disease, and HIV seropositivity may be an independent risk factor for Alzheimer's disease itself. Second, as one ages, there is an increased risk of developing diseases that increase the risk for dementia, particularly dyslipidemias, hypertension, and diabetes mellitus. Diabetes mellitus was recently found to be independently associated with HAD.[21] Third, these high-risk comorbid medical conditions are also a consequence of HIV treatment, particularly protease inhibitors. Fourth, higher viral loads at time of diagnosis, which often occurs in older adults, and CD4 cell counts below 200 cells/µl are associated with increased risk of HAD. Finally, intravenous drug use, which causes microglial activation, coinfection with hepatitis C virus, and a history of alcohol abuse and dependence are all associated with increased risk for development of HAD.

SYMPTOMS

HAD is a spectrum of disorders, ranging from subtle cognitive difficulties with minimal impairment of activities of daily living (minor cognitive motor disorder) to dementia with impaired social and occupational functioning. The symptoms may remain stable or progress rapidly, and fall into three broad categories:

- *Motor:* Slowness of fine motor movements, poor coordination, lower extremity weakness, loss of balance, tendency to drop things, worsening handwriting, loss of bladder/bowel control, paralysis of lower limbs.
- *Cognitive:* Difficulty with concentration and shortened attention span, inability to complete routine tasks, memory loss, slowed processing of information, difficulty comprehending instructions, increased latency of response, loss of sense of humor.
- *Behavioral:* Personality change (irritability, apathy, loss of motivation, social withdrawal), mood swings, impulsivity, disinhibition, psychosis.

DIFFERENTIAL DIAGNOSIS

Many of the symptoms of HAD can also occur with other dementias and in the older adult are often attributed to aging or concomitant medical conditions, before HIV is even considered. An accurate diagnosis of HAD requires a comprehensive medical evaluation in order to identify risk factors for HIV infection. Once HIV seropositivity is established, other diseases commonly seen in AIDS populations, including toxoplasmosis, CNS lymphoma, and cryptococcal meningitis must be ruled out. Neuropsychological testing is helpful in localizing and quantifying the cognitive deficits. The Executive Interview (EXIT25)[22,23] is a useful bedside tool to identify HAD. Neuroimaging can also rule out vascular lesions, masses, and structural neuronal damage.

COURSE AND OUTCOME

In the pre-HAART era, the mean time to death after diagnosis of HAD was 6 months, but currently the average is 44 months, although progression of disease is highly variable. A history of intravenous drug use and prominent psychomotor slowing is associated with more rapid neurologic progression. It has been suggested that as a result of HAART, the course of HAD has been altered into two subtypes—an inactive form with fixed deficits and a chronic, gradually progressive form.

TREATMENT

Treatment approaches consist of antiretrovirals, psychopharmacologic management of psychiatric symptoms, and psychosocial treatments. Antiretroviral combinations that include drugs that penetrate the blood–brain barrier, particularly zidovudine, have been shown in some small studies to lead to cognitive improvement or a partial return of functioning. The strongest clinical evidence exists for zidovudine; however, didanosine and abacavir may have some effect. Experimentally, improvements in neuropsychological performance correlated with declines in cerebrospinal fluid (CSF) HIV ribonucleic acid (RNA) levels, so this may prove to be a biologic marker to monitor. In vitro, microglial activation has been shown to be attenuated by galantamine. Similarly, neurotoxicity caused by HIV proteins can be blocked by memantine. In patients with comorbid Alzheimer's disease and HIV, galantamine and memantine are thus first-line treatments.

Psychopharmacologic management of psychiatric symptoms is similar to that previously described, with a few added considerations. An association has been reported between the use of some atypical antipsychotics (risperidone, olanzapine, and aripiprazole) and cerebrovascular events ranging from syncope to strokes in older adults, with behavioral disturbances and dementia. The incidence of these events was low, ranging from 1% to 4% of actively treated subjects (compared to 0.4% to 2% on placebo) and occurred in subjects with risk factors for vascular disease. The subjects were frail older adults, mostly nursing home residents, in their 70s and 80s. No such association has been found for younger, nondemented patients. There is currently no information regarding the potential risk of cerebro-vascular adverse events (CVAEs) in older adults with HAD. The benefits of instituting treatment with these medications must be weighed against potential risks. Minimally, risk factors for vascular disease should be evaluated and medical management optimized to reduce this risk (daily aspirin; control of hypertension, diabetes, dyslipidemias, etc.). Psychosocial treatments include providing orienting clues (large clock, calendar, maintaining regular routine and "sameness" to environment); dividing tasks into small, successive steps; treating pain; stating instructions one at a time to allow for longer processing time; providing reassurance, comfort, and explanations; distraction with conversation; written instructions; use of pill boxes.

SUMMARY

The proportion of older adults living with HIV is growing at a rapid pace. Seniors, especially ethnic minority older adults, have the same exposure risk as do younger adults, but may be more vulnerable to HIV infection and its complications. Older HIV-positive adults are at risk for high rates of psychiatric disorders, but psychopharmacologic and psychosocial interventions are effective treatments to improve clinical outcomes and quality of life. Age-related pharmacokinetic changes and comorbid medical conditions are important considerations in the choice of psychopharmacologic agent and effective doses. Future research will investigate age-specific HAART drug actions, drug–drug and drug–disease interactions, and adverse events. Neuropsychopharmacologic research will focus on interventions that may alter the course of, and ideally prevent, HIV-related CNS disease.

REFERENCES

1. Mack KK, Ory M. HIV/AIDS and older Americans at the end of the 20th century. *J Acquir Immune Defic Syndr.* 2003;33:S68–S75.
2. Kilbourne AM, Justice AC, Rabeneck L, et al. General medical and psychiatric comorbidity among HIV-infected veterans in the post-HAART era. *J Clin Epidemiol.* 2001;54:S22–S28.
3. Hammerlein A, Derendorf H, Lowenthal DT. Pharmacokinetic and pharmacodynamic changes in the elderly: clinical implications. *Clin Pharmacokinet.* 1998;35:49–64.
4. Goodwin JS, Searles RP, Tung KSK: Immunological responses of a healthy elderly population. *Clin Exp Immunol.* 1982;48:403–410.
5. Nokes K, Holzemer W, Corless I, et al. Health-related quality of life in persons younger and older than 50 who are living with HIV/AIDS. *Res Aging.* 2000;22:290–310.
6. Crystal S, Akincigil A, Sambamoorthi U, et al. The diverse older HIV-positive population: a national profile of economic circumstances, social support and quality of life. *J Acquir Immune Defic Syndr.* 2003;33:S76–S83.
7. Patterson TL, Lacro J, McKibbin CL, Moscona S, Hughs T, Jeste DV. Medication management ability assessment: results from a performance-based measure in older outpatients with schizophrenia. *J Clin Psychopharmacol.* 2002;22:11–19.
8. Buchanan RJ, Wang S, Huang C. Analyses of nursing home residents with HIV and dementia using the minimum data set. *J AIDS.* 2001;26:246–255.
9. American Diabetes Association, American Psychiatric Association, American Association of Clinical Endocrinologists, North American Association for the Study of Obesity. Consensus development conference on antipsychotic drugs and obesity and diabetes. *Diabetes Care.* 2004;27:596–601.
10. Kwiatkowski CF, Booth RE. HIV risk behaviors among older American drug users. *J Acquir Immune Defic Syndr.* 2003;33:S131–S137.
11. Justice AC, McGinnis KA, Atkinson JH, et al. Psychiatric and neurocognitive disorders among HIV-positive and negative veterans in care: Veterans Aging Cohort Five-Site Study. *AIDS.* 2004;18:S49–S59.
12. Hinkin CH, Castellon SA, Atkinson JH, Goodkin K. Neuropsychiatric aspects of HIV infection among older adults. *J Clin Epidemiol.* 2001;54:S44–S52.
13. Bartels SJ, Coakley E, Oxman TE, et al. Suicidal and death ideation in older primary care patients with depression, anxiety, and at-risk alcohol use. *Am J Geriatr Psychiatry.* 2002;10:417–427.
14. Kroenke K, Spitzer RL. The PHQ-9: a new depression diagnostic and severity measure. *Psychiatric Ann.* 2002;32:1–7.
15. Yesavage JA, Brink TL, Rose TL, et al. Development and validation of a geriatric depression screening scale: a preliminary report. *J Psychiatr Res.* 1983;17:37–49.
16. Alexopoulos GS, Abrams RC, Young RC, et al. Cornell Scale for Depression in Dementia. *Bio Psychiatry.* 1988;23:271–284.
17. Repetto MJ, Evans DL, Cruess DG, Gettes DR, Douglas SD, Petitto JM. Neuropsychopharmacologic treatment of depression and other neuropsychiatric disorders in HIV-infected individuals. *CNS Spectr.* 2003;8:59–63.
18. Goodkin K, Heckman T, Siegel K, et al. Putting a face on HIV/AIDS in older adults: a psychosocial context. *J Acquir Immun Defic Syndr.* 2003;33:S185–S184.
19. Arean PA, Ayalon L, Hunkeler E, et al. Improving depression care for older, minority patients in primary care. *Med Care.* 2005;43:381–390.
20. Jannssen RS, Nwanyanwu OC, Selik RM, et al. Epidemiology of HIV encephalopathy in the US. *Neurology,* 1992;42:1472–1476.
21. Valcour VG, Shikuma CM, Shiramizu BT, et al. Diabetes, insulin resistance, and dementia among HIV-1-infected patients. *J Acquir Immune Defic Syndr.* 2005;38;31–36.
22. Royall DR, Mahurin RK, Gray KF. Bedside assessment of executive cognitive impairment: the executive interview. *J Am Geriatr Soc.* 1992;40:1221–1226.
23. Berghuis JP, Uldall KK, Lalonde B. Validity of two scales in identifying HIV-associated dementia. *J Acquir Immune Defic Syndr.* 1999;21:134–140.

CHAPTER 27

HIV/AIDS Among Women

Isabel T. Lagomasino, Gustavo Rodriguez

The first case of acquired immunodeficiency syndrome (AIDS) among women was reported at the start of the epidemic in 1981.[1] By 2002, human immunodeficiency virus (HIV) disease was the fifth leading cause of death for women 25 to 34 years old in the United States and the sixth leading cause for women 35 to 44 years old, accounting for approximately 5% of deaths among women 25 to 44 years old.[2] Women now make up approximately 27% of HIV infection and AIDS cases in the United States, and the majority are exposed through heterosexual contact.[2] Several biologic and social risk factors place women at greater risk for HIV infection, and their disease burden is compounded by the risk for vertical transmission. Multifaceted treatment and prevention programs must be developed and implemented to address the specific needs of women at risk and infected with HIV.

EPIDEMIOLOGY

Over the past two decades, women have accounted for an increasing proportion of new HIV infections and AIDS diagnoses. Within the United States, ethnic minority women are disproportionately affected. Compared to White women, for example, African Americans have 25 times the rate of AIDS diagnoses and Latinos 6 times the rate.[2] In 2002, HIV disease was the leading cause of death for African-American women 25 to 34 years old, accounting for 14.7% of deaths.[2] Younger women are also at greater risk; teenagers account for 50% of new infections, of whom 61% are females and more than half are African American.[3] Heterosexual women acquire HIV at an earlier age than heterosexual men, likely due to infection by older sex partners.[4]

By 1995, heterosexual contact surpassed intravenous drug use as the major mode of HIV transmission for women.[5] The 2003 HIV/AIDS Surveillance Report estimates that 79% of HIV infection and AIDS cases among women were due to heterosexual contact; 19% to intravenous drug use; and 2% to other causes, including hemophilia, blood transfusions, perinatal exposure, and unknown or unidentified risks.[2] Five states—New York, Florida, New Jersey, Texas, and North Carolina—accounted for 52% of newly reported cases of HIV infection.[2] Although HIV infection and AIDS cases among women were originally concentrated among intravenous drug users in the Northeast, increasingly, women infected thorough heterosexual contact reside in the South and rural areas.[2] Those infected through intravenous drug use often use cocaine and amphetamines rather than heroin, both of which have been associated with increased needle sharing.[6] Use of crack cocaine, although not a direct mode of transmission, has been reported to increase the risk of heterosexual spread through increases in high-risk behaviors, including higher numbers of sex partners and the exchange of sex for drugs.[7]

RISK FACTORS

Both biologic and social risk factors may increase the risk of HIV infection among women. The odds of male-to-female heterosexual transmission has been estimated to be as much as 20 times higher than that of female-to-male transmission.[8] Susceptibility increases when biologic factors are present that provide direct viral access to the bloodstream, that cause inflammation or immune activation that results in greater numbers and susceptibility of target cells, or that facilitate the survival of HIV in mucosa.[9] In addition to viral HIV load, risk factors thus include receptive anal intercourse, cervical ectopy, genital ulcer disease or other sexually transmitted disease, use of hormonal contraceptives, and pregnancy.[9,10] Cervical ectopy refers to the extension of columnar epithelium from the endocervix to the proximal portion of the cervix, immediately adjacent to squamous epithelium. Characteristic of cervical immaturity, the area of ectopy is fragile and promotes easy access to blood and lymphatic systems.[11] Although not clearly understood, contraceptive hormones may increase cervical ectopy or produce thinning of vaginal epithelia. Pregnancy is similarly a time of increased progesterone levels and ectopy.[12]

Numerous social factors place women at risk for HIV infection. Cultural norms and attitudes may discourage sexual education or the use of safe-sex methods, while promoting acceptance of promiscuity among men.[13] Poverty may increase risk for women through multiple mechanisms. In the midst of multiple issues related to survival, the need to negotiate safe sex practices may be perceived as less important and women may feel less empowered to engage in such discussions. They may be forced to rely on men who engage in high-risk sexual behaviors and are more likely to exchange sex for gifts or money.[13] Violence may result directly in unwanted sexual acts. Women exposed to early childhood traumas may also be more likely to engage in high-risk behaviors, and those fearing violence may be less able to negotiate barrier methods of protection. Commercial sex workers are at especially high risk, as are incarcerated women, who may have high-risk partners, engage in unprotected sex and sex exchange, and use intravenous drugs.[13]

In an interesting exploration of racial disparities in rates of sexually transmitted infections, differences between the sexual networks of Blacks and Whites are theorized to also contribute to elevated risks for African Americans.[14] Compared to Whites, Blacks are more likely to report having overlapping sexual partners and to have more closed sexual networks. The low male-to-female ratio that results from high mortality and incarceration rates among Black men results in low marriage rates, greater tolerance by women of high-risk behaviors by men, and increased high-risk behaviors among women. The marginal economic status of many African-American men contributes to fewer long-term partnerships, and high rates of incarceration promote further risk for infection for individuals and their sexual networks.[14]

HIV ILLNESS

Although disease progression of HIV infection appears to be similar for women and men, several studies have reported lower survival rates among women. Differences have mostly been attributed not to biologic factors but to disease stage, socioeconomic factors, and access to care.[5] A large cohort study from the late 1980s found that 3-fold differences in mortality rates from HIV infection were mostly accounted for by disease stage (56% of excess risk), age

(12%), ethnicity (11%), mode of transmission (8%), gender (8%), and interactions among these variables (5%).[15] A subsequent large-scale, multisite, multicity study examined mortality rates for women and men infected with HIV in each of six CD4 strata, adjusting results for age, ethnicity, mode of transmission, history of intravenous drug use, and Karnofsky score. Disease progression was found to be similar for both genders, but the mortality rate was higher among women, especially for African-American women and those using intravenous drugs, although deaths were mostly from non–HIV-related causes.[16] The excess mortality was postulated to be secondary to socioeconomic factors, including poverty, homelessness, domestic violence, substance abuse, lack of social support, and limited access to care.[16]

Gender differences in biologic markers of HIV infection, including CD4 counts and plasma HIV ribonucleic acid (RNA) levels, have been reported but are of unclear significance. Uninfected women have higher CD4 counts than uninfected men, and infected women maintain higher counts than infected men throughout much of their disease course.[17] Women have also been found to have lower HIV RNA levels than men at the same CD4 counts, although this difference seems to equalize when CD4 counts fall below 200×10^6/L.[18] Disease progression and survival at given CD4 counts or HIV RNA levels have not consistently been found to be different for women and men, however; thus recommendations for initiating antiretroviral therapy are no different for genders. Some studies report, however, that women may progress to AIDS at higher CD4 counts and lower viral levels, suggesting that perhaps they should be treated earlier in the course of HIV infection.[18] Additional research is required in this area.

The occurrence of HIV-related illnesses appears to be similar for women and men. Common manifestations that appear equally in both genders include *Pneumocystis jiroveci* (formerly *carinii*) pneumonia, esophageal candidiasis, mycobacterial infections, bacterial pneumonias, and non-Hodgkin's lymphomas. Gynecologic infections, especially bacterial vaginosis, may be common among HIV-infected women, although rates may be similarly high among women not infected but at high risk secondary to demographic and behavioral risk factors.[5] HIV-infected women have been found to have increased risk for cervical cancer, leading to the inclusion of cervical cancer as an AIDS-defining condition in 1993. They have extremely high rates of human papillomavirus (HPV), the sexually transmitted DNA virus responsible for most cases of cervical cancer, and increased rates of squamous cervical lesions.[19] HPV infections have been associated with low CD4 counts and elevated HIV RNA levels.[19] Among women with HIV, HPV infections are more persistent than among those without, and infection may be more likely to extend outside the cervix to the vagina and vulva. Infections with HPV-16 and HPV-18, the strains most associated with cervical cancer, may also be more common.[20]

SEXUALITY AND PREGNANCY

PREGNANCY AND CONTRACEPTION

Pregnancy does not appear to influence disease progression among HIV-infected women.[21] Overall, obstetric outcomes for women with HIV appear to be similar to those of noninfected women, although lower CD4 percentages have been associated with low-birth-weight infants and a trend toward preterm births.[22] However, in the absence of HIV-specific interventions, the risk of vertical transmission from infected mother to infant in industrialized countries such as the United States is roughly 25%.[23] HIV may be transmitted in utero, at birth, or through breast feeding.

Among HIV-infected women who do not breast feed, approximately one third of vertical transmissions occur in utero (95% of them in the 2 months before delivery) and two thirds occur around the time of delivery.[23] Transmission is more likely in the presence of elevated maternal HIV RNA levels or decreased CD4 counts. Obstetric complications that increase risk include prolonged rupture of membranes, chorioamnionitis, and in some studies, amniocentesis, maternal sexually transmitted infections, intrapartum maternal hemorrhage, and use of intrapartum fetal scalp electrodes or sampling.[24] Preterm infants and those with a birth weight less than 2500 g may be more likely to become infected. Rates of HIV transmission though breast feeding are estimated to be 15% to 16%.[25] Risk factors for transmission through breast feeding similarly include low CD4 counts and elevated viral loads, as well as the mother being recently infected with HIV or having breast pathology (i.e., cracked nipples, mastitis) or the infant having oral thrush.[26]

Fortunately, antiretroviral agents dramatically reduce the risk of vertical transmission. Two large cohort studies found that rates of transmission were reduced from 20% among women not receiving antiretroviral therapy to 5% to 10% for those on zidovudine and to 1% to 2% for women taking multiagent regimens.[27] The benefits of these antiviral combinations must be weighed against their potential risks, however, which include the development of resistant mutations in the mother or infant, maternal complications (possible hepatic failure, gestational diabetes, and preeclampsia), and effects on the fetus (possible preterm delivery, very low birth weight, and mitochondrial dysfunction). Elective cesarean delivery at 38 weeks' gestation also appears to reduce the risk of infection. A meta-analysis of 15 prospective cohort studies found that HIV-infected women undergoing cesarean section had roughly half the odds of vertical transmission.[28] The association held even for women receiving antiretroviral therapy before or during delivery and for whose neonates received antiretrovirals. More recent work has not shown a protective effect for cesarean section among women with low HIV RNA levels and has called attention to the morbidity associated with cesarean section among HIV-infected women.[29] Similarly, although women in industrialized countries who have access to sanitary breastmilk substitutes have been encouraged not to breastfeed, the risks and benefits must be more carefully weighed in developing countries.[26]

SEXUALITY AND WOMEN WITH HIV/AIDS

The majority of women infected with HIV continue to be sexually active, but their effective use of contraceptive and safe sex methods is limited.[30] Although hormonal contraception offers excellent protection against unwanted pregnancy, it has been linked to greater cervical HIV shedding (and thus infectivity), as well as higher HIV RNA levels and greater viral diversity (thus potentially hastening disease progression). Hormonal contraceptives may also offset condom use, and their metabolism may be induced by concurrent use of antiretrovirals.[23] Although male condoms offer a high degree of protection against HIV, they are frequently used incorrectly and their failure rate as a contraceptive is estimated to be 12%;[30] women are thus encouraged to use male condoms in conjunction with another effective contraceptive method. The female condom is less likely than male condoms to break or leak during intercourse, but shares a high failure rate as a contraceptive. The sole use of diaphragms or Vimule cervical caps or other caps by HIV-infected women is not recommended, because these devices all leave large areas of the vaginal mucosa exposed; these also require concomitant use of nonoxynol-9 spermicide, which may cause epithelial disruption and increase the risk of viral transmission.[30] Finally, a growing number of women infected with HIV may be choosing to become pregnant, given improved outcomes with antiretroviral treatments and cesarean sections. A growing body of literature has started to address the ethics and science of providing assisted reproduction techniques for those infected or for serodiscordant couples, both for infertility treatment and for prevention of HIV transmission to sexual partners.[31]

PSYCHIATRIC COMPLICATIONS

HIV disease and mental illness are frequently associated with one another, either because HIV places persons at risk for psychiatric sequelae or because those with psychiatric illness may have greater risk for HIV infection. In general, the co-occurrence of psychiatric and substance abuse disorders with HIV illness has been found to reduce adherence to complicated medication regimens, to negatively affect health services use, and to impair health outcomes and quality of life. Mental health conditions are also associated with high-risk behaviors that may increase the likelihood of HIV transmission and with significant social burden and health care costs.[32]

DEPRESSION

Significant depressive symptoms have been reported in as many as 30% to 60% of infected women, compared to 20% or less of infected men. Although women in general are more likely to suffer from depression than are men, those infected with HIV often have serious risk factors for depression, including low socioeconomic status, exposure to violence, lack of social support, and high rates of substance abuse.[33] In a compelling analysis of 765 HIV-infected women that were followed for 7 years, 42% reported chronic, persistent depressive symptoms. These women were more than twice as likely to die during the follow-up period than women with no or limited depressive symptoms, after controlling for sociodemographics, substance use, and clinical features.[33] Depressive symptoms were associated with greater decline in CD4 counts, especially among those with lower counts and higher viral titers. Potential mechanisms for these effects include that depression produces harmful neuroendocrine and immunologic changes; promotes harmful behaviors, such as smoking and alcohol use; and lessens adherence to medication regimens. The latter has implications for viral resistance and treatment failure.[33]

ANXIETY

Rates of specific anxiety disorders among HIV-infected women have been less frequently studied. However, some studies have estimated rates of post-traumatic stress disorder to be as high as 30% to 40% among women with HIV infection secondary to their alarmingly high rates of violence exposure during childhood and adulthood.[34] Among a national sample of 1,288 HIV-infected women, 66% reported a lifetime history of domestic violence, defined as physical or sexual abuse or coercion by an intimate partner or spouse.[35] One quarter of the women reported domestic abuse in the past year, and 31% reported a history of childhood sexual abuse. Similar to results from other studies, childhood sexual abuse was strongly associated with a lifetime history of domestic violence and high-risk behaviors, including having more than 10 male sexual partners and having high-risk male partners; using drugs; and exchanging sex for drugs, money, or shelter.[35] The authors comment that HIV-infected women may have a continuum of risk, in which sexual abuse as a child leads to repeated abuse and violence as an adult, which confers increased HIV risk. A history of trauma may certainly affect choice of partners or the ability to negotiate safe-sex methods. Notably, there have also been reports of partner violence resulting from women's disclosure of their HIV status. Among a sample of 257 women, the majority of whom were African American and half of whom had used intravenous drugs, 4% reported being sexually or physically assaulted as a result of their disclosure; 24% reported losing friends, 23% reported being insulted or sworn at, and 21% reported being rejected by family.[36]

SUICIDE

Increased rates of depression and violence among women with HIV may place them at increased risk for suicide. In an urban sample of 611 mostly African-American women, the majority of whom used drugs and half of whom were HIV-positive, half reported problems with depression and 26% with anxiety, although only just over half of those reporting depression and anxiety had received mental health treatment. In the past month, 31% had had suicidal thoughts and 16% had attempted suicide.[37] Women with both HIV disease and violence exposure were at particularly elevated risk for depression, anxiety, and suicidal thoughts and behavior; 38% of them had thought about suicide, and 24% had made an attempt.[37] Those recently diagnosed were more likely to contemplate suicide. These findings were remarkably similar to those in another study of 207 HIV-infected women in New York, 26% of whom had attempted suicide since their diagnosis, almost half of them within the first month.[38]

PSYCHOSOCIAL FACTORS

Women with HIV infection frequently suffer from the effects of poor social support, stigma, and multiple losses. These women are often unlikely to receive social support from their families, partners, or friends and are often the caregivers for infected family members or for children.[39] Among women with HIV disease or AIDS in the Unites States, more than half have children 16 years of age or younger for whom they are often the primary providers of economic and social support.[40] In one four-site study, 35% of the 871 HIV-infected women had a family member also infected with HIV; Latina and African-American women were especially likely to have infected family members.[41] In a moving report of interviews with 21 HIV-infected persons in a Southern city, subjects reported "chronic sorrow" related to illness, fear of death, poverty, and social isolation.[39] Women, the majority of whom were African American and living with children, were especially likely to report isolation, mostly as a result of stigma. They were avoided by friends and communities because of their association with "dirty sex," contagion, and moral threat.[39] Stigma may be especially magnified for pregnant women, who are seen as vectors for the virus to their innocent children, and for prostitutes, who may be blamed for spreading HIV.[42]

TREATMENT

Treatment guidelines currently recommend similar antiretroviral care for women and men, based on clinical, immunologic, and viral status. Large-scale trials to date support the effectiveness of antiretrovirals for preventing HIV disease progression, regardless of gender.[43] Fortunately, women are increasingly being represented in clinical antiretroviral trials; however, their absolute numbers in these trials remains small, limiting the power to detect any potential gender differences in efficacy and toxicity.[5] Available data suggest that the pharmacokinetics of antiretrovirals do not generally differ by gender, although they may differ by body mass and composition, metabolism, and hormonal milieu. Several drugs (e.g., nelfinavir, ritonavir, amprenavir, and efavirenz) may induce the metabolism of hormonal contraceptives, thus reducing their efficacy. Efavirenz may be teratogenic if given in the first trimester of pregnancy, and indinavir may cause hyperbilirubinemia and nephrolithiasis if given late in pregnancy.[44]

Some studies have reported that women are more likely to have adverse effects from antiretrovirals than men. One large Italian cohort study of more than 1,000 women and 2,000 men found that women were 1.4 times as likely as men to discontinue at least one retroviral agent secondary to toxicity (27% of women versus 20% of men), after adjusting for sociodemographic and clinical variables and for weight and body mass index.[45] Women were less likely to have gastrointestinal and hepatic toxicities and more likely to report hypersensitivity reactions and lipodystrophy (a syndrome characterized by redistribution of body fat from the extremities and face to the trunk). Indeed, several studies have noted that women may be at increased risk for lipodystrophy, which may promote insulin resistance and dyslipidemias.[43]

Although antiretroviral treatments may be effective for both genders, women may be less likely to receive them, often because they are more likely to be African American, injection drug users, and less educated about appropriate treatments. Studies have consistently found racial disparities in the receipt of antiretrovirals and other appropriate HIV treatments. One group examined variations in medication use and service utilization in a national probability sample of HIV-infected adults in the United States in 1996 to 1997, following the establishment of highly active antiretroviral therapy (HAART) as the standard of care.[46] After adjusting for CD4 counts, women received less quality care than men, Blacks and Latinos less care than Whites, uninsured and Medicaid-insured less care than privately insured, and other risk/exposure groups less care than men who had sex with men. Some of the poor care received by women was related to their lack of insurance coverage and ethnic status.[46] As recently as 2001, in a sample from 10 sites, HIV-infected persons who were women, African American, drug users, less educated, younger, and uninsured continued to be less likely to receive appropriate antiretroviral treatment.[47]

Women may have less access to regular health services and more barriers to care. In addition to lacking insurance, women may have multiple competing needs that prevent them from timely health care use. For example, among a national sample of HIV-infected persons in treatment, more than one third reported going without or postponing medical care as a result of needing the money for food, clothing, or housing; not having transportation; not being able to get time off from work; and being too sick.[48] Having at least one of these four needs was associated with less access to care, emergency room visits, and not receiving antiretrovirals. Women were more likely to report having at least one of these four needs and to report a lack of transportation and being too sick as reasons for going without care.[48] A subsequent analysis of this dataset found that women were 1.6 times as likely as men to postpone care, and that persons with a child in the home were 1.8 times as likely, as a result of caregiver responsibilities.[39]

In addition to insurance status and practical barriers to care, other patient, provider, and system factors may likely play a role in care disparities for HIV disease. In a national telephone survey, compared to Whites, Latinos were two thirds as likely, and African Americans about half as likely, to know that there are medical treatments for HIV disease.[49] African Americans with HIV infection have been found to have less access to providers with HIV-related expertise and to experience greater delays in receiving antiretroviral care when their providers are racially discordant.[50] Among providers who seriously consider patient adherence in their decision to prescribe, early antiretroviral therapy is less likely for women, Latinos, and the poor, even after adjusting for patient demographics and clinical characteristics and for provider demographics and HIV-related knowledge and experience.[51] Regardless of provider attitudes concerning adherence, African Americans are less likely to receive early treatment.[51]

PREVENTION

Successful risk reduction strategies for preventing HIV infection with have been targeted at the individual, couple, group, community, and social policy and structural levels. Several have been tested among, or tailored for, women and have been found to be effective in decreasing occurrence of unprotected sex and increasing condom use during intercourse. Typically, interventions have been based on models of risk reduction that emphasize the influence of risk education, skills, attitudes, and normative supports as determinants of behavior change. Accordingly, programs thus educate about risk, teach skills such as safe-sex negotiation and condom use, promote risk reduction attitudes, and reinforce efforts toward changing behavior. They frequently consist of peer-led, multiple intervention sessions and for women ideally emphasize gender-related differences.[52] More recent work is further tailoring existing approaches or developing new, gender-specific approaches for younger and minority women.

One notable group level intervention was developed by a task force from the National Institute of Mental Health (NIMH) in response to the need to reach understudied, disadvantaged populations in the United States with best-practices risk reduction strategies.[53] The NIMH Multisite HIV Prevention Trial enrolled 3,706 high-risk persons (23% women) from 37 public health and primary care clinics and randomized them to a 1-hour education session about AIDS or to a small-group, coed, 7-session program led by peers using a protocol. Patients in the group reported fewer unprotected sexual acts and had higher levels of condom use over a 12-month period.[53] Although there were no differences in rates of sexually transmitted disease, group participants reported fewer symptoms from these conditions. The efficacy of the intervention did not differ by age, gender, ethnicity, education, recent alcohol or drug use, commercial sex, unwanted sexual activity, or mental health services use.[53]

An interesting community-level intervention for minority women randomized 18 low-income housing developments in five cities.[54] Women in control communities received an AIDS brochure and condom coupon, while those in intervention communities had access to a program that included HIV risk reduction workshops and HIV prevention events that were implemented by women who were popular opinion leaders.[54] Two months later, although women in the control condition reported little behavior change, the proportion of women in intervention communities reporting they had engaged in unprotected intercourse declined from 50% to 38% and the percentage of condom-protected acts of intercourse rose from 30% to 47%.[54]

Interventions at the social policy/structural level to address the social and economic factors that place women at risk might be expected to reach large numbers, but have seemingly not been fully developed or evaluated for their effects on high-risk behaviors or HIV disease. Programs might include increasing access to educational or employment opportunities, improving services for domestic violence, reducing gender stereotypes in the media, reducing HIV-related stigma, and enhancing partnerships between faith-based organizations and HIV prevention efforts.[52] There is also a need to develop relapse prevention strategies, because many existing prevention programs for women lose effectiveness 3 to 6 months after completion. Additional strategies for existing programs might include group booster sessions to promote group norms and enhance social support, as well as cognitive-behavioral techniques that specifically address relapse.[52]

Finally, although prevention programs have focused on preventing new HIV infections (primary prevention), interventions also are needed to prevent the spread of HIV from infected to noninfected individuals and to reduce the risk of disease progression among infected persons (secondary prevention). Only 60% of HIV-infected women report using condoms during vaginal sex, and fewer use condoms during other sexual activities,[30] placing them at risk for infecting their partner and also for being exposed to other strains of HIV or sexually transmitted infections. Most secondary prevention programs have been developed for gay men, but others have been developed for both genders and specifically for women. Often delivered in 4 or 5 group sessions, these programs emphasize motivation and resiliency, coping skills, communication skills, problem-solving, and social networks.[55]

SUMMARY

In summary, women account for an increasing proportion of HIV infection and AIDS cases in the United States. Younger, ethnic minority women, particularly African Americans, are most at risk and are most frequently exposed through heterosexual contact. Numerous biologic and social factors contribute to HIV risk among women; cultural norms, poverty, and violence play a large role in perpetuating the epidemic. Although HIV disease progression appears to be similar for women and men, women may suffer higher mortality rates from other causes and are prone to gynecologic infections, especially with HPV. In the United States, vertical transmission of the infection through pregnancy, labor, and breast feeding has fortunately been dramatically reduced with antiretroviral therapies, cesarean sections, and supplemental feedings. Women with HIV disease have significant mental health needs, given their high rates of depression, violence exposure, and suicidal thoughts; they may be particularly prone to suffering from a lack of social support and stigma. Although women benefit from antiretroviral treatment as do men, they are less likely to receive timely care, often secondary to factors related to their ethnicity and socioeconomic status. Common barriers to care include lack of insurance, money, or transportation; childcare responsibilities; and illness. Several prevention strategies are effective in reducing high-risk sex behaviors among infected and noninfected women, although large percentages of women continue to engage in unsafe practices.

Women who are most at risk or infected with HIV frequently fall into not one, but several vulnerable, disadvantaged groups. They are commonly poor, ethnic minority, single mothers who have significant socioeconomic, medical, and mental health needs. These vulnerable groups must continue to be included in efficacy and effectiveness trials of HIV/AIDS treatments and interventions. Future treatment efforts may need to be more comprehensive and multifaceted to address the multiple needs of those infected and may need to be offered in alternative settings. Similarly, prevention efforts must be targeted at multiple tiers to address the numerous factors that place women at risk.

REFERENCES

1. Centers for Disease Control and Prevention. Follow-up on Kaposi's sarcoma and *Pneumocystis* pneumonia. *MMWR Morb Mortal Wkly Rep*. 1981;30:409–410.
2. Centers for Disease Control and Prevention. Cases of HIV infection and AIDS in the United States, 2003. Available: http://www.cdc.gov/hiv/stats/2003SurveillanceReport.htm. Accessed August, 2005.
3. Centers for Disease Control and Prevention. Young people at risk: HIV/AIDS among America's youth. Available: http://www.cdc.hiv/pubs/facts/youth.pdf. Accessed August, 2005.
4. Lindegren ML, Hanson C, Miller K, Byers RH Jr, Onorato I. Epidemiology of human immunodeficiency virus infection in adolescents, United States. *Pediatr Infect Dis J*. 1994;13:525–535.
5. Hader SL, Smith DK, Moore JS, Holmberg SD. HIV infection in women in the United States: status at the millennium. *JAMA*. 2001;285:1186–1192.
6. Chu SY, Wortley PM. Epidemiology of HIV/AIDS in women. In Minkoff H, DeHovitz JA, Duerr A, eds. *HIV Infection in Women*. New York: Raven Press; 1995:1–12.
7. Edlin BR, Irwin KL, Faruque S, et al. Intersecting epidemics: crack cocaine use and HIV infection among inner city young adults. Multicenter Crack Cocaine and HIV Infections Study Team. *N Engl J Med*. 1994;331: 1422–1427.
8. Padian NS, Shiboski SC, Jewell NP. Female-to-male transmission of human immunodeficiency virus. *JAMA*. 1991;266:1664–1667
9. Royce RA, Sena A, Cates W Jr, Cohen MS. Sexual transmission of HIV. *N Engl J Med* 1997;336:1072–1078.
10. Miller CJ. Host and viral factors influencing heterosexual HIV transmission. *Rev Reprod*. 1998;3:42–51.
11. Moscicki AB, Ma Y, Holland C, Vermund SH. Cervical ectopy in adolescent girls with and without human immunodeficiency virus infection. *J Infect Dis*. 2001;183:865–870.
12. Quinn TC, Overbaugh J. HIV/AIDS in women: an expanding epidemic. *Science*. 2005;308:1582–1583.
13. Logan TK, Cole J, Leukefeld C. Women, sex, and HIV: social and contextual factors, meta-analysis of published interventions, and implications for practice and research. *Psychol Bull*. 2002;128:851–885.
14. Adimora AA, Schoenback VJ. Social context, sexual networks, and racial disparities in rates of sexually transmitted infections. *J Infect Dis*. 2005;191(suppl 1):S115–S122.
15. Rothenberg R, Weolfel M, Stoneburner R, Milberg J, Parker R, Truman B. Survival with the acquired immunodeficiency syndrome: experience with 5833 cases in New York City. *N Engl J Med*. 1987;317:1297–1302.
16. Melnick SL, Sherer R, Louis TA, et al. Survival and disease progression according to gender of patients with HIV infection. The Terry Beirn Community Programs for Clinical Research on AIDS. *JAMA*. 1994; 272: 1915–1921.
17. Prins M, Robertson JR, Brettle RP, et al. Do gender differences in CD4 cell counts matter? *AIDS*. 1999;13: 2361–2364.
18. Sterling TR, Lytes CM, Vlahov D, Astemborski J, Margolick JB, Quinn TC. Sex differences in longitudinal human immunodeficiency virus type I RNA levels among seroconverters. *J Infect Dis*. 1999:180:666–672.

19. Strickler HD, Burk RD, Fazzari M, et al. Natural history and possible reactivation of human papillomavirus in human immunodeficiency virus-positive women. *J Natl Cancer Inst.* 2005;97:577–586.
20. Sun XW, Kuhn L, Ellerbrock TV, Chiasson MA, Bush TJ, Wright TC Jr. Human papillomavirus infection in women infected with the human immunodeficiency virus. *N Engl J Med.* 1997;337:1343–1349.
21. Burns DL, Landesman S, Minkoff H, et al. The influence of pregnancy on human immunodeficiency virus type 1 infection: antepartum and postpartum changes in human immunodeficiency virus type 1 viral load. *Am J Obstet Gynecol.* 1998;178:355–359.
22. Stratton P, Tuomala RE, Abboud R, et al. Obstetric and newborn outcomes in a cohort of HIV-infected pregnant women: a report of the women and infants transmission study. *J Acquir Immune Defic Syndr Hum Retrovirol.* 1999;20:179–186.
23. Cohan D. Perinatal HIV: special considerations. *Top HIV Med.* 2003;11:200–213.
24. Mandelbrot L, Mayaux MJ, Bongain A, et al. Obstetric factors and mother-to-child transmission of human immunodeficiency virus type 1: the French perinatal cohorts. SEROGEST French Pediatric HIV Infection Study Group. *Am J Obstet Gynecol.* 1996;175:661–667.
25. Nduati R, John G, Mbori-Ngacha D, et al. Effect of breastfeeding and formula feeding on transmission of HIV-1: a randomized clinical trial. *JAMA.* 2000;283:1167–1174.
26. Coutsoudis A. Breastfeeding and HIV. *Best Pract Res Clin Obstet Gynaecol.* 2005;19:185–196.
27. Cooper ER, Chararut M, Mofenson L, et al; Woman and Infants' Transmission Study Group. Combination antiretroviral strategies for the treatment of pregnant HIV-1 infected women and prevention of perinatal HIV-1 transmission. *J Acquir Immune Defic Syndr.* 2002;29:484–494.
28. The International Perinatal HIV Group. The mode of delivery and the risk of vertical transmission of human immunodeficiency virus type 1: a meta-analysis of 15 prospective cohort studies. *N Engl J Med.* 1999;340:977–987.
29. Read JS. Cesarean section delivery to prevent vertical transmission of human immunodeficiency virus type 1: associated risks and other considerations. *Ann N Y Acad Sci.* 2000;918:115–121.
30. Mitchell HS, Stephens E. Contraception choice for HIV positive women. *Sex Transm Infect.* 2004;80:167–173.
31. Drapkin L A, Anderson J. Human immunodeficiency virus and assisted reproduction: reconsidering evidence, reframing ethics. *Fertil Steril.* 2001;75:843–858.
32. Bing EG, Burnam MA, Longshore D, et al. Psychiatric disorders and drug use among human immunodeficiency virus-infected adults in the United States. *Arch Gen Psychiatry.* 2001;58:721–728.
33. Ickovics JR, Hamburger ME, Vlahov D, et al. Mortality, CD4 cell count decline, and depressive symptoms among HIV-seropositive women: longitudinal analysis from the HIV Epidemiology Research Study. *JAMA.* 2001;285:1466–1474.
34. Brief DJ, Bollinger AR, Vielhauer MJ, et al.; HIV/AIDS Treatment Adherence, Health Outcomes and Cost Study Group. Understanding the interface of HIV, trauma, post-traumatic stress disorder, and substance use and its implications for health outcomes. *AIDS Care.* 2004;16(suppl 1):S97–S120.
35. Cohen M, Deamant C, Barkan S, et al. Domestic violence and childhood sexual abuse in HIV-infected women and women at risk for HIV. *Am J Public Health.* 2000;90:164–168.
36. Gielen AC, Fogarty L, O'Campo P, et al. Women living with HIV: disclosure, violence, and social support. *J Urban Health.* 2000;77:480–491.
37. Gielen AC, McDonnell KA, O'Campo PJ, Burke JG. Suicide risk and mental health indicators: do they differ by abuse and HIV status? *Womens Health Issues.* 2005;15:89–95.
38. Cooperman NA, Simoni JM. Suicidal ideation and attempted suicide among women living with HIV/AIDS. *J Behav Med.* 2005;28:149–156.
39. Lichtenstein B, Laska MK, Clari JM. Chronic sorrow in the HIV-positive patient: issues of race, gender, and social support. *AIDS Patient Care STDS.* 2002;16:27–38.
40. Stein MD, Crystal S, Cunningham WE, et al. Delays in seeking HIV care due to competing caregiver responsibilities. *Am J Public Health.* 2000;90:1138–1140.
41. Fiore T, Flanigan T, Hogan J, et al. HIV infection in families of HIV-positive and 'at-risk' HIV-negative women. *AIDS Care.* 2001;13:209–214.
42. Bunting SM. Sources of stigma associated with women with HIV. *Adv Nurs Sci.* 1996;19:64–73.
43. Prins M, Meyer L, Hessol NA. Sex and the course of HIV infection in the pre- and highly active antiretroviral therapy eras. *AIDS.* 2005;19:357–370.
44. Centers for Disease Control and Prevention. Report of NIH panel to define principles of therapy of HIV infection and guidelines for the use of antiretroviral agents in HIV-infected adults and adolescents. *MMWR Morb Mortal Wkly Rep.* 1998;47:1–82. Available: http://www.hivatis.org. Accessed August, 2005.
45. Murri R, Lepri AC, Phillips AN, et al. Access to antiretroviral treatment, incidence of sustained therapy interruptions, and risk of clinical events according to sex: evidence from the I. Co. N. A. study. *J Acquir Immune Defic Syndr.* 2003;34:184–190.
46. Shapiro MF, Morton SC, McCaffrey DF, et al. Variations in the care of HIV-infected adults in the United States: results from the HIV Cost and Services Utilization Study. *JAMA.* 1999;281:2305–2315.
47. Gebo KA, Fleishman JA, Conviser R, et al.; HIV Research Network. Racial and gender disparities in receipt of highly active antiretroviral therapy persist in a multistate sample of HIV patients in 2001. *J Acquir Immune Defic Syndr.* 2005;38:96–103.
48. Cunningham WE, Andersen RM, Katz MH, et al. The impact of competing subsistence needs and barriers on access to medical care for persons with human immunodeficiency virus receiving care in the United States. *Med Care.* 1999;37:1270–1281.

49. Ebrahim SH, Andersen JE, Weide P, Purcell DW. Race/ethnic disparities in HIV testing and knowledge about treatment for HIV/AIDS: United States, 2001. *AIDS Patient Care STDS*. 2004;18:27–33.
50. Heslin KC, Andersen RM, Ettner SL, Cunningham WE. Racial and ethnic disparities in access to physicians with HIV-related experience. *J Gen Inter Med*. 2005;20:283–289.
51. Wong MD, Cunningham WE, Shapiro MF, et al.; HCSUS Consortium. Disparities in HIV treatment and physician attitudes about delaying protease inhibitors for nonadherent patients. *J Gen Intern Med*. 2004;19:366–374.
52. Wingood GM. Feminization of the HIV epidemic in the United States: major research findings and future research needs. *J Urban Health*. 2003;80(4 supp 3):iii67–iii76.
53. The NIMH Multisite HIV Prevention Trial. Reducing HIV sexual risk behavior. The National Institute of Mental Health (NIMH) Multisite HIV Prevention Trial Group. *Science*. 1998;280:1889–1894.
54. Sikkema KJ, Kelly JA, Winett RA, et al. Outcomes of a randomized community-level HIV prevention intervention for women living in 18 low-income housing developments. *Am J Public Health*. 2000;90:57–63.
55. Kalichman SC, Rompa D, Cage M. Group intervention to reduce HIV transmission risk behavior among persons living with HIV/AIDS. *Behav Modif*. 2005;29:256–285.

CHAPTER 28

HIV/AIDS Among Men Who Have Sex with Men

Milton L. Wainberg, Kenneth B. Ashley

The impact of human immunodeficiency virus (HIV) around the world in the last 25 years is indescribable. Some countries face losing a sizable proportion of their most productive and reproductive age-groups, which will affect their economies for years to come and generate an orphan problem of significant magnitude. Psychiatric vulnerability has been documented, with the severely mentally ill being at considerable risk for infection; having any mental disorder increases HIV transmission, morbidity, and mortality. In the United States, communities of color, injection drug users, and gays have been the hardest hit. Early in the acquired immunodeficiency syndrome (AIDS) epidemic, gay men were stigmatized in various ways, including labeling the epidemic a "gay-plague"; many religious leaders justifying it as "God's punishment"; and the medical community initially naming the syndrome "Gay-Related Immune Disorder" (GRID) when gays were not the only affected group (e.g., people with hemophilia or from Haiti). As a consequence, homosexuals faced more discrimination in the social arena, employment, housing, and medical care. The then United States President, Ronald Reagan, waited six years in office to mention the word AIDS and modeled the slow treatment and prevention efforts. AIDS reinforced and spread the already existing homophobia/anti-homosexual bias, yet strengthened the gay civil rights movement. Through the advocacy and protest efforts of a gay community–based organization, the AIDS Coalition To Unleash Power (ACT-UP; "Silence = Death"), easier access to medications in clinical trials and expedited approval of medications by the Food and Drug Administration (FDA) ensured the current faster availability of newer medications to the public in the United States. Community-based organization (e.g., Gay Men Health Crisis [GMHC]; God's Love We Deliver) and fundraising (e.g., AIDS Walks) models developed in response to the AIDS crisis have been replicated by advocacy groups for other diseases. Where possible, community activism worldwide brought about changes to medical services and ethical responses to all affected by the disease (e.g., surgery, pregnancy, transplants).

This chapter focuses mainly on the impact of HIV disease and AIDS on men who have sex with men (MSM), one of the first groups to be affected with the disease and a group that continues to be significantly affected by the HIV infection and AIDS epidemic. This chapter targets clinical issues around HIV disease prevention and treatment specific to MSM. The diversity among MSM, just like the diversity among other groups (e.g., heterosexuals), implies that there is not a "gold standard" HIV infection prevention or treatment intervention for MSM. MSM is used as a descriptive term that includes all men of various identities and social contexts who engage in sexual behavior with other men, regardless if they engage in sex with women or not or their self-identification as gay, bisexual, or straight. Even though in some sections references will be made to the lesbian, gay, bisexual (LGB), and/or transgender (LGBT) population, this chapter will mostly address issues to consider in working with the MSM population; other chapters in this book will address issues for women who have sex with women and the transgender population.

PROVIDING CARE TO MEN WHO HAVE SEX WITH MEN

Although the American Psychiatric Association removed homosexuality from its list of psychiatric disorders in 1973, negative attitudes within the mental health community persist and continue to affect the treatment provided to MSM.[1] Many MSM patients report nondisclosure of their sexual orientation to providers despite feeling that disclosure is important for their optimal care. As a result, many MSM individuals do not seek care or fear disclosing their sexual orientation to providers to avoid rejection, discrimination, or poor care. Unfortunately, many studies confirm their fears.[1] Harm from "reparative" or "conversion" interventions (treatments with the goal of changing an individual's sexual orientation) has been demonstrated, and there is a body of work on homophobia showing that health care providers' negative attitudes can be hazardous to their patients.[2] The mental health care clinician should create a safe, affirming, and nonjudgmental environment that encourages patients who are MSM to disclose their sexual identity and sexual orientation and to discuss their sexual behavior with the clinician. The following strategies might be used to create an office environment free of heterosexism (the expectation of heterosexuality) and homophobia, which will encourage open dialog between the clinician and patient and therefore better health outcomes. For example, one should use intake forms that do not assume heterosexuality and offer the option of "significant other, partner, or other," in addition to "married, single, or divorced."[3] Similar assumptions should be avoided when interviewing patients. In hospitals or clinics, one should display a nondiscrimination statement that includes sexual orientation and any distribution of health education materials should include language referring to and pictures of same-sex couples and transgendered individuals with information about local community resources.[3] Assumptions about sexual behavior based on an individual's sexual orientation, whether heterosexual, homosexual, or bisexual should be avoided. Clinicians should routinely ask whether sexual partners are male, female, or both. Research shows that many self-identified gay men have been sexually active with women. Clinicians who are not comfortable discussing different sexual behaviors with MSM patients and ways to reduce the risk of sexually transmitting HIV should seek training or supervision to enhance their comfort level and their clinical skills.

There are social and cultural disincentives to being attracted to people of the same sex: violence, discrimination, marginalization, illegal status, youth homelessness (runaways/throw-aways), imprisonment, individual and social abuse, and less than equal status in relation to public services.[2] Meyer discusses how minority stress—stigma, prejudice, and discrimination—create a hostile and stressful social environment that causes mental health problems, possibly explaining why MSM may have a higher prevalence of mental disorders than heterosexuals.[4] The experience of prejudice, expectations of rejection, hiding, concealing, and internalized homophobia may worsen coping processes. Internalized homophobia has been found to be a predictor of mental health problems, intimacy problems, and AIDS-related risk-taking behavior and is not uncommon even among self-identified gay and bisexual men who report acceptance of their homosexual orientation.[4] Rates of domestic violence in same-gender relationships are the same as in heterosexual relationships, and screening should be performed accordingly. However, accessing services tends to be more difficult for MSM victims of domestic violence.

Earlier in the epidemic, the gay community was ravaged by death and a sense of hopelessness; many lost partners and friends to AIDS. This resulted in a chronic state of bereavement, with survivor guilt and/or loss of support system. HIV-negative partners in serodiscordant couples (one HIV-positive and one HIV-negative) desiring sexual intimacy ("normal sex" is unsafe), driven by survivor guilt, wanting to offer support to their infected partner, or not wanting to feel left out, may have chosen not to engage in safer sex and therefore risk becoming HIV-infected. The lack of government responses and the devastating impact of HIV disease among MSM obliged the organized gay community efforts to focus on the needs of their HIV-infected members, leaving the non-HIV infected members to potentially perceive themselves as outsiders within their own gay community. Further, some HIV-negative young MSM (YMSM; aged 15 to 22) felt isolated in their coming out process, because their potential mentors seemed unavailable. Wanting to belong to the community drove some of these YMSM not to take the precautions necessary to avoid infection. For the current generation of YMSM the specter of AIDS has diminished. They did not lose their cohort of gay friends and did not attend multiple memorials—for some of them the first person they had any connection with who died of AIDS was Pedro Zamora from MTV's "The Real World." It is important when working with uninfected MSM, particularly YMSM to consistently remind them of the risks of HIV infection and other sexually transmitted infections (STI) and encourage safer behaviors using skills described later on in this chapter.

Until the 1990s, there was a void in the research, professional training, media presence, and recommendations for medical and mental health care of YMSM.[1,5] Their invisibility increased their vulnerability. YMSM face the same developmental needs and health and mental health challenges as their heterosexual peers, with the addition of social and health challenges associated with having a stigmatized sexual orientation or identity. Stigma, not deficit, is what separates YMSM from their heterosexual peers, and some gay youth, such as ethnic and racial minorities, are stigmatized even more.[1,5] Documented consequences of homophobia include suicide among young homosexual men and women.[2]

Providers should encourage all adolescents to postpone sexual activity, while respecting them by providing appropriate information and discussing their choices. For youth who are intent on sexual exploration, providers should discuss a range of safer sex options—explaining the continuum of sexual behaviors from "outercourse" (nonpenetrative massage, petting, and mutual masturbation) to the use of barriers (condoms or dental dams) when exchange of fluids is possible. Providers should clearly explain the risks (HIV, sexually transmitted infections [STIs], Hepatitis B and C, pregnancy) of unprotected oral, anal, and vaginal intercourse and should demonstrate the proper use of latex or polyurethane condoms, including female condoms.[1,5]

HIV EPIDEMIOLOGY AMONG MEN WHO HAVE SEX WITH MEN

Worldwide, AIDS cases among MSM are under-recognized, under-reported, or ignored.[6] Inadequate surveillance systems and the stigma associated with same-sex behavior contribute to the lack of data; this situation worsens in less developed countries.[6] The trend of HIV incidence among MSM for much of the world is unknown. Latin America, particularly Brazil, has the largest number of AIDS cases among MSM in emerging nations. An increasing HIV prevalence among MSM in Eastern Europe may point to a rising epidemic. Little can be understood about the trends of HIV incidence among MSM in North Africa; the Middle East; East, Central, and South Asia; and sub-Saharan Africa because of the virtual absence of MSM focus in the surveillance and epidemiologic data.[6] Currently, in the United States, about 70% of new HIV infections occur among men.[7] Among the newly infected men, 60% became infected through homosexual sex and 25% through injection drug use (which includes MSM who use injection drugs).[7] MSM represent 40% of all new AIDS diagnoses.[7] However, MSM are less likely than women and heterosexual men to receive prevention counseling and only 10% of the U.S. HIV prevention outcome studies have focused on MSM.[8]

HIV PREVENTION FOR MEN WHO HAVE SEX WITH MEN

Systematic reviews of HIV prevention research provide evidence that behavioral interventions can decrease sexual risk behavior of MSM. Studies of the AIDS epidemic in the early 1980s documented remarkable reductions in sexual high-risk behaviors among gay and bisexual men. Studies in the late 1980s began to describe the difficulty in sustaining risk reduction over longer periods.[6] These prevention messages targeted the educated, White, middle-class, outer segment of the gay community. Many MSM (often men of color) did not identify with the gay community, did not consider that they were gay, did not think the early messages applied to them, and, therefore, thought they were not at risk. Efforts have been made to develop interventions that specifically target different community groups.

Rates of high-risk sexual behavior are increasing among MSM in major European, Australian, Canadian, and U.S. cities since the late 1990s, when antiretroviral treatment became available. HIV infection risk taking may have increased because of the optimism brought about by treatment and decreased worry about HIV disease, with a shift of some community norms making unsafe sex more acceptable.[9] Internet sexually specific websites have opened the door for easier access to sex, both safer and risky. Recent data suggest that prevalence of sexual risk behavior and HIV infection and other STI rates among MSM is increasing.[7,10] Some correlates of high-risk behavior include mental health states, substance abuse, violence, childhood sexual abuse, social marginalization, social dislocation, migration, and poverty. In some areas, seroprevalence estimates indicate 33% of African-American MSM between the ages of 22 and 29 are HIV-positive.[11] MSM from other racial and ethnic groups also have high rates of infection, with an average across all groups of over 13% for those aged 22 to 29 years.[7]

Ample evidence exists that behavioral interventions reduce high-risk sexual behaviors and promote safer practices. Interventions have reliably reduced risk in primary care and community settings. However, it is only through community approaches embraced by the government that the HIV incidence can be slowed. These policy interventions remain underutilized in the United States, but have been used successful in other countries, such as in Brazil and Australia, where a national HIV prevention strategy reduced HIV seroprevalence.[12] Effective new medical treatments have produced significant declines in progression from HIV infection to AIDS (i.e., AIDS incidence) and in AIDS deaths, but these declines are slowing, indicating that much of the benefit of new therapies has been realized. Because HIV is transmitted through sexual and drug-use behaviors that encompass issues of human identity, pleasure, and need, making changes to prevent exposure to HIV can be difficult to initiate and sustain. As with any other behavior change, relapse is the norm. Behavioral scientists and mental health care providers have brought their expertise and experience to the task of developing, testing, and implementing a vast array of prevention interventions. Mental health providers can have a very important role in all of these levels of prevention, from community efforts to work in their individual offices.

CLINICAL PRACTICE: AN OUNCE OF PREVENTION IS WORTH A POUND OF CURE

Good prevention efforts must be individualized to appropriately target the individual's needs and personalized risks. Assessing risk behaviors must be conducted in a nonjudgmental environment, with empathy, especially in the presence of high-risk behaviors. Patients share more if they do not feel criticized; otherwise, they give the answers that will prevent criticism and shame. Risk assessment after assessing satisfaction with sex and sexual activities frames the evaluation in a more empathic way; sex is a healthy activity and "normal" sex is unsafe. Further, questions about sexual behavior may be asked in the context of healthy human functions such as diet/appetite, exercise, sleeping patterns, and relationships instead of within the context of tobacco, alcohol, and drug use. The following illustrates some of the issues:

Provider: "How is your sex life?"
Patient: "OK . . ."
Provider: "Are you enjoying it?"
Patient: "Sort of, yeah!"
Provider: "Good. What about condoms? Are you using them?"
Patient: "Sometimes."
Provider: "So, sometimes you use them. But sometimes you don't. Let's figure out what helps you use them and what stands in the way of your using them."

Without compromising one's role, one can create an open environment and stimulate communication. It is important to adjust the language to ensure comprehension and clarity. Technical terms hamper communication; intercourse may not be understood as sex, and many consider intercourse only one type of sex. Also, asking for definitions of slang is important, because meanings and usage may change among individuals. When assessing risk behaviors it is important to focus on risky behaviors and not identified risk groups. Not all MSM will identify as being gay. In some communities it is only the receptive partner who may be identified as gay.

Knowledge about HIV disease does not necessarily lead to safer behaviors. In creating goals for behavior change, it is helpful to keep them simple and realistic and not to assume that intervening once is enough. Repetition and maintenance intervention with positive reinforcement are key to achieve and sustain the newly acquired behavior change. Regardless of the prevention model one prefers (e.g., motivational interviewing, cognitive behavioral therapy), the goal is to move the behavior to a safer place. Any movement to healthier, safer, or less risky behavior is a move in the right direction. It is important to remember that it is normal that people who have adopted safer behaviors can relapse. Community peer influences are strong factors in encouraging behavior change in either direction. Thus it is important to understand the context of each individual; one size does not fit all. One must be pragmatic and consider the individual's situational context before proscribing a standard prevention intervention.

HIV ANTIBODY TESTING AND COUNSELING

Testing for HIV antibodies may be the first instance when MSM report same-sex activity. Regardless of the test result, testing can offer providers the opportunity for HIV prevention efforts promoting healthier self-perception of their sexual orientation. The relief of a negative antibody result offers the opportunity to engage MSM in a prevention plan tailored to meet patients' individual needs; they also should be reminded that the current test could not identify HIV infection that occurred within the previous two months. For some MSM, testing HIV-positive may coincide with their coming out or being "outed" as a gay man. A healthier outcome requires separating their difficulties with their sexual orientation from the risky sexual behavior that led to their becoming HIV infected; otherwise, they would associate their homosexuality with illness.

HIV DISCLOSURE

An open discussion about HIV status needs to be encouraged among all those engaging in sexual behavior. Some gay community peer norms consider low risk to be when HIV-positive MSM engage in unsafe sex with other HIV-positive men (e.g., seroconcordant), overlooking potential superinfection with another HIV strain or medical complications from acquiring another STI. This issue is on the background of the work with Mr. B, described in the following case:

> Mr. B is a 38-year-old, HIV-positive gay man who is well controlled with psychiatric medication to treat his symptoms of depression and anxiety, and perfectly adheres to antiretroviral medication. Mr. B enjoys sex and having others find him sexually attractive; he looks healthy. Mr. B understands the different degrees of risky sexual activity and engages mostly in unprotected oral sex. Having an undetectable viral load, he feels "less contagious." He assumes that with all the information about HIV infection in the gay community and in the media, if a sex partner does not ask about his HIV status, it is likely that he is also infected as well or he understands the risk he is taking.

Mr. B. illustrates a widespread assumption made by HIV-infected MSM that if a man does not ask about HIV status when having sex, it is because he is also infected and there is no need to use condoms. The opposite is assumed by HIV-negative MSM; if another man does not ask about HIV status or does not disclose being HIV-positive when having sex, it is because he is HIV negative and condoms are not needed. Therefore not talking about or disclosing HIV status leads to unsafe sex on the incorrect belief that it is with someone of their own HIV status and thus not risky.

Even though the general assumption is that disclosure is a healthy step, the therapeutic work of helping an HIV-positive MSM disclose "the secret" requires careful review of the individual context to ensure specific solutions that fit.

MENTAL HEALTH TREATMENT OF HIV-POSITIVE MEN WHO HAVE SEX WITH MEN

MSM HIV-infected patients are at increased risk for mental health and substance use disorders, possibly as a result of society's prejudice, internalized homophobia, and lack of support; preexisting mental health and substance use disorders may have put them at risk for contracting HIV. In general, people with HIV disease are even more likely to experience emotional distress or mental illness. Depression, anxiety, post-traumatic stress disorder, and cognitive impairment are among the most common disorders among people with HIV disease. Psychosis is more common among patients with HIV infection who abuse substances, particularly stimulants, than in the general population. Because of the known negative consequence of untreated mental health problems among HIV-infected people, providers working with them must help to prevent, identify, or treat psychiatric illness, including substance use disorders, and maximize patients' psychological health. Because of denial and the stigma of mental illness, patients may mask their psychological symptoms or may not ask for help. Patients may be unaware of treatment options. The issue of the stigma of mental illness may play a greater role for racial/ethnic minority MSM who already may feel stigmatized and marginalized by their sexuality, their racial/ethnic minority status, and their HIV status. It may be important to focus on how their symptoms may be impairing their function and explain that the reason for treatment is to improve their functioning.

As with the care of any HIV-infected person, communication between the HIV primary provider and mental health care provider (as well as any other members of the treatment team) is fundamental to enhance intervention and maintain updated information about diagnoses, medications, and other medical or psychiatric issues.

Several themes emerge during therapy sessions that underscore the complex interaction of biological, psychological, and social factors associated with AIDS and symptomatic HIV infection. Besides the shame about contracting HIV, themes include AIDS as a punishment for being gay and guilt about the possibility of infecting others. The appearance of new symptoms of physical illness or changes in disease markers (e.g., CD4 count, viral load) can be associated with relapse into depression, with cognitive distortions (e.g., "my life is over;" "why continue this life"). HIV-positive friends becoming ill may trigger hopelessness and fear. The sense of having lost value or attractiveness to others may interfere with the formation of new relationships with noninfected gay men. Forming relationships with other HIV-positive men may bring up the despair of having to pair with someone who can get ill and die. However, for some, the infection offers an opportunity to explore and improve their lives (i.e., "how will I live my life, as long as possible or as fully as possible?"). Concerns about dying were common before antiretroviral therapy; with this new possibility for treatment, patients' underlying assumptions about the immediacy of death has shifted. The resulting hopefulness can allow patients to focus more constructively on their treatment and their lives.[13]

The clinician should explore the MSM HIV-infected patient's support system, understanding that a broad and inclusive definition of family is necessary. The clinician should encourage the patient to involve a member of his or her support system in treatment planning. MSM patients may have less of a support system than heterosexual patients. Their support system may not fit the narrow, traditional family construct. Questions such as "Who is important to you?" or "Who would you turn to in an emergency?" allow patients to define their support system. Selection (or identification) of a health care proxy, important for everyone, is especially important for MSM patients because unmarried partners, even in long-standing, committed relationships may not be afforded the same rights as their married counterparts, which may include hospital visitation rights.

DISCUSSING SEX AND RISK BEHAVIORS WITH HIV-POSITIVE MEN WHO HAVE SEX WITH MEN

Clinicians should evaluate and discuss sexual health, including sexual function/dysfunction, with all HIV-infected patients, including MSM. Common physiologic causes of sexual dysfunction in HIV include, but are not limited to, a low testosterone level, diabetes, and medication side effects. After excluding physiologic causes for sexual dysfunction, clinicians should evaluate possible psychological causes. Besides the common psychiatric causes for sexual dysfunction, such as depression or anxiety, one must assess psychological factors that can interfere with sexual functioning. Some common issues that may be present are difficulty with intimacy, fear of infecting sex partners, and low self-esteem; however, occasionally MSM who acquire HIV via same-sex sexual activity may carry guilt and shame about their sexuality.

Once sexual health is discussed, condom use and risk behaviors must be explored nonjudgmentally. Unsafe sex is the "normal" sex; none of us, HIV-positive, HIV-negative, or unknown status fantasize having sex with condoms, and many of us do not use condoms when having sex. Beginning with this premise may help providers engage HIV-positive people into discussing safer sex behaviors. Also, we may be one of many discussing safer sex with them, besides their own conscience. Several therapeutic models have been used to engage HIV-positive patients to reduce their risky ("normal") sex (e.g., motivational interviewing); they are not within the scope of this chapter.

Patient: "My boyfriend and I do not use condoms anymore. I don't think he can get HIV from me. We have had sex many times and he is still HIV-negative. He even got tested regularly, but not anymore because it was always so scary and intrusive in our lives."

Provider: "Maybe the fact that you can handle it so well means that you have become comfortable that he can never get HIV from you, because he has not so far. He even got tested regularly, perhaps doubting his luck. Yet, it was such a reminder of what could go wrong that you have opted for not finding out anymore, so you worry about it. Now you avoid worrying by not getting tested and not having to think about the clear risks you both take. So, deep inside you probably know that partners can get HIV after years of having unsafe sex. The reality is unpredictable."

TREATMENT FOR MEDICATIONS' AND RECREATIONAL DRUGS' INDUCED SEXUAL DYSFUNCTION

Several HIV infection medications, antidepressants (selective serotonin reuptake inhibitors [SSRI]-containing agents), and several other prescribed medications have sexual side effects, including decreased libido and erectile dysfunction. Erectile dysfunction can be treated with phosphodiesterase inhibitors (sildenafil, tadalafil, vardenafil). Alcohol initially can "improve" sexual functioning by decreasing anxiety and inhibitions and increasing impulsivity. With time, alcohol negatively affects the ability to get and maintain a penile erection. Similarly, crystal methamphetamine (Crystal, Tina) initially drastically enhances interest in sexual activity but causes a phenomenon known as "crystal dick" in which the erectile dysfunction is severe and achieving and maintaining an erection is very difficult. MSM with erectile dysfunction caused by prescribed medications or alcohol and drugs may remain sexually active by becoming the anal receptive partner (i.e., bottom). By doing so, an HIV-negative MSM is at higher risk of acquiring HIV infection, because unprotected receptive anal intercourse is the riskiest sex act. In the case of an HIV-infected MSM experiencing sexual dysfunction, the transmission risk decreases, unless treatment with phosphodiesterase inhibitors are prescribed, and insertive anal intercourse (i.e., top) can be resumed. Clinicians must understand these complexities, including sexual activity and condom use as described earlier in this chapter, before deciding to prescribe medications that can cause sexual dysfunction or whether to treat medication-, alcohol-, or drug-induced sexual dysfunction. Even though there is no correct answer, careful considerations must be taken. Deciding never to treat sexual dysfunction, whatever the cause, in an HIV-infected man whose preferred sexual act is unprotected anal intercourse may follow public health recommendations. However, besides the fact that phosphodiesterase inhibitors are easily bought in the street or via the Internet, refusing to treat while missing the opportunity to openly and nonjudgmentally discuss sexual activity and risky behaviors and offer treatment as a plan to work on prevention and condom use may passively contribute to HIV transmission.

RACIAL/ETHNIC MINORITY MEN WHO HAVE SEX WITH MEN

Just as there is no single gay community, neither is there a uniform community of racial/ethnic minority MSM; rather there is a collection of communities. Racial/ethnic minority MSM must deal with their sexuality and their racial/ethnic minority status, which on the most basic level involves both anti-homosexual bias/heterosexism and racism. How the individual integrates the various aspects of his personality will play a role in how he interacts with his environment. The sense of invisibility many racial/ethnic minority MSM experience within the larger gay community or nonidentification with the gay community has resulted in many of the HIV infection prevention messages directed at the gay community being ignored. More recently, as the increased rates of HIV infection among African-American and Latino MSM have been acknowledged, more culturally appropriate HIV prevention messages and interventions have been developed. Ethnic minorities MSM have also developed their own support organizations (e.g., Gay Men of African Descent—GMAD), and ethnic/culturally focused AIDS organizations have been developed (e.g., Asian Pacific Islander Coalition on HIV/AIDS—APICHA).

When working with the racial/ethnic minority MSM with HIV disease it is important to recognize that anti-homosexual bias/homophobia, heterosexism, and racism are issues that preceded the medical condition and be aware that some aspect of these issues may present at times during the course of treatment. It is important to get to know the individual issues of each patient, understand that the issues may arise in different ways depending on the situation. Often there may be a distrust of institutions—the government, the health care system, and the pharmaceutical industry. These issues often come up around the issue of medications—fears that the medications are poison, beliefs about the pharmaceutical companies and the government having a cure but wanting to sell medications for profit, concerns that HIV is not the cause of AIDS, refusal to enroll in clinical trials for fear of being a "guinea pig," or as a legacy of Tuskegee. Recent data from the Institute of Medicine and other studies indicating the racial/ethnic disparities in health care in the United States seems to warrant some of such concern.

There is a perception that within racial/ethnic minority communities there is greater anti-homosexual bias/homophobia. Racism within the gay community is also present, however there is no reason to believe that it is any greater than that in the general culture, and it might be lower (in the overall sense), given the focus on inclusion in the LGBT community. It is important, however, to understand how the individual identifies with the various communities to understand his support systems.

Given that each person has various identities, rather than expecting that there is some formula to understand people coming from a particular background, it is more important to work with individuals to understand how they have integrated their various identities and what role that plays in how they function in the world. There may be some key issues to think about as possible factors (e.g. racism, anti-homosexual/homophobia bias, AIDS phobia); however, ultimately it comes down to the individual, and it is the goal of providers to understand the unique person that they are working with in treatment.

DRINKING AND DRUG USE IN THE MSM COMMUNITY

Problem drinking occurs at a rate of 12% to 13% in urban MSM.[14] Some studies indicate that recreational drug use, moreover, occurs at substantially higher rates among MSM than among other men, and both alcohol and drug use are regarded with a greater degree of acceptability among MSM than in the general population. Among MSM, alcohol and drug use are often regarded as integral parts of gay life, and their use is often intermingled such that neither behavior can be considered in isolation. Lifestyle differences between heterosexuals and MSM, including greater reliance on bars as social outlets and lower abstinence rates among peers, may inhibit treatment seeking if the treatment is perceived as being abstinence-oriented or unresponsive to the unique needs of MSM. Alcohol and drugs may affect risky sex, adherence to medications, depression and other mental health problems, finances, relationships, and the ability to obtain a better life. HIV risk behavior is associated with alcohol and some recreational drug (e.g., crystal methamphetamine, cocaine, poppers) consumption, although the exact nature of the relationship is unclear. Thus problem-drinking or drug-using MSM comprise a group at uniquely elevated risk for contracting and transmitting HIV infection, and interventions addressing these two health risk behaviors in MSM have potential to serve the important public health goals of alleviating substance use problems and reducing HIV transmission.

YMSM are at particularly elevated risk for alcohol use and sexual risk behaviors. Although YMSM do not always differ from heterosexual peers on lifetime prevalence of substance use, the frequency and quantity of tobacco, alcohol, and illicit drug use are elevated among YMSM.[15] Sexual risk behaviors also are elevated among YMSM compared with heterosexual peers.[16] A high number of YMSM in U.S. urban areas engage in illegal drug use, with some using three or more drugs or using drugs once a week or more.[17]

Several studies have documented that LGB youths who attend schools with non–gay-sensitive instruction report more substance use, high-risk sexual behaviors, suicidal thoughts or attempts, and personal safety issues than heterosexual or LGB youth that attend schools with gay-sensitive instruction. LGB youths who attend schools with gay-sensitive instruction have similar risk behaviors than those of heterosexual youth.[18]

The goals of substance abuse treatment interventions are to build specific behavioral and cognitive skills needed to effect behavior change while increasing individual knowledge about HIV and influencing intrapsychic factors thought to mediate risk behavior.

SUMMARY

Even though AIDS reinforced and spread the already existing homophobia, it also strengthened the gay community and HIV-infected communities' civil rights movement. Individual work in HIV disease prevention and treatment must parallel this hopeful and positive outcome in the face of adversity and loss. AIDS is not about to disappear, and neither is homophobia, real or internalized. A safe, caring, nonjudgmental and productive environment created by a mental health care clinician encourages MSM patients to be healthier and freer, be open for the needs of the individual and health promotion, be comfortable with their sexual identity and sexual orientation, be responsible about their lives and sexual activity, and exhibit better adherence to medical care. Clinicians who are not comfortable working with MSM or HIV-infected individuals can, and should, seek training or supervision to enhance their comfort level and allow them to provide appropriate care.

The challenges of working with MSM patients may be many, but the rewards of offering care are enormous. MSM, especially if requiring mental health care, may be at increased risk for acquiring or transmitting HIV infections and another STIs, for developing substance use disorders and therefore for having adherence to treatment problems. The situation often becomes more complex if the individual also belongs to a racial/ethnic minority. These variables must be taken into consideration in the course of treatment and prevention education. Providers have responsibilities in their offices; they can also be advocates in professional, civil, political arenas. The heterosexualization of the AIDS epidemic, with increasing numbers of women being infected, should ensure efforts to target all those affected, without disregarding the impact of AIDS in the gay community by diverging funds.

REFERENCES

1. Futterman DC. HIV and AIDS in adolescents. *Adolesc Med Clin.* 2004;15:369–391.
2. Wainberg ML, Bux DA Jr, Carballo-Diéguez A, et al. Science and the Nuremberg Code: a question of ethics and harm—peer commentaries on Spitzer. *Arch Sex Behav.* 2003;32:455–457.
3. AIDS Institute. *Mental Health Guidelines: Special Populations.* New York: New York State Department of Health AIDS Institute, Mental Health Guidelines Committee; 2006 In press.
4. Meyer IH. Prejudice, social stress, and mental health in lesbian, gay, and bisexual populations: conceptual issues and research evidence [review]. *Psychol Bull.* 2003;129:674–697.
5. Ryan C, Futterman DC. *Lesbian and Gay Youth: Care and Counseling.* New York: Columbia University Press; 1998.
6. Stall RD, Hays RB, Waldo CR, et al. The gay '90s: a review of research in the 1990s on sexual behavior and HIV risk among men who have sex with men. *AIDS.* 2000;14 (suppl 3): S104–S114.
7. Centers for Disease Control and Prevention. *Cases of HIV infection and AIDS in the United States: 2003 HIV/AIDS Surveillance Report.* Vol. 15. Atlanta: U.S. Department of Health and Human Services, Centers for Disease Control and Prevention; 2004.
8. Johnson WD, Hedges LV, Diaz RM. Interventions to modify sexual risk behaviors for preventing HIV infection in men who have sex with men. *Cochrane Database Syst Rev.* 2003;CD001230.
9. Crepaz N, Hart TA, Marks G. Highly active antiretroviral therapy and sexual risk behavior. *JAMA.* 2004;292:224–236.
10. Catania JA, Osmond D, Stall RD, et al. The continuing HIV epidemic among men who have sex with men. *Am J Public Health.* 2001;91:907–914.
11. Valleroy LA, MacKellar DA, Karon JM, et al. HIV prevalence and associated risks in young men who have sex with men: Young Men's Study Group. *JAMA.* 2000;284:198–204.
12. Carey MP. Prevention of HIV infection through changes in sexual behavior. *Am J Health Promot.* 1999;14:104–111.
13. Mayne TJ, Vittinghoff E, Chesney MA, et al. Depressive affect and survival among gay and bisexual men infected with HIV. *Arch Intern Med.* 1996;156:2233–2238.

14. Stall R, Paul JP, Greenwood G, et al. Alcohol use, drug use, and alcohol-related problems among men who have sex with men: the Urban Men's Health Study. *Addiction*. 2001;96:1589–1601.
15. Russell ST, Driscoll AK, Truong N. Adolescent same-sex romantic attractions and relationships: implications for substance use and abuse. *Am J Public Health*. 2002;92:198–202.
16. Garofalo R, Wolf RC, Kessel S, et al. The association between health risk behaviors and sexual orientation among a school-based sample of adolescents. *Pediatrics*. 1998;101:895–902.
17. Thiede H, Valleroy LA, MacKellar DA, et al. Regional patterns and correlates of substance use among young men who have sex with men in 7 US urban areas. *Am J Public Health*. 2003;93:1915–1921.
18. Blake SM, Ledsky R, Lehman T, et al. Preventing sexual risk behaviors among gay, lesbian, and bisexual adolescents: the benefits of gay-sensitive HIV instruction in schools. *Am J Public Health*. 2001;91:940–946.

CHAPTER 29

HIV/AIDS Among Women Who Have Sex with Women

Alison R. Jones, Cynthia L. Hoyler

In 1997, The Institute of Medicine (IOM) Committee on Lesbian Health Research Priorities concluded the following:

> There is no standard definition of lesbian. The term has been used to describe women who have sex with women, either exclusively or in addition to sex with men (i.e., behavior); women who self-identify as lesbian (i.e., identity); and women whose sexual preference is for women (i.e., desire or attraction).[1]

Sexual orientation has been described as occurring along continua that include behavior, desire, and identity.[1] "That is, women may exhibit differing degrees of same-sex sexual behavior, desire, or identity in combinations that vary from person to person."[1] To appreciate the concept of continua in female sexuality, this chapter will examine the psychiatric aspects of human immunodeficiency virus (HIV) disease and acquired immunodeficiency syndrome (AIDS) in lesbians and expand the focus to include all women who have sex with women (WSW).

INCIDENCE AND RISK FACTORS FOR HIV/AIDS IN WOMEN WHO HAVE SEX WITH WOMEN

Women are now the population with the fastest growth of new infections with HIV.[2] Currently, the greatest risk for HIV in women throughout the world is heterosexual intercourse.[1] The CDC regards the highest level of risk for HIV infection to occur through unprotected anal sex, although risk in unprotected vaginal sex is also high. The National Lesbian and Bisexual Women's Health Survey reported that 16% of the 6,146 women surveyed were currently having sex with both male and female partners.[1,2] Compared to their exclusive cohorts (homosexual or heterosexual), behaviorally bisexual women had higher rates of HIV seroprevalence.[1]

Although considered to be low, the incidence for HIV infection through female-to-female transmission has not been established.[1,3] Although there are limited case reports of female-to-female transmission, these have not been substantiated through large-scale, longitudinal studies.[4] Controversial evidence does exist regarding female-to-female transmission for other sexually transmitted infections (STIs) (i.e., bacterial vaginosis, trichomonas vaginalis, human papillomavirus, herpes simplex virus, hepatitis A, and syphilis).[2,4–6] Reports concerning data regarding female-to-female transmission of HIV infection are conflicting at best.[5] The lack of consistent definitions for WSW and the fact that the Centers for Disease Control and Prevention (CDC) has no HIV reporting category for lesbians limits reliability of data regarding transmission rates.[1,3] The prospective study cited most often regarding female-to-female transmission for HIV was done in Italy. It followed 18 HIV-discordant, partnered lesbians in which no incidence of HIV occurred in the uninfected partner after 10 months.[1,4,5]

Although WSW have risk factors similar to those in all women, some are unique. Studies indicate that WSW engage in higher rates of injection drug use, sex with gay or bisexual men, sex with injection drug users (IDUs), sex with an HIV-infected partner, and sex for secondary gain (i.e. money, drugs, etc.). Although this may be an effect of sampling that included high rates of women involved in sex work, these findings were comparable throughout most studies.[1,2,6,7] Other factors that influence risk for WSW include their specific sexual practices, their attitudes regarding risk, and their limited use of risk-reducing behaviors. Sexual practices in WSW include, but are not limited to, the following: oral sex (receptive, active), vaginal penetration (digital, sex toy), mutual masturbation, genital–genital (perineal) contact, anal penetration (digital, sex toy), fisting (hand-vagina or anus), rimming (mouth-anus), and sadomasochistic activity. For any of these activities, sex during menses may also apply.[1,3,5,6] Practices of highest risk are those with the potential for tearing (i.e., fisting, use of sex toys, sadomasochistic activities) and exchange of bodily fluids (oral sex, genital–genital contact, rimming, and sex during menses). As is true for heterosexual practices, not all WSW engage in all practices cited. An additional risk for WSW seeking motherhood is donor insemination.[5]

As indicated earlier, many WSW have past or present histories of sex with men, particularly men in higher risk categories. These women, regardless of their sexual orientation, are also unlikely to use safe sex practices already established for heterosexual intercourse. One U.S. study with a sample of 7,929 total respondents from all 50 states found that of the 6,935 self-identified lesbians, 70.5% had a lifetime history of vaginal intercourse with a man and 17.2% had lifetime history of anal sex. The rates of lesbians with histories of vaginal intercourse without a condom were significantly high—88.2% compared to 63.9% of all respondents. Rates for anal sex without a condom were 15.8% for all respondents. Older lesbians (greater than age 50) were more likely to report sexual histories without a condom.[4] A United Kingdom study consisting of 803 lesbian and bisexual women from two lesbian health clinics and 415 lesbian and bisexual women from a fairly diverse community found similar results. With a breakdown of 90% lesbian, 8% bisexual, and 2% other, 85% had reported past or present sex with men and 12% in past year. Rates for use of condoms or female condoms for vaginal intercourse were 23% always, 45% occasionally, and 32% never. With anal intercourse, rates were 29% for always, 29% occasionally, and 42% never.[6] Both studies denote minimal risk-reducing practices for high-risk heterosexual contact.

Use of safe-sex practices between women is also low. Although there are currently no safe-sex guidelines for prevention of HIV infection in lesbians, there are methods to reduce risk.[1,8] The use of dental dams during oral sex, latex gloves with penetration, and washing or placing condoms on sex toys between uses are all known precautions that are seldom practiced.[3,6] Even in high-risk groups of WSW, safer sex practices when having sex with women are infrequently used. In one study of 871 HIV-infected women, 67 had a female partner at some time during the 3½-year period. Of those 67 HIV-infected WSW, 44 had a steady female partner. Thirty-five of the 44 reported engaging in receptive oral sex in which barriers were used always at 26% of the time, sometimes at 31%, and never at 43%. Surprisingly, HIV serostatus of their partner did not affect the use of barriers. Couples reported use of barriers as always (23% concordant, 27% discordant) and sometimes or never (77% concordant, 73% discordant).[8]

Another study involving women who were IDUs or crack cocaine users who engaged in having sex with women 30 days before interview reported use of barrier protection when giving oral sex only 6% and only 3% while receiving oral sex.[9] Factors that influence the use of risk-reducing behaviors in WSW include their attitudes regarding vulnerability to risk, especially for lesbians.

There seems to be a myth within society and WSW that female-to-female sexual activity is protective against HIV infection. This attitude is also reflected in the medical community, addressed later in this chapter. The fact that there are no established guidelines regarding HIV prevention in WSW supports this misperception.[1,8] Lesbians are assumed to be at low risk because of lack of heterosexual intercourse.[1] Their relationships are commonly assumed to be monogamous and long term, with low rates of outside sexual partners.[1] Self-identified lesbians who have the perception of "lesbian immunity" consider themselves not at risk for HIV infection.[3] One study reported that although 82% of lesbians surveyed believed HIV infection was a problem in their community, only 30% were worried about contracting HIV infection and 53% believed they were at low risk.[3] Another study found that 39% of lesbians surveyed did not perceive that they had any risk for contracting HIV.[3] Part of the problem in self-assessment of risk may be due to insufficient education and communication within the lesbian community. Something unique to lesbians compared to other WSW that may hinder education and communication is their level of disclosure in the coming out process.

COMING OUT

Addressing the psychiatric aspects of WSW, and specifically lesbians, demands a discussion of the "coming out" process. This process of disclosure and self-acceptance can begin at any age and may continue for many years of a woman's life. Many adult lesbians continue to live a "hidden life" and have not negotiated this disclosure process. The following section describes the stages of coming out and addresses some reasons many women continue to live hidden lives.

There have been many theories and stages of the coming out process presented in the literature. Richard Niolon[10] presents a concise model that includes self-recognition, disclosure to others, socialization with other gays, positive self-identification, and integration and acceptance. As with other human emotional processes, the stages are fluid and a woman can move back and forth as she negotiates the process of becoming accepting of her sexual orientation and identity.

Initially a woman becomes aware of her physical and emotional attraction to other women.[10] This awareness may be associated with feelings of guilt, shame, and anxiety and a sense of being abnormal compared to her family or peers.[10] This internal awareness can be denied and repressed for months or years.[10] If a young girl fears rejection of her family, on whom she is dependent on for food, shelter, and love, this repression may be part of her survival.[10] Even if an adolescent has support from her family, there is often ridicule and marginalization from her peers. Pressures exist to conform to "the norm," and many women who later identify themselves as lesbian will attempt relationships with the opposite sex because of the need for social acceptance.

Disclosing oneself as lesbian usually occurs first to a close friend or family member.[10] If there is a response of rejection or ridicule, a woman may return to the initial stage and question her sexual orientation or identification or choose to keep her awareness of being lesbian to herself, sensing a shameful connection with her identification.[10,11] This shame is not only at her "behavior," but a feeling of shame that her "being" is not acceptable and should remain hidden. Religion often judges the homosexual "as a contaminant to be condemned, permanently distanced, and inexorably punished."[11] The homosexual is seen as one who will "contaminate others who are healthy and pure."[11] If a woman internalizes this view, or experiences judgment on this harsh level, she may find it impossible to tolerate the "coming out" process because it would be attached to a proclamation of disease and disgust.[11] This process of disclosing to others can last many years and often occurs in stages. A woman may disclose to her family and close friends, but stay "closeted" in her school, work, or church setting. Kaufmann and Rapheal[11] in their book *Coming Out of Shame* describe self-disclosure as a form of self-exposure that inherently has the risk of shame. "Coming out to someone who doesn't know you're gay or lesbian risks not only rejection, but disgust, contempt, and possibly the loss of the relationship."[11]

Once a woman has begun to "come out" to others she often seeks the company of others who are identified as gay or lesbian.[10] This socialization helps give her a sense of not being alone and a place for freedom to begin being herself. Learning how to live as a lesbian occurs as she observes modeling from others at various stages of their disclosure process and relationship commitments.[10]

The next stage incorporates positive self-images and self-esteem. This positive self-identification includes feeling comfortable with being gay and the development of positive and fulfilling relationships (both friendships and romantic relationships).[10] Lesbians who accept their identity are more likely to have "increased self-esteem, better psychological adjustment, greater satisfaction, and less depression or stress than experienced by (those) who are at conflict with their identity."[1] As mentioned, this coming out process can last a lifetime, can occur in one particular setting and not another, is often associated with much internal distress, and affects a woman's psychological well-being. It is important to note that this process, as with all other psychological development, is influenced by cultural factors that can shape individuation.

PSYCHIATRIC ASPECTS OF HIV IN WOMEN WHO HAVE SEX WITH WOMEN

To date there are no studies specifically addressing psychiatric morbidity in HIV-infected WSW; however, it may be possible to extrapolate hypotheses from existing reports of psychiatric issues for lesbians, other WSW, women in general, and HIV-positive individuals. The National Comorbidity Survey (NCS) reported data from a survey of 8,098 persons by telephone interview.[12] Of this cohort, those who had a positive result on screening for a mental disorder based on *Diagnostic and Statistical Manual of Mental Disorders (DSM-III-R)* criteria (n = 5,877) were further surveyed about sexual activity, preference, and risk behaviors.[12] Fifteen females reported same-sex behavior exclusively, and 36 females reported both same-sex and opposite-sex behavior.[12] "Women in the same-sex subsample (n = 51) had higher 12-month prevalences of 11 of 12 disorders assessed than did women in the opposite-sex subsample; in three instances (major depression, simple phobia, and post-traumatic stress disorder [PTSD]), the differences were statistically significant."[12] Although not statistically significant, the prevalence of suicidal thoughts and plans were higher among the same-sex women subsample compared to the exclusively opposite-sex women subsample.[12] This survey also found that the age of onset of alcohol use disorders occurred earlier for women with same-sex partners compared to those with opposite-sex partners.[12] Consistent with these findings, the 1996 National Household Survey on Drug Abuse reported higher 1-year prevalence rates of substance dependency for homosexually active women, but not for anxiety or depressive disorders, compared to heterosexually active women.[13] In contrast to these findings, a recent study compared lesbian physicians (n = 115) with heterosexual physicians (n = 4,177).[14] There were no statistically significant differences in this study between lesbian and female heterosexual physicians when looking at recent or current alcohol use.[14] Although the lesbian cohort were more likely to report histories of depression and sexual abuse, the relationship between sexual abuse history and sexual orientation was evident only for those born in the United States and those who identified their race as White.[14]

Although some population-based studies have found elevated risk for mood, anxiety, and substance use disorders in homosexually and bisexually active individuals, these were based on sexual partner history rather than sexual identity. Recent data collected from the 1995 MacArthur Foundation National Survey of Midlife Development in the United States (MIDUS) were utilized by Cochran, Sullivan, and Mays[13] to study the associations of sexual orientation and psychological morbidity. The MIDUS was a population-based study by random telephone sampling of over 3,000 adults in the United States aged 25 to 74. From the final sample 2,917 answered a single question regarding their sexual orientation, either heterosexual (n = 2,844), homosexual (n = 41), or bisexual (n = 32).[13] Additional questions included 1-year prevalence of mental health disorders and other mental health indices.[13] Questions regarding major depressive disorder (MDD), generalized anxiety disorder, and panic disorder were based on *DSM-III-R* criteria, whereas alcohol dependence and drug dependence based on *DSM-IV* criteria. Only 2.2% of the female respondents classified themselves as homosexual or bisexual, and none of them reported HIV or AIDS treatment in the 12 months preceding their interview. Of the five mental health disorders assessed, generalized anxiety disorder was more prevalent in lesbian and bisexual women compared to their heterosexual cohorts.[13] Comorbidity rates for lesbian and bisexual women were three to almost four times higher than in heterosexual women. In general, minority sexual orientation was associated with an increased use of mental health services.[13]

In the National Lesbian Health Case Survey (NLHCS) from 1988, three fourths of respondents reported receiving counseling services for mental health issues that were common to women in general. Unfortunately, this survey did not have control groups for all women or heterosexual women; therefore specific conclusions regarding lesbians could not be made.[1] Comparisons of NLHCS to studies involving women in general reveal similar rates for depression and physical or sexual abuse.[1] From the National Comorbidity Survey (NCS) 30.5% of women reported a lifetime history of an anxiety disorder (primarily social or simple phobia), with 22.6% occurring in the past year. For affective disorders (primarily depression), women reported a lifetime history of 23.9%, with 14.1% occurring in past year. Prior history of MDD occurred in 21.3% of women; 12.9% within the past year.[1] Although there were no HIV-positive women in the NCS, the data from the HIV-positive males found a positive and significant association between HIV-positive serostatus and anxiety, mood, and substance disorders.[12] There appears to be a general increased risk of anxiety, mood, and substance use disorders, though not consistently reaching statistical significance. Reaching statistical significance is difficult because there are relatively small numbers of homosexual individuals in each of the studies, which diminishes the power for hypothesis testing.[12] As previously stated, there are no studies to date identifying the relationship between HIV infection and psychological disorders in WSW. However, there are some studies regarding HIV-positive individuals. One recent meta-analysis of 10 existing studies of HIV-positive individuals found prevalence rates of major depressive disorder almost twice as high as in HIV-negative individuals, regardless of sexual orientation or disease stage. These data were still heavily weighted to gay and bisexual men because 6 of the 10 studies assessed only this population.[15] In addition to MDD, PTSD has also been associated with HIV-positive individuals.

PTSD has been documented to occur following a diagnosis of HIV infection. In a study of 61 homosexual/bisexual men who were diagnosed with HIV infection, 30.2% met *DSM-III-R* criteria for PTSD in response to HIV infection (PTSD-HIV).[16] The sample included resolved as well as current diagnosis of PTSD. Onset of PTSD symptoms within 1 month of diagnosis of HIV infection occurred in 52.1% and within 6 months in 60.9%. Delayed onset of PTSD (i.e., greater than 6 months) occurred in 37%.[16] Before HIV diagnosis, certain psychiatric conditions were more prevalent in the PTSD-HIV cases, but the only statistically significant difference was for anxiety disorders.[16] After HIV diagnosis, 21% of PTSD-HIV cases developed depression compared to only 3% of non-PTSD-HIV cases. Previous PTSD diagnosis from any trauma was the strongest predictor of developing the disorder after diagnosis of HIV infection.[16] In comparing other studies, rates of PTSD were higher in response to HIV disease than other medical illnesses, even cancer.[16]

In the general population, the traumatic life event most likely to trigger PTSD is rape, especially if it occurs in childhood or adolescence.[17] Women are more often the victims of rape. For incarcerated women, PTSD is the second most common diagnosis within this group, following substance abuse, and occurs in approximately one third of this population.[17] HIV infection rates from national surveys of women prisoners range from 2.5% to 20%, which is significantly higher than the 0.15% for women in general. In a 1997 study of 177 incarcerated women from a Maryland correctional facility, 58 met criteria for a lifetime history of PTSD and 27 for a current PTSD diagnosis.[17] Among these women prisoners, rape before 16 years of age was the most commonly reported precipitating event for PTSD.[17] A lifetime occurrence of PTSD in these women was associated with a history of anal sex or sex work and possibly contributed to risky sexual behavior before incarceration. PTSD appears to be associated with higher risk for HIV infection.[17]

These studies highlight the notion that a diagnosis of PTSD following a single traumatic event is more likely if a person has a prior history of PTSD or trauma, as well as a history of an anxiety disorder(s). Factors that place WSW at more risk for PTSD and MDD may include histories of sexual abuse, rape, and discrimination. The factor that is different for WSW compared to women in general is discrimination based on homosexual behavior.

Homosexuals are frequently exposed to discrimination in America, and research on other forms of discrimination (i.e., racial) has clearly shown that exposure to such discriminatory behavior is associated with psychological distress and mental disorders.[12] The MIDUS as studied by Mays and Cochran[18] found that homosexual and bisexual adults more often than heterosexual adults report experiences with discrimination. Discrimination was based on sexual orientation solely or in part for 42% of the respondents. For the total sample there was a positive association between perceived discrimination and negative effects on quality of life, as well as indicators of psychiatric morbidity.[18]

There is evidence to suggest that the adolescent population may be more susceptible to these assaults. The literature has conflicting conclusions on whether adolescent individuals identified as gay or lesbian are at a higher risk of mental health problems and self-harm behaviors. A study of over 1,000 youth in New Zealand over a 21-year period examined the subpopulation identified as GLB for mental illness and suicidal behavior.[19] This study found that youth identified as GLB had an odds ratio between 1.9 and 6.2 times higher for several psychiatric disorders (MDD, generalized anxiety disorder, conduct disorder, nicotine dependence, other substance abuse or dependence) than their heterosexual cohort.[19] The odds ratio for suicidal behavior or having multiple psychiatric disorders was over 5 for the group of GLB youth.[19] Another study compared 104 GLB high school students with 4,055 students identified as heterosexual and found the rates of suicide attempts were 3.5 higher for the GLB youth.[19] Another study from 1998 comparing 394 GLB high school students with 336 heterosexual controls found the odds of suicide attempt 7.1 times higher for the GLB group and the odds 3.6 times higher for suicidal intent for this same group.[19] A 1997 study of 82 homosexual or bisexual men compared with 668 heterosexual men found rates of suicidal behaviors nearly 14 times higher for the homosexual men.[19] "The weight of evidence from these studies clearly supports the view that GLB sexual orientation acts as a risk factor for suicidal behaviors."[19] Although causality of differences in prevalence and patterns of mental health disorders and utilization of services has not been determined, this area of study is growing. One may attribute these differences to the stigma society places on homosexuality, which manifests as discrimination[13] (i.e., homophobia) and creates barriers to health care.

ACCESS TO HEALTH CARE

There are many barriers to receiving adequate health care for lesbians. One of the most pervasive barriers is assuming that everyone is heterosexual. This is seen in the clinical setting, where forms for health histories, insurance information, and educational materials are exclusive to heterosexuals.[1] Additionally, counseling for STDs typically assumes sex with male partners; thus all WSW are often neglected by the health care system. "Lesbians, like other marginalized groups of women, underutilize health care services."[20]

"The term 'lesbian' has negative connotations because of homophobia."[20] "There is no stereotypical profile to easily identify lesbian patients. Lesbians are found in every ethnic group and socioeconomic class. They are single, celibate, divorced, mothers, teenagers, and senior citizens."[20] A survey of 711 members of the Gay and Lesbian Medical Association found 59% of physicians had a personal experience with discrimination and 52% observed their colleagues providing suboptimal care to patients based on their sexual orientation.[20] "Many lesbians are no longer willing to disclose their sexual identity after having negative encounters with physicians that led to suboptimal care. Health care personnel and medical students should be educated that lesbianism is within the normal range on the continuum of human sexual behavior."[20] If medical interviews consist of nonjudgmental acceptance and gender-neutral questions and language, lesbian patients may be more willing to disclose their sexual identity and access care for their health.[20]

Barriers to receiving adequate health services include: "(1) structural barriers (e.g., availability of services, organizational configuration of health care providers); (2) financial barriers (e.g., insurance coverage); and (3) personal and cultural barriers (e.g., attitudes of patients and providers)."[1] "Structural barriers that affect health care for lesbians include potential barriers presented by managed care systems and the fact that lesbian relationships are often not afforded the same legal standing as heterosexual marriages."[1] The IOM in their book *Lesbian Health* suggests several of these potential barriers posed by the managed care health care system.[1] They suggest that the pressure to keep medical visits short may deter the development of a trusting environment in which a woman may feel comfortable to disclose her sexual orientation and sexual behaviors. They also suggest that it is more difficult for women to choose lesbian-friendly providers when their access is restricted to providers on a particular insurance plan. Because most lesbians do not have the option of coverage under their partner's health insurance plan, it is difficult to see the same providers and enjoy family-focused health care.[1] Finally, hospitals and health care providers often refuse to honor the lesbian partner of a patient in discussions about treatment or in visitation. This even occurs when the patient has designated her lesbian partner as her health care proxy.[1]

The financial barriers to access were also addressed in *Lesbian Health*.[1] "Since insurance coverage is the primary gateway to health care in this country, lesbians are at a distinct disadvantage relative to married heterosexual women because of the common prohibition against spousal benefits for unmarried partners."[1] Because spousal benefits do not apply for lesbians, many do not have health insurance.[1]

The final barriers to health care are personal and cultural barriers. Cultural competency is described as a set of skills that providers hold that allows them to give culturally appropriate and high-quality services to patients from cultures differing from their own.[1]

> Providers who are culturally competent with respect to lesbians would be expected to understand the reasons lesbians might be reluctant to seek medical care and the impact

of homophobia on the provision of services to lesbians; to be aware of the range of health problems experienced by lesbians as well as their health care risks; to avoid making heterosexual assumptions in the gathering of medical and social health information from patients; and to be willing to involve partners of lesbian patients in discussions about their health care.[1]

A lack of training to address these cultural differences propagates discriminatory practices such as "reluctance or refusal to treat, negative comments during treatment, or rough handling during examination."[1] Most medical school curricula devote minimal time to the study of homosexuality and bisexuality, in some cases as little as 2.5 hours over 4 years.[1]

Another barrier for lesbians is that the focus of primary care and public funding for women tends to be organized around reproductive health needs such as family planning and prenatal care; and these issues tend to be less salient for lesbians than for heterosexual women.[1] This is likely to change as more lesbians pursue motherhood. Women who are not sexually active with men may be unlikely to believe health information about routine care applies to them and may feel their individual health needs would not be understood.[1] Keeping in mind the continua of sexuality, these factors would likely be present for all WSW and especially for women who are heterosexual but have sex with women, because negating assumptions might be more difficult.

Although it potentially sounds simple, it is important to remember that lesbians are first of all women and thus are at risk for the same types of health problems as other women.[1] Cardiovascular disease is the major cause of death for women, whether heterosexual, bisexual, or lesbian. Therefore education and preventive care is of prime importance but may not reach the population of WSW for the barriers mentioned in this section. These same barriers are likely to reduce identification of WSW who are HIV-positive before symptom development.

An example of how the health care system may be more sensitive and responsive to lesbians needs can be found in The Mautner Project for Lesbians with Cancer. This project is dedicated to dissolving the barriers that exist to keep lesbians from receiving regular cancer screenings and treatment.[21] This project focuses on educating lesbians and health care providers and conducts research on health issues of lesbians related to cancer.[21] There is a training program entitled Removing the Barriers that, though focused on cancer screening and prevention, may be instructive to raise awareness of the issues of limited access to health care and may provide insight into how to dismantle these barriers for other health care issues specific to lesbians.[21]

SUMMARY

In conclusion, WSW have lower incidence rates of HIV infection and AIDS but higher risk factors than exclusively heterosexual women. Lack of well-defined categories of study and limited study populations hinder identifying incidence and psychiatric morbidity of HIV disease and AIDS specific to WSW. Research collected from other populations suggests mood, anxiety, and substance use disorders are more probable in WSW who are HIV-positive. Health information and research questionnaires are needed that are sensitive to the continua of human sexuality, addressing not only sexual identity but also sexual partner histories and behavior. There needs to be a move away from labels and toward understanding. Researchers, educators, and clinicians in the field should become leaders in conducting assessments that are unbiased and tolerant and that recognize the racial, ethnic, and socioeconomic diversity of WSW. Funding from both the public and private sector is needed to support research and education regarding WSW health needs. Conferences should be held to gather and disseminate this information.[1] These efforts would greatly assist in collecting data to better direct research, dissolve barriers that exist for women who do not fit "the norm," and benefit society at large by decreasing morbidity.

REFERENCES

1. Solarz AL. *Lesbian Health: Current Assessment and Directions for the Future.* Washington, DC: National Academy Press; 1999.
2. Marrazzo JM, Koutsky LA, Handsfield HH. Characteristics of female sexually transmitted disease clinic clients who report same-sex behaviour. *Int J STD AIDS.* 2001;12:41–46.
3. Fishman SJ, Anderson EH. Perception of HIV and safer sexual behaviors among lesbians. *J Assoc Nurs AIDS Care.* 2003;14:48–55.
4. Diamant AL, Schuster MA, McGuigan K, et al. Lesbians' sexual history with men: implications for taking a sexual history. *Arch Intern Med.* 1999;159:2730–2736.
5. Dolan KA, Phillip WD. Nuances and shifts in lesbian women's constructions of STI and HIV vulnerability. *Soc Sci Med.* 2003;57:25–38.
6. Bailey JV, Farquhar C, Owen C, et al. Sexual behaviour of lesbians and bisexual women. *Sex Transm Infect.* 2003;79:147–150.
7. Fethers K, Marks C, Mindel A, et al. Sexually transmitted infections and risk behaviours in women who have sex with women. *Sex Transm Infect.* 2000;76:345–349.
8. Kennedy M, Moore J, Schuman P, et al. Sexual behavior of HIV-infected women reporting recent sexual contact with women [letter]. *J Am Med Assoc.* 1998;280:29–30.
9. Kral AH, Lorvick J, Bluthenthal RN, et al. HIV risk profile of drug-using women who have sex with women in 19 United States cities. *J Acquir Immune Defic Syndr Human Retrovirol.* 1997;16:211–217.
10. Niolon R. The stages of coming out. Gay/Lesbian Resources. Available: http://www.psychpage.com/learning/library/gay/comeout.html. Accessed March 26, 2005.
11. Kaufman G, Raphael L. *Coming Out of Shame: Transforming Gay and Lesbian Lives.* New York: Doubleday; 1996.
12. Gilman SE, Cochran SD, Mays VM, et al. Risk of psychiatric disorders among individuals reporting same-sex sexual partners in the National Comorbidity Survey. *Am J Public Health.* 2001;91:933–938.
13. Cochran SD, Sullivan JG, Mays VM. Prevalence of mental disorders, psychological distress, and mental health services use among lesbian, gay, and bisexual adults in the United States. *J Consul Clin Psychol.* 2003;71: 53-61.
14. Brogan DJ, O'Hanlan KA, Elon L, et al. Health and professional characteristics of lesbian and heterosexual women physicians. *J Am Med Womens Assoc.* 2003;58:10–19.
15. Ciesla JA, Roberts JE. Meta-analysis of the relationship between HIV infection and risk for depressive disorders. *Am J Psychiatry.* 2001;158:725–730.
16. Kelly B, Raphael B, Judd F, et al. Posttraumatic stress disorder in response to HIV infection. *Gen Hosp Psychiatry.* 1998;20:3345–3352.
17. Hutton HE, Treisman GJ, Hunt WR, et al. HIV risk behaviors and their relationship to posttraumatic stress disorder among women prisoners. *Psychiatr Serv.* 2001;52:508–513.
18. Mays VM, Cochran SD. Mental health correlates of perceived discrimination among lesbian, gay, and bisexual adults in the United States. *Am J Public Health.* 2001;91:1869–1876.
19. Fergusson DM, Horwood LJ, Beautrais AL. Is sexual orientation related to mental health problems and suicidality in young people? *Arch Gen Psychiatry.* 1999;56:876–880.
20. Carroll NM. Optimal gynecologic and obstetric care for lesbians [clinical commentary]. *Obstet Gynecol.* 1999;93:611–613.
21. Centers for Disease Control and Prevention. Lesbians face many barriers to good health care. *Chron Dis Note Rep.* 2002;15. Available: http://www.cdc.gov/nccdphp/cdnr/cdnr_fall0206.htm. Accessed March 26, 2005.

CHAPTER 30

HIV/AIDS Among the Homeless

Jacqueline Maus Feldman, Stephen Mark Goldfinger

Approaches to the treatment of people with human immunodeficiency virus (HIV) and acquired immunodeficiency syndrome (AIDS), homelessness, and mental illness is constantly evolving. The incidence of HIV infection and AIDS is increasing in the United States, affecting a variety of demographics differently. Many of those with HIV disease or AIDS are living longer, although their lives are often fraught with multiple challenges. Recipients and providers of care must address a multitude of issues: stigma, adherence, physical and psychiatric complications, limited resources, and competing political agendas. A variety of strategies have proven effective in people with HIV infection and AIDS, homelessness, and mental illness; these include education; advocacy; federal, state, and local involvement and funding of research and services; utilization of evidence-based practice and translational research; cultural sensitivity; collaboration and partnerships; integration of services; inclusion of family and significant others; aggressive outreach; provision of a spectrum of housing solutions; and movement to person-centered treatment. Although significant gains have been achieved, further challenges exist for those committed to quality care.

HIV/AIDS, HOMELESSNESS, AND POVERTY

The lives of those with HIV disease or AIDS become much more complicated if they are also affected by homelessness and poverty; the process of treatment becomes exponentially more difficult, and the quality of life diminishes. Of those living with HIV disease or AIDS, 65% report that housing stability is their second largest need, behind health care.[1] In 2004, seroprevalence in urban indigent adults in San Francisco was reported as 10.5%, five times greater than in the San Francisco general population. Of these, almost 30% were men who have sex with men (MSM), over 7% were non-MSM injection drug users (IDUs), and 5% were non-MSM non-IDU. For those MSM with HIV disease or AIDS, risk factors include sex trade among Whites, non-White race, recent receptive anal sex, and syphilis. For non-MSM IDUs with HIV disease or AIDS, risk factors included syphilis, lower education, prison, syringe sharing, and transfusions. For non-MSM, non-IDUs with HIV disease or AIDS, risk factors included having had five recent sexual partners and female crack users who exchanged sex for drugs.[2]

One third to half of all people living with AIDS are "either homeless or in imminent danger of losing their homes." Of those who are homeless, 15% are infected with HIV.[3] The

Substance Abuse and Mental Health Services Administration (SAMHSA), the Health Resources and Services Administration (HRSA), and the National Institutes of Health (NIH) reported that of those who are HIV-positive, 5% are homeless.[4] Of those diagnosed with AIDS, 18% were homeless in 2003. Urban settings with inordinately high housing prices are particularly difficult housing environments for those who are HIV-positive. Their average income is $575 per month, only 21% are employed, 32% receive public assistance, and only 13% have private health insurance. Of those in the CARES program, 50% lived below the federal poverty level, less than 10% had private health insurance, and only slightly more than 25% had Medicaid. The poverty level in 2002 was $18,100 for a family of four, and treatment and cost of antiretroviral medication was approximately $14,000.[4] Those with HIV disease or AIDS are not only at risk for poverty and homelessness, but death as well. "HIV disease is the most predictive condition for mortality among all homeless people."[5]

HIV/AIDS AND MENTAL ILLNESS

The rate of HIV infection appears elevated in those with serious mental illness. A 2002 report reflected that patients with schizophrenia spectrum disorder were 1.5 as likely to have a diagnosis of HIV infection, and those with a diagnosis of affective disorder were 3.8 times as likely to have a diagnosis of HIV infection.[6] Sexually transmitted infections (STIs) are common among psychiatric patients who are homeless,[7] which might reflect a variety of challenges within those settings.

HIV/AIDS, HOMELESSNESS, AND MENTAL ILLNESS

The combination of homelessness and mental illness increase the risk for becoming HIV-positive. One third of those with mental illness are homeless; they often struggle with nonadherence, are frequently sexually active, and appear particularly vulnerable to physical and sexual violence.[8] A study in 2001 of homeless shelters in Philadelphia reflected a rate of HIV-positive status nine times that of the general population, with increased risk correlated to substance abuse in males and a history of serious mental illness.[9] Of those occupying homeless shelters, about 20% have psychiatric problems.[7] It has been noted that those who are homeless and have mental illness are particularly vulnerable to HIV infection because of cognitive deficits, vulnerability to coercion by others, and desperate need for money. Those with mental illness and who are homeless often belong to high-risk groups engaging in intravenous (IV) drug abuse, with histories of incarceration, other substance abuse, and involvement in sex trade.[10]

A review of these demographics highlights that the incidence of HIV infection and AIDS continues to increase, especially across ethnic/racial minorities; women in particular bear an increasing burden in terms of mortality. The interface between HIV disease, homelessness, and mental illness has been demonstrated to produce particularly vulnerable populations. The challenges then are identification, education, prevention, treatment, and support.

CHALLENGES

Those struggling with HIV disease and AIDS, homelessness, and mental illness, along with those who provide their care and those who create and fund policy and health care systems must grapple with a particularly burdensome set of challenges.[11] They are as follows:

a. Identification and Acceptance of Illness

As noted earlier, perhaps 20% of those who are HIV-positive are unaware of their status, and another 20% do not receive any medical care. Susser et al.[7] noted that patients with serious mental illness were reluctant to admit their sexual activity, much less demonstrate willingness to be tested. Acceptance of the illness and need for treatment are often closely tied to perceptions of stigma (see "e" below) and fear of being diagnosed with at best a chronic medical illness or at worst a potentially fatal disease.

b. Complicated Medical Problems

Complicated medical problems necessitate rapid and consistent access to medical care, medication, and nutrition. According to a study reported by the Department of Housing and Urban Development (HUD), two thirds of those who are homeless suffer from a chronic illness; nearly 25% of the study participants indicated that they needed to see a doctor within the last year but could not.[12] It has also been reported that homeless people with HIV disease or AIDS are less likely than HIV-infected populations on the whole to receive antiretroviral medications.[12] By 2002 the CARES program was funding or providing enormous amounts of medical care; access to medical care was four times greater than any service besides case management.[3,13] Increased rates of immunosuppression, opportunistic infections such as tuberculosis (TB), Hepatitis B and C [HBV, HCV], *Bartonella quintana* (the bacterium that causes bacillary angiomatosis peliosis)[5] pneumonia, and influenza, along with cancer, malnutrition, infestations, neurologic problems, and dental problems plague those with HIV disease and homelessness.[1] Homeless people with HIV infection who sleep in a shelter are twice as likely to have TB as the general shelter population. Injection drug use and lack of insurance can affect health care use as well.[14] Klinkenberg et al.[15] studied a population of whom 6% were HIV-positive, 33% of whom were HBV-positive, and 30% of whom were HCV-positive. These illnesses were often thought to be the result of substance abuse, especially intravenous drug abuse (IVDA).[15] Homeless persons with HIV disease or AIDS are believed to be more ill than those with stable housing. One study notes location of services and inclusion of aggressive outreach and minimization of barriers to access to care in treatment planning.[12]

c. Access to Mental Health Care and Medication

Those with HIV infection or AIDS have an illness that may also affect them psychiatrically; "depression, mania, dementia, and other direct effects on the CNS" become manifest.[16] Psychological factors of stress, anxiety, cognitive impairment, and psychosis can also contribute to denial or avoidance of treatment.[12]

d. Unstable Housing

Approximately 15% of those who are homeless are HIV-positive.[17] Homelessness contributes to nutritional problems and exposure to elements and extremes in weather.[12] Housing, once attained, can be tenuous because of cost or may be difficult to access and sustain because many of these individuals carry a history of criminal behavior or of being poor tenants. Unstable housing may encourage transient interpersonal sexual relationships (e.g., crowding or strangers as roommates, little privacy, or poor interpersonal skills of those with serious mental illness).

e. Stigma

Those diagnosed as HIV-positive are aware that the diagnosis is disproportionately represented in gay, minority, and substance-using subpopulations, which may be a source of stigma. They may experience "fear, shame, distrust, rejection, exile, guilt, isolation, hopelessness, helplessness, alienation, lack of self worth, powerlessness, and aloneness."[12]

f. Nonadherence

Adherence to a treatment plan is tempered by multiple factors: acceptance of illness, provider–patient relationship, establishment of a positive risks/benefits ratio (positive effect of medication outweighs the side effects of medication), access to and cost of medicine, and ease of use of medicine regimen (pill versus liquid, once per day versus 4 times per day,

1 type of medicine versus 10 different medicines). "As it is believed that decreased adherence is the single best predictor of protease inhibition failure and the primary cause of medication resistance, this problem has grave personal and public health implications."[14] Treatment regimens for HIV disease and AIDS, combined with treatment regimens for serious mental illness, within the context of the chaos of homelessness (no place to store medications, no refrigeration, inconsistent meal schedules, limited access to clean water, inconsistent schedules, no privacy) make the chances of adherence very low.

g. Risk Reduction
Multiple factors contribute to impaired judgment, impulsivity, and risk-taking behavior such as participating in unprotected sex, frequenting shooting galleries, exchanging sex for money or drugs, and nonadherence. Poverty may prevent the purchase of condoms.[7] Substance abuse, poor nutrition, or untreated medical and emotional problems might inflame problems with judgment and behavioral control.[2]

h. Substance Use, Abuse, and Dependence
By 2000, injection substance abuse was responsible for 25% of all new AIDS cases (although this reflected a decrease of 17% since 1998).[18] It has been suggested that non-IV drugs (cocaine, alcohol, 3,4 methylenedioxymethamphetamine [MDMA], methamphetamines) enhance risk-taking behavior, impair judgment (and hence adherence), and may exacerbate disease progression.

i. Inadequate Infrastructure
Systems of care are often complex, fragmented, and uncoordinated. Without someone to help them identify, advocate for, and broker services, without transportation, or without resources to purchase services, identified patients are at high risk for inability to surmount barriers to care.

j. Limited Resources, Rising Health Costs, and Cutbacks in Entitlements
As noted before, many of these patients have significantly limited employment capacity, few financial resources, and little or no insurance. Medications can be profoundly expensive (one year of antiretroviral medication can cost over $14,000), and threatened cutbacks in Medicaid are a constant reminder of the tenuousness of these patients treatment plans.

k. Lack of Skills Development for Independent Living and Possible Employment
Lack of information and underdeveloped interpersonal skills can exaggerate risk behavior. Without assertiveness training, many succumb to peer pressure. Often, people with homelessness, mental illness, or HIV disease or AIDS feel disenfranchised, feel inadequate in vocational skills, and lack the capacity to effectively perform activities of daily living, communicate, or make decisions.[12]

l. Identification of Culturally Sensitive Services
Often services are provided by clinicians who lack understanding and respect for a wide variety of experiences, value systems, and beliefs. Exploration of reasons for undeveloped adaptational skills is neglected. Therapeutic alliances can be crushed by clinician prejudgment. A lack of understanding and acceptance of different educational levels, sexual orientation, socioeconomic status, and physical disability can affect clinician perceptions and make treatment that much more challenging to patients.[12]

m. Funding Agency Support for Research and Clinical Services
Although tremendous strides have been made locally, regionally, and at the federal level in funding services and research, much more is needed to adequately house and support those in need. In particular, research into the most effective treatments for those with HIV disease or AIDS, homelessness, and mental illness is imperative.

STRATEGIES FOR SUCCESS

A variety of programs have been developed for those with HIV infection or AIDS, homelessness, and mental illness that have been successful in ameliorating medical conditions, offering psychiatric interventions, and stabilizing infrastructure by providing multiple levels of support. These programs all share common guidelines, including treatment, prevention, education regarding adherence, risk reduction, collaboration, and integration of services.

Eleven demonstration projects funded by the Department of Health and Human Services, NIH, HRSA, and SAMHSA offered 10 core principles of care[2]:

1. Unencumbered access to comprehensive mental health and substance abuse services
2. Services should be flexible and person centered
3. HIV, mental health, and substance abuse treatment should be coordinated and integrated with communication between providers
4. Services should be culturally sensitive (staff should be trained)
5. Attention to stigma is paramount; self-respect and dignity must be preserved
6. Services should enhance behavior that is healthy
7. Barriers to care must be reduced
8. Services should be evidence-based
9. Decision making should flow from therapeutic partnerships, and involve consumers and advocates
10. HIV-infected "communities" should be encouraged, with programs and individuals working in full partnerships providing comprehensive services and systems of support

Several extant reports offer specific practical guides for establishing housing for persons with special needs. In this book, treatment of HIV/AIDS is elaborated upon in other chapters. However, special notice should be taken of the need to focus on those parameters that affect adherence (for *no* treatment is effective if the patient chooses to not participate). Desai and Rosenheck[19] note that "depression, fear, economic status, magical beliefs, and denial" all play a role in adherence. They report that patients are more likely to return for HIV testing results if they have a history of multiple tests and greater social support and are less like to return if they have a history of sexual victimization. Those with less severe HIV illness were less likely to access services; people living in the northeast United States were more likely to receive services.[17]

Prevention is predicated on education of consumers. Risk assessment (including establishing a baseline of risk tolerance) for each patient is a key issue in each evaluation and in the development of an effective treatment plan. Risky sexual behavior may be extrapolated from information garnered on unwanted pregnancies, therapeutic abortions, contraception use, and the presence of or history of sexually transmitted diseases. In addition, empathic acceptance of a patient's life circumstances is imperative; risk-taking behavior must be understood within the context of a patient's psychosocial realities.[8]

It is important that health care providers offer treatment, education, and services within the context of a therapeutic alliance, with an emphasis on developing and displaying multicultural sensitivity.[12] An understanding and acceptance of culturally based behavior is imperative for effective treatment. Broadening of one's own treatment perspective can be helpful as well (e.g., part of the *engagement* process is acceptance into treatment programs of patients with co-occurring disorders who are not sober). Asking patients to formulate their *own* treatment goals will empower them and enhance adherence. It will honor and recognize the importance of their input in decisions regarding their life. Inclusion of family members or significant others (with patients' consent) may expand understanding of the patients' strengths and challenges and may serve to reengage necessary supports.

SUCCESSFUL PLANNING AND SUCCESSFUL PROGRAMS

An example of successful collaborative planning is reflected in the report from the Tenderloin (in San Francisco) Collaborative Work Group (TCWG), which focused on residents with HIV infection and AIDS, as well as substance abuse, mental illness, medical problems, and homelessness; low-income residents at risk for developing HIV infection or AIDS were included, as well. Aware of the importance of mental health supports, the TCWG Proposition 63 position paper noted the following[3]:

> ... As with disparities in access to medical care, the issues of unavailable services, poverty, cultural competence, discrimination based on race, against individuals who are not proficient in English, have undocumented immigration status, or are members of minorities based on gender identity and sexual identity are the *same* disparities in access to mental health services. Although unlike other medical conditions, mental illness and its subsequent care *are* stigmatized, thereby creating an additional barrier due to the lack of understanding mental illness.
>
> The lack of decent safe, affordable, and integrated housing is one of the most significant barriers to full participation in community life for people with mental illnesses. The shortage of affordable housing and accompanying support services causes people with unaddressed mental illnesses to cycle among jails, institutions, shelters, and the streets or to live in seriously substandard housing. People with serious mental illness represent a large portion of those who are repeatedly homeless or who are homeless for long periods of time. In fact, people with serious mental illnesses are overrepresented among the homeless, especially among the chronically homeless. Of the more than 2 million adults in the United States who have at least one episode of homelessness in a given year, 46% report having had a mental health problem within the previous year, either by itself or in combination with substance abuse. Homeless people with mental illnesses are likely to experience the following[3]:

- Have acute and chronic physical health problems
- Use alcohol and drugs
- Have escalating ongoing psychiatric symptoms
- Become victimized and incarcerated

The Tenderloin holds 10% of the city's population, is ethnically diverse, and has become the epicenter of the HIV-positive population in San Francisco. Of its homeless population, 10% are HIV-positive. The mentally ill, substance abusing HIV-positive population served by the TCGW consortium typically lives on a very low income; few are employed, and many have no insurance. Vigorous advocacy and case management help them obtain necessary resources, although their income is woefully insufficient for housing in San Francisco and their backgrounds (poor history as tenant, substance abuse, and history of incarceration) make access to housing that much more difficult. The Tenderloin project began with commitment to integrated care (mental health, medical, and substance abuse), treating individuals as whole persons, collaborating with consumers, providing support in accessing resources, ensuring employment if capable, establishing and maintaining housing, and preventing unjust incarceration.[3]

Of the 400 referrals to the Tenderloin Outpatient Clinic, 69% had co-occurring disorders, 44% had criminal histories, 34% were homeless, and 51% had medical problems beyond their HIV or AIDS status (e.g., TB, HCV, diabetes mellitus, and cardiovascular disease). There were increasing numbers of street-based sex industry trade workers. Failure of prior attempts to serve this population occurred because of failure to adapt services to address the norms, values, beliefs, or actual life conditions of homeless people; "adherence to rigid treatment requirements often proves impossible and individuals either drop out of care all together or find themselves excluded from options afforded to more stable residents."[3] Clinicians often failed to realize that fear, aggression, and suspicion were all normal responses to that with which the homeless person must deal; "ultimately this creates a vicious cycle of client distrust, provider frustration, perceptions of discrimination, and actual discrimination and deterioration of health and inaccessibility of care."[3]

Other programs have been successful in working with those who are affected by HIV disease or AIDS, homelessness, and mental illness; the core issue addressed must always be housing.

> For people struggling with the disabling and impoverishing effects of HIV/AIDS, housing is the cornerstone of health and stability. Maintaining health and stability is essential when managing HIV. For people living with HIV/AIDS, housing *is* healthcare"... "Homelessness, HIV disease, and access to healthcare are fundamentally interconnected. Stable housing, coupled with supportive services responsive to their complex needs, increases the ability of persons living with HIV/AIDS, particularly those who are low income, to access and adhere to life sustaining HIV/AIDS treatment. Without stable housing, persons with HIV/AIDS cannot access the complex treatment and care vital to survive. Access to clean water, bathrooms, refrigeration and food, and the ability to take medications on a routine schedule can be severely impaired, resulting in declining health. Further, research indicates that stable housing for people living with HIV/AIDS saves Medicaid expenditures and is a crucial component of efforts to control rising healthcare cost throughout the nation."[1]

Multiple housing projects exist. The aforementioned CARES program is a federally funded program designed to maximize innovative and vigorous HIV disease and AIDS care, including housing, risk prevention, substance abuse treatment, and social supports.[13] Another example is Housing Opportunities for People with AIDS (HOPWA). HOPWA offers multiple resources, including short-term assistance with rent, mortgages, and utility costs. HOPWA ensures not only stable housing, but also wraparound services as well, including medical care and public subsidies. To date, this program is available only to low-income populations (families earning less than $1,000 per month).[1]

RECOMMENDED STRATEGIES FOR SUCCESS

It is recommended that the following comprehensive, integrated services should be included when considering, planning, and funding development of systems of care for those with HIV disease or AIDS, homelessness, and mental illness[3]:

- HIV testing and counseling
- Access to medical, mental health, and substance abuse care, including hiring of staff that are trained in the neuropsychiatric presentations found in HIV/AIDS
- Evaluations that include assessment for risk behavior, including a comprehensive sexual behavior history
- Prevention services that focus on educational presentations that are clear, simple, and repetitive and include role playing and suggestions for alternative sexual activity (including abstinence and behavior without exchange of body fluids)
- Services offered by nonjudgmental, accepting staff with multicultural sensitivities, tolerance of "transient" behavior (coming and going from sessions); for example, "tolerance of alternative lifestyles and sensitivity to the despair often experienced by individuals with HIV infections"[12]

- Needle exchange
- An array of stable housing situations with available, integrated services, including multi-disciplinary teams that both broker and provide services

SUMMARY

The incidence of HIV infection and AIDS is increasing, affecting a variety of demographics. Enhancing the quality of the lives of these individuals is a daunting goal. When HIV disease and AIDS intersect with poverty, homelessness, and mental illness, those affected face serious challenges. Systems of care must work to provide easy access to medical, mental health, and substance abuse treatment, focus on patient education, ensure staff understanding and cultural sensitivity, provide a spectrum of stable housing, and commit to rapid response partnerships and integrated care. Models of care for this unique population should be identified and subject to research, and effective programs should be funded and replicated.

REFERENCES

1. 2005 Advocates guide to housing and community development policy. Housing Opportunity for People with AIDS. Available: http://www.nl.hc.org/advocated/hopwa.htm. Accessed August 15, 2005.
2. Robertson MJ, Clark RA, Charlebois ED, et al. Research and practice: HIV sero-prevalence among homeless and marginally housed adults in San Francisco. *Am J Public Health*. 2004;94:1207–1217.
3. Tenderloin Collaborative Work Group: *Tenderloin Collaborative Work Group Final Report*. San Francisco: San Francisco Community Foundation; 2004.
4. Farber EW, McDaniel JS. Clinical management of psychiatric disorders in patients with HIV disease. *Psychiatr Q*. 2002;73:5–16.
5. Song J. *HIV/AIDS and Homelessness: Recommendations for Clinical Practice and Public Policy*. Washington, DC: Bureau of Primary Health Care and the HIV/AIDS Bureau, Health Resources and Services Administration; 2000.
6. Blank MB, Aiken C, Hadley TR. Co-occurrence of serious mental illness among Medicaid recipients. *Psychiatr Serv*. 2002;53:868–873.
7. Susser E, Valencia E, Miller M, et al. Sexual behaviors of homelessness at risk for HIV. *Am J Psychiatry*. 1995;152:583–587.
8. Goldfinger SM, ed. Psychiatric aspects of AIDS/HIV infection. In: *New Directions for Mental Health Services*, San Francisco: Jossey-Bass; 1990.
9. Culhane DP, Gollub E, Kuhn R, et al. The co-occurrence of AIDS and homelessness: results from the administrative databases for AIDS surveillance and public shelter utilization in Philadelphia. *J Epidemiol Community Health*. 2001;55:515–520.
10. Goldfinger SM, Susser E, Roche BA, et al. *HIV, Homelessness, and Serious Mental Illness: Implications for Policy and Practice*. Washington, DC: National Resource Center on Homelessness and Mental Illness, Policy Research Association, Center for Mental Health Services; 1998.
11. Hals, K. *Put Your House in Order: Securing Your Supportive Housing Program's Future Through Effective Asset Management*. Seattle: AIDS Housing of Washington; 2002.
12. Aruff C. *Mental Health Care for People Living with AIDS: A Practical Guide*. Research Triangle Park, NC: Research Triangle Institute, 1999.
13. The AIDS epidemic and the Ryan White CARES Act: past successes and future challenges. Available: http://hab.hrsa.gov/tools/progress05/part-three.html. Accessed August 15, 2005.
14. Coalition in Homelessness and Housing in Ohio. AIDS/HIV and Homelessness. Available: http://www.cohhio.org/resources/factsheets/AIDSfactsheet.html. Accessed August 15, 2005.
15. Klinkenberg WD, Caslyn RJ, Morse GA, et al. Prevalence of HIV, hepatitis B, and hepatitis C among homeless persons with co-occurring severe mental illness and substance use disorders. *Compr Psychiatry*. 2003;44:293–302.
16. Centers for Disease Control and Prevention. *HIV/AIDS Surveillance Report, 2002*. Atlanta: Centers for Disease Control and Prevention; 2003.
17. Burnham MA, Bing MA, Morton SC, et al. Use of mental health and substance abuse treatment services among adults with HIV in the United States. *Arch Gen Psychiatry*. 2001;58:729–736.
18. Fullilove MT, Fullilove RG III. What's housing got to do with it? *Am J Public Health*. 2000;183:183–184.
19. Desai M, Rosenheck R. *Mental Health AIDS Spring 2005 Newsletter;* 2005. Available: http://mentalhealthaids.samhsa.gov/Spring2005/assessment1.asp.

CHAPTER 31

HIV/AIDS Among Prisoners

Wade C. Myers, Glenn Catalano, Deborah L. Sanchez, Meghan M. Ross

The state and federal prison systems have grown significantly since 1980, with the federal prison population and the correctional systems of 18 states actually doubling in size by 1993.[1] This dramatic increase in the incarcerated population has occurred at roughly the same time as the striking rise in those diagnosed with human immunodeficiency virus (HIV) and acquired immunodeficiency syndrome (AIDS). It seems that each of these epidemics has affected the other.[2]

A check of the ethnic backgrounds of prison inmates in the state and federal systems reveals a much higher representation of persons of color (five times higher) and Latinos (two times higher) than the general population.[1] These groups are at increased risk of contracting HIV because of the high-risk behaviors they engage in before incarceration.[3] These minority groups that are over-represented in the prison populations are the very groups that are hardest hit by HIV, and they have less access to health care in their outside communities.[2] It is for these reasons that prisons and jails bear a disproportionate share of the infectious disease burden in the United States. Although it is true that the great majority of inmates' HIV infections are obtained in the community before incarceration,[3] it is still the responsibility of the prison system to provide appropriate health care to its inmate population. From inmates' perspectives, one of the few positive aspects to incarceration might be that they are able to experience complete dental and medical evaluations while in prison. This includes access to care from a certified HIV health care provider and HIV education and prevention information.[3]

Although most inmates that are infected with HIV have become infected through high-risk behaviors in the community,[2] high-risk behaviors occur in prisons and jails as well.[4] However, discussions of said high-risk behaviors have remained somewhat taboo in the United States.[4] Still, because the preincarceration lifestyles of many inmates include such HIV risk factors as unprotected intercourse and substance abuse, it would not be surprising if inmates continue their high-risk activities during their incarceration.[3]

PREVALENCE

Patients with HIV disease or AIDS are commonly seen in the prison population. However, there is much variability in prevalence between states, regions of the country, and even countries. In 1993, rates of HIV seropositivity in prisons ranged from 0.6% (Oregon and

Wisconsin) to 17% (New York).[1] In a study of inmates serving a sentence at the Adult Correctional Institution (ACI) in Rhode Island, 4% of men and 12% of women were HIV-seropositive.[1] In fact, in 1990, 40% of all the newly identified cases of HIV infection in the entire state of Rhode Island were diagnosed at the ACI. In the Florida prison system there have been significant problems with HIV infection. From 1987 to 1992, AIDS was the leading cause of death in Florida prisons.[5] In 1992, of all the inmates in the Florida prison system who died, 52.3% died of conditions secondary to AIDS. This was four times as many as died from either cardiovascular causes or cancer.[5] At the end of 1994, the rate of confirmed AIDS cases was seven times higher in the state and federal prison systems than in the general population. Up to one quarter of those people with HIV infection in the United States pass through a U.S. correctional facility each year. In a study of female inmates in Quebec, 6.9% of all female inmates were seropositive for the HIV antibody.[6] Female inmates who were injection drug users (IDUs) (13.0%) or prostitutes (12.9%) had increased rates of HIV seropositivity as well. However, other available information is quite variable, depending on the country and population studied. It is difficult to compare the data that are available secondary to the different methodologies and samples used.

Considering that over 22 million people pass in and out of correctional institutions each year,[4] public health experts are focusing on the HIV situation in this population. People who are incarcerated form a new community that is ethically entitled to appropriate medical care. The majority of individuals in this population are only temporarily removed from their respective communities.[7] Thus, improving the HIV health care and educational programs available in prisons is of the utmost importance.[1]

As noted previously, for some inmates, incarceration can often be a rare opportunity for those participating in high-risk behaviors to have access to quality health care.[2] It may also be the only time that they are exposed to specialized HIV medical care along with HIV education and prevention information.[1] Incarceration is also felt to be a time when inmates can come to terms with imprisonment and acknowledge that the behaviors that led to the incarceration may also have placed them at risk for HIV infection.[2] For many inmates, incarceration is an opportune time for intervention, because they may be most amenable at this point to reception of HIV prevention information and the institution of the HIV treatment.

BARRIERS TO DIAGNOSIS AND TREATMENT

Although common sense would suggest that the prison system is an ideal venue to diagnose HIV infection, begin treatment, and educate inmates about prevention, there are still many barriers to this course of action. To begin, many prisons are hesitant to embrace the HIV prevention message that they feel directly contradicts prison policies.[3] They express the rationale that it is unnecessary to provide clean syringes and condoms when sex between prisoners and drug abuse are prohibited in prison. At this time, only a small number of U.S. prisons have policies allowing prisoners access to HIV risk-reduction tools.[4]

Limited financial resources are problematic to attempts to stem the epidemic of HIV infection in prisons. Many departments of corrections are facing budget cuts, which means that lower priority activities (such as HIV education programs) are often eliminated.[3] Also, many prisons have a set pharmaceutical budget to provide medications to all prisoners. With the high cost of retroviral agents, many prisons have begun to administer these agents under direct observation to ensure that the doses are actually taken.[2] Although this may seem a good way to ensure compliance, it may deter many inmates from taking medications because they fear they will be labeled as HIV-positive because they are waiting in long lines to take medications under direct observation.[2] Inmates often do not trust correctional facility staff and may refuse to participate in HIV treatments because they feel that their confidentiality may be breeched. The high prevalence of the mental illness in prisons also has been a barrier in the attempts to control HIV infection in prisons, because these patients may pose challenges regarding compliance with HIV treatments.[2] Another major barrier to HIV infection education efforts is that there is often a lack of explicit information about specific preventive behaviors.[7]

The educational materials and activities used to target those at risk cannot be "one size fits all." No standardized format of AIDS education is likely to meet the needs of all high-risk groups.[7] There needs to be an understanding of the diverse beliefs and backgrounds of the inmates, along with their appreciation and perceptions about HIV disease. It has been noted that the behavioral interventions should be "gender specific, developmentally appropriate, and culturally competent."[7] Prevention education requires that the educators have an understanding of the specific risk behaviors in their treatment population and the "contexts and conditions that sustain them."[7] For example, for many African-American inmates, same-sex sexual encounters are felt to be situational in nature and do not mean that they are gay or bisexual. Therefore these inmates may not respond to HIV educational programming that targets bisexual or gay men.[3] Therefore different educational programming may be necessary in this and other populations.

Finally, another barrier to controlling the HIV epidemic in prisons is the different mission of each of the parties involved. The department of corrections is dedicated to the security and custody of the inmates, whereas the public health system is most interested in disease prevention.[3] For the prison system, above all else, maintaining a secure environment is the most important job, even if this means having some apathy toward inmate health and well-being.[3] Although this attitude may be more cost effective for the prison system, it is very likely that there will be higher public health expenditures in the long term, after inmates are released back into their community if their care has been less than optimal.[7]

DISEASE CONTROL

There are many different ideas regarding the control of HIV infection in the prison population. Some infectious disease specialists recommend that inmates with HIV disease be clustered together to allow for the coordination of educational efforts and to concentrate the provision of expert HIV medical care.[2] From a logistical standpoint, inmates should be easier to reach with education and prevention information because they have fewer demands on their time than when they were in the community.[3] When incarcerated they also may be evaluating their life choices and therefore be more amenable to listening to the HIV educational message. HIV educational activities should address inmate concerns by increasing their awareness of the illness, especially in the context of avoiding postrelease high-risk behaviors.[3] These educational activities should include a general AIDS education program for both the inmates and the correctional officers.[1] This education should also stress the importance of disease prevention and risk avoidance. Incarceration is also a time when the inmate is supposedly encountering fewer situations of risk, so there is the opportunity to stop further spread of the virus.[3] It is also helpful that the inmate has access to comprehensive medical care.[3] Inmates thus have an opportunity to have medical problems addressed and treated so that their HIV status can be managed in the best manner possible. For example, in a patient with viral hepatitis and HIV, the hepatitis may need to be treated with antivirals before the patient may begin highly active antiretroviral therapy (HAART).[2] In female patients with HIV, it is imperative that pregnancy be detected promptly so antiretroviral therapy can be initiated to avoid vertical transmission of the virus.[2]

In the past, the concern had been that the prison system is a reservoir of HIV infection, and that once released the inmates would spread the infection into the general population. This view is felt to be unsupported based on the evidence currently available. Although intra-prison spread is a concern, extra-prison spread is more of a concern because high-risk behaviors are more common in the community than in prison.[2] Therefore the risk for HIV transmission increases rather than decreases when an inmate is released from prison. HIV risk-reduction programs are important because they teach inmates how to maintain safe behaviors so they can avoid acquiring HIV infection upon release from prison.[2] Prevention work with inmates gives public health workers the chance to address prevention in the larger community outside of prisons. This can be done through the education of family members, friends, and contacts.[7] Careful discharge planning is of the utmost importance if the inmate is going to maintain the health care gains made while incarcerated. In fact, a face-to-face meeting between the inmate and the community health care provider while the inmate is still incarcerated improves follow-up rates.[2] Prerelease counseling is a final important opportunity to reinforce in those inmates about to be released ways to reduce the risk of acquiring HIV upon returning home to high-risk environments.[7] The most effective HIV infection and AIDS prevention program is one that links correctional facilities, public health agencies, and community organizations in an attempt to design a network of support and prevention services.[7]

HIV/AIDS PREVENTION PROGRAMS

There is no consensus regarding the ideal HIV infection and AIDS prevention program, and approaches have varied between systems. In Rhode Island, the AIDS Education and Management Program was initiated in the Adult Correctional Institution.[1] This program had four objectives: to begin HIV education programs, to have widespread HIV testing (with appropriate counseling) in the facility, to aggressively manage the medical issues of HIV-positive patients, and to institute prerelease counseling and postrelease medical follow-up of HIV-seropositive individuals.[1] Others note that the ideal HIV infection and AIDS prevention program would begin with both the staff and the inmates receiving HIV educational programming that acknowledges that high-risk sexual activity and drug use occur behind bars.[4] Some members of the public health community recommend that to reduce the risk of HIV transmission among inmates there should be mandatory testing in state prisons to reveal the numerous undiagnosed cases and facilitate subsequent treatment.[3] They also recommend an increase in initiatives that will provide continuity of care for HIV-infected inmates returning to their community. Finally, they recommend improved access to incarcerated populations for AIDS service organizations and community-based organizations that deliver HIV infection and AIDS education.

Overall, there are many reasons to identify and treat as many cases of HIV infection and AIDS as possible in correctional facilities. The most important one is likely that early intervention in the correctional institution, linked to continuity of care in the community, will allow for the prevention or early treatment of many opportunistic infections. This will then avoid many costly hospitalizations and poor outcomes.[1] In turn, each inmate will be given the opportunity to live the healthiest life possible.

TRANSMISSION AND SEXUAL BEHAVIOR

As mentioned previously, many HIV-positive inmates become infected through high-risk behaviors in the community.[2] Studies of risk behaviors have compared behaviors in incarcerated populations to those in the general population. These studies have indicated that inmates tend to initiate sexual intercourse at an earlier age, have higher numbers of recent and lifetime sexual partners, inconsistently use disease and pregnancy prevention, and have a higher frequency of sexual risk behavior.[8]

There is a pervasive belief that sex in prisons is rarely consensual.[2] A wide range of sexual behaviors, both consensual and nonconsensual, occur between prisoners and between prisoners and correctional personnel.[4] This is despite laws in 14 states prohibiting sexual acts between corrections staff and inmates.[4] According to male and female focus groups that included currently and previously incarcerated individuals, prisoners exchange sex for a variety of reasons: access to services, for protection, and to receive goods.[4] Male-on-male prison rape occurs with some frequency and can involve men who do not identify themselves as homosexual. Male focus groups describe a code of silence between male inmates not to talk about sex in prison to outsiders or even among themselves. They depict a high prevalence and complexity of nonconsensual sex between men. These include tricking or coercing new prisoners into accepting goods and then demanding sexual payment and a form of sexual slavery under which the dominant male lends out his "slave" to other prisoners for goods such as cigarettes and drugs.[4] According to female inmate focus groups, women lack the ability to say no to sex with corrections officers, for fear of retribution or loss of privileges.[7] A prisoner's ability to truly consent to sexual activity with staff is obviously severely compromised because of incarceration status. Among females, when consensual sex occurred, it typically took place in showers, bathrooms, and cell blocks, usually under great time pressures. Sex between male prisoners also occurred in short time spans, in whatever place was available, most commonly in the showers. Reported consensual sexual behaviors among the women included oral sex, mutual masturbation, and using and sharing sex toys such as dildos; men reported oral sex, rectal sex, and mutual masturbation.[4]

It has been suggested that if high-risk sexual activity increases rates of HIV transmission among prisoners, they should be given condoms to help prevent its spread. However, there are virtually no studies that have assessed sexual behavior before and during imprisonment among a representative sample of inmates.[9] Focus groups of both former and current inmates note that some prisoners would use condoms and dental dams during consensual sex if they were confidentially and anonymously distributed.[4] In the absence of such services, inmates are left to their own devices to find ways to practice safer sex. Female inmates reported stealing surgical gloves from the prison health clinic, which they cut and used for barrier protection with other female partners.[4] Others reported similar activities with plastic gloves and plastic wrap; however these devices were often reused multiple times. Male inmates reported using the fingers of plastic gloves to attempt to prevent HIV transmission, and often used hand lotion for lubricants. The reuse of primitive latex barriers and the use of water-based lubricants are insufficient methods for confidently decreasing the risk of sexual transmission of HIV infection.

In studies of intra-prison transmission of HIV, it was unclear whether sex, tattooing, or intravenous drug abuse was the cause for many cases.[2] However, the concentration of drug users in correctional institutions is associated with a high prevalence of HIV infection among inmates.[7] In one study of HIV in prisons, 35% of male cases and 69% of female cases were associated with intravenous drug abuse.[1] This high-risk group for HIV infection often does not receive adequate HIV disease education and health care services. One impediment to targeting services to these individuals is that although offenders with a history of injection drug abuse have a higher risk of developing HIV disease, the crime for which they are jailed may not identify them as drug users.[2] Of interest, there are more IDUs in correctional facilities than in treatment centers,[1] which suggests this as a logical target for public health efforts.

Focus groups of both former and current prisoners in New York City and New York State revealed that 30% of group participants were HIV-positive. Of those who were HIV-positive, 40% had AIDS. Eighty percent had been arrested for a drug-related crime, 44% had a history of injection drug use, and 30% had shared injection drug equipment.[4] Participants reported that an array of illegal drugs (including glue, heroin, cocaine, and marijuana) entered their facility via staff, visitors, and personal mail.[4] Syringes are relatively difficult to find in jail; therefore they are almost always shared. Inmates sometimes are able to scavenge dirty syringes out of the medical clinic trash and reuse them. Inmates also create makeshift syringes using such improvised devices as pens, pieces of broken light bulbs, and the needles used to inflate basketballs. Injection drug use is the predominant risk factor for HIV infection among female inmates, and needle use practices contribute substantially to the risk of HIV infection among this group.[6] However, no domestic correctional system distributes bleach or clean needles to prisoners.[4]

ASSOCIATED CONDITIONS

As previously noted, there have been concerns that correctional facilities may serve as reservoirs for infectious diseases and could possibly amplify their spread to the community as prisoners who become infected while in prison or jail are released.[10] Such diseases include tuberculosis (TB), hepatitis B (HBV), hepatitis C (HCV), and other sexually transmitted infections (STIs). Many HIV-infected convicts harbor TB and continue to be vectors of transmission. The treatment of these infectious diseases is complicated by the frequent movement of inmates between facilities and their rapid turnover in the correctional facility, which makes completion of TB treatment and other conditions challenging.[2] One study of prevalence and within-prison incidence of HIV, HBV, and HCV infections among male prisoners of the Rhode Island Correctional Institute found high prevalence of HBV and HCV at intake (20.2% and 23.1%, respectively), which was consistent with reported rates in other U.S. prison settings.[10] The most common AIDS-defining opportunistic infections at Rhode Island adult correctional facilities in 1991 were *Pneumocystis jiroveci* (formerly *carinii*) pneumonia, candida esophagitis, toxoplasmosis encephalitis, and progressive multifocal leukoencephalopathy.[1] In addition, many incarcerated women have engaged in commercial sex work, predisposing them to STIs. Unprotected sex may increase risk of HIV-infected women for diseases such as chancroid, syphilis, herpes, gonorrhea, and chlamydia infection.[2]

TESTING ISSUES

HIV testing can help to prevent the problem of HIV transmission and improve treatment in the prison system. Testing allows for the treatment of individual prisoners and provides social benefit by improving preventive and, ultimately, therapeutic efforts. However, a difficult question exists regarding mandatory versus voluntary testing for all prisoners. The World Health Organization states that "compulsory HIV testing is unethical . . . should be prohibited . . . [and] HIV policies for inmates should be congruent with policies accepted in the community."[11] However, as of 1994, 15 state prison systems and federal prisons required mandatory testing of inmates.[12] Obtaining consent for such testing is a difficult issue facing correctional facilities. Attempts to increase the number of inmates who consent to have voluntary HIV testing have not led to satisfactory results, and researchers seek to understand the primary deterrents to testing. Problems of voluntary testing arise in part because inmates are concerned that showing interest in HIV infection and AIDS education will be, in essence, admitting that they are engaging in drug activity or homosexual behavior.[3] One strategy proposed to increase compliance with voluntary HIV testing was to routinely offer testing to all inmates regardless of crime committed or history of risky behaviors.[4]

Another deterrent against voluntary HIV infection and AIDS testing is that prisoners fear that their HIV status will become public knowledge and fear segregation from HIV-negative inmates. In 1986, the California Legislature passed Proposition 96, which allowed correctional staff access to the HIV status of inmates.[12] The correctional officers' union in multiple states has lobbied to mandate disclosure of inmates' HIV status, citing their possible risk of exposure.[2] However, the Centers for Disease Control and Prevention (CDC) have found no cases of HIV infection or AIDS in correctional staff due to work-related transmission.[13] This mandate could actually serve to worsen the overall exposure risk of the correctional staff by providing a false sense of security to the officers. Many correctional officers ignore universal precautions when dealing with inmates who are supposedly HIV-negative, thereby increasing their risk of exposure to HBV, HCV, and other, not yet diagnosed, cases of HIV infection.[2] Another reason stated for prison systems needing to know an inmate's HIV status is to allow for possible segregation of these individuals. However, segregation of HIV-positive prisoners has become much less commonplace, such that, from 1985 to 1993, the percentage of U.S. prisons that segregated its prisoners with HIV disease and AIDS decreased from 42% to 8%.[12] This movement toward mainstreaming has improved the success of voluntary testing by removing the associated stigma and segregation that comes with being HIV-positive.[14] In fact, all but one of the U.S. prisons that required mandatory HIV testing did not segregate HIV-positive inmates.[15]

Confidentiality of HIV testing results is a major factor in determining the success of voluntary testing programs within the prison system. In Maryland, where results remain confidential, about 50% of inmates consented to HIV testing. In Oregon and Washington state, where the incidence of HIV is lower overall, studies have found that 65% to 71% of inmates consent to voluntary testing. Another study found that over 90% of Rhode Island inmates have agreed to voluntary testing upon entry.[2]

CONDOM AND SYRINGE DISTRIBUTION

Correctional institutions provide a unique opportunity to optimize HIV prevention and treatment strategies for the individual, which, on a broader scale, can provide social benefit.[4,16] Several studies have outlined specific recommendations to maximize voluntary testing. The first recommendation is that testing be confidential. Ideally, it should be completely anonymous, although anonymity may be logistically difficult to accomplish in the prison setting.[12] Also, testing should be carried out by non–correctional staff to prevent discrimination or a possible breach of confidentiality. Further, prisoners should be provided counseling, education, and appropriate medical treatment upon receiving test results. Finally, interventions to decrease transmission of disease should be made available, the most important of which is condom distribution.[1]

Although condom distribution provides a simple method to help control the problem of HIV infection within the prison system, as of 2003 only two state prison systems (Mississippi and Vermont) and four city or county jails had condoms available to inmates.[3] In one study's inmate focus group, a majority of participants felt that condom distribution was not equal across their institution and, instead, depended on a number of variables, including which programs an inmate was enrolled in and what staff members the prisoner knew.[4] Anonymous distribution of latex barriers appears to be critical to compliance for both men and women in this study's focus group. The focus group of imprisoned men voiced the importance of anonymous distribution of condoms to prevent HIV-related violence and homophobic reactions. The group reported that any expressed interest in HIV prevention implied homosexuality.[4] This same study noted the importance of having universal barrier protection (condoms, dental dams, etc.) available to female prisoners as well. This was especially important in light of their reported frequent relations with male correctional officers.[4] One inmate suggested that correctional institutions add latex barriers into daily allotments of toiletries.[4] Making condoms readily and anonymously available at sites where sexual activity usually occurs, such as having bowls available in showers, was further recommended as a logistically simple approach to disease prevention.

The ultimate goal is to educate inmates about effective prevention strategies for use upon release from the prison system. Making condoms and dental dams available to inmates at release as well as during incarceration can provide a logistically viable disease prevention strategy.[4] This knowledge gained during imprisonment can benefit the individual as well as provide a broader social benefit to the community upon the inmate's release.

LEGAL ISSUES

Various types of lawsuits have arisen at the crossroads of HIV infection and prison life. Legal issues raised by inmates have included breaches of confidentiality, inadequate medical and mental health care, HIV testing without consent, lack of HIV testing, improper diagnosis, and lack of HIV education. Additionally, prisoners have sued over allegedly contracting HIV infection while in prison on the grounds that the institution did not afford them adequate protection from sexual assault. On the other hand, HIV-positive inmates have been tried or sued for a host of aggressive acts, such as allegedly biting, spitting, or throwing blood during skirmishes with prison personnel.

One area with the potential to have an impact on inmate mental health has been the practice of some prisons to segregate HIV-positive inmates from the general population. This leads to a loss of confidentiality regarding their HIV status and also stigmatization. Inmates who have sued to reverse these policies have generally not prevailed. Moreover, the U.S. Supreme Court in January 2000 refused to consider an appeal by Alabama prisoners who challenged their segregation both residentially and in other programs such as in classrooms and workplaces. The 11th Circuit Appeals Court 1999 decision in this case, *Davis v. Hopper*, was allowed to stand. The Appeals Court ruled that these segregation practices did not violate the Americans with Disabilities Act or the Rehabilitation Act of 1973. The court agreed with prison officials that due to the unpredictable behavior of prisoners and AIDS being a fatal disease, HIV-positive inmates presented a "direct threat" to other inmates and corrections officers and thus could be segregated from prison programs.

Safety issues for inmates in prison environments remain a crucial issue. One major area of risk is sexual assault. Advocacy groups, such as *Stop Prison Rape*, have long tried to draw attention to what is viewed as a major problem in prisons both within and outside the United States. The figure of 1 in 10 inmates becoming a victim of rape is often quoted as an estimate of the extent of this problem. An undetermined number of inmates, male and female, have contracted HIV infection and other diseases from having been sexually assaulted behind bars. This figure can never be reliably determined without having preincarceration and postincarceration HIV testing and universal surveys on the prevalence of sexual assault for all prisoners.

The following are updates on recent legislative activity nationwide as it relates to HIV disease and AIDS in prisons. As will be seen, there is growing momentum by state and federal government to address the issues of sexual assault and HIV diagnosis and treatment in penal institutions in a more serious manner.

U.S. JUSTICE DEPARTMENT STUDY

A recent study by the Justice Department found that there were 8,210 acts of alleged sexual violence in 2004,[17] and an acknowledgment was made that this figure is likely a significant underestimate. The dynamics of underreporting were explained as follows[17]:

> Administrative records cannot alone provide reliable estimates of sexual violence . . . . Due to fear of reprisal from perpetrators, a code of silence among inmates, personal embarrassment, and lack of trust in staff, victims are often reluctant to report incidents to correctional authorities.

Of these 8,210 alleged sexual assaults, only 2,090 could be substantiated. These figures come from a report that was mandated by the 2003 Prison Rape Elimination Act (P.L. 108-79), which was signed into law on September 4, 2003 by President George W. Bush. One of the requirements of the legislation was to have the Bureau of Justice Statistics collect data on the incidence and prevalence of sexual violence in correctional facilities (details are in the BJS Report[17]). Some other findings were that 90% of victims and perpetrators of inmate-on-inmate nonconsensual sexual acts in prison and jail were male, and over 40% of allegations of sexual violence implicated staff sexual misconduct.

2005 TEXAS CLASS ACTION LAWSUIT

The seriousness of the HIV transmission risk among prisoners was highlighted by a recent federal lawsuit in Texas against prison officials who were accused of violating a prisoner's constitutional right against cruel and unusual punishment. The plaintiff, Roderick Johnson, testified he had been made a slave of prison gangs for 18 months during his incarceration and was raped by 49 different men. At times he was rented out to other inmates at a cost of $3.00 to $7.00. His pleas for help, protection, and medical attention were reportedly met by officials with indifference, ridicule, or scorn. The jury, to the dismay of many advocacy groups, ultimately ruled for the six prison official defendants from the Texas Department of Criminal Justice.

2005 CALIFORNIA LEGISLATIVE ACTION

The Sexual Abuse in Detention Elimination Act (AB 550) in California was signed into law in September of 2005 by Governor Arnold Schwarzenegger. California has the largest penal system in the country. This act is further evidence of the nation's growing concern about the risks facing prisoners, and it in all probability will significantly lower the number of cases of HIV transmission in California's prisons. It seeks to protect all inmates and wards from sexual abuse while incarcerated in institutions operated by the Department of Corrections and the Department of the Youth Authority. These agencies will be required to develop and implement protocols and procedures designed to specifically protect inmates from sexual assault. An Office of the Sexual Abuse in Detention Ombudsperson will be created to increase accountability of institutions and to ensure compliance with the federal Prison Rape Elimination Act.

2005 ILLINOIS LEGISLATIVE ACTION

Another law passed in 2005 addressing HIV and prisons was The African American HIV/AIDS Response Act (P.L. 94-0629). This law focuses on preventing HIV transmission in blacks in Illinois, especially those who are incarcerated. It requires the Illinois Department of Corrections (DOC) and state jails to offer free HIV antibody tests and HIV infection and AIDS counseling to all inmates when they arrive at prison, during their imprisonment, and before they are released at the end of their sentences. Moreover, HIV-positive inmates are entitled to medical care throughout their incarceration. Prison officials must also provide transitional case management and arrange treatment and support services referrals for all HIV-positive inmates upon their release. Even all visitors to the Illinois DOC are to be offered written material on HIV disease and AIDS and informed of how to get public health counseling if they desire it. To make sure the above provisions of the Act are carried out, a nine-member panel housed in the governor's office was established; three of the members are required to be representatives of HIV/AIDS organizations.

ETHICAL ISSUES

The medical profession's *Principles of Medical Ethics* has seven of its nine sections that can be considered to have particular importance to psychiatrists' and other physicians' work in prisons with HIV-infected and at-risk inmates.[18] They are paraphrased below:

Section 1: The provision of competent medical care with compassion and respect for human dignity and rights

Section 3: Recognize a responsibility to seek changes in those laws that are contrary to the best interests of the patient

Section 4: Safeguard patient confidences and privacy within the constraints of the law

Section 5: Make relevant information available to patients . . . use the talents of other health professionals when indicated

Section 7: Responsibility to participate in activities contributing to improvement of the community and betterment of public health

Section 8: While caring for a patient, regard responsibility to the patient as paramount

Section 9: Support access to medical care for all people

Space constrictions prevent examining each these sections in depth regarding their application to HIV issues. However, it is not hard to imagine an entire book devoted to the ethical challenges for health care practitioners that arise within the HIV disease prison spectrum. The provision of medical care in correctional settings raises many ethical challenges for physicians given the unique circumstances brought about by the imprisonment of people within a closed environment that also has the mission of segregation from society and punishment for its tenants. Examples of the difficulties that can arise when striving to practice ethical medicine in prison settings are discussed in the following section.

Perhaps one of the greatest ethical challenges physicians face in treating prison patients is in maintaining confidentiality of their medical records. It can be particular hard to keep medical information such as HIV status confidential in the confines of a prison medical clinic. The importance of confidentiality may not be taken as seriously because the patients are prisoners, with fewer civil rights. Word travels fast in the closed system of a prison when leaked. Furthermore, there are pressures from prison personnel who believe they have a need to know, for example, in order to allow themselves and officers to best protect themselves during inmate management. Imagine the ethical predicament physicians were placed in when California voters passed Proposition 96 in 1988. This proposition allowed court-ordered HIV testing of persons charged with sex and assault crimes, and prison and jail doctors were required to provide lists of suspected or known HIV-positive prisoners to prison staff.

Another ethical issue practitioners in prison health clinics face is the question of whether condoms should be distributed to inmates. Most prison administrators have not supported condom distribution to inmates. Many public and prison health groups advocate that inmates have access to condoms to help stem the spread of HIV and other sexually transmitted diseases. This issue was recently addressed in Tennessee. The Tennessee Department of Corrections (DOC) responded in the negative to calls for inmate condom access by saying such action on their part would "send the wrong message," given that sexual contact among inmates is prohibited, and might even increase sexual activity. It was further pointed out by prison officials that they did not have any evidence HIV was being spread from prisoner to prisoner to support such a policy. Of interest, an average of 800 disciplinary actions are meted out yearly in the Tennessee DOC for inmate sexual behavior, which to the authors sounds like sufficient evidence, given that this figure is in all likelihood the tip of the iceberg when it comes to the actual frequency of sexual contacts among inmates.

Physicians took contrasting positions on this issue, this in itself an indication of the presence of complex ethical and political issues (and in perhaps this case religious issues as well). For example, a medical director for the private contractual agency providing health care to the DOC cited the lack of epidemiologic data showing HIV was being spread from prisoner to prisoner, closely following the party line. Public health physicians, on the other hand, supported inmate condom access, and the recommendation was even made that HIV-positive inmates should be segregated from the general prison population. The impressive potential savings to taxpayers for every infection avoided was also raised. Meanwhile, the Tennessee DOC will be spending roughly $2 million this year—one third of their state pharmacy expenditures—for HIV disease and AIDS medications for the known infected inmates in their system, about 1% of their prison population. This percentage is an under-representation of actual infected inmates, because HIV testing is largely voluntary in this system.

In contrast to Tennessee, other jurisdictions, such as Mississippi, Vermont, the District of Columbia, Los Angeles, New York City, Philadelphia, San Francisco, Australia, Brazil, Canada, and many European countries permit condom distribution to their inmates.

SUMMARY

There is a growing recognition that HIV infection and its many ramifications are a serious problem in our prisons. It is estimated that the rate of HIV infection in prisoners is three to six times higher than in the general population, and 20% to 25% of persons who are HIV-positive and living in the United States will be in a correctional institution during a given year.[19] This is not all bad news in that correctional institutions actually can serve as key points of contact for HIV prevention and treatment interventions. Greater emphasis needs to be placed on the prevention of HIV transmission among inmates, along with increased efforts to provide appropriate diagnosis and treatment for those who are HIV-positive. Additionally, large increases in U.S. incarceration rates in turn are leading to large numbers of persons released from custody, and a not insignificant number of them will be HIV-positive. Many such persons will transition to poverty-stricken urban areas with limited options for health care and monitoring and poor psychosocial support. The need for ongoing case management and support services for these people is crucial—not only for the maintenance of the former inmates' health but to also help prevent transmission to others in the community—and this topic needs to be a priority for lawmakers and community service providers. Appropriate interventions to help these persons with multiple vulnerabilities adjust and receive necessary care following release can have a major influence on their postrelease outcomes in the community.

REFERENCES

1. Dixon PS, Flanigan TP, DeBuono BA, et al. Infection with the human immunodeficiency virus in prisoners: meeting a health care challenge. *Am J Med*. 1993;95:629–663.
2. Spaulding A, Stephenson B, Macalino G, et al. Human immunodeficiency virus in correctional facilities: a review. *Clin Infect Dis*. 2002;35:305–312.
3. Braithwaite RL, Arriola KRJ: Male prisoners and HIV prevention: a call for action ignored. *Am J Public Health*. 2003;93:759–763.
4. Mahon J. New York inmates risk behaviors: the implications for prevention policy and programs: *Am J Public Health*. 1996;86:1211–1215.
5. Amankwaa AA: Causes of death in Florida prisons: the dominance of AIDS. *Am J Public Health*. 1995;85:1710–1711.
6. Hankins CA, Gendron S, Handley MA, et al. HIV infection among women in prison: an assessment of risk factors using a nominal methodology. *Am J Public Health*. 1994;84:1637–1640.
7. Gaiter J, Doll LS. Improving HIV/AIDS prevention in prison is good public health policy [editorial]. *Am J Public Health*. 1996;86:1201–1203.
8. Seal DW. HIV-related issues and concerns for imprisoned persons throughout the world. *Curr Opin Psychiatr*. 2005;18:530–535.
9. McKee KJ, Power KG. HIV/AIDS in prisons. *Scott Med J*. 1992;37:132–137.
10. Macalino GE, Vlahov D, Sanford-Colby S, et al. Prevalence and incidence of HIV, hepatitis B virus, and hepatitis C virus infections among males in Rhode Island prisons. *Am J Public Health*. 2004;94:1218–1223.
11. Global Programme on AIDS. *WHO Guidelines on HIV Infection and AIDS in Prisons*. Geneva: World Health Organization; 1993.
12. Diamond J. HIV testing in prison: what's the controversy? *Lancet*. 1994;344:1650–1651.
13. Centers for Disease Control and Prevention. *HIV/AIDS Surveillance Report 1994*. Atlanta: Centers for Disease Control and Prevention; 1995.
14. Harding TW. AIDS in prison. *Lancet*. 1987;2:1260–1263.
15. Hammett TR, Harold L, Gross M, et al. *1992 Update: HIV/AIDS in Correctional Facilities*. Washington, DC: US Department of Justice, National Institute of Justice; 1994.
16. Glaser JB, Greifinger RB. Correctional health care: a public health opportunity. *Ann Intern Med*. 1993;118:139–145.

17. Beck AJ, Hughes TA: Sexual Violence Reported by Correctional Authorities, 2004. Bureau of Justice Statistics Special Report: July 2005, NCJ 210333.
18. American Psychiatric Association. *The Principles of Medical Ethics with Annotations Especially Applicable to Psychiatry*. Washington, DC: American Psychiatric Association; 2001.
19. Hammett TM, Harmon P, Rhodes W. *The Burden of Infectious Disease Among Inmates and Releases from Correctional Facilities, in the Health Status of Soon-to-be-Released Inmates*. Report to Congress National Commission on Correctional Health Care, Chicago; 2002.

CHAPTER 32

HIV/AIDS and the Patient's Family

James L. Griffith, Michael Golder

Most often, human immunodeficiency virus (HIV) and acquired immunodeficiency syndrome (AIDS) have been regarded by clinicians either as a public health concern or an infection borne by an individual. Neither of these perspectives sufficiently accounts for the roles families play in HIV disease and AIDS. As chronic illnesses, HIV infection and AIDS heavily affect the well-being of couples and families. Likewise, the communications, organization, and quality of relationships in couples and families heavily influence the risk for infection and the severity of illness. Primary prevention programs that have successfully imputed accurate knowledge about AIDS have failed to reduce adolescent sexual risk-taking when family and peer influences were omitted from the programs.[1] The role of families in HIV disease and AIDS is bypassed by either a public health focus on society as a whole or upon individual patients.

Efforts to understand the mediating effects of families in HIV disease and AIDS have led to the following three domains of investigation:

1. As illnesses, how do HIV infection and AIDS affect families? In what ways are these similar or different from other chronic illnesses?
2. In what ways do families bear influences that may be harmful? How can these factors be attenuated? Harmful factors include both those that amplify risk of HIV infection and those that compromise the care of ill family members.
3. In what ways do families bear influences that are salutatory for health? How can these factors be amplified? Salutatory factors include both those acting to prevent HIV infection and those that support optimal care of ill family members.
4. What are the health consequences of social stigma in HIV disease and AIDS? How can the adverse effects of stigma be countered? HIV disease and AIDS have been unique during recent decades as laden with social stigma, both moral and related to contagion. The stigma associated with HIV infection has given rise to special relational problems for couples and families with an infected member. These stigma-associated relational problems have been most pronounced for gay couples.

For a clinician, these four domains provide the structure for a systematic assessment of couples and families coping with HIV disease or AIDS and help organize interventions that can help families and their ill members prevail against threats from HIV disease and AIDS.

THE IMPACT OF HIV/AIDS ON COUPLES AND FAMILIES

The initial diagnosis of HIV infection commonly precipitates a family crisis. There are concerns that a partner or parent might die, worries about the future of the family, and guilt over responsibility for the infection.[2] As the sense of crisis dissipates, a family begins assessing and responding to its new reality.

The subsequent impact of HIV disease and AIDS depends in great part on expected disease outcome, whether that of a chronic illness still permitting normal functioning in daily life or a progressive illness with deteriorating medical and mental health ending in death.[3] Worldwide, HIV disease and AIDS largely remain fatal, with a high level of stigma. In the United States, however, effective antiviral medications, elimination of perinatal HIV transmission, and educational campaigns have partially shifted perceptions of HIV infection toward that of a chronic, but manageable, medical illness.[4] In this regard, HIV disease and AIDS in the United States bear increasing similarities to other slowly progressive chronic diseases, such as cancer and heart disease.

A major stressor in nearly all cases is the inevitable shift from a lifestyle organized about usual family concerns to one organized around doctor visits, diagnostic tests, medications, and costs of medical care.[2] This stress is particularly severe for single mothers, whose fatigue and other medical symptoms both hinder parenting and limit family income. A 1996 Canadian study of 91 families with HIV infection or AIDS found two generations infected in 42% of the families, compounding the challenges in managing the illness.[2] This study identified the following as dominant themes of family stress among families with HIV infection or AIDS:

- Parents confronting "a web of personal, health, and family concerns"
- Financial pressures
- Dilemmas around disclosure
- Social challenges for the HIV-infected person.

The primary clinical strategy with families coping with HIV-related stresses is to partner with the couple or family in composing a plan that simultaneously accepts the reality of HIV infection or AIDS as a permanent presence in the couple or family and works to minimize the amount of time, energy, and other resources that HIV disease and AIDS take away from family life.

A family-centered approach to care of HIV disease and AIDS assumes that the impact of disease will largely result from the natural course of HIV infection and AIDS intersecting with the following domains of family life[3]:

- Family members' levels of scientific knowledge about the illness and its treatments
- Developmental tasks that concern individual family members and the family unit as a whole, according to stages of the life cycle
- The organizational structure of the family
- Communication processes
- Members' beliefs about health and illness

An assessment of family members' levels of scientific knowledge is an initial concern because an understanding of the natural course of HIV disease and AIDS is vital not only for the immediate crisis but for the family's plans over the next decade. Developmentally, HIV disease and AIDS have most affected the 25- to 44-year-old age generation in families, who normally should be parenting the next generation.[4] Identifying specific developmental tasks that need to occur helps family members to avoid secondary effects from the illness on children and other well family members. Assessment of family structure helps clarify the state of readiness for managing a long-term drain on family resources from HIV disease and AIDS, particularly when there are comorbid medical disorders, substance abuse, or HIV-related cognitive or mood disorders. This drain is heaviest when the HIV-infected member is a single parent or the primary wage earner. Assessment of communication processes gauges whether dialog that can ameliorate suffering and facilitate problem-solving is possible. Assessment of family beliefs focuses on issues of stigma both within the family and between family and community. Families can hesitate to provide needed support for an ill member when they fear contagion, blame the HIV-infected member for contracting the virus, or fear shunning by their surrounding community.

FAMILY FACTORS THAT ADVERSELY AFFECT HEALTH

A family assessment prioritizes identification of competencies, resources, and practical wisdom within families that can be brought to bear on the adversities of HIV disease and AIDS. However, it is important that the assessment screen not only for strengths, but also for specific family factors that can speed disease progression or place family members at risk. The culture of a family can adversely affect the health of its members when it hinders transmission of information about HIV infection and AIDS, fails to parent effectively adolescents at risk for infection, or produces neglect of family members ill with AIDS.

The following family factors have been demonstrated to increase risk of infection among adolescents[4]:

1. Poor parent–child communication
2. Family dysfunction that fosters early or impulsive sexual behavior
3. Limited parental monitoring of adolescent sexual behavior
4. Family stigma contributing to unsafe sexual practices and avoidance of HIV testing

Adolescents who engage earlier in sexual behaviors are those with low levels of parental support or greater emotional distance from their families.[4] When recognized, any of these factors should become a focus of preventive intervention. They have become the impetus for community primary prevention programs, discussed below.

Family members with AIDS fare poorly in a family culture that intensifies affects of blame, shame, guilt, fear, and despair. Psychosomatic research has raised concerns whether negative emotional arousal can directly impair physiologic resistance to HIV infection and AIDS disease progression via stress hormones, autonomic nervous system dysregulation, and attenuation of immune competence.[5] Aside from direct physiologic effects, such an emotional climate disables family members' capacities to communicate and to team effectively in managing the challenges of a chronic medical illness. For ill family members, it fosters demoralization that can lead to self-neglect and nonadherence to medical treatment. Family beliefs promoting a family climate of negative emotional arousal require clinical intervention.

Other deleterious effects result from secrecy. Research on family factors has shown that family knowledge about and attitudes toward HIV infection operate as independent factors separable from stigma generally present in society. Secrecy about HIV status damages intimacy and effective problem-solving in couples and families. A "double crisis" can ensue when the family discovers unsuspected homosexuality, bisexuality, infidelity, or drug use at the same time that they learn that a family member is infected. The family member must then cope with the ensuing family crisis at the same time as new health problems and death and dying issues are arising.[4]

FAMILY FACTORS WITH SALUTATORY EFFECTS ON HEALTH

Families can both decrease the risk of HIV transmission and also provide vital support for infected family members. To maximize positive family contributions, the National Institute of Mental Health (NIMH) Office of AIDS has adopted the definition of a "network of mutual commitment" to connote the often improvised social networks that subserve the traditional roles of family members for people with HIV disease or AIDS.[4] HIV infection and AIDS are disproportionately represented in poor and minority communities, where intact nuclear families are the exception rather than the rule. Families at risk, or who have HIV disease or AIDS, often have nontraditional family structures, with friends or lovers fulfilling traditional roles of family members. Differentiation between "family of choice" and "family of origin" has been particularly useful in conceptualizing the families of gay couples.[4]

A number of parent-oriented preventive interventions have been developed by members of the NIMH Consortium on Families and HIV/AIDS. Families are regarded as the single most influential force in the life of children and adolescents. Parent–child communication about sex decreases HIV-risk behaviors. Adolescents who believe that they have a close relationship with their parents are less likely to engage in early sexual intercourse. These research findings have led to family-based interventions that impart education about HIV infection and AIDS and build parental competencies that can influence adolescents' behaviors. These programs have emphasized the sexual education role of parents, strengthening of parent–child communication, amelioration of family dysfunction fostering risk-taking behaviors outside the home, improving parental monitoring of adolescent activities.[4]

The CHAMP Family Program developed by McKay et al.[1] has exemplified a family-based preventive program focused on fourth and fifth grade children in a poor urban community with high rates of substance abuse and HIV disease, with an intent to delay adolescent sexual behavior. Preadolescent children were targeted in the belief that they are exposed to situations of sexual possibility but are not yet sexually active. Family communications regarding information, values, and beliefs were therefore more likely to have an impact than with older adolescents who already were sexually active. The CHAMP program sought to strengthen family relationships and to enhance peer influences with training in social problem-solving and peer negotiations. The content and form of the intervention were designed in collaboration with families from the neighborhoods of concern. Families met for twelve 90-minute sessions that began with a multifamily group discussion focusing on a particular topic (e.g., "Talking and listening to each other," "Rules keep kids safe," "What we need to know about HIV/AIDS"). Separate parent- and child-only groups then focused on in-depth exploration of the topic and skill-building. The last 30 minutes of each session consisted of a family practice activity conducted within the multifamily group. Compared to control families, those completing the intervention demonstrated statistically significant strengthening of parental decision-making, increased comfort in family communications regarding sensitive topics, and increased parental knowledge about HIV infection and AIDS.

Other family-based prevention programs have been implemented. Krauss et al.[6] developed a prevention program for mothers and fathers to use with preadolescent children to help parents become experts in their child's eyes. Paikoff[7] combined both parent-only groups and child-only groups with multifamily groups. This intervention has promoted comfort and communication about information and values related to puberty, early sexual behavior, and HIV infection and AIDS. Dilorio et al.[8] have developed a prevention program for mothers and their adolescents. This approach has fostered family involvement in the sexual health of adolescents, including delay of sexual intercourse, acquisition of information about HIV infection and AIDS, and the enactment of HIV risk-reduction practices. Jemmot et al.[9] developed an intervention designed to help African-American mothers teach sons about sex to decrease risky behavior. Internationally, Weine and Agani[10] have developed in Kosovo an eight-session multifamily group intervention for reducing HIV infection and AIDS risk behaviors among at-risk 14- to 16-year-olds, the Kosovar Families Addressing Risk in Youth (KFARY).

Family-based interventions also have been designed to aid families in adapting to HIV infection and in caring for dying family members. Rapkin et al.[11] developed an intervention to enhance AIDS-affected families' abilities to problem-solve. Mitrani et al.[12] designed an intervention to improve the quality of social relations and supports of African-American seropositive women. Wingood and DiClemente[13] developed the WiLLOW program to create HIV disease support networks for women in semirural areas.

Two prevention programs have developed community-based prevention programs for AIDS orphans. Bauman et al.[14] developed Project Care as a preventive intervention to improve the psychological functioning of children who survive the death of a parent from AIDS. Rotheram-Borus and Lightfoot[16] designed a program to help parents to make decisions regarding disclosure and custody and to maintain positive daily routines.

SPECIAL ISSUES FOR GAY COUPLES

Ambiguity in the sociolegal status of gay couples and the impact of the AIDS epidemic in gay communities together have created unique clinical issues for gay couples. The social marginality of gay couples has magnified the significance of HIV disease stigma. These psychological impacts have added complexity according to the couple's serologic status—whether seronegative (both partners HIV-negative), serodiscordant (mixed HIV status), or seropositive (both partners HIV-positive). Discussion of these issues is detailed in Chapters 28 and 29.

COUPLE OR FAMILY ASSESSMENT AND INTERVENTION

A clinician helping a couple or family to cope with HIV disease or AIDS can provide assessment and interventions within the scope of a limited number of family meetings. This collaborative, family-centered care is grounded both in empirical family studies and family systems theory.

The first step is building a collaborative, strength-focused therapeutic relationship with a couple or family. This often is better facilitated by referring to gatherings as "family meetings," rather than "family therapy," implying the strengths-competencies-resilience focus of the work to follow. A key decision is who to include in the meetings, which often is best answered by asking: "During the next stretch of time, who do you most wish to be involved in coping with the challenges of this illness?" This question points to "the network of mutual commitment" as "family," rather than traditional bloodline or legal definitions. A genogram is a useful tool to display visually everyone who is "like family."[16]

The second step consists of one to four meetings that systematically assess the following[3,16]:

1. What levels of scientific understanding do family members have about HIV infection and AIDS, its prevention, and its treatments?
2. What are the anticipated developmental tasks that likely will be concerns for each family member during the duration of the illness? For example, who may be leaving for college, planning to retire, changing jobs, moving across the country?
3. What are the anticipated developmental tasks of the couple or family, according to its life cycle? For example, are there young children to be parented, teenagers to be launched into adulthood, midlife issues of the couple around intimacy?
4. What are the qualities of communications within the family? For example, are communications open and direct? Are any family members excluded from important discussions? Can practical issues be fully discussed? Can emotional problems be fully discussed?

5. How will the organizational structure of the family respond to the challenges of HIV disease or AIDS? For example, are problem-solving skills adequate? Are privacy and intimacy for the couple sufficiently protected? Is any one family member likely to become overburdened with caretaking responsibilities? Are the practical tasks reasonably distributed for managing doctor visits, monitoring medications, and securing sufficient family income? Is the well-being of any healthy family member neglected due to a family focus on the HIV disease or AIDS?
6. How do family beliefs about HIV infection and AIDS influence care of the patient or well-being of the family? What are family members' beliefs about etiology, illness transmission, prognosis, treatment, and relative roles of patient, family members, and health care professionals in its management? How have family members derived their beliefs (i.e., popular press, scientific readings, health care professionals, having known someone with HIV infection or AIDS)?

If the second step has emphasized identification of family strengths, competencies, and resources that can be employed therapeutically, then the third step is identification of specific factors that may impede needed medical treatment, erode family well-being, or amplify the patient's suffering. These include an absence of accurate knowledge about HIV infection and AIDS; paucity of family problem-solving skills; family beliefs that mobilize blame, shame, guilt, or fear, or despair; poor parent–child communication or failures in parental oversight of adolescents at risk for HIV exposure.[3,16]

The fourth step is negotiation of an action plan with the family. This action plan is constituted by practical steps members can take to amplify and extend their competencies for coping and to attenuate factors threatening to weaken coping or to place family members at risk of harm. This action plan also can connect the family with advocacy groups, community family-based HIV disease and AIDS prevention programs, or other community resources. Subsequent follow-up meetings can be arranged as appropriately fit the plan for action. In an outpatient setting, this most often constitutes a brief family-centered psychotherapy conducted within 4 to 20 sessions.

Confidentiality regarding both HIV status and mode of infection must be addressed when planning a couple or family meeting, as illustrated in the following vignette:

> Barbara was a middle-aged woman for whom psychiatric consultation had been requested because of her difficulties in coping with AIDS-related polyneuropathy and myoclonic seizures. When the consultant entered the room, three female family members who had been feeding and bathing her left so that she could speak alone with the consultant. During the interview, Barbara mentioned that other family members and friends, as well as her pastor, had visited during her hospitalization. The consultant wondered whether it would be possible to meet together with her family and other close supportive relationships. "I need to be able to communicate better with them," she said. "But there is something I can't tell them." She paused in silence, then said, "I have AIDS." She told how she feared that people would become angry with her or would avoid her for fear of catching it. She most feared their response if it were learned that for years she had been keeping her HIV status secret. "I was having unprotected sex." She wept as she spoke about her guilt that she may have spread the virus to others. She nodded in agreement as the consultant articulated her dilemma—secrets separate people; she wanted to be close and open, but if she were so, some indeed likely would leave her while others would stay.

An agreement about therapist confidentiality—"what can be discussed with whom, in which conversation"—must be negotiated explicitly with the patient when planning a family meeting. This negotiation should address both the clinician's duty to protect (clinician may refuse to keep secret HIV status if others are at active risk of infection) and the patient's right to privacy (patient may insist on protection from moral or contagion stigma). If subsequent psychiatric treatment is conducted in a "split therapy" model between a psychiatrist and non–psychiatric psychotherapist, this negotiation also must cover issues of disclosure between the psychiatrist and psychotherapist. Before initiating formal couple therapy, a clear agreement must be established regarding confidentiality of information that either couple partner reveals to the therapist in private communications, including revelations about infidelity. If either partner expresses discomfort with such confidentiality, a contract for full disclosure is generally recommended for all information privately revealed by either partner. When a patient's desire for confidentiality about HIV status is paramount, individual psychotherapy that also addresses relational and family systems issues can be a more prudent alternative to couple or family therapy.

The above therapeutic principles can be implemented in even a single couple or family meeting, as illustrated in the following two contrasting vignettes from a general hospital psychiatric consultation-liaison service:

> David was a 34-year-old architect for whom psychiatric consultation was requested because of his attending physician's concerns that he was depressed. David was HIV-positive and infected with a chronic bacterial infection that was proving difficult to eradicate with antibiotics. Although he indeed had some depressive symptoms, his overall score on a Hamilton Depression Scale was only moderately elevated. Further, his intensity of regret for never honestly talking with his family about his sexual identity suggested that grief and demoralization might better account for his dispirited state than a mood disorder. Now he feared telling his family that he was not only gay, but also had AIDS. The psychiatric consultant obtained his consent for a family meeting, in addition to recommending a psychostimulant for brightening his mood and subsequent bedside psychotherapy.
>
> Three days later, David's mother and two siblings arrived from out of town. Sensitive to David's ambivalence about meeting with them, the consultant inquired slowly and carefully about what they already understood and what they were ready to address in this meeting. The mother, however, responded curtly: "We are from New York. We get right to the point." Taking this cue, the consultant turned to David and asked: "In your gut, how much time does it feel that you have left. Is it measured in days, weeks, months, or years?" "A few weeks," David responded. This opened a frank discussion in which David asked his family's forgiveness that he had not told them he was gay. Should he have only a few weeks until death, he wanted to spend it near his family. Not surprisingly, his sister told David that they had known that he was gay, but had not spoken about it with him out of respect, because he had not brought it up. The ensuing conversation revealed that the following:
>
> 1. All family members were knowledgeable about AIDS and had known someone who had suffered with the illness.
> 2. No judging beliefs were evident that would validate David's guilt.
> 3. They could team together in practical ways to address the challenges of David's illness, albeit with concerns about his mother's heart disease if she were to provide his nursing care alone at home.
> 4. David was viewing the direness of his situation due to his concrete interpretation of a doctor's comment that "There is nothing more we can do...."
>
> The consultant responded that this interpretation was going too far without first clarifying what were the facts. The family agreed that the next step should be a family conference with his doctor to learn what precisely was David's medical condition and prognosis. They would then proceed with plans to help him move him near his family home.

In another case, Raffie was a 38-year-old musician for whom psychiatric consultation was requested "to evaluate and treat depression." Raffie had known that his partner had been HIV-positive for 9 years, but the partner had never shown signs of AIDS. They had carefully followed safe-sex guidelines for 3 years. Raffie had his HIV status checked several times, and it had never been found to be positive. On this hospital admission, however, he had been diagnosed with *Pneumocystis* pneumonia, and his CD4 cell count was low. He was HIV-positive and had AIDS. Raffie had responded to the diagnoses with so much despair that his medical team was concerned he could become suicidal.

Raffie told how he was the son of a Baptist minister. He said he knew from the Bible that homosexuality was a sin. He had never been able to acknowledge to his family that he was gay. Although he had been promiscuous and used drugs as a teenager, he had never stopped feeling the pull of his family. He had stopped the recreational drug use years earlier and had settled into a long-term, committed relationship with his partner. However, he had never felt peace about their relationship. Six months earlier, he had decided to stop having a sexual relationship, in his belief that to continue doing so was evil. Recently, he had considered returning to church. He viewed the Bible as authoritative and absolute: homosexuality was evil, and he was evil as long as he engaged in it. He felt he had been the prodigal son who had gone into a foreign land, where he had lived licentiously.

Raffie was reluctant to involve his partner in a discussion of his illness. Both had known friends who had died from AIDS. Both feared AIDS as if a death sentence. Weighed down with the heaviness of emotion, they could not at this time talk together about practical challenges that might lie ahead with this illness. Raffie's partner was in psychotherapy already and asked that Raffie join him there as a couple. Raffie shook his head silently.

The consultant responded by acknowledging and respecting Raffie's refusal of couple therapy. However, he also noted the commitment and endurance of their relationship in confronting past adversities. He also summarized in broad strokes recent research pointing to the importance that well-being in one's close relationships played in helping the body to be immunologically strong. The interview ended with the consultant gently suggesting they rediscuss in a few days whether meeting together as a couple might be worth considering. In his recommendations to Raffie's primary care physician, the consultant stated the following:

1. Raffie's current distress was best conceptualized as traumatic grief in its dimensions of sorrow and shock, rather than a major depressive disorder.
2. The role of antidepressants or other medications was presently unclear and best reevaluated during subsequent weeks as an outpatient.
3. Raffie's acute distress was opening the fissures of unresolved conflicts in Raffie's relational world, as commonly occurs in couples and families reeling from traumatic stress. The consequences of these changes were alarming. Raffie was leaving precipitously his primary sustaining relationship in an act of allegiance to the religion of his birth family, whom he was now frantically trying to rejoin. Rejoining his family's church presumably would necessitate his renouncing his homosexuality, which would be at high risk for failure over time.
4. Although Raffie did not currently show indicators of acute suicidal risk, the loss of his partner and/or rejection or humiliation by his family or their church plausibly could propel future suicidal impulses. He needed close and regular follow-up during coming weeks, with a low threshold for psychiatric consultation should worsening demoralization, depression, or suicidal thoughts be noted.
5. Outpatient consultation with a systemic family therapist was recommended to help Raffie, his partner, and his primary care physician navigate these complexities of Raffie's relational dilemmas.

These cases are clinically similar in their medical and psychiatric aspects, yet stand in stark contrast in how their family relations were conferring resilience or vulnerability. In David's family, the family meeting found his family members to be knowledgeable about HIV disease and AIDS. Their family organizational structure would be able to respond to the demands of a life-threatening medical disorder. A key developmental event (the mother's declining health) was noted and factored into planning. Family communications were open and direct throughout the meeting. David's belief about his prognosis was noted to generate despair and helplessness, and a plan was formulated for the family to join him in determining its validity.

In contrast, it seemed likely that Raffie's family of origin had little scientific understanding of HIV infection and AIDS. Rather, their religious convictions likely would lead to a moral view of his illness as a punishment imposed by God for his sinfulness. Should he rejoin their church and embrace its faith, the risk might be substantial that his sense of shame, guilt, and humiliation would escalate. Raffie's traumatic response to the news of AIDS so dominated the couple meeting that no inquiry could be made about other developmental concerns that might also be priorities for Raffie, his partner, or their relationship. At this time, the couple's organizational capacities for problem-solving were paralyzed and ineffective. The consultant listed these concerns and articulated recommendations that emphasized the high level of risk for Raffie and need for close and frequent monitoring after hospital discharge.

These contrasting cases illustrate the efficiency and power of couple and family assessments in delineating either family resilience factors, which can bolster effectiveness of other medical or psychiatric treatments, or family risk factors, which can render impotent other treatments. Couple- or family-centered care often can best position a clinician for providing effective biopsychosocial treatment of HIV disease and AIDS.

REFERENCES

1. McKay MM, Chasse KT, Paikoff R, et al. Family-level impact of the CHAMP Family Program: a community collaborative effort to support urban families and reduce youth HIV risk exposure. *Fam Process*. 2004;43:79–93.
2. DeMatteo D, Wells LM, Goldie S, et al. The "family" context of HIV: a need for comprehensive health and social policies. *AIDS Care*. 2002;14:261–278.
3. Rolland J. *Families, Illness, & Disability*. New York: Basic Books; 2004.
4. Pequegnat W, Szapocznik J. The role of families in preventing and adapting to HIV/AIDS. In: Pequegnat W, Szapocznik J, eds. *Working with Families in the Era of HIV/AIDS*. Thousand Oaks, Calif: Sage Publications; 2000:3–26.
5. Ironson G, Antoni MH, Schneiderman N, et al. Stress management and psychosocial predictors of disease course in HIV-1 infection. In: Goodkin K, Visser AP, eds. *Psychoneuroimmunology: Stress, Mental Disorders, and Health*. Washington, DC: American Psychiatric Press; 2000:317–356.
6. Krauss BJ, Godfrey C, Yee D, et al. Saving our children from a silent epidemic: The PATH program for parents and preadolescents. In: Pequegnat W, Szapocznik J, eds. *Working with Families in the Era of HIV/AIDS*. Thousand Oaks, Calif: Sage Publications; 2000:89–112.
7. Paikoff RL. Early heterosexual debut: situations of sexual possibilities during the transition to adolescence. *Am J Orthopsychiatry*. 1995;65:389–401.
8. Dilorio C, Resnicow K, Denzmore P, et al. Keepin' it R.E.A.L.! A mother-adolescent HIV prevention program. In: Pequegnat W, Szapocznik J, eds. *Working with Families in the Era of HIV/AIDS*. Thousand Oaks, Calif: Sage Publications; 2000:113–132.
9. Jemmott LS, Outlaw N, Jemmott JB, et al. Strenthening the bond: The mother-son health promotion project. In: Pequegnat W, Szapocznik J, eds. *Working with Families in the Era of HIV/AIDS*. Thousand Oaks, Calif: Sage Publications; 2000:133–151.
10. Weine S, Agani F. R01 Proposal to the National Institute of Mental Health, 2005.
11. Rapkin B, Bennett JA, Murphy P, et al. The Family Health Project: Strengthening problem solving in families affected by AIDS to mobilize systems of support and care. In: Pequegnat W, Szapocznik J, eds. *Working with Families in the Era of HIV/AIDS*. Thousand Oaks, Calif: Sage Publications; 2000:213–242.
12. Mitrani VB, Prado G, Feaster DJ, et al. Relational factors and family treatment engagement among low-income, HIV-positive African American mothers. *Fam Process*. 2003;42:31–45.
13. Wingood GM, DiClemente RJ. The WiLLOW program: Mobilizing social networks of women living with HIV to enhance coping and reduce sexual risk behaviors. In: Pequegnat W, Szapocznik J, eds. *Working with Families in the Era of HIV/AIDS*. Thousand Oaks, Calif: Sage Publications; 2000:281–298.

14. Bauman LJ, Draimin B, Levine C, et al. Who will care for me? Planning the future care and custody of children orphaned by HIV/AIDS. In: Pequegnat W, Szapocznik J, eds. *Working with Families in the Era of HIV/AIDS*. Thousand Oaks, Calif: Sage Publications; 2000:155–188.
15. Rotheram-Borus MJ, Lightfoot M. Helping adolescents and parents with AIDS to cope effectively with daily life. In: Pequegnat W, Szapocznik J, eds. *Working with Families in the Era of HIV/AIDS*. Thousand Oaks, Calif: Sage Publications; 2000:189–211.
16. Bray JH, Fruge E. Assessment and evaluation of HIV/AIDS families: Applications to prevention and care. In: Pequegnat W, Szapocznik J, eds. *Working with Families in the Era of HIV/AIDS*. Thousand Oaks, Calif: Sage Publications; 2000:3–26.

SECTION VI

Special Issues

CHAPTER 33

Ethical, Forensic, and Legal Considerations

James Satriano

HIV AND PRISONS

As of mid-2004 there were 2.1 million people incarcerated in jails and prisons in the United States.[1] At the end of 2002, the latest year for available data, 3.0% of all female inmates and 1.9% of all male inmates were infected with human immunodeficiency virus (HIV).[2] The number of known HIV-positive inmates totaled just below 24,000 nationally. The national HIV infection rate in jails and prisons is six times higher than that among the general population.[3] About a quarter of all people living with HIV disease or acquired immunodeficiency syndrome (AIDS) in the United States have been incarcerated at one time.[4] The incidence of HIV infection in jails and prisons closely follows the pattern of injection drug use by region. A study of prison AIDS cases compared to total U.S. AIDS cases found that 61% of prison cases had injection drug use histories compared to only 27% of national cases.[5] As a result, New York State accounted for more than a fifth of all inmates (5,000) known to be HIV-positive. The most common HIV risk behaviors reported before incarceration for female inmates were crack cocaine use and the resulting sex exchange for drugs, intravenous drug use, and sex with intravenous drug users.[6] For male inmates, HIV risk behaviors before incarceration included intravenous drug use, high-risk sex associated with the use of alcohol and other noninjection drugs, and homosexual behavior.[7] Drug use and sexual activity continue following incarceration, but inmates have less chance to procure clean needles or barrier protective methods to prevent HIV transmission. Inmates reported using improvised devices, such as stolen surgical gloves to serve as condoms or purloined plastic wrap in place of dental dams.[8] Nonconsensual sex with inmates and coerced sex with corrections officers further contribute to the problem.

MENTAL ILLNESS IN PRISONS

The prevalence of psychiatric disorders among incarcerated persons is also greatly elevated. The most common psychiatric disorder among inmates is personality disorder, with the antisocial type being by far the most common. This is of little surprise, because criminal behavior is one of the diagnostic criteria of this disorder. However, highly elevated rates of serious mental illness have also been reported.[9] Serious mental illness is a term used to describe people with diagnoses of schizophrenia and other psychotic disorders, as well as bipolar disorder and major depression. Published reports put the rate of serious mental illness in city and county jails at between 6% and 15% and in state prisons at between 10% and 15%.[10]

It is not news that prisons have replaced mental hospitals as the repository of people with severe mental illness. A report on the National Institute of Corrections' website cites estimates that over 250,000 people with mental illness are currently incarcerated in the nation's jails and prisons and that an additional 500,000 are being supervised on probation. Contrast those statistics with the fact that in 1959 over 550,000 persons with mental illness resided in state mental hospitals, whereas today that number is less than 60,000. The situation has commanded so much attention that Human Rights Watch, an independent, nongovernmental not-for-profit agency, issued a 215-page report on the problem, and the *New York Times* has run front page stories on the issue.

Also well established are the elevated rates of HIV infection among people with mental illness. Rates of HIV infection among the mentally ill have been reported to range from 4% to almost 23%, depending on the subgroup of the population studied.[11] Little is known about the number of HIV-positive mentally ill individuals in correctional facilities in this country and the treatment that they receive. This chapter examines the reasons that so many people with mental illness are in jails and prisons, looks at the implications of having so many mentally ill persons incarcerated, considers the impact of HIV-positive mentally ill detainees, and discusses the integration of mental health and medical treatment within the prison system for the HIV-infected mentally ill.

THE SITUATION IN THE CORRECTIONAL SYSTEM

How did so many people with serious mental illness end up in correctional institutions? First and foremost, it began with the widespread deinstitutionalization of the mentally ill. The deinstitutionalization of people in state psychiatric facilities that began in the 1950s was a result of many converging factors.

Drastic change in psychiatric treatment occurred with the introduction of psychotropic medications in the mid-1950s. Before the introduction of these medicines, treatment consisted of talk therapy, various forms of "cures" and "shock" treatments and psychosurgery, mostly to little effect. The administration of these medications allowed many institutionalized mentally ill people to be discharged from state hospitals. The first of these drugs introduced to the market was chlorpromazine. Within the first year after its introduction in 1954, the drug was being administered to more than 2 million patients in the United States.[12] During the following decade, so many patients were administered chlorpromazine that it became known as the "drug that emptied the state metal hospitals."[13] The problem with discharging mentally ill patients on antipsychotic medication is that many are frequently discharged into unstable environments, are unlikely to continue treatment without support, and may discontinue treatment because the drugs have negative side effects.[14]

This period also saw tremendous changes in civil commitment law. Riding the wave of change that had begun in the civil rights movement in the 1960s, the first major change in civil commitment procedures established the criteria of dangerousness as necessary to involuntary confine an individual.[15] Thus, although based on a civil libertarian idea of preventing unnecessary detention, the ruling took the idea of commitment from a therapeutic concept to one that is protective of society. Those found to represent less than an imminent threat were to be treated in the least restrictive environment.

Also at this time, conditions for institutionalized individuals at their most abhorrent condition began to receive media attention. Perhaps the greatest example of the mistreatment of the mentally ill was the 1967 film *Titicut Follies* by Frederick Wiseman. This documentary exposed abject neglect and outright abuse by staff of the inmates at the Massachusetts Correctional Institution for the Criminally Insane at Bridgewater. What is so glaring about the film is the utter lack of concern by the staff for having their actions filmed. In a review of the film in the *New Republic*, the psychiatrist Robert Coles[16] stated "After a showing of *Titicut Follies* the mind does not dwell on the hospital's ancient and even laughable physical plant, or its pitiable social atmosphere. What sticks, what really hurts is the sight of human life made cheap and betrayed." The uproar following such exposés further fueled support for the deinstitutionalization of the mentally ill. Also occurring at this time was the antipsychiatry movement, most closely associated with Thomas Szasz and R. D. Laing. These psychiatrists believed mental illness to be a myth and viewed psychosis to be a reactive response to a bad situation. Many of their criticisms sprang from inhumane treatment of the mentally ill and damaging effects of long-term institutionalization, which lent more fuel to the fire to begin to empty the asylums. Also, reported abuses of psychiatry in the Soviet Union and the misuse of psychotropic drugs by the U.S. Central Intelligence Agency helped to bolster this movement.

As a result of deinstitutionalization, people with severe mental illness make up a disproportionate number of the homeless. A recent study found that a full 15% of patients who were treated for serious mental illness in a large urban public mental health system were homeless.[17] Although there are few data on the incidence of HIV infection among the homeless mentally ill, a study of psychiatric patients in a New York City shelter for men reported a 19.4% rate of infection.[18] An HIV infection rate of 10.6% was reported for patients aged 18 to 39 years admitted for inpatient psychiatric care who were homeless before admission.[19] Given the disproportionate number of people with mental illness who are infected with HIV and the high number of the mentally ill in our jails and prisons, we can expect that many of those incarcerated are infected with HIV.

Substance abuse is also rife among these patients. Among 20,000 people interviewed in the National Institute of Mental Health Epidemiological Catchment Area Program for those with a mental disorder, the lifetime prevalence of having some addictive disorder was about 29%.[20] Homeless adults with serious mental illness are reported to have even higher rates of co-occurring substance abuse. A federal demonstration project conducted by the Center for Mental Health Services[21] examined the mentally ill at five different homeless shelters and found that levels of co-occurring substance abuse to be 58%.

In spite of the massive discharge of patients from public psychiatric facilities, the promised rise in community mental health care failed to materialize. This significant dumping of psychiatric patients, with inadequate treatment available in community settings, inevitably led to contact for these patients with the criminal justice system. Community law enforcement officials, under pressure to get these people off of the streets, began to enforce "quality of life" crimes against the mentally ill. The mentally ill began to be arrested for reasons such as disorderly conduct. The vast majority of the mentally ill incarcerated in jails and prisons are arrested for nonviolent crimes. This trend led to the coining of the term *criminalization of the mentally ill*. Police began speaking in terms of mercy arrests, simply to get the homeless mentally ill off of the streets and into shelter.[22] As a result, the Los Angeles County Jail and Rikers Island Jail in New York are the two largest psychiatric inpatient treatment facilities in the country.[23] These factors have resulted in the prisons becoming our new asylums.

Do these mentally ill inmates get mental health treatment during incarceration? A report issued by the U.S. Department of Justice stated that only 6 of 10 mentally ill detainees receives mental health treatment while incarcerated and just over half of mentally ill probationers reported receiving treatment.[24]

TREATING PSYCHIATRIC ILLNESS IN JAILS AND PRISONS IN THE CONTEXT OF HIV/AIDS

What is the association of HIV infection and psychiatric illness in the correctional setting? To date, little work has been done to investigate this association. One comprehensive cross-sectional study of all inmates in Texas jails and prisons over a 3-year period reveals a significantly higher rate of psychiatric illness among HIV-positive inmates for all diagnoses examined.[25] The study found that HIV-infected inmates were significantly more likely to have been diagnosed with major depression, dysthymia, bipolar disorder, schizophrenia, schizoaffective disorder, and nonschizophrenic psychotic disorders.

This is not surprising, because a number of studies have reported elevated rates of HIV risk behavior among people with even severe mental illness such as schizophrenia and bipolar disorder. These risk behaviors include having sex with multiple partners, having sex under the influence of substances, elevated rates of male homosexual activity, having reported to have engaged in sex with a prostitute, engaging in the exchange of sex for some commodity, low levels of reported condom use, having sex with strangers, increased reports of engaging in anal intercourse, and elevated rates of injection drug use.[26] These elevated risk behaviors have been ascribed to a number of characteristics found among people with severe mental illness, including poor impulse control, high rates of substance abuse, difficulty maintaining stable sexual relationships, and the high rate of sexual victimization.[27,28]

SUMMARY

Given that such high rates of co-occurring mental illness and HIV infection exist in the prison population, all individuals entering a correctional facility with a history of mental illness should be carefully screened for a history of HIV risk behavior. Those found to have positive risk histories should be encouraged to undertake voluntary HIV testing. Those testing positive should have an integrated health and mental health care program designed that would optimize adherence to both antiretroviral and psychopharmacologic treatments, with special concern about drug interactions. Clearly, these patients will require special planning when released from custody, and intensive case management should be set up before leaving the correctional setting.

But those recommendations do not consider the issue of how to keep these patients out of correctional settings to begin with. Clearly, those who are mentally ill and commit violent crimes have been to a large extent abandoned by the public mental health system and have become the responsibility of the criminal justice system. These "lost souls" will get the mental health treatment that they need only when behind bars. That treatment should be delivered in the most humane way possible. For example, treating agitated patients with serious mental illness by placing them in solitary confinement is probably counterproductive to their well-being. Similar methods of isolation used in a psychiatric setting, separating those who represent a danger, should be adopted in the correctional setting. Those placed in isolation should be closely monitored and released as soon as they can be stabilized.

But how can we keep these individuals from becoming inmates in the first place? The first thing that we can do is to make police officers more aware of the symptoms of mental illness in the hope of avoiding inappropriate arrest. The establishment of a mental health team and specialized training of officers are needed to prevent the criminalization of the mentally ill. For those who do enter the criminal justice system and have not committed violent crimes, prison diversion programs should be established. One such program in the Bronx was established though the district attorney's office and requires that the patient plead guilty to the crime and agree to enter and continue in mandated mental health treatment or be remanded to jail. The project includes mental health professionals and is associated with several established mental health care settings in the community. Given the high rates of HIV in this population, HIV risk intervention and HIV testing are being integrated into the program.

An attempt has been made to deal with potential crises for people with serious mental illness through assisted outpatient treatment or outpatient commitment. As of March 2005, 42 states had adopted assisted outpatient treatment statutes. These statutes allow a judge to order that a person with a history of mental illness comply with outpatient treatment or face involuntary confinement. The patient must have a history of noncompliance with treatment and be judged to be unlikely to follow recommended treatment plans. A few studies of the effectiveness of assisted outpatient treatment to reduce arrests reported a 74% to 83% drop in contact with the criminal justice system.[29,30] This form of treatment remains controversial, and detractors decry the abridgement of civil liberties and the right to refuse treatment. For programs of this type to be truly effective a greatly enhanced system of community mental health care is required. Perhaps as an increasing number of patients are mandated to receive outpatient treatment, the courts will rule that the community must comply and provide funding for the services that the courts have deemed necessary. These programs require patients who most likely had been lost to the mental health system to be in contact with that system. They provide an opportunity to assess risk for HIV, refer those with a positive risk history for voluntary HIV testing, and connect those who test HIV-positive with the health care that they need.

REFERENCES

1. Harrison PM, Beck AJ. Prison and jail inmates at midyear 2004. *Bur Just Stat Bull*. April 2005.
2. Maruschak LM. HIV in prisons and jails. *Bur Just Stat Bull*. December 2004.
3. Braithwaite RL, Hammott TM, Mayberry RM. *Prisons and AIDS: A Public Health Challenge*. San Francisco: Jossey-Bass; 1996.
4. Hammett TM, Harmon P, Rhodes W. The burden of infectious diseases among inmates and releasees from correctional facilities, in the health status of soon-to-be-released inmates. Report to Congress. National Commission on Correctional Health Care. Chicago; March 2002.
5. Dean-Gaitor HD, Fleming PL. Epidemiology of AIDS in incarcerated persons in the United States. *AIDS*. 1999;3;13:2429–2435.
6. Bond L, Semaan S. At risk for HIV infection: incarcerated women in a county jail in Philadelphia. *Womens Health*. 1996;24:27–45.
7. Grinstead O, Zack B, Faigeles B. Reducing postrelease risk behavior among HIV seropositive prison inmates: the health promotion program. *AIDS Educ Prev*. 2001;13:109–119.
8. Mahon N. New York inmates' HIV risk behaviors: the implication for prevention policy and programs. *Am J Public Health*. 1996;86:1211–1215.
9. Singleton N, Meltzer H, Gatward R. *Psychiatric Morbidity Among Prisoners in England and Wales*. London: Stationary Office; 1998.
10. Lamb HR, Weinberger LE. Persons with mental illness in jails and prisons: a review. *Psychiatr Serv*. 1998;49:483–492.
11. Cournos F, Bakalar N. *AIDS and People with Severe Mental Illness: A Handbook for Mental Health Professionals*. New Haven, Conn: Yale University Press; 1996.
12. Isaac RJ, Armat VC. *Madness in the Streets: How Psychiatry and the Law Abandoned the Mentally Ill*. New York: Free Press; 1990.
13. Kramer PD. *Listening to Prozac*. New York: Penguin; 1993.
14. Engstrom F. Psychotropic drugs: modern medicine's alternative to purgatives, straightjackets and asylums. *Postgrad Med*. 1997;101:198–207.
15. Lessard v. Schmidt. 379 F Supp 1078 (ED Wis 1872).
16. Coles R. "Titicut Follies" (film review). *New Republic*. 1968;Jan. 20.
17. Folsome DP, Hawthorne W, Lindamer L, et al. Prevalence and risk factors for homelessness and utilization of mental health services among 10,340 patients with serious mental illness in a large public mental health system. *Am J Psychiatry*. 2005;162:370–376.
18. Susser E, Valencia E, Conover S. Prevalence of HIV infection among psychiatric patients in a New York City men's shelter. *Am J Public Health*. 1993;83:568–570.
19. Empfield M, Cournos F, Meyer I, et al. HIV seroprevalence among street homeless patients admitted to a psychiatric inpatient unit. *Am J Psychiatry*. 1993;150:47–52.
20. Regier DA, Farmer DS, Rae BZ, et al. Comorbidity of mental disorders with alcohol and other drug abuse: results from the Epidemiological Catchment Area (ECA) Study. *J Am Med Assoc*. 1990;264:2511–2518.
21. Center for Mental Health Services. Making a difference: interim status report of the McKinny research demonstration program for homeless mentally ill adults. Washington, DC: Center for Mental Health Services; 1994.

22. Butterfield F. Asylums behind bars: prisons replace hospitals for the nations mentally ill. *New York Times*. March 5, 1998.
23. Sharfstein S. The impact of the mentally ill offender on the criminal justice system. Testimony for the U.S. House Subcommittee on Crime, House Judiciary Committee, September 21, 2000. Available: http://www.psych.org/advocacy_policy/leg_res/apa_testimony/testimonysubcrimeposted91800.cfm. Accessed July 14, 2005.
24. Ditton PM. *Mental Health and Treatment of Inmates and Probationers: Bureau of Justice Statistics Special Report*. Washington, DC: US Department of Justice; 1999.
25. Baillargeon J, Ducate S, Pulvino J, et al. The association of psychiatric disorders and HIV infection in the correctional setting. *Ann Epidemiol*. 2003;13;9:606–612.
26. McKinnon K. Sexual and drug use risk behavior. In: Cournos F, Bakalar N, eds. *AIDS and People with Severe Mental Illness*. New Haven, Conn: Yale University Press; 1996.
27. Steiner J, Lussier R, Rosenblatt W. Knowledge about and risk factors for AIDS in a hospital population. *Hosp Community Psychiatry*. 1992;43:734–735.
28. Aruffo J, Coverdale J, Chacko R, et al. Knowledge about AIDS among women psychiatric outpatients. *Hosp Community Psychiatry*. 1990;41:326–328.
29. New York State Office of Mental Health. *Kendra's Law: Final Report on the Status of Assisted Outpatient Treatment*. New York: Office of Mental Health; 2005.
30. Swanson JW, Borum R, Swartz MS, et al. Can involuntary outpatient commitment reduce arrests among persons with severe mental illness? *Crim Just Behav*. 2001;28:156.

CHAPTER 34

Religious and Spiritual Considerations

Daniel W. Hicks, Francis G. Lu

The course of human immunodeficiency virus (HIV) disease has changed dramatically due to scientific research that has led to the discovery of remarkable new treatments and medications. Now, instead of being considered an automatic death sentence, HIV disease is considered a chronic and manageable illness for most people. Corresponding to this tremendous growth in data-based biomedical research, there has also been increasing interest and research into holistic treatment of the patient: body, mind, and spirit. The National Center for Complementary and Alternative Medicine was established in 1998 at the National Institute of Health, to focus on and study nontraditional treatment approaches, including "mind-body" methods. Research on religion and spirituality in medical illness has shown that faith plays a significant role in wellness and healing for most patients.[1] Despite the supposed secular nature of the country and the separation of church and state, U.S. citizens are known to be very religious, with the majority reporting belief in God and regular attendance at religious services.[2] Persons who endorse that spirituality is an important part of their lives have been shown to have decreased anxiety and depression, better health, and greater longevity.[1] Religious beliefs have been shown to help people find meaning in suffering from their illness and help them move toward acceptance. It also provides a buffer against depression, hopelessness, and desire for hastened death.[3]

Treating persons with HIV infection and acquired immunodeficiency syndrome (AIDS) brings up issues related to sexuality, serious illness, and death, and these subjects intersect with religion and spirituality. Religion dictates our sexual mores, and religious or spiritual beliefs are essential in coping with and understanding serious illness and death.[4] Being diagnosed with HIV disease exposes a person to multiple stressors: living with a potentially life-threatening disease, accommodating a complicated medical regimen with multiple side effects, and uncertainty about the future. In addition, there are also many psychosocial stresses, including the stigma of AIDS, possible social rejection or isolation, discrimination in work, housing or medical care, the threat of transmission of the disease, and preexisting issues such as wrestling with sexuality and substance abuse. This emotional turmoil can lead to what is termed "spiritual distress," a disturbance in a person's belief system.

This spiritual crisis can lead to questioning of the meaning of life, death, and suffering; doubts about one's beliefs; a sense of detachment from others; a feeling of spiritual emptiness;

and feeling that life is not worth living.[5] Irving Yalom[6] has written about the four existential issues that we all face: death, meaninglessness, isolation, and freedom. An existential crisis may lead a person to search for spiritual answers, which can be a source of strength and provide a sense of meaning for their struggle. As Victor Frankl[7] discovered in the concentration camps, one can endure incredible suffering if a sense of meaning and purpose can be found. The AIDS epidemic has caused many people to face their own mortality at an early age rather than late in life, and many have embraced spirituality.[8]

The North American Nursing Diagnosis Association (NANDA International) defines spiritual distress as a disruption in the life principle that, when intact, suffuses a person's entire self, integrating and transcending one's biologic and psychosocial aspects.[9] The *Diagnostic and Statistical Manual of Mental Disorders (DSM-IV-TR)*, in the section entitled "Other Conditions That May Be a Focus of Clinical Attention," has a similar diagnostic category of "Religious or Spiritual Problem." "This category can be used when the focus of clinical attention is a religious or spiritual problem. Examples include distressing experiences that involve loss or questioning of faith, problems associated with conversion to a new faith, or questioning of spiritual values that may not necessarily be related to an organized church or religious institution."[10] In this chapter, several examples of spiritual distress or "Religious or Spiritual Problem" are discussed. Awareness of these diagnoses is critical to addressing this aspect of the patient's distress in the treatment plan and depends on the clinician's comfort with discussing religion and spirituality with their patients.

RELIGION VERSUS SPIRITUALITY: DISTINCTIONS

Religion and spirituality are often thought to be synonymous, especially by health care providers, yet the distinction is most important in working with patients with HIV and AIDS who may have been traumatized by their church. A clinician usually asks patients about their faith only as a means to establish their religion so that the appropriate clergy can be contacted. Most psychotherapists are trained to use rational, evidence-based therapy methods, and are inexperienced and uncomfortable in asking questions about faith or religious beliefs. But in working with persons with HIV and other serious illnesses, helping patients explore their spirituality is one of the most important tools the therapist can offer.

Religion and spirituality have been described as two sides of the same experience—spirituality as the inward, individual experience of the transcendent and religion as the external, collective manifestation of the experience.[2] Spirit means breath, life, and soul, "the animating or vital principle" in a person. In the modern Western world, the body is thought to contain the spirit, but more ancient wisdom sees the spirit as the highest evolution of consciousness and containing the body.[11] Spirituality is thought of as a basic human need,[4] which Jung called a natural search for something beyond ourselves.[2] Frankl[7] believed that spirituality was vital to psychological health and well-being. Spirituality has been defined to include transcendence, the experience of moving beyond the self and the material world; connection to a greater power or force (the Divine); uniting with all other beings; and finding meaning in life and hope for the future.[4] Spirituality can be expressed through meditation, prayers, visualization, and relationship to others; it is expressed in love, community, and connection to others and to God. Religious rituals and worship can also be a means to connect to the divine, either through organized religion or individual practices.[10]

Before the advent of modern medicine and modern psychology, people often turned to spiritual leaders (such as shamans, medicine women, and clergy) to help with serious life and death matters. In many cultures, spirituality is thought to be an intrinsic energy or life force, such as *ch'i* in China, *prana* in Eastern India, and *ki* in Japan. Hindus speak of the Self in everyone and in all. Buddhism describes *nirvana* as "the peace supreme that is in me." This life force flows though us and connects us to all of nature. Jesus spoke of the human spirit as "the Kingdom of Heaven is within you." Plato stated that "If the head and body are to be well, you must first begin by curing the soul."[11]

Early Christianity and some modern practitioners believe that healing can occur through laying on of hands, or the "healing touch." The Japanese martial art of *aikido* is based on harnessing *ki* energy by using breath power, which unites one to the indestructible power of the universe.[12] The spirit is a part of the person, like the mind or the pancreas.

Organized religion is a manmade, formalized way to connect the individual to the holy. Religion consists of a creed, or set of beliefs; a cult, or set of established rituals and practices; and community, involving authority, law, and membership. It is recognition of a higher power that controls man's destiny and must be obeyed, revered, and worshiped.[11] Because it is a human institution, it can be subject to distortion, appropriating the holy to justify one's prejudices, as has been done to justify slavery and war. Sanctity often mixes with self-interest in most organized religions. Religion and religious practices can unite persons with the holy, but unfortunately it can also alienate them from those they love.[13]

It is essential to distinguish between spirituality and religion when working with persons with HIV and AIDS. Most organized religions do not recognize and honor sexual minorities, including gay, lesbian, bisexual, and transgender people. Some fundamentalist denominations actively fight against rights for homosexuals and their families and preach that AIDS is God's retribution for sin. Drug abusers, sex workers, and other high-risk groups have been judged and rejected by most organized religions. Churches also continue to dishonor nonmarital relationships by calling for abstinence or teaching against basic life-saving safe-sex practices such as using condoms. Therefore many persons with AIDS have been and continue to be deeply wounded by religion and are either very angry at the church or find it irrelevant to their lives.[14] Just as many people with addictions have benefited tremendously from Alcoholics Anonymous and other 12-step programs, others cannot benefit from the program until they can separate their own past painful experiences with organized religion from the important spiritual guidance found in these programs. Persons with HIV and persons with addictions must separate the damage done to them by manmade religions from their own innate spirituality in order to move toward healing.

Not all churches and organized religions are equally to blame for causing this emotional damage. Some individual churches, some denominations, and some clergy have been on the forefront of the fight against AIDS. In Indianapolis, a retired Canon from the Episcopal Church negotiated with the Catholic Archdiocese and arranged for them to donate and renovate one of their buildings. This became the Damien Center, the first organized response to AIDS in Indiana, which housed support groups, buddy programs, and educational and social services that served the entire state. (No condoms could ever be distributed from the building, however). In city after city, the Catholic church and other denominations organized to offer direct help to AIDS patients and their families, through ministry, counseling, housing, food, and medications.[15] Volunteers, often faith based, demonstrating a true inward spirituality, did much of the supportive work in HIV and AIDS through establishing support groups and buddy programs. Meanwhile, most of the major religions are still struggling with recognizing and supporting gay and lesbian people and their families. This is evidenced in the battle within the Anglican Church over the ordination of a gay man as bishop and the Pope calling for members of the Catholic Church to fight against gay marriage.

African-American churches have been leaders in their communities for years, playing a major role not only in ministry, but also socialization, education, and political mobilization.[16] However, many black churches have been silent about AIDS and still preach against homosexuality, bisexuality, and drugs, while AIDS is rapidly spreading in the black community, which has the highest rate of new infections. Fortunately, many other black churches have

RESEARCH ON RELIGION AND SPIRITUALITY AND HEALTH/MENTAL HEALTH

Several studies have demonstrated the importance of religion and spirituality for persons with life-threatening illness, including AIDS. As some studies point out, a critical distinction was made between intrinsic and extrinsic religiosity.[17] Extrinsic religiosity corresponds to outward behaviors of attending church and practicing the rituals of organized religion, whereas intrinsic religiosity deals more with the incorporation of these beliefs into daily life and spiritual practices. Most of these studies found an inverse relationship between intrinsic religiosity and depression; in other words, spirituality protected against depression. Extrinsic religiosity was found to have no correlation with depression. In a study by Nelson et al.,[17] terminally ill patients with cancer and AIDS were assessed using the Functional Assessment of Cancer Therapy (FACIT) Spiritual Well-Being Scale and the Hamilton Depression Rating Scale (HDRS). They also found that those who scored higher on the spirituality scale, especially the meaning and peace subscale (having an internal sense of inner peace and meaning in your life), had lower rates of depression. Those who scored high on extrinsic religiosity showed no effect or even a higher incidence of depression. Their interpretation was that the ability to find meaning in suffering through spirituality was helpful to people with terminal illnesses, but the external rituals and practices of religion did not in themselves bring meaning or comfort and so could increase distress.

Targ[1] reviewed the literature on using prayer, or "distant healing," and showed significant findings in many of the studies, including one that showed prayers reduced morbidity in coronary care patients. A placebo-controlled study of 40 AIDS patients who were anonymously prayed for by healers for 6 months showed improved health as reflected by fewer AIDS-defined illnesses, hospitalizations, and doctors' visits.[18] The healers were from a variety of backgrounds, including Christian, Jewish, Buddhist, and Native American and had a great deal of experience using distant healing. They were randomly matched to patients, given only a packet of information about the patient, and asked to pray for 1 hour daily, 6 days per week. The patients were rotated weekly between healers to control for differing effectiveness among healers. These results showed an impressive effect of prayer and have led to studies to replicate and expand these findings.

Kendall[19] interviewed 29 gay men with varying stages of HIV disease to look at factors that helped them cope well with their illness and from this devised a concept called "wellness spirituality." The group defined illness as a lack of inner peace, with emotional and spiritual pain, fear, and isolation. This could lead to a focus on illness and symptoms and a sense of hopelessness and fatalism. Wellness involved physical survival, holistic understanding of mind-body connections, and transcendence over the physical. The author pointed out that most of the subjects began talking about wellness in more spiritual terms. Even the patients who were in later stages of AIDS tended to focus less on their physical symptoms and more on a transcendent view of wellness. From this came the concept of wellness spirituality, which involved an appreciation and understanding of life, fulfillment of a purpose, and meaningful connections with others. This sense of well-being came from emotional intimacy with others, finding purpose and meaning in life, and an inner sense of peace and self-acceptance.

Below is the summary of a case which illustrates how re-discovering spirituality helped lead to self-acceptance, recovery, and improved well-being.

> Michael was a 35-year-old HIV-positive attorney. He grew up in a small midwestern town and was active in his church. He did well in school and went away to college,

where he discovered he was gay. He went to law school in a large city and enjoyed the freedom of exploring his sexuality. He was no longer active in his faith because they rejected homosexuality. Michael worked hard after school and was very successful, but he started going to circuit parties and using crystal methamphetamine to enhance his pleasure. This led to multiple unsafe sexual encounters, until he was finally diagnosed as HIV-positive. He became bitter and angry, and his drug use crept into his daily life. Friends and colleagues staged an intervention, and Michael went into a gay-affirmative treatment program. He was treated for depression and in recovery rediscovered his spirituality. He found a gay-affirming church and became very active, started a new relationship, and became a leader at his work and in his community. He credited his success to his new-found faith.

In interviews of 15 terminally ill cancer and AIDS patients, Fryback and Reinert[20] explored the role of spirituality. One of the critical factors was a belief in a higher power, in something greater than oneself. Some of them found strength and peace in their church. Some of the people were angry at organized religion because of bad experiences or felt rejected by their church because of their lifestyle choices. Some were angry with God because of their illness and how it was affecting their loved ones. This anger did not stop the patients from looking for spiritual answers, including the sense of transcendence beyond the physical body. Facing death often leads to a deepening spirituality and movement toward accepting death as an inevitable part of life. This acceptance was much more difficult for younger people to accept, because it forced them to give up the illusion of immortality. This change in focus led to a greater appreciation of life, to enjoying each day fully, including precious time with family and loved ones, joy in the beauty of nature, and living in the moment instead of delaying gratification. Finding self-love and meaning in life and their illness were part of the spiritual journey. Byock[21] highlighted the importance for people at the end of life to be able to communicate to their loved ones these important messages: "1. I love you; 2. Please forgive me; 3. I forgive you; 4. Good-bye."

Hall[15] also interviewed 10 persons with advanced AIDS who identified that spirituality had helped them deal with their disease. She found that many referred to God or a higher power, but related this more to personal faith than to a church. She found the following three major themes in her subjects:

1. Purpose in life emerged from the stigmatization of their disease, as well as from prior rejections by family, church, and others due to their sexuality, their drug use, or their lifestyle choices. All but one had left their original childhood religion, but found a different, more personally authentic spirituality. Many were able to reconnect to family and faith in new and stronger ways.
2. Opportunities for meaning arise from an incurable disease. Some substance abusers went into treatment and got clean for the first time. Others left jobs or relationships that were not fulfilling to find more satisfying ones. They used the opportunity to learn about their illness and take control of their lives, to appreciate the time they had left, and to value their relationships.
3. After suffering, spirituality helped frame their lives. They learned to accept themselves, clarify their beliefs about life and death, and find new purpose and meaning. They reached out to others and were open to giving and receiving love.

Studies have shown that HIV-positive substance abusers want spirituality incorporated into their addiction treatment, to help them with their addiction. In addition, they felt it would also help them cope with their HIV disease, be more compliant with their medication, and control the risk behavior that could cause transmission of the virus.[22,23]

The following case summary helps illustrate the importance of spirituality and religion in recovery, as well as improved health and functioning.

> Paulette is a 38-year-old single African American with two young children. She grew up in a single-parent home, and the church was a large part of her life. Unfortunately, a family friend sexually abused her. She became rebellious as a teenager and experimented with drugs and alcohol, which led to addiction. She had two children, but they were taken away from her because of her drug use; and she had multiple arrests for drug-related charges and eventually ended up in prison. There she found out that she was HIV-positive and became despondent. A church ministry reached out to her, and she reestablished her connection to her faith. She started going to a 12-step program and became one of the leaders. The prison ministry helped her transition out of prison, where she became active in her church, found a stable job, and was able to obtain custody of her children. She maintains HIV saved her life, allowing her to recover from her addiction and return to her faith.

COMMUNICATION ABOUT SPIRITUALITY

These studies make it clear that spirituality can be enormously helpful for persons with HIV and AIDS, and it is important that caregivers learn how they can help their patients on this journey. Health care providers tend to be uncomfortable discussing religious and spiritual issues. There is often lack of time, and certainly there is lack of experience and training in this area. There is also concern about invasion of privacy and fear that discussing religion will be seen as proselytizing.

The important point to remember is that every person has a right to his or her own unique belief system, and it may not be based on any particular religion. Caregivers should not discuss their own belief systems, because it usually is not relevant. The goal of these discussions is to foster hope and help patients integrate meaning through their spiritual beliefs.[3] One effective tool to help frame or lead this discussion is the FICA Brief Spiritual Screening Instrument, illustrated in Table 34.1.[24]

THERAPEUTIC INTERVENTIONS

One approach to care is termed integrative, combining existential and religious approaches to spirituality.[10] The religious aspect is defined as the belief that a divine influence operates inside a person and guides behavior, using prayer, worship, readings, and other rituals. The existential perspective focuses on individual concerns, knowledge of self, interaction with others, and sense of purpose, utilizing meditation, visualization, guided imagery, and information gathering. The goal of both approaches is to achieve self-transcendence, hope, and meaning in life. Providers can promote hope by the following four steps:

1. They can encourage obtaining support from family, friends, support groups, and a faith community with tolerance and outreach to HIV-positive patients. Working collaboratively with sympathetic pastoral counselors, ministers, and chaplains may be essential, either when patients request this or when clinicians feel they have reached their limit in knowledge and skills.

TABLE 34.1	FICA Brief Spiritual Screening Instrument
F	Is religious **f**aith an important part of your daily life? This could be followed with important questions about formal religious identity and involvement.
I	How do your beliefs **i**nfluence your daily life, and have you had important spiritual experiences in the past?
C	Are you a member of a religious **c**ommunity, and can they be helpful to you now?
A	How do you want me to **a**ddress your spiritual needs, and can this be part of your treatment plan?

2. In addition, health care providers can help the patient focus on enjoying each day by finding meaningful activity through work or hobbies.
3. They can provide education about HIV, its transmission, its treatment, medications, and the importance of regular medical follow-up. In addition, patients can be educated about the importance of exercise, proper nutrition, adequate rest, and avoiding substance abuse.
4. Patients can be empowered to help others with HIV; to use meditation, visualization, and prayer; to become involved in research through drug trials; and to put their legal affairs in order, such as setting up a will and living will. As Kushner[25] stated, finding spiritual meaning in illness comes from moving beyond "Why me?" to "What can I do about it?"

Spiritual needs of terminally ill patients include finding meaning in life and death, giving and receiving love, and finding a sense of forgiveness and hope.[11] The caregiver, by listening and forming a nurturing relationship, can provide compassion and caring. By exploring patients' spiritual beliefs and history, one can encourage patients to practice new rituals that may be helpful or use ones that may have been helpful in the past. Exploring their thoughts about God, life, and death can help patients reconnect to their spirituality. If patients have unresolved conflicts with their religious faith, they may be willing to discuss their spirituality with local spiritual leaders or clergy who are more open and accepting. Facilitating connection with loved ones, encouraging prayer or meditation, helping them do a "life review" to find meaning in their life, all can help create a sense of hope.

Persons with HIV and AIDS have multiple stressors that require special attention and care from health care providers. Basic skills such as taking time to be with patients, listening empathically, and forming a trusting relationship are important tools. Understanding their history and background may help them uncover strengths and skills that helped them overcome adversity in the past and reframe their illness. Nonjudgmental acceptance and positive affirmation can help overcome uncertainty and self-doubts. Spirituality is also a basic need of all humans and is not separable from the biologic, social, or psychological state of health. Physicians, nurses, and therapists must become comfortable and proficient in helping patients explore their spirituality. Being open to questions and conversations about their beliefs can encourage them to seek out answers. The goal of care should be not cure of the disease but spiritual wellness for the person with the disease—through finding meaning in life, transcendence, and hope.

REFERENCES

1. Targ E. Healing HIV: mind, body and spirit. *Focus*. 2002;17:1–4.
2. Hopcke RH. The place of religion and spirituality in HIV counseling. *Focus*. 2004;19:1–4.
3. Breitbart W, Gibson C, Chochinov HM. Palliative care. In: Levenson JL, ed. *Textbook of Psychosomatic Medicine*. Arlington, Va: American Psychiatric Publishing; 2004.
4. Pargament K. *The Psychology of Religion and Coping*. New York: Guilford Press; 1997.
5. Relf M. Illuminating meaning and transforming issues of spirituality in HIV disease and AIDS. *Holist Nurs Pract*. 1997;12:1–8.
6. Yalom I. *Existential Psychotherapy*. New York: Basic Books; 1980.
7. Frankl V. *Man's Search for Meaning*. Boston: Beacon Press; 1963.
8. Matousek M. Savage grace. *Comm Bound*. 1993;11:22–31.
9. Sparks SM. *Nursing Diagnosis Reference Manual*. Springhouse, Pa: Springhouse; 1998.
10. Turner RP, Lukoff D, Barnhouse RT, et al. Religious or spiritual problem: a culturally sensitive diagnostic category in the DSM-IV. *J Nerv Ment Dis*. 1995;183:435–444.
11. Kearney M, Mount B. Spiritual care of the dying patient. In: Chochinov, Breitbart, eds. *Handbook of Psychiatry in Palliative Medicine*. New York: Oxford Press; 2000.
12. McCormick DP, Holder B, Wetsel MA, et al. Spirituality and HIV disease: an integrated perspective. *J Assoc Nurs AIDS Care*. 2001;12:58–65.
13. Peri TAC. Promoting spirituality in persons with AIDS. *Holist Nurs Pract*. 1995;10:68–76.
14. Dunphy R. Helping persons with AIDS find meaning and hope. *Health Progr*. 1987:68:58–63.
15. Hall B. Patterns of spirituality in persons with advanced HIV disease. *Res Nurs Health*. 1998;21:143–153.
16. Coleman CL, Holzemer WL. Spirituality, psychological well-being, and HIV symptoms for African Americans living with HIV disease. *J Assoc Nurs AIDS Care*. 1999;10:42–50.

17. Nelson CJ, Rosenfeld B, Breitbart W, et al. Spirituality, religion, and depression in the terminally ill. *Psychosomatics*. 2002;43:213–220.
18. Sicher F, Targ E, Moore D, et al. A randomized double-blind study of the effect of distant healing in a population with advanced AIDS. *West J Med*. 1998;169:356–363.
19. Kendall J. Wellness spirituality in homosexual men with HIV infection. *J Assoc Nurs AIDS Care*. 1994;5:28–34.
20. Fryback PB, Reinert BR. Spirituality and people with potentially fatal diagnoses. *Nurs Forum*. 1999;34:13–22.
21. Byock I. *Dying Well*. New York: Riverhead Books; 1997.
22. Arnold RM, Avants SK, Margolin A, et al. Patient attitudes concerning the inclusion of spirituality into addiction treatment. *J Substance Abuse Treat*. 2002;23:319–326.
23. Avants SK, Marcotte D, Arnold R, Margolin A. Spiritual beliefs, world assumptions and HIV risk behavior among heroin and cocaine users. *Psychol Addict Behav*. 2003;17:159–162.
24. Puchalski CM. *Spirituality in Principles and Practices of Palliative Care and Supportive Oncology*. 2nd ed. Philadelphia: Lippincott; 2002.
25. Kushner HS. *When Bad Things Happen to Good People*. New York: Avon; 1981.

CHAPTER **35**

Psychotherapeutic Strategies

Claire Zilber

Human immunodeficiency virus (HIV) affects all spheres of a person's life, forcing physical, psychological, social, and spiritual adaptation. Mental health challenges to individuals with HIV infection include grief, stigmatization, the need to adapt to a chronic and life-threatening illness, neuropsychiatric disorders, and fundamental changes in identity. Preexisting psychiatric and substance abuse disorders are often present, as are social marginalization and poverty. A person's adjustment to HIV disease is affected by his or her coping style, the quality of social support, and the presence of other life stressors. Psychotherapy promotes adaptation to the neuropsychiatric and psychosocial challenges associated with HIV infection and acquired immunodeficiency syndrome (AIDS).

This chapter describes the challenges associated with HIV infection and AIDS that are most amenable to psychotherapy. Specific individual and group therapy techniques with demonstrated efficacy in the treatment of those infected with HIV are presented. Psychotherapeutic principles of transference, countertransference, and boundaries are reviewed, because they require special consideration in working with HIV-infected patients. Prevention of burnout is also addressed.

CHALLENGES AMENABLE TO PSYCHOTHERAPY

RESPONSE TO INITIAL INFECTION

Mr. A., a 26-year-old gay White man, requested HIV testing after learning that a former partner was ill with AIDS. For the first 6 months after receiving the positive test result, Mr. A. went about his life as if nothing had changed. Eventually, with persistent encouragement by a friend, he made an appointment with an infectious disease specialist. The week before his first appointment he experienced the first in a series of panic attacks.

Denial and avoidance are common responses to learning one's HIV status. Persistent denial may have major implications, such as ongoing high-risk behaviors that involve exposure to HIV, hepatitis, and other sexually transmitted infections (STIs) and the delay of medical care. Denial may be a defensive alternative to emotional flooding. Despite widespread public knowledge of treatment advances, it is not uncommon for newly diagnosed individuals to fear that death is imminent. As denial erodes, new symptoms of anxiety or depression may emerge.

Other common responses to one's initial awareness of HIV serostatus are anger, outrage, and feelings of betrayal. Transient suicidal or homicidal feelings may develop. Effective pretest and post-test counseling helps patients anticipate and cope with their initial responses to HIV infection. Pretest counseling may identify individuals who would benefit from psychotherapy to shore up psychosocial functioning before HIV testing. Similarly, post-test counseling provides an opportunity for referral to a mental health provider.

PREEXISTING PSYCHIATRIC DISORDERS

There is a high rate of HIV infection among people with chronic mental illness. The risk of exposure to HIV is increased by the impulse control difficulties and hypersexuality present with mania, the poor reality testing associated with psychosis, the low self-esteem and poor self-care common to depression, and the impaired judgment that accompanies substance abuse disorders. Some patients may already be in mental health care when they become seropositive. Entry into the health care system for HIV disease care may encourage other patients to seek mental health care for preexisting but untreated psychiatric disorders. Psychiatric treatment is often a necessary precursor for adherence to the complexities of medical treatment. In addition, psychoeducation to convey the importance of and enhance the skills required for safe sex and safe needle use is important for both patient safety and public health. The combination of psychotherapy and psychopharmacology has repeatedly been demonstrated to be more effective than psychopharmacology alone for a variety of chronic psychiatric conditions, including schizophrenia, bipolar disorder, major depression, and anxiety disorders.

ADJUSTMENT TO MEDICAL ILLNESS

Psychotherapy plays a vital role in adjustment to medical illness. Psychosocial variables that have been demonstrated to predict a higher level of well-being and a lower level of depressed mood in HIV-infected patients include social support, problem-focused coping, and the attribution of positive meaning (i.e., appraising HIV as having created an opportunity for personal growth).[1] Consider the following case example of Ms. B.

> Ms. B., a 34-year-old mother of two with major depression who had abused cocaine for 12 years, entered both mental health and substance abuse treatment after learning she was HIV-positive. Twelve months into treatment, abstinent and euthymic, she declared, "HIV is the best thing that has happened to me. It scared me into treatment because I realized I had to get my act together. Now I'm a happier person and a better mother."

GRIEF

People living with HIV disease mourn the loss of their health, appearance, mobility, career and financial security, and ultimately the loss of life. Many have experienced the HIV-related deaths of spouses, partners, children, friends, and other members of their social network. "Bereavement overload" occurs when a fresh loss interrupts the grieving process, making it impossible to grieve each loss completely.[2] Multiple losses may alter a person's ability to trust or to form new relationships and may affect the ability to engage in psychotherapy. Therapists will be faced with talking about loss and death and will encounter their own grief.

STIGMATIZATION

The social isolation of people living with HIV disease or AIDS, which stems mostly from stigma, is a psychological death experience that precedes the physical death.[2] HIV infection often is associated with gay men and intravenous drug users, groups that are often judged negatively and rejected by others. Patients are frequently afraid or ashamed to disclose their serostatus, and when they do reach out they are vulnerable to discrimination and rejection, as well as others' irrational fears of infection.

TREATMENT ADHERENCE

In the 1980s and early 1990s, the psychiatric literature on HIV disease and AIDS focused on depression, dementia, death, and dying. At that time, most people with HIV infection expected to die within 2 to 3 years. After protease inhibitors became available in 1996, HIV infection shifted from a fatal illness to a chronic illness for many, but not all, patients. Survival is contingent upon strict, lifelong adherence to complex multidrug regimens, and patients are subjected to chronic anxiety that their regimens may fail. Psychotherapy may help patients identify and ameliorate the environmental and psychological barriers to adherence.

Ms. C., a 40-year-old woman with dysthymia and HIV infection, was referred to a therapist by her primary care provider because of repeated refusal to take antiretroviral medication despite a falling CD4 count, rising viral load, and mounting fatigue. In therapy she recognized that her chronic low self-esteem and feelings of hopelessness were worse every time she came to the clinic or thought about her HIV status. She believed that taking medication twice daily would represent an intolerable reminder of her seropositivity and that she would become suicidal. She also worried that the antiretrovirals would not work for her, in which case she would feel more despair than she could endure. To her, to not take antiretrovirals and become ill seemed better than to fail the antiretroviral therapy having tried to stay well. With psychotherapy and antidepressants, she tentatively agreed to a trial of antiretroviral medication. Pleased with the improvement in her energy level brought about by suppressed viral replication, she found it easier to commit to ongoing antiretroviral therapy.

CHANGES IN IDENTITY

Long-term survival exerts other stressors besides those associated with medication adherence. HIV seropositivity forces an adjustment of self-concept as the serostatus is integrated into one's identity. This is reflected in patients' language, such as when they say, "I am HIV." Whether a patient can accept the challenge of this crisis and achieve successful integration depends on ego strength, which is determined in part by early childhood experiences involving separation. One of the therapist's tasks is to explore earlier experiences with loss, learn how the individual coped with those losses, and help mobilize the patient's inner resources to adapt to the current challenge to his or her integrity.

CHANGES IN DEVELOPMENTAL PROGRESSION

In addition to coping with adjustments in identity, HIV-positive patients may experience an acceleration of the usual stages of psychological development. HIV infection challenges young people in the first half of life to take on the developmental tasks of the second half of life. Adolescence and early adulthood are concerned with the developmental issues of separation, identity, independence, establishing relationships, gaining status in society through work, and learning to create and enjoy a meaningful life. HIV infection disproportionately affects people in the first half of life and thrusts them into a confrontation with the tasks of later adulthood and old age. In the second half of life there is a gradual letting go, a decline of aims and ambitions, reflection, awareness and acceptance of the choices and limitations in one's life, and a passing on to the next generation the experiences and wisdom one has acquired. Erik Erikson's final stage of development, Integrity versus Despair, is the fulfillment of the successful negotiation of prior stages, resulting in a sense of having lived a productive and worthwhile life. Some HIV-positive patients achieve remarkable self-understanding and self-acceptance as they accelerate their progression through the developmental stages.

> Mr. D., a 37-year-old man who developed multidrug resistance, has run out of antiviral treatment options and knows that death is approaching. He initiates therapy to cope with his anxiety and because he has a goal to "live his dying." In therapy he resolves his hurt and anger about adolescent and adult encounters with homophobia, achieving a new compassion and understanding for people with narrower views of human behavior. He also develops new compassion for himself, understanding the forces that propelled him to seek community and thus engage in high-risk behaviors. He deepens his relationship with his sister, to whose home he moves to live his last months of life. He and his sister both understand this is a gift they are giving to each other, sharing the intimacy of dying.

Although this process may result in positive growth for some, the challenge of prematurely facing the developmental tasks of old age may overwhelm some patients' ego capacity. Conversely, an internal renegotiation may be required for those patients who have confronted and accepted their deaths, only to be restored to better health by new treatment options.

SPIRITUALITY

An individual's religious or spiritual belief system may help or hinder the adjustment to a potentially fatal illness. Spiritual beliefs are important determinants of one's outlook on death. Many patients with HIV infection feel alienated by religious institutions that are intolerant of alternative lifestyles. In the absence of a safe spiritual community, patients may lack opportunities to understand and modify their beliefs about illness and death. In therapy, patients may explore their feelings about God and religion and assess how HIV disease affects their spiritual development.

> Mr. E., a 45-year-old man raised as a Mormon, entered therapy because of intolerable feelings of anger, depression, and guilt. He struggled with childhood indoctrination that homosexuality is evil and that HIV infection is his punishment from God. The resulting guilt and shame coexisted with anger at his religion's belief system, which he rejected at an intellectual level. Psychotherapy helped him reframe the meaning of his HIV infection and reduced his feelings of shame and anger.

SPECIFIC TECHNIQUES

Therapists who work with HIV-positive patients should be comfortable using a variety of techniques to foster mental health. The majority of the literature concerning specific psychotherapeutic strategies for people with HIV infection is descriptive, case-based reporting that offers a detailed view of how the therapist intervenes with intrapsychic and environmental forces to facilitate mental health. A variety of prospective, controlled, outcome-based studies testing specific techniques have been reported. These are organized in the following sections according to treatment modality. In practice, patients are likely to require several modalities, either in combination or sequence, according to changes in their clinical status, psychological health, and social support systems.

COGNITIVE-BEHAVIORAL THERAPY

Cognitive-behavioral therapy (CBT) is a short-term, collaborative treatment that was specifically designed to alleviate major depression, but its techniques are equally effective in the treatment of anxiety disorders, insomnia, habit reversal, eating disorders, and other conditions. CBT includes a range of interventions that promote changes in thinking or behavior to alter mood or other symptoms. It includes objectively examining patients' perception of their problems and by doing so altering their interpretation and response. By simply addressing patients' perception of their situation with HIV, their response may begin to change. In addition to formal CBT, a variety of CBT-based techniques have been developed, including forms of arousal reduction (biofeedback, guided imagery, progressive muscle relaxation, hypnosis) and coping effectiveness training. Many of these techniques have been studied in men and women with HIV infection and found to reduce stress, anxiety, and depression and improve markers of immune function.[3,4] In addition to reducing psychological distress, CBT diminished pain intensity, pain-related interference with functioning, and measures of distress in patients with HIV disease or AIDS with peripheral neuropathy.[5] A CBT intervention was used successfully to improve antiretroviral medication adherence.[6]

INTERPERSONAL THERAPY

Interpersonal therapy (IPT) is a short-term (12 to 20 weeks) therapy technique originally designed for the treatment of dysthymic disorder and modified for the treatment of other conditions, including major depression, bereavement, panic disorder, bulimia nervosa, body dysmorphic disorder, and coping with HIV infection. IPT addresses problems in the present while acknowledging the exacerbating role of long-standing interpersonal dysfunction. The four areas of interpersonal difficulties specifically addressed by IPT are grief, interpersonal role disputes, role transitions, and interpersonal deficits. HIV infection and AIDS may have an enormous impact on a person's various roles (spouse/partner, parent, employee, bread-winner, student, etc.), and IPT may assist in the resulting renegotiation of identity and relationships. Its specific modification for and efficacy in the treatment of men and women with HIV have been described.[7] A study that compared IPT, CBT, supportive therapy, and imipramine in conjunction with supportive therapy for the treatment of HIV-positive patients suffering from depression revealed that IPT and imipramine plus supportive therapy yielded the most robust antidepressant responses.[8]

PSYCHODYNAMIC PSYCHOTHERAPY

Psychodynamic psychotherapy focuses on the exploration and resolution of internal conflicts that interfere with optimal functioning. Because of the difficulty in scientifically assessing psychodynamic treatment, the literature is composed of case reports and discussions of methodology. For example, Nuttall[9] presents the cases of two gay men who engaged in brief psychoanalytically informed psychotherapy. Using an object relations paradigm, he discusses his work with the defensive systems of patients whose illness and approaching death (the rejecting object) are experienced as coming from sexual behavior (the libidinal object).

Many changes in technique are required of the psychodynamic therapist treating HIV-positive patients. These include attending to the patient's external as well as internal reality; working with the special emotional stresses and discomforts associated with the uncertainties of HIV infection; listening to and being receptive to the stigma incurred by the HIV-positive patient and, by association, the therapist; and examining the therapist's own values and conceptions about life and death. The therapist must be willing to explore potentially uncomfortable topics such as sexuality and sexual orientation, substance abuse, death and dying, religion, and spirituality. Reduction in shame is an important therapeutic task, achieved through the experience of being accepted by the therapist.[10]

Psychodynamic therapists help patients to reconceptualize their intrapsychic world, incorporating the trauma of HIV infection that "threatens to endanger psychic life in a way that is isolating, immobilizing, and akin to a kind of psychic death."[11] The therapist's tasks are to restore mental aliveness by containing the traumatizing process and support the patient in the search for meaning and fulfillment in a life with HIV disease.

EXISTENTIAL AND SPIRITUAL THERAPIES

Existential therapy explores patients' beliefs, feelings, and experiences involving isolation, meaning, and death. HIV infection serves as an existential stressor, raising fears of unworthiness, uncleanliness, sinfulness, and punishment. Existential concerns and psychological themes surrounding isolation and meaninglessness, death, and freedom are explored in therapy.[12] A therapy approach that emphasizes the moral integrity of the person and explores the significance of one's contributions as a human being may help to transcend suffering.

Spiritual therapy focuses on themes of power and powerlessness, life and death. To promote psychological integration and well-being, spiritual therapy explores the individual's ideas about God, religion, prayer, and what happens after death. A spiritual approach to therapy helps resolve conflicts stemming from rejecting or punitive experiences within organized religion, and encourages patients to live in the present and deal with their fear of death[13] (refer to Chapter 34).

GROUP THERAPIES

Reports of group therapy techniques for people with HIV infection and AIDS abound. Because of the isolation and shame that many HIV-positive patients experience, the opportunity to work through problems in a group setting may be particularly valuable. Groups for HIV-positive patients are used for a range of treatments, such as substance abuse recovery, stress management, skills training in cognitive coping strategies, support for medically ill inpatients, and bereavement. For example, a 12-week AIDS-related bereavement coping group resulted in significant reduction in psychiatric distress compared to a control condition in which subjects received individual therapy on request. Women in the group intervention also showed significant reductions in grief and depressive symptoms compared to men in both interventions and women in the control group.[14] In addition, psychoeducation groups for people with AIDS-related dementia, couples groups for HIV-positive patients and their partners, and treatment groups for sexually addicted gay men are among the many applications for group therapy in this population.

FAMILY AND COUPLES THERAPIES

HIV infection has a profound effect on spouses, partners, children, parents, siblings, friends, and extended families. In addition to anxiety, feelings of helplessness and grief that may be expected when any illness is introduced into a couple or family, HIV infection brings additional stigma, isolation, and fear of contagion. Family and couples therapy assists with adaptation to the HIV-positive patient's illness, which in turn improves the patient's social support.

The majority of HIV-positive women in the United States are African American, mostly from urban, low-income communities. The family is a crucial source of support for inner-city African-American women. Pivnick[15] describes the role of a women's center for HIV-positive women and their children, family members, and friends as a prerequisite for family therapy.

The safety and practical support offered by the women's center promotes a willingness to participate in formal treatment. Similarly, Structural Ecosystems Therapy (SET) is a family therapy model specifically designed to reduce distress, decrease family conflicts, and increase family support for HIV-positive African American women. SET has been shown to be more effective than individual counseling in reducing psychological distress. SET has also been shown to be superior in reducing family conflicts, but did not appear to have an advantage in increasing support, perhaps because the families enrolled in the study already provided good support.[16]

CULTURALLY SPECIFIC THERAPIES

Just as family therapy techniques have been developed to address specific HIV-positive populations, other psychotherapy techniques may require modification to accommodate the needs of people from distinct subcultures. HIV disproportionately affects people from minority sexual, racial, and ethnic cultures who may have different values than the logic-based, individualistic, well-to-do, heterosexual European and American patients for whom psychotherapy was developed.

The error of assuming that well-established forms of psychotherapy can be applied to diverse populations is illustrated by a surprising finding in a study by Markowitz et al.[17] In a controlled clinical trial, HIV-positive patients were randomized into four treatment modalities: IPT, CBT, supportive therapy, and imipramine plus supportive therapy. African-American subjects assigned to CBT had significantly poorer outcomes than Latino or White subjects. This study requires replication and further elaboration to understand why ethnicity may matter in CBT efficacy.[17]

To provide culturally competent treatment, the therapist must examine his or her own cultural biases and must appreciate cultural differences in interpersonal relationships. In addition to careful self-examination, the therapist must learn about each patient's culture. Is it acceptable to share personal or family problems with a stranger? Is it acceptable to identify as a homosexual? What confers dignity and respect in the culture? Does a particular homosexual patient primarily identify with his ethnic minority group, gay culture, or the majority culture? With which culture does a multiethnic patient most identify?

Many ethnic minority patients present with concrete problems. To promote trust and respect, a therapist may initially take a direct, problem-solving approach rather than delving into feelings and life histories. Chazin et al.[18] describe the use of the strengths perspective paradigm, in which the focus of treatment is on strengths rather than pathology. This respects cultural differences and avoids pathologizing culturally diverse populations.[18]

TRANSFERENCE, COUNTERTRANSFERENCE, BOUNDARIES, AND BURNOUT

TRANSFERENCE

Although most patients with HIV disease or AIDS are not receiving psychodynamic psychotherapy, their treatment may still benefit from the mental health provider's consideration of transference and countertransference. Transference refers to how the patient experiences the therapist, including unconscious projections based on earlier relationships. Countertransference refers to how the therapist experiences the patient, including unconscious responses to the patient's projections.

Therapists working with HIV-infected patients may be challenged by special vulnerabilities elicited in the transference. Many people with HIV have histories of childhood physical and sexual abuse. They may experience HIV infection as a perpetrator and fear the return of the abuse. Such a patient may long for the therapist to be the good, rescuing parent and simultaneously fear that the therapist will inflict abuse, neglect, or shame. HIV-positive patients may also struggle with mistrust, fears of abandonment, shame, anger, and concern that the therapist will be overwhelmed or overburdened by the patient. A skilled therapist will work to recognize transference-based responses in patients and incorporate this understanding into the treatment.

> Mr. F., a 22-year-old heterosexual man with intravenous cocaine dependence, HIV infection, hepatitis C infection, and bipolar disorder had a pattern of being demanding and verbally abusive with the clinic staff but charming and friendly with his infectious disease doctor and psychiatrist. The psychiatrist knew that Mr. F. was emotionally abused and neglected by his parents and understood that Mr. F. was projecting his early rageful and entitled feelings because he unconsciously expected to be neglected by the staff. With his physicians he was more conciliatory because he perceived them to be the longed-for nurturing parents upon whom his survival depended. Although the psychiatrist did not make this interpretation to Mr. F. at the outset of treatment, she used it to inform her treatment approach.

COUNTERTRANSFERENCE

Patients with HIV infection may elicit intense feelings among providers. Therapists may make moral judgments about nonadherence to medical care or about risk behaviors such as substance abuse, sexual practices, and exchanging sex for drugs or money. Therapists may harbor feelings of racism, anger at the disadvantaged urban poor, or hopelessness about making a difference. Conversely, a therapist may have fantasies of rescuing patients, which may lead to over-involvement. All of these responses may interfere with effective treatment.

Similarly, a therapist who is uncomfortable talking about death in a direct manner may develop unhelpful responses such as avoidance or denial when patients raise this important topic. Countertransference responses may also be related to irrational fears of contamination. A therapist may feel insecure about his or her ability to make a difference in patients with chronic illness or may feel overwhelmed by anger at the patient, the illness, or the "system."

Therapists may also develop countertransference responses based on identification with their patients. For example, a gay male therapist working with a gay male patient with HIV disease or AIDS will have to deal with his personal fears of or experience with infection and his personal grief related to partners, friends, and colleagues who have succumbed to AIDS. Gay therapists may also have to attend to guilt feelings related to being more privileged than their patients—privileged in having been raised in a family or community that is accepting of homosexuality, privileged in not having HIV infection, or privileged in having a loving partner or social support system. Likewise, a therapist who is also a mother of young children may have a strong countertransference response when working with an HIV-infected mother of young children, perhaps experiencing great anxiety or horror at the prospect of leaving one's children orphaned. These countertransference responses through identification with the patient may lead to over-involvement and rescue attempts or to withdrawal and avoidance. Although all of these countertransference responses are common and expected, treatment success hinges on appropriate management of the countertransference.[11] Peer support and supervision are indispensable when working with HIV-infected patients.

BOUNDARIES

Patients with AIDS sometimes need their therapists to extend the therapy beyond the ordinary treatment frame. Therapists may visit patients in the hospital or make home visits, may facilitate medical decision-making, may meet with family members and partners, and may provide case management. The therapist must consider whether each intervention has a deliberate purpose in the treatment and is not merely a gratification of a patient's wish and ensure that the treatment remains ethical. The treatment plan must remain flexible to adjust to the progression of a patient's experience and needs, from first testing to, potentially, death. Stable, compassionate continuity of care is more important than adhering to any one modality of therapy.[19]

BURNOUT

Psychotherapists necessarily become involved in the lives of their patients. A balance must be achieved between over-identification with the patient's struggles concerning hope and despair, and the erection of defensive armor to ward off feelings of impotence and loss. Attention to setting clear goals and expectations of treatment helps protect against rescue fantasies or feeling overwhelmed by hopelessness. Therapists of patients with HIV infection or AIDS experience multiple losses and must actively attend to their own mourning, finding strategies to assist their personal grieving process. Therapists in this field may also struggle with stigma for working with this population, with frustration about limited resources, and with survivor guilt.

All these stressors require therapists to engage in rigorous self-care. Peer supervision and support help therapists cope with transference, countertransference, boundary crossings, and burnout. Therapists who examine their own spiritual and existential beliefs, and confront their own fears about death, may be able to remain more consistently available to their patients. Creating a balance between professional and personal lives is crucial to long-term survival in this field. These challenges lead to the internal and professional growth experienced by many therapists who work with patients with HIV infection and AIDS.

SUMMARY

Psychotherapy is an indispensable part of the psychiatric treatment of patients with HIV disease or AIDS. In addition to helping patients manage underlying psychiatric disorders, psychotherapy assists with the response to initial infection, adjustment to illness, adherence to medical treatment, grief, stigmatization, changes in identity, and changes in adult development brought on by HIV infection and AIDS. Many treatment modalities have demonstrated efficacy in treating patients with HIV disease and AIDS, including CBT, IPT, psychodynamic psychotherapy, existential therapy, and spiritual therapies. Group, couple, and family therapies also have a valuable role in the care of these patients. When working with this population, therapists may find self-examination, supervision, and support particularly useful for coping with transference, countertransference, boundaries, and burnout.

REFERENCES

1. Farber E, Mirsalimi H, Williams K, et al. Meaning of illness and psychological adjustment to HIV/AIDS. *Psychosomatics*. 2003;44:485–491.
2. Elia N. Grief and loss in HIV/AIDS work. In: Winiarski MG, ed. *HIV Mental Health for the 21st Century*. New York: New York University Press; 1997;67–81.
3. Lutgendorf S, Antoni MH, Ironson G, et al. Cognitive-behavioral stress management decreased dysphoric mood and herpes simplex-type 2 antibody titers in symptomatic HIV-seropositive gay men. *J Consult Clin Psychol*. 1997;65:31–43.

4. Lechener S, Antoni M, Lydston D, et al. Cognitive-behavioral interventions improve quality of life in women with AIDS. *J Psychosom Res.* 2003;54:253–261.
5. Evans S, Fishman B, Spielman L, et al. Randomized trial of cognitive behavioral therapy versus supportive psychotherapy for HIV related neuropathic pain. *Psychosomatics.* 2003;44:44–50.
6. Weber R, Christen L, Christen S, et al. Effect of individual cognitive behavioral intervention on adherence to antiviral therapy: prospective randomized trial. *Antiviral Ther.* 2004;9:85-95.
7. Weissman M. Interpersonal psychotherapy: current status. *Keio J Med.* 1997;46:105–110.
8. Markowitz J, Kocsis J, Fishman B, et al. Treatment of depressive symptoms in human immunodeficiency virus-positive patients. *Arch Gen Psychiatry.* 1998;55:452–457.
9. Nuttall J. Fairbairnian object relations: the challenge to the moral defense in gay men with HIV. *Psychodynam Counsel.* 1998;4:445–461.
10. Schaffner B. Modifying psychoanalytic methods when treating the HIV-positive patient. *J Am Acad Psychoanal.* 1997;25:123–141.
11. Cartwright D, Cassidy M. Working with HIV/AIDS sufferers: when good enough is not enough. *Am J Psychother.* 2002;56:149–166.
12. Farber E. Existential treatment with HIV/AIDS clients. In: Kaslow FW, ed. *Comprehensive Handbook of Psychotherapy: Interpersonal/Humanistic/Existential.* Vol. 3. New York: John Wiley & Sons; 2002;303–331.
13. Conforti P. Spirituality. In: Winiarski MG, ed. *HIV Mental Health for the 21st Century.* New York: New York University Press: 1997;52–66.
14. Sikkema K, Hansen N, Kochman A, et al. Outcomes from a randomized controlled trial of a group intervention for HIV positive men and women coping with AIDS-related loss and bereavement. *Death Studies.* 2004;28: 187–209.
15. Pivnick A. The women's center: feminism in the treatment of AIDS. In: Silverstein LB, Goodrich TJ, eds. *Feminist Family Therapy: Empowerment in Social Context.* Washington, DC: American Psychological Association; 2003;281–290.
16. Szapocznik J, Feaster D, Mitrani V, et al. Structural ecosystems therapy for HIV-seropositive African American women: effects on psychological distress, family hassles and family support. *J Consult Clin Psychol.* 2004;72:288–303.
17. Markowitz J, Spielman L, Sullivan M, et al. An exploratory study of ethnicity and psychotherapy outcome among HIV-positive patients with depressive symptoms. *J Psychother Pract Res.* 2000;9:226–231.
18. Chazin R, Kaplan S, Terio S. The strengths perspective in brief treatment with culturally diverse clients. *Crisis Interven Time Limit Treat.* 2000;6:41–50.
19. Ruiz P. Living and dying with HIV/AIDS: a psychosocial perspective. *Am J Psychiatry.* 2000;157:110–113.

CHAPTER **36**

Complementary and Holistic Medicine

Janet Konefal, Jessica Lillisand

Complementary and alternative medicine (CAM) can be defined as "those practices that aren't part of the politically dominant medical system of a country."[1] In the United States, this means those practices that are not usually taught in medical schools; not available in most hospitals, clinics, and private practices; and often not reimbursed by insurance or otherwise routinely accessible.[1] This encompasses an amazingly wide range of practices, including, but not limited to, the following general categories:

1. *Alternative medical systems* are comprehensive systems of care that may have evolved from a non-Western philosophical tradition, such as Traditional Chinese Medicine (TCM) or Ayurveda, or that may have evolved concurrently with conventional Western medical approaches, such as homeopathy and naturopathy. The essential element of these systems is a complete methodology for treatment based on an underlying theory or philosophy.
2. *Mind-body interventions* involve a variety of techniques designed to promote the mind's capacity to affect body functions and symptoms. This includes a wide array of practices, from cognitive-behavioral therapy to meditation and prayer.
3. *Biologically based therapies* use substances found in nature, such as herbs, foods, vitamins, and other dietary supplements.
4. *Manipulative and body-based methods* involve hands-on manipulation and/or movement of one or more parts of the body—for example, chiropractic or osteopathic manipulation or massage.
5. *Energy therapies* involve the use of energy fields of two basic types—biofield and bioelectromagnetic. Biofield therapies affect energy fields, which hypothetically surround and permeate the body. Examples of these are Qigong, Reiki, and Therapeutic Touch. Bioelectromagnetic-based therapies use electromagnetic fields such as pulsed fields, magnetic fields, or alternating current or direct current fields in unconventional and not yet scientifically validated ways.

The debate that has surrounded the uses of CAM health care practices has been politically charged for many years, because in the early years there were few, if any, scientifically valid studies demonstrating the efficacy of these therapies. CAM has been criticized because most of the information about its effectiveness has been anecdotal and gathered from treatments that are generally individualized, rather than standardized, thus not lending themselves to the requirements of the scientific method. Even though much of Western medicine was itself developed from anecdotal information, the current standard for evaluation of a Western medical treatment is a double-blind, placebo-controlled trial. In recent years, there has been an increasing effort to apply the scientific method to the evaluation of CAM practices, with mixed results. A number of factors have contributed to the difficulty of this endeavor. For example, many alternative practices, such as massage therapy, do not lend themselves to the possibility of a double-blind design. Also, pure substances, a requirement of a controlled drug trial, are often not available, or are undesirable for treatment.

As an indication of the slowly changing relationship of CAM to the mainstream medical world, in 1992 the National Institute of Health (NIH) became involved in CAM research and by 1998 established the National Center for Complementary and Alternative Medicine, or NCCAM with a budget of $123 million. NCCAM has defined its 5-year (2000 to 2005) plan, with priorities in the areas of research, training of practitioners, expanding outreach, and facilitating integration. These recent developments are evidence of a dramatic expansion of interest in CAM.

The list of what is considered to be CAM continually changes because complementary and alternative therapies, because they are proven to be safe and effective, are adopted into conventional practices and, at the same time, new and complementary approaches to health care are constantly emerging. For example, scientists have found that folic acid prevents certain birth defects and that a regimen of vitamins and zinc can prevent age-related macular degeneration (AMD), and thus these are now used in mainstream or conventional medicine.

Even within the class of CAM practices, there is also some confusion about correct terminology. Complementary medicine refers to practices that are used in conjunction with conventional medicine. For example, aromatherapy is a complementary therapy that may be used to lessen a patient's discomfort following surgery. Alternative medicine is also used in place of conventional medicine. For example, the practice of using a special diet to treat cancer as an alternative to undergoing surgery, radiation, or chemotherapy recommended by a conventional doctor. Integrative medicine, on the other hand, combines mainstream medical practices with CAM therapies for which there is some valid scientific evidence of efficacy and safety.

The focus of this chapter is on complementary medicine, specifically with regard to its use with patients with human immunodeficiency virus (HIV) disease and AIDS. Patients with HIV or AIDS typically receive conventional treatment. However, more and more, persons living with HIV disease or AIDS are seeking CAM treatments for symptoms and side effects from the antiretroviral drug therapies they receive, as well as for the disease itself. Most of these treatments are designed to augment, not replace, the conventional treatments patients with HIV disease and AIDS receive.

PREVALENCE OF CAM USE IN HIV/AIDS

Although there is some debate over the extent to which it is happening, there is no question that patients with HIV disease or AIDS have also increasingly been seeking CAM treatments. This trend came about largely after 1996, when the efficacy of highly active antiretroviral therapy (HAART) was first presented, and patients with HIV disease and AIDS began to view their illness as something that might become a chronic controllable condition. Initially, lack of understanding of the disease motivated interest in CAM. Taking high doses of vitamin C was one of the first types of CAM that was widely used by those with HIV infection and AIDS. Dinitrochlorobenzene (DNCB), a chemical used in developing color photographs, applied to the skin in the hopes of stimulating cellular immunity, was another treatment that was used in the early years of the disease. Others included dextran sulfate, hypericin (St. John's wort), hyperthermia, ribavirin, and compound Q. Most of these therapies have fallen out of favor in recent years. Since the advent of a broad array of new antiretroviral drugs, CAM use has dramatically changed. Many individuals who are HIV-positive or have AIDS and who use CAM today do so to reduce the side effects of prescribed medications, improve or sustain well-being, or increase their energy. CAM is therefore more likely now to be used in a more complementary fashion. Today, many patients with HIV disease or AIDS are also interested in CAM as a way to treat conditions that do not respond to HAART, such as wasting syndrome.

The use of CAM in patients with HIV disease or AIDS was recently extensively studied by Standish et al.,[2] who reported on 1,675 HIV-positive individuals and found that they had used 1,600 different types of CAM and 1,210 CAM substances, visited 119 types of CAM providers, and used 282 CAM therapeutic activities. Most of the participants in this study were using CAM in conjunction with antiretroviral drug therapy (63%) and thus could be characterized as using integrated medicine. Only 3.5% of the subject pool reported seeing only alternative providers. The most frequently used modalities were biologically based therapies such as vitamins and herbal supplements (63%). Massage therapists (49%), acupuncturists (45%), nutritionists (37%), and psychotherapists (35%) were also employed, and the activities most commonly used were aerobic exercise (63%), prayer (58%), massage (53%), and meditation (46%).

CAM use is also associated with several sociodemographic variables. A study by Gore-Felton et al.[3] concluded that HIV-positive women and Whites were both four times more likely to use CAM. CAM use is also higher among homosexuals, persons with a college education, persons with greater incomes, and persons with poorer health status.[4]

REASONS FOR CAM USE IN HIV/AIDS

It appears that HIV-positive individuals turn to CAM for a variety of reasons. Some of these reasons include, but are not limited to, the desire to take an active role in one's own health care, the treatment of side effects caused by conventional medications, and the desire to improve general well-being and stress levels, boost immunity, and lower viral load.

Individuals with HIV infection or AIDS generally use the same types of CAM as the population as a whole, with therapies such as acupuncture, massage, herbs, and nutritional supplementation used most frequently. In a study by Sparber et al.,[5] postdiagnosis therapies that were increasingly used were imagery, relaxation, spiritual, herbal, weight gain, acupuncture, massage, and high-dose vitamins. However, many different techniques are employed by those with HIV infection or AIDS in the treatment of a variety of conditions. The following sections discuss these methods and the symptoms they are used to treat, as well as the efficacy of the treatments, both as perceived and as tested.

BIOLOGICALLY BASED SYSTEMS

By far the most commonly used CAM modality for patients with HIV disease or AIDS is biologically based systems. This includes herbs, foods, vitamins, and other dietary supplements. Herbs are used by naturopaths, herbalists, homeopaths, acupuncturists, and practitioners of Ayurvedic, Chinese, and Native American medicine. Chinese herbs in particular are often used in combination, such as Composition A, to provide a tonic for general health or to cure a specific ailment. The study by Gore-Felton et al.[3] found that 50% of their sample reported that they took more one or more multivitamins, 17% reported taking mineral supplements, 12% reported using Chinese herbs, and 12% reported using botanicals. One of the most common reasons that patients with HIV disease or AIDS take herbs is to support the immune system and help it repair damage caused by the virus. Unfortunately, herbal remedies have not generally been rigorously or effectively studied for use with these patients. Most of the knowledge about herbal immune therapies, therefore, comes from herbs that were previously used for cancer. Some herbs that are used as immune therapies include ginseng, greater celandine, cat's claw, atractylodes, astragalus, ashwagandha, and shatvari, shitake, and maitake mushrooms.

Herbs are also taken as antimicrobial therapies, to prevent AIDS-related infections or to treat mild infections. These herbs include garlic, goldenseal, neem, propolis, sanguinaria, and tea tree. Various herbs have also been found to have some moderate anti-HIV impact, usually in combination. Herbal combinations have several benefits, including fewer side effects than drug "cocktails" and less likelihood that the virus will mutate to evade the attack. Herbs such as bitter melon, curcumin, glycyrrhizin, and SPV-30 have been used to treat HIV with some claimed effectiveness. However, although a few small clinical trials have been done on antiretroviral herbs, no herbal treatment has been found to be as effective as antiretroviral drugs in stopping the replication of HIV. Herbs are also used to treat HIV-related conditions, such as ginkgo for dementia, aloe vera for skin problems, St. John's wort for depression, marijuana for wasting, greater celandine for Kaposi's sarcoma, and lemon balm for insomnia and herpes simplex. Patients with HIV and AIDS produce high levels of free radicals; herbs such as ginger, ginkgo, milk thistle, and turmeric can be used for their antioxidant properties. Herbs are also used to treat the side effects of antiretroviral drug therapy, though they must be used carefully because dangerous herb–drug interactions can occur that might weaken the effectiveness of treatment, increase side effects, or cause drug resistance. For short-term side effects, herbs such as ginger or marijuana for nausea, and peppermint or psyllium husks for diarrhea can be used. High cholesterol and triglyceride values, seemingly associated with the use of antiretroviral drugs, are also being treated with herbs such as garlic, ginger, ginseng, and guggul.

Standish et al.[2] reported that the most commonly used CAM substances in their 2001 survey were vitamins and herbs, including multivitamin supplements, vitamin C, vitamin E, garlic, beta-carotene, and vitamin B_{12}. Substances such as ginseng, *Echinacea*, and acidophilus were also employed at a high rate. Vitamin C is a powerful antioxidant, useful for increasing immune function and neutralizing free radicals. Vitamin C has been shown in vitro to suppress HIV replication in CD4 cells, but there is a dearth of rigorously controlled studies conducted to test its true efficacy. A daily multivitamin has also been shown to reduce the risk of AIDS and lower CD4 count in HIV-positive men.[6] One of the downsides to using vitamin and mineral supplements in high dosages is possible gastrointestinal distress, along with several other, nutrient-specific side effects. For example, high dosages of zinc carry the risk of impaired immune function. Whole food supplement extracts reduce the risks of high dosage.

ALTERNATIVE MEDICAL SYSTEMS

Alternative medical systems, such as TCM and Ayurveda, also use herbs as a key part of their treatment of HIV disease. TCM has become a popular complementary treatment for patients with HIV disease and AIDS. Unlike Western herbs, Chinese herbs are generally combined, using herbs that complement and balance one another, thus reducing risk of toxicity. However, TCM also employs a wide range of therapies in addition to herbal medicine, including acupuncture, massage, bone adjustment, dietary therapy, and energy therapies such as Qigong. Acupuncture points may be affected by needles, heat, finger pressure, suction, scraping, and laser and electrical stimulation. The points may also be stimulated using massage to affect the energetic system manually. Dietary therapy in TCM is extensive and complex and is not discussed in detail here. However, when a practitioner of TCM is consulted for treatment of HIV disease, most of these therapies will be employed in a synergistic way.

The fundamental aim of Ayurvedic treatments is the balance of the *tridosha*, which is the name for the combination of the forces, or humours, that make up the body: *vata* (wind), *kapha* (phlegm), and *pitta* (bile). Ayurveda aspires for optimal health by balancing the factors that influence the mind, body, and spirit. Oil baths and massage are often employed, as well as the use of several Ayurvedic herbs, including guggul and ashwaganda, for the treatment of HIV disease. Homeopathy is a more Western, and more recent, medical system that also employs a holistic approach to care. Homeopathic remedies are highly individualistic and are chosen by matching a cure to the unique characteristics of the person being treated. Homeopathic remedies are often very dilute, highlighting homeopathy's second key principle—that the more dilute a remedy is, the stronger it is. Very little has been published about the effects of and experiences with homeopathy by HIV-positive people, but a recent publication in *The Lancet* concluded that the effects of homeopathy could not be attributed to placebo effect. Flower essences are also used in homeopathy. They are designed to address emotional and mental states, and may be useful in the treatment of anxiety and depression in HIV-positive individuals. Both homeopathy and flower essences are too subtle to interact with prescription medications and are safe for use in the HIV-positive patient.

Naturopathy, a more Western approach, involves the use of the body's natural abilities to heal itself. Naturopaths use a wide variety of approaches, including but not limited to acupuncture, dietary recommendations, herbal remedies, homeopathy, TCM, exercise therapy, and counseling. The goal for a naturopathic practitioner is to evoke a lifestyle change in patients by teaching proper diet, exercise, relaxation, and eating techniques.

MANIPULATIVE, OR BODY-BASED, TECHNIQUES

Another commonly used modality in HIV and AIDS therapy is manipulative, or body-based, CAM. This includes practices such as massage, acupuncture, and chiropractic manipulation. Standish et al.[2] reported that 52.5% of respondents used massage, 45.4% used acupuncture, 12.1% used acupressure, 25.7% used chiropractic manipulation, and 8.6% used spinal manipulation. American practices of acupuncture incorporate medical traditions from China, Japan, Korea, and other countries. Acupuncture has been claimed to affect the immune response dramatically in the treatment of patients with HIV disease, including the ability to reduce fever, increase production of antibodies, and increase resistance to disease. Although there are no similar studies of its effectiveness in patients with HIV disease, it has been shown to increase CD4+ cells in cancer patients. Acupuncture has also been used to treat generalized symptoms such as fatigue and pain and localized symptoms such as neuropathy.

Massage is also a widely used therapy for patients' HIV disease and AIDS. Massage is the manipulation of body tissues by a therapist. The tissues that are manipulated can be muscles, such as with Swedish massage, or bones and joints, such as with chiropractic massage and osteopathy. Considerable research on touch therapies such as massage have indicated positive results in the treatment of HIV-positive individuals. Therapeutic massage has been used to treat a variety of physical symptoms, including chronic pain, peripheral neuropathy, stress, and fatigue. A 1996 study demonstrated that HIV-positive adults receiving a 45-minute massage five times a week for 1 month showed an increase in natural killer cell production and activity, as well as a decrease in anxiety and depression.[7] Massage techniques are used in the treatment of discomfort relating to Kaposi's sarcoma and associated lesions and to ease difficulty breathing after bouts of *Pneumocystis jiroveci* (formerly *carinii*) pneumonia (PCP) by reducing muscular and chest tension. Massage has also been effective in increasing circulation, improving lymphatic drainage, and relieving pain or restriction following opportunistic infections or serious HIV infection symptoms. These benefits are in addition to the psychoneurologic benefits of increased mood and improved outlook and self-esteem that touch can give.

ENERGY THERAPIES

Another form of touch therapy that does not involve direct, manipulative stimulation is energy work, which includes biofield practices such as Therapeutic Touch, Reiki, and Qigong. Biofield therapies are very closely related to massage because they deal with touch, but focus on the energy fields that are hypothesized to surround each person's body. In the study by Standish et al.,[2] energy therapies were employed by 14.5% of respondents. Other forms of energy therapies include bioelectromagnetic techniques, such as the use of cranio-electrical stimulation, crystals, and electromagnetic therapy, are used to a lesser extent by patients with HIV or AIDS. They also reported that crystals were the medium most often employed in this category, used by 11.2% of respondents. However, there are not many studies documenting the effectiveness of these types of therapies in the treatment of HIV-positive individuals.

One type of therapy that straddles the fence between massage and energy work is Therapeutic Touch, developed by Dolores Krieger, Ph.D., R.N., and Dora Kunz. It is based on a number of ancient healing practices and aims to redirect the flow of energy in the body. This can be done without touching the physical body, because it is thought that a person's energy field extends beyond the surface of the skin. There has been some indication that Therapeutic Touch significantly reduces pain and accelerates the healing process, particularly with PCP, and, to a lesser extent, with Kaposi's sarcoma, but rigorous research is lacking. Qigong and tai'chi may be useful in replenishing the energy drained from fighting HIV infection and AIDS.

MIND-BODY INTERVENTIONS

Mind-body techniques recognize the undeniable connection between the mind and the body and the ability for mental states to influence the promotion or deterioration of a person's health. This modality incorporates a wide range of practices, including cognitive-behavior therapy, visualization, biofeedback, yoga, prayer, and meditation. These techniques are increasingly utilized by patients with HIV disease and AIDS. The study by Gore-Felton et al.[3] reported that 28% of its participants engaged in meditation to treat their illness. Standish et al.[2] reported that mind-body techniques were employed quite often, with 58.5% of respondents engaging in prayer, 45.9% in meditation, and 33.7% in breathing exercises. Furthermore, 44.1% of respondents participated in support groups and 34.7% in psychotherapy.

An HIV-positive diagnosis is a devastating event and takes its toll on the person emotionally and physically. The field of psychoneuroimmunology has identified that emotions can be associated with specific chemical processes not only in the brain, but throughout the entire body. These processes affect all systems of the body, including the immune system. Emotions such as anger, fear, guilt, and hopelessness, often experienced by patients with HIV disease and AIDS, can significantly weaken the immune system. Studies have shown that patients with these diseases who practice mind-body techniques such as meditation and visualization live longer and require fewer pain medications.

Meditation and breathing techniques can be used to increase resistance to stress and reduce anxiety and fatigue. Meditation teaches awareness through the practice of noticing one's breath and can lead to a greater sense of control over one's life and an increased sense of well-being in general for patients with HIV and AIDS. However, studies have produced inconclusive results as to the effectiveness of these therapies.

Jon Kaiser has developed an extensive manual for treating HIV disease and AIDS and utilizes several mind-body techniques as an integral part of his program. Dr. Konefal has developed mind-body processes using neurolinguistic psychology to address specific psychological issues that often cause stress in patients with HIV disease or AIDS. These include creating a positive visual image for the future, changing negative self-talk, and enhancing the will to live.

TREATMENT EFFECTIVENESS STUDIES FOR CAM MODALITIES: PROBLEMS AND OUTCOMES

Researchers in the conventional medical community, for example Ernst,[8] comment that there is as yet little evidence that CAM has any specific value beyond a placebo effect as a treatment for HIV disease and AIDS and that longitudinal data do not indicate any affect on disease progression or mortality. However, the placebo effect, indicated by perceived effectiveness, potentially leads to increased feelings of well-being or quality of life, which in turn could influence clinical outcomes.

Despite the increasing popularity and medical acceptance of CAM outlined in the previous sections, scientific research has been curiously lacking, and the outcomes of existing studies often raise more questions than they resolve. Adequate effectiveness studies of specific complementary therapies in the treatment of all HIV-related conditions are "a rarity in scientific literature." She notes that most studies of complementary medicine have been anecdotal reports, surveys, case studies, or ratings of perceived effectiveness or have involved small sample size in the studies.

On the other hand, when patients' perceptions of the effectiveness of CAM modalities to improve life quality, increase energy level, or enhance patients' sense of control over their life and disease, was used as the outcome measure, many studies suggested the positive efficacy of several different CAM treatments.[9]

COLLABORATION BETWEEN CONVENTIONAL MEDICINE AND CAM PRACTICTIONERS

Standish et al.[2] observed that, despite the considerable overlap between conventional (antiretroviral) medicine use and use of CAM modalities, there was little evidence of any collaboration or communication between the treating physicians and CAM practitioners. On the other hand, despite the apparent lack of collaborative teamwork between physicians and CAM providers, Duggan et al.[10] reported that physicians' acceptance of CAM (or at least patients' perception of physician acceptance) may be increasing in recent years. These investigators found that about 65% of patients who used CAM indicated that their physicians knew about, and tolerated, their use of complementary medicine, and in fact that the medical community was the major source of CAM information.

OUTCOMES FOR BIOLOGICALLY BASED METHODS

Langewitz et al.[11] found patients' ratings of the perceived effectiveness of CAM ranged from 64 (of 100) for Bach flower remedies to 83 for dietary treatments. Burack et al.[12] stated that HIV-positive patients treated with Chinese herbs reported a reduction in neurologic, gastrointestinal, and respiratory symptoms and sleep disturbance compared to placebo controls. At the same time, no differences between groups were found in terms of symptom severity, weight, CD4 cell count, anxiety, or depression. With regard to the effectiveness of vitamins and other nutritional supplements, several studies were inconsistent in demonstrating any medical improvement following treatment with a variety of vitamins or mineral supplements. Pichard et al.[13] studying 64 HIV-infected outpatients randomly assigned to receive daily supplements of vitamins, trace elements, and minerals, or the same supplements plus arginine and omega three fatty acids, found no positive change, or difference between the groups in CD4 and CD8 lymphocyte counts, viremia, and tumor necrosis factor soluble receptors, while at the same time body weight increased in *both* groups. Studies of vitamin A supplementation showed no positive effects on HIV-infected patients, and inconclusive results were found for vitamin C supplementation.

Min et al.[14] investigated the effectiveness of a variety of Korean plants in promoting the inhibition of RNA-dependent DNA polymerase (RT) and ribonuclease H (RNaseH) activities of HIV-1 reverse transcriptase and HIV-protease, and anti–HIV-1 activity. *Agrimonia pilosa* was also active against RNaseH activity. *Agrimona pilosa, Atractylodes japonica, Clematis heracleifolia* and *Syneilesis palmate* components were also active against recombinant HIV-1 protease, and *Crinum asiaticum* var. *japonicum* showed significant anti–HIV-1 activity.

Although more Americans are using herbs to treat a variety of illnesses, and patients with HIV disease and AIDS are using biologicals (vitamins, herbs, and nutritional supplements) in increasing numbers, there are relatively few rigorous clinical studies, and even fewer have looked at the herbs in conjunction with HIV antiretroviral therapy. Some estimates indicate that more than 75% of herbal plants might possess anti–HIV-positive potential, but have unassessed levels of toxicity to humans. Thus careful research on drug interactions is essential to assess both the benefits and dangers of herb use in patients receiving more conventional Western medical treatments.

OUTCOMES FOR MANIPULATIVE AND BODY-BASED INTERVENTIONS

With regard to the effectiveness of manipulative, or body-based, CAM treatments, Beal and Nield-Anderson,[15] in a pilot study of 11 HIV-positive participants, using a sham-acupuncture control group, demonstrated that experimental subjects perceived acupuncture as effective and reported improvements in symptoms and quality of life. A 1998 study by Shlay et al.[16] demonstrated that a standardized acupuncture regimen had little or no specific effect on HIV-related peripheral neuropathy pain. Thus acupuncture may be helpful for some conditions and not helpful for other conditions.

With regard to massage therapy, a 1996 study by Ironson et al.[7] found that daily massage for 1 month did demonstrate reductions in natural killer cells and CD8 counts, as well as reported reductions in HIV-related symptoms, but not in CD4 counts. A study by Shor-Posner et al.[17] of children with HIV infection or AIDS compared a group who received massage therapy with a friendly visit control group. The control group children were found to be more at risk for CD4 count decline, as well as lymphocyte loss, indicating that massage-treated children may maintain immunocompetence better, perhaps giving hope to children worldwide who lack antiretroviral access.

Henrickson[18] used an innovative methodology to evaluate both clinical outcomes and patient perceptions of acupuncture and massage therapies in patients with HIV. Three treatment groups were used: acupuncture-only, massage-only, and acupuncture massage. These were compared to nontreatment controls, using a quasi-experimental retrospective case-control design. Treatment groups showed improvement compared to the nontreatment controls in premeasures and postmeasures of CD4 counts. The participants' ratings of subjective experience of the treatments was high for all treatment groups.

Several studies have suggested that massage therapy, particularly in combination with other CAM modalities, can actually improve immune system function. For example, Birk et al.[19] found that massage therapy alone did not enhance immune measures such as change in peripheral blood level of CD4 lymphocytes, CD8 lymphocytes, CD4/CD8 lymphocyte ratios, and natural killer cells. Massage therapy in combination with stress management did, however, result in favorable perceptions of health status and thus to less utilization of health care resources and improved assessment of quality of life.

OUTCOMES FOR MIND-BODY INTERVENTIONS

With regard to mind-body and psychological treatment methodologies, several studies indicate that stress management techniques, meditation, and cognitively-based psychological interventions may lead to both improved subjective outcomes, such as sense of well-being and increased energy and mental focus, and measures of enhanced immune system function. For example, Robinson et al.,[20] in a quasi-experimental, prepost, nonrandomized design study of participants in a Mindfulness-Based Stress Reduction (MBSR) Program, compared to nontreatment controls, found that natural killer cell activity and number increased in the treatment group, suggesting that MBSR may improve immunity in HIV-infected individuals. Rucklidge and Saunders[21] studied the efficacy of hypnosis in the treatment of pruritus in patients with HIV disease or AIDS, using a time-series analysis methodology. Although anecdotal reports had suggested that hypnosis might be useful in reducing itching, and thus distress, there had been no previous empirical evaluation of these conjectures. The study by Rucklidge and Saunders,[21] albeit flawed by small sample size and lack of appropriate controls, did obtain significant reductions in daily itch severity and extent of sleep disturbance resulting from the pruritus.

Other mind-body interventions that are widely used, although not so widely evaluated, in the treatment of patients with HIV disease or AIDS are imagery, meditation, prayer, spiritual practices, cognitive restructuring, psychological counseling, and psychotherapy. Guillory et al.[22] studied the meaning and use of spirituality in a group of women infected with HIV and women who had AIDS and concluded that the acceptance of spirituality as an essential element of health and quality of life might lead to the development of new strategies of treatment and care that could return a sense of dignity and self-worth to the chronically or incurably ill. Carson[23] demonstrated a positive relationship between the long-term survival of patients with HIV disease or AIDS and their perceptions of their physical, emotional, and spiritual health, their participation in prayer and meditation, and their use of exercise and special diet programs as health-promoting behaviors.

Studies on the use of stress management techniques with patients with HIV disease and AIDS have yielded some positive results. Taylor[24] evaluated the effectiveness of a stress management program that included progressive muscle relaxation training, EMG-biofeedback assisted relaxation training, meditation, and hypnosis and found significant improvement in anxiety, mood, and self-esteem among the treatment group, as well as improved T cell count, compared to untreated controls. However, the study suffered from some of the usual methodologic flaws, for example, small sample size and absence of double-blind design or appropriate comparison groups.

Lutgendorf et al.[25] reported decreases in dysphoria, anxiety, and total distress in a group treated with cognitive-behavioral stress management training. There was also a reduction in herpes simplex virus (HSV-2) immunoglobulin G antibody titers in the treatment group, although no significant change in HSV type 1 antibody titers and CD4+/CD8 cell counts were noted when the two groups were compared.

ALTERNATIVE MEDICAL SYSTEMS

Earlier studies on the various techniques of TCM in the prophylaxis and treatment of AIDS have indicated that AIDS has been treated by acupuncture and moxibustion, with results indicating improved immune function and resistance to disease, as well as significant improvement in Karposi's sarcoma and signs of hemorrhage. Studies on the use of Chinese herbal medicine in the treatment of patients with AIDS have also shown some positive results. For example, Li et al.[26] demonstrated an in vitro inhibitory effect of baicalin—a flavonoid component purified from the Chinese herbal medicine plant *Scutellaria baicalensis Georgi*, against HIV-1–infected H9 cells, and the enzymatic activity of purified recombinant HIV-1/RT. In an in vivo study, Maek-a-nantawat et al.[27] found no significant change in log viral load and CD4 count after 6 months of treatment with Jin-Huang Chinese herbal medicine, but reported that patients felt that quality of life was improved in terms of subjective reports of appetite, sleep habits, and general health improvements, with no serious adverse effects documented. However, sources of information on Chinese traditional medicines urge caution in the reporting of research on the effectiveness of various substances and warn of the need to control medicine quality, perform detailed observations in a clinical setting, and utilize objective and valid indicators of efficacy.

PROBLEMS AND DILEMMAS IN CAM RESEARCH

As already mentioned, research on the effectiveness of CAM modalities has been plagued with many problems over the years, particularly because of the pressure to apply the research design of conventional medicine to CAM. To gain credibility and acceptance (as well as research funding), CAM studies must resolve problems such as the need to create placebo groups, individualization of treatment, and appropriate outcome measures. For example, some complementary therapies, such as massage, are resistant to defining a comparable placebo group, as well as to the impossibility of creating a double-blind research design. In addition, whereas conventional medicine uses a standardized treatment protocol for all experimental subjects, which lends itself well to research design and statistical analysis, complementary medicine, to be effective, is often specifically tailored to each individual.[9] For example, acupuncture patients being treated for the same condition may be managed differently (e.g., different techniques, or different needle placements) based on their constitution, physical signs, personal needs, lifestyle, or emotional status. With regard to the problem of outcome measures, conventional medicine relies on physiologic measures that indicate the course of the disease process, whereas CAM tends to rely on self-report measures, such as increased quality of life, decreased pain or fatigue, or subjective assessments of psychological or physical well-being.

In addition, CAM research is often plagued with the problems caused by small sample size, subject attrition, and little follow-up data, thus limiting the generalizability of the results. Small sample size also interferes with appropriate research design, especially the creation of control groups, double-blind design, and randomization, often the result of limited funding. Properly designed research and increased follow-up are necessary to demonstrate the efficacy and safety of CAM treatments. More empirically based research is needed to examine the toxicities, interactions, and health benefits or risks of supplements among patients with HIV disease and AIDS, so that both patients and physicians can make informed decisions about appropriate and effective treatments.

There is a pressing need for controlled outcome studies among large, diverse samples of people living with HIV disease and AIDS. Clinical research must include ethnically diverse populations that are gender-balanced and must avoid the "one method suits all" view that has been prevalent in Western medicine. Research studies must take into account the cultural values, practices, and belief systems of the patients, as well as the physiologic and cultural gender-based and age-based differences between men and women and between children, adults, and the elderly. Western medicine must integrate subjective outcome measures such as quality of life indicators into their research protocols. Finally, longitudinal controlled designs are necessary, in both conventional and CAM research, to accurately assess the safety and cost-benefit status of interventions.

RISKS, WARNINGS, AND DANGEROUS INTERACTIONS

CAM treatment modalities are often promoted and accepted as harmless by CAM practitioners and patients alike. Many people use CAM because they perceive it as helpful and without side effects, because they see it as their only remaining alternative, or because they wish to leave no stone unturned in their fight to prolong life, improve health, or ameliorate quality of life. However, some CAM treatments have been associated with adverse effects, complications, dangerous interactions with conventional treatments, and even fatalities. Ernst[8] comments that the safety of CAM has been greatly under-researched—a situation that is gradually changing in recent years, despite ongoing problems in developing adequate research methodologies.

Several studies have shown that the use of herbal remedies, vitamin and mineral supplements, and other natural health products may be linked to negative interactions with HIV medications, which could potentially contribute to drug failure. Mills et al.[28] reviewed nine studies for different herbal medicines (St. John's wort, garlic, golden seal, and milk thistle), and one vitamin (vitamin C). Their review found that there may be important drug-level changes when megadoses of vitamins and herbal products are combined with HIV medications. Methodologic considerations limit the generalizability of the studies reviewed, but do not lessen the urgent need to come up with more precise evaluations of CAM substances and their interactions with conventional medications used in HIV infection and AIDS treatments. Given the prevalence of polypharmaceutical treatments, investigation of potentially detrimental interaction effects is critical. Recent studies indicate that almost all patients with HIV disease or AIDS using CAM do so in conjunction with conventional techniques such as HAART. However, combining complementary therapies with conventional drugs raises the possibility of adverse interactions. These interactions can lead to increased side effects or toxicity. They can also reduce the effectiveness of HAART, possibly leading to drug resistance and treatment failure. It is therefore essential for patients to discuss the use of CAM with their medical doctor and for doctors to ask about CAM usage. Herbs such as chaparral, germander, comfrey, mistletoe, skullcap, Kombucha tea, pennyroyal, yerba tea, margosa oil, Gordolobo, and some types of maté teas have been associated with toxicity and sometimes death.

Primary care physicians, their patients, and the public at large need high-quality information to guide both their decision to use CAM substances and to justify the financial expenditure on these treatments. Herb–drug interactions may have the potential to improve health, reduce the side effects of conventional medication, or to reduce the effectiveness of conventional treatment. A few may even increase the side effects of conventional medications, perhaps contributing to their toxicity. It may be possible that a specific herbal product may decrease the therapeutic effect of medications, thereby contributing to treatment failure, or (in the case of HAART) the interaction may lead to drug resistance, thus reducing future options for treatment. Herb–drug interactions may also modify the action of drugs, leading to unexpected complications, or they may potentiate the therapeutic effects of the medication, leading to overmedication. The Canadian AIDS Treatment Information Exchange (CATIE) recommends caution when mixing herbs and drugs if the herbal therapy can change digestion or affect kidney or liver function; if it has similar side effects to the drug therapy; if both are used to treat the same condition; or if there is underlying damage to, or impairment of, the stomach, liver, or kidneys as a result of illness or adverse drug reactions.

In addition, literature sources warn that St. John's wort should not be taken with any protease inhibitor or non-nucleoside reverse transcriptase inhibitor (NNRTI). Garlic in large quantities (whether raw or processed) should not be used with any protease inhibitor. Milk thistle may also interact with protease inhibitors and NNRTIs to alter levels of antiretroviral drugs in the blood. Patient with HIV disease or AIDS may be taking other conventional drug therapies for AIDS-related illnesses or infections, as well, for other conditions such as high blood pressure and diabetes. Care should be taken to avoid herb–drug interactions with these non–AIDS-related medications. For example, combining ginkgo biloba with anticoagulants may potentiate the anticoagulant effect; the use of St. John's wort may be dangerous with some antidepressants, particularly monoamine oxidase (MAO) inhibitors and may diminish the therapeutic function of oral contraceptives, anticoagulants, and transplant medications. Kava-kava should not be used with alcohol or in patients with compromised liver function. Ginseng, or dong quai, can interact in a negative or harmful way with warfarin. Hawthorn (*Crataegus* species) is contraindicated with antihypertensive medications, digoxin, or antidepressants.

Finally, a study by Leonard et al.[29] reported that HIV-positive individuals felt strongly about their desire to utilize CAM substances for health maintenance and to provide a sense of empowerment in their own health care, but that their access to safe, accurate, and well-validated information about interactions was quite limited. Respondents in this study had major concerns about safety issues, but had difficulty evaluating the quality of the information obtained from sources such as their CAM providers, their primary care physicians, the Internet, health food stores, and books and articles. There is a pressing need for research on the dissemination and evaluation of information on safety and efficacy of medication interactions in a vulnerable and needy population.

SUMMARY

Although there may be disagreement about the efficacy of many types of CAM therapy, people with HIV disease and AIDS are using it and in increasing numbers. Even so, stigmas still persist today in the conventional medical community, though this is slowly changing. However, whether or not doctors find CAM acceptable or scientifically valid seems irrelevant when they must care for patients who believe in its effectiveness and use it. It is necessary, therefore, for medical doctors caring for HIV-positive patients to keep hostile lines of communication open and nonhostile and ask their patients about their use of CAM therapies. If the use of CAM is discouraged by the patients' doctors, it may simply lead to patients using of CAM without full disclosure and at the risk of their health. Although physicians who wish to practice medicine conscientiously may have reservations about the uncorroborated claims of CAM practices, their patients are best served by an open discussion of the strengths and limitations of such therapies. As CAM becomes increasingly used in the population with HIV disease and AIDS, what is needed now is a push for more funding for research on the efficacy of various techniques and an effort to disseminate the most accurate and ethical information to the public who wish to use CAM.

REFERENCES

1. Jonas W. One kind of medicine or many: the view from NIH. *Contemp Obstet Gynecol*. 1998;43:123–145.
2. Standish LJ, Greene KB, Bain S, et al. Alternative medicine use in HIV positive men and women: demographics, utilization patterns and health status. *AIDS Care*. 2001;13:197–208.
3. Gore-Felton C, Vosvick M, Power R, et al. Alternative therapies: a common practice among men and women living with HIV. *J Assoc Nurs AIDS Care*. 2003;14:17–27.
4. Berg MA, Hatch RL, Neims AH. Lifetime use of alternative therapies: a study of Florida residents. *South Med J*. 1998;91:1126–1131.
5. Sparber A, Wooten JC, Bauer L, et al. Use of complementary medicine by adult patients participating in HIV/AIDS clinical trials. *J Altern Complement Med*. 2000;6:415–422.
6. Hanna, L. Complementary and alternative medicine: exploring options and making decisions. *Bull Exp Treat AIDS*. 1998;Apr:36–42.
7. Ironson G, Field T, Scafidi F, et al. Massage therapy is associated with enhancement of the immune system's cytotoxic capacity. *Int J Neurosci*. 1996;84:205–217.
8. Ernst E. Complementary AIDS therapies: the good, the bad and the ugly. *Int J STD AIDS*. 1997;8:281–285.
9. Ozsoy M, Ernst E. How effective are complementary therapies for HIV and AIDS? A systematic review. *Int J STD AIDS*. 1999;10:629–635.
10. Duggan J, Peterson WS, Schutz M, et al. Use of complementary and alternative therapies in HIV-infected patients. *AIDS Patient Care STD*. 2001;15:159–167.
11. Langewitz W, Rüttimann S, Laifer G, et al. The integration of alternative treatment modalities in HIV infection: the patient's perspective. *J Psychosom Res*. 1994;38:687–693.
12. Burack JH, Cohen MR, Hahn JA, et al. Pilot randomized controlled trial of Chinese herbal treatment for HIV-associated symptoms. *J AIDS Hum Retrovirol*. 1996;12:386–393.
13. Pichard C, Sudre P, Karsegard V, et al. A randomized double-blind controlled study of 6 months of oral nutritional supplementation with arginine and omega-3 fatty acids in HIV-infected patients. *AIDS*. 1998;12:53–63.
14. Min BS, Kim YH, Tomiyama M, et al. Inhibitory effects of Korean plants on HIV-1 activities. *Phytother Res*. 2001;15:481–486.
15. Beal MW, Nield-Anderson L. Acupuncture for symptom relief in HIV-positive adults: lessons learned from a pilot study. *Altern Ther Health Med*. 2000;6:33–42.
16. Shlay JC, Chaloner K, Max M, et al. Acupuncture and amitriptyline for pain due to HIV-related peripheral neuropathy. *JAMA*. 1998;280:1590–1595.
17. Shor-Posner G, Miguez MJ, Hernandez-Reif M, et al. Massage treatment in HIV-1 infected Dominican children: a preliminary report on the efficacy of massage therapy to preserve the immune system in children without antiretroviral medications. *J Altern Complement Med*. 2004;10:1093–1095.

18. Henrickson M. Clinical outcomes and patient perceptions of acupuncture and/or massage therapies in HIV-infected individuals. *AIDS Care*. 2001;13:743–748.
19. Birk TJ, McGrady A, MacArthur RD, et al. The effects of massage therapy alone and in combination with other complementary therapies on immune system measures and quality of life in human immunodeficiency virus. *J Altern Complement Med*. 2000;6:405–414.
20. Robinson FP, Mathews HL, Witek-Janusek L. Psycho-endocrine-immune response to mindfulness-based stress reduction in individuals infected with the human immunodeficiency virus: a quasiexperimental study. *J Altern Complement Med*. 2003;9:683–694.
21. Rucklidge JJ, Saunders D. The efficacy of hypnosis in the treatment of pruritus in people with HIV/AIDS: a time-series analysis. *Int J Clin Hypn*. 2002;50:149–169.
22. Guillory JA, Sowell R, Moneyham L, et al. An exploration of the meaning and use of spirituality among women with HIV/AIDS. *Altern Ther Health Med*. 1997;3:55–60.
23. Carson VB. Prayer, meditation, exercise and special diets: behaviors of the hardy person with HIV/AIDS. *J Assoc Nurs AIDS Care*. 1993;4:18–28.
24. Taylor DN. Effects of a behavioral stress-management program on anxiety, mood, self-esteem and T-cell count in HIV positive men. *Psychol Rep*. 1995;76:451–457.
25. Lutgendorf SK, Antoni MH, Ironson G, et al. Cognitive-behavioral stress management decreases dysphoric mood and herpes simplex virus-type 2 antibody titers in symptomatic HIV-seropositive gay men. *J Consult Clin Psychol*. 1997;65:31–43.
26. Li BQ, Fu T, Yan YD, et al. Inhibition of HIV infection by baicalin—a flavonoid compound purified from Chinese herbal medicine. *Cell Mol Biol Res*. 1993;39:119–124.
27. Maek-a-nantawat W, Pitisuttithum P, Bussaratid V, et al. 6-month evaluation of JinHuang Chinese herbal medicine study in asymptomatic HIV infected Thais. *Southeast Asian J Trop Med Public Health*. 2003;34:79–84.
28. Mills E, Montori V, Perri D, et al. Natural health product-HIV drug interactions: a systematic review. *Int J STD AIDS*. 2005;16:181–186.
29. Leonard B, Huff H, Merryweather B, et al. Knowledge of safety and herb-drug interactions amongst HIV+ individuals: a focus group study. *Can J Clin Pharmacol*. 2004;11:227–231.

CHAPTER 37

Biopsychosocial Aspects

Cheryl Gore-Felton, Cheryl Koopman, David Spiegel

As the medical management of human immunodeficiency virus (HIV) disease continues to improve, patients living with HIV disease or acquired immunodeficiency syndrome (AIDS) are experiencing the disease as a chronic stressor that shares similarities to other chronic life-threatening illnesses in relation to psychological functioning. Patients with chronic or terminal illnesses often experience a number of psychosocial problems that can exacerbate their medical condition, including alienation, anxiety, and depression. For patients living with HIV disease or AIDS, psychosocial problems are often exacerbated by the physical demands of dealing with medication side effects and the course of the illness. The biopsychosocial burdens on patients can be overwhelming and adversely affect health outcomes. Fortunately, more than two decades of research provides evidence that many of the psychosocial problems that chronically ill patients experience respond to psychotherapeutic intervention.

THE INTERACTION OF PSYCHOSOCIAL ASPECTS OF HIV/AIDS AND PHYSIOLOGY

DISCLOSURE

Persons living with HIV disease are faced with a number of challenges, including whether or not to inform people in their social network about their seropositive status. Prevention experts have identified disclosure as a key factor in reducing HIV transmission. Disclosure to potential sexual and needle exchange partners allows for informed decisions about engaging in practices known to increase risk of HIV infection. In addition to reducing risk of viral transmission, disclosure of serostatus is often necessary in order to access health and social services. Nevertheless, deciding who to tell, when to tell, and how to tell can be a stressful process. Furthermore, it may be dangerous in certain relationships or circumstances to disclose one's serostatus because of the possibility of becoming the target of physical violence. Factors that inhibit disclosure vary across individuals, but fear of negative responses and breach of confidentiality are common concerns. The social stigma associated with HIV disease prevents individuals from getting tested. For those who know their status, stigma can be a barrier to seeking treatment and care, which often results in individuals being seen for the first time by a physician during advanced stages of disease.

DEPRESSION

Depression is one of the most common mental health disorders reported among individuals with chronic illnesses, and depression among adults living with HIV is well documented.[1] There is a relationship between the chronic effect of depression and HIV disease such that depressive symptoms predict an increased risk of developing AIDS.[2] There is also recent evidence that some of the association between depression and disease progression is due to a "protective" effect of positive affect or mood, such that positive affect is associated with decreased AIDS progression among persons infected with HIV.[3] Moreover, research with symptomatic HIV-positive men that examined a cognitive behavioral stress management (CBSM) intervention identified the reduction of depression as a likely mediator of the therapeutic effects on reconstituting immunity.[4]

STRESSFUL LIFE EVENTS

Traumatic and other stressful life events are highly prevalent among persons who become HIV-positive. Childhood sexual abuse and other traumatic life events appear to be risk factors for sexual risk behavior and injecting and other drug use associated with HIV infection.[5] Clinical evidence suggests that stressful life events predict more rapid HIV disease progression. Indeed, research has found that for every severely stressful life event per 6-month interval, the risk of early HIV disease progression doubles.[6] Among persons recently notified of HIV-positive serostatus, post-traumatic stress disorder (PTSD) symptoms of avoidance and intrusion have been associated with greater distress and avoidance was associated with lower CD4+ percentages.[7] Furthermore, both general perceived stress and the chronic stress of living in unstable housing conditions have been positively associated with physical health status in HIV-positive persons in the Deep South of the United States.[8]

SOCIAL SUPPORT

The lives of HIV-positive persons are often complex, and their social as well as psychological needs often go unmet. There is substantial need for social support in the face of life-threatening illness. Under normal circumstances, social support can help individuals to mobilize their psychological resources, master their emotional burdens, obtain tangible resources like money or shelter, and acquire skills to handle situations optimally. Studies have shown that the mere perception that adequate support is available can serve to buffer situational stress as much as the actual social support itself.[8]

HIV-infected patients are confronted with high levels of stress related to their health status, and their social support systems are often burdened and impaired. An AIDS diagnosis is frequently linked to a decrease in the number of supportive contacts or a change in the pattern of those contacts. For example, AIDS patients report lower levels of practical and emotional support from family members.[9] In fact, many AIDS patients report greater availability of emotional support from friends than from family members.

Problems with inadequate social support may have physiologic as well as psychological consequences. In general, greater social support has been associated with better immune system function. Among HIV-positive persons, those with more available social support had significantly less deterioration in CD4+ cell count.[10] Consistent with the research suggesting that more social support is associated with better immune function, bereavement (i.e., grieving the loss of an important source of social support) has been associated with two functional measures of a decrement in immune function, namely, decreased natural killer cytotoxicity and decreased lymphocyte proliferative response to phytohemagglutinin.[11]

Social support is an important factor in attenuating the stress experienced by HIV-positive individuals. An explanation as to how this may occur can be found within the theoretical framework of the stress-buffering hypothesis of social support. The stress-buffering hypothesis of social support[12] refers to protection that social support provides against the effects of stressful events and situations. This protective effect of social support is thought to operate by both contributing to the resources available to individuals to cope with the stressor and reducing the stress response to the stressor.[12]

PHYSIOLOGICAL STRESS RESPONSE

Through allostasis, the autonomic nervous system, the hypothalamic-pituitary-adrenal (HPA) axis, and the cardiovascular, metabolic, and immune systems protect the body by responding to internal and external stress. However, cumulative stress can disrupt this complex interactive system. McEwen's model of stress and health[13] incorporates a considerable body of research, suggesting that chronic elevation of cortisol caused by stress, as well as other factors, can lead to immunity problems as a function of allostatic load, which is the cumulative effect of stress on the body. In healthy individuals, cortisol levels are usually highest before awakening and decrease over the course of the day.[14]

Experiencing chronic stress or enduring major traumatic life events may result in raising cortisol above its usual levels. HIV-positive individuals often have evidence of HPA axis dysregulation,[15] which may contribute to disease progression. Indeed, excessive activation of the HPA axis can influence immunologic processes that are related to HIV pathogenesis and disease resistance.[16] Moreover, HIV-positive patients are more likely to have hypercortisolemia (i.e., chronic elevation of cortisol).[17] This is problematic because there is evidence suggesting that chronic elevation of cortisol is immunosuppressive and may increase HIV viral replication.[17] Recent research further indicates an association among depressive symptoms, cortisol, and disease progression among HIV-positive men.[18] Further support of these relationships was established by a psychosocial intervention (i.e., CBSM therapy) that demonstrated that decreases in depression and cortisol lead to immune system reconstitution.[4]

IMPLICATIONS FOR DISEASE MANAGEMENT AND CLINICAL PRACTICE

Although there has been a great deal of progress in understanding the life cycle of HIV that has resulted in the development of highly active antiretroviral therapy (HAART), at present there is no cure for AIDS or a vaccine against HIV infection and none seem imminent. HAART is responsible for prolonging life and slowing the disease progression among many persons with HIV infection or AIDS; however, not everyone has been helped by the HAART regimen.[19]

Support groups and other psychosocial interventions have a role to play in enhancing the quality of life for HIV-positive persons. Research has found in some, but not all, studies that psychosocial interventions may enhance survival among persons with cancer and may have similar effects on individuals living with HIV infection or AIDS.[20] In a study examining changes in immunologic status among 25 HIV-infected men randomly assigned to a 10-week stress management intervention or to a wait-list control, men receiving stress management had higher CD4(+), CD45RA(+), and CD29(+) cell counts over a 12-month period post intervention.[21] It is important to note that this difference was found independent of the individual's number of naïve T cells and HIV virus load. Thus, there is evidence that stress management is an efficacious method of immunologic reconstitution among HIV-infected men. These findings are consistent with results found in a 10-week bereavement support group research trial for HIV-positive individuals that demonstrated health benefits such that greater CD4+ cell count, lower plasma cortisol levels, and fewer number of physician visits was found among the treatment group compared to the control group.[22] The clinical implications of such immune function benefits are continuing to be investigated. Given the importance of immune function in HIV disease and AIDS, further research on the psychoimmunology of psychosocial interventions is likely to lead to clinically useful results.

In addition to reducing HIV risk behavior, cognitive-behavioral group interventions have been successful at reducing stress symptoms. For example, cognitive restructuring and developing adaptive coping skills have produced marked improvement in reducing "reexperiencing" and "avoidance" symptoms. This is an extremely important clinical finding in light of the fact that the most frequently experienced symptoms in PTSD are reexperiencing and autonomic arousal symptoms.[23] A body of evidence over the past decade indicates that when different treatment modalities are compared, cognitive-behavioral interventions are the most effective in alleviating trauma symptoms.[24] Notably, cognitive-behavioral interventions that have been successful in reducing PTSD symptoms have also been successful at reducing comorbid psychological distress.[25]

Fortunately, group interventions that provide social support and the ability to learn adaptive coping skills have been successful in helping patients manage their anxiety and depression.[26] It is clear from the literature that distress, PTSD symptoms, social network exposure, and drug abuse can complicate the course of HIV disease and may predispose vulnerable individuals to engage in risk behavior. It is also clear that psychosocial interventions, particularly those conducted within a group format, have consistently demonstrated efficacy in reducing risk behavior, alleviating psychological distress, and improving health outcomes. Incorporating psychosocial approaches to the standard treatment and care of patients with HIV disease or AIDS may promote better health outcomes by reducing morbidity and mortality.

SUMMARY

Transforming how medicine views psychosocial factors within the context of chronic illness undoubtedly means treating HIV infection from an interdisciplinary approach, which focuses appropriate attention on the psychosocial influences that affect disease course. As individuals live longer with HIV disease, becoming middle- or older-aged, it will be necessary to consider developmental influences on psychosocial functioning within the context of a chronic, life-threatening disease that continues to be socially stigmatized. The research suggests that disclosure, depression, social support, and stress are four important psychological domains that will need to be considered through this developmental lens as health providers intervene to improve HIV-related health outcomes.

ACKNOWLEDGMENTS

Manuscript preparation was supported, in part, by the following research grants: NIMH, R01 MH54930 (PI, David Spiegel), NIMH R03 MH63643 (PI, Cheryl Gore-Felton), and NIMH Center grant P30-MH52776.

REFERENCES

1. Komiti A, Judd F, Grech P, et al. Depression in people living with HIV/AIDS attending primary care and outpatient clinics. *AIDS*. 2003;37:70–78.
2. Leserman J. HIV disease progression: depression, stress, and possible mechanisms. *Biol Psychiatry*. 2003;54:295–306.
3. Moskowitz JT. Positive affect predicts lower risk of AIDS mortality. *Psychosom Med*. 2003;65:620–626.

4. Antoni MH, Cruess DG, Klimas N, et al. Increases in a marker of immune system reconstitution are predated by decreases in 24-h urinary cortisol output and depressed mood during a 10-week stress management intervention in symptomatic HIV-infected men. *J Psychosom Res*. 2005;58:3–13.
5. Gore-Felton C, Koopman C. Traumatic experiences: harbinger of risk behavior among HIV-positive adults. *J Trauma Dissoc*. 2002;3:121–135.
6. Evans DL, Leserman J, Perkins DO, et al. Severe life stress as a predictor of early disease progression in HIV infection. *Am J Psychiatry*. 1997;154:630–634.
7. Lutgendorf SK, Antoni MH, Ironson G, et al. Cognitive processing style, mood, and immune function following HIV seropositivity notification. *Cogn Ther Res*. 1997;21:157–184.
8. Stewart KE, Cianfrini LR, Walker JF. Stress, social support and housing are related to health status among HIV-positive persons in the Deep South of the United States. *AIDS Care*. 2005;17:350–358.
9. Sarna L, Van Servellen GL, Padilla G. Comparison of emotional distress in men with acquired immunodeficiency syndrome and in men with cancer. *Appl Nurs Res*. 1996,9:209–212.
10. Theorell T, Blomkvist V, Jonsson H, et al. Social support and the development of immune function in human immunodeficiency virus infection. *Psychosom Med*. 1995;57:32–36.
11. Goodkin K, Feaster DJ, Tuttle R, et al. Bereavement is associated with time-dependent decrements in cellular immune function in asymptomatic human immunodeficiency virus type 1-seropositive homosexual men. *Clin Diagn Lab Immunol*. 1996;3:109–118.
12. Cohen S, Wills TA. Stress, social support, and the buffering hypothesis. *Psychol Bull*. 1985;98:310–357.
13. McEwen BS. Protective and damaging effects of stress mediators. *N Engl J Med*. 1998;338:171–179.
14. Posener JA, Schildkraut JJ, Samson JA, et al. Diurnal variation of plasma cortisol and homovanillic acid in healthy subjects. *Psychoneuroendocrinology*. 1996;21:33–38.
15. Biglino A, Limone P, Forno B, et al. Altered adrenocorticotropin and cortisol response to corticotropin-releasing hormone in HIV-1 infection. *Eur J Endocrinol*. 1995;133:173–179.
16. Cole SW, Kemeny ME. Psychobiology of HIV infection. *Crit Rev Neurobiol*. 1997;11:289–321.
17. Swanson B, Zeller JM, Spear GT. Cortisol upregulates HIV p24 antigen production in cultured human monocyte-derived macrophages. *J Assoc Nurs AIDS Care*. 1998;9:78–83.
18. Leserman J, Petitto JM, Golden RN, et al. Impact of stressful life events, depression, social support, coping, and cortisol on progression to AIDS. *Am J Psychiatry*. 2000;157:1221–1228.
19. Deeks SG, Smith M, Holodniy M, et al. HIV-1 protease inhibitors: a review for clinicians. *JAMA*. 1997;277:145–153.
20. Spiegel D. Effects of psychotherapy on cancer survival. *Nat Rev Cancer*. 2002;2:383–389.
21. Antoni MH, Cruess DG, Klimas N, et al. Stress management and immune system reconstitution in symptomatic HIV-infected gay men over time: effects on transitional naïve T cells (CD4(+)CD45RA(+)CD29(+)). *Am J Psychiatry*. 2002;159:143–145.
22. Goodkin K, Feaster DJ, Asthana D, et al. A bereavement support group intervention is longitudinally associated with salutary effects on the CD4 cell count and number of physician visits. *Clin Diagn Lab Immunol*. 1998;5:382–391.
23. Resnick HS, Kilpatrick DG, Dansky BS, et al. Prevalence of civilian trauma and posttraumatic stress disorder in a representative national sample of women. *J Consult Clin Psychol*. 1993;61:984–991.
24. Gore-Felton C, Gill M, Koopman C, et al. Acute stress reactions among victims of violence: implications for early intervention. *Aggress Viol Behav*. 1999;4:293–306.
25. Zoellner LA, Fitzgibbons LA, Foa EB. Cognitive behavioral approaches to PTSD. In: Wilson JP, Friedman MJ, Lindy JD, eds. *Treating Psychological Trauma & PTSD*. New York: Guilford Press; 2001:159–182.
26. Markowitz JC, Klerman GL, Perry SW. Interpersonal psychotherapy of depressed HIV-positive outpatients. *Hosp Community Psychiatry*. 1992;43:885–890.

CHAPTER **38**

Suicide and End-of-Life Care

Mary Ann Cohen

This chapter addresses two of the most challenging aspects of the care of persons with human immunodeficiency virus (HIV) and acquired immunodeficiency syndrome (AIDS)—suicide and end-of-life care. Although there are commonalities, each of the topics is presented separately. Some of the precipitants of suicide are also issues at the end of life in patients with HIV disease and AIDS. For example, intractable pain, severe pruritus, end-stage renal disease, and depression, as well as other psychiatric disorders, lead to high levels of distress in persons with AIDS long before the end of life. Each of these symptoms and illnesses alone may be risk factors in vulnerable individuals. These are also important factors to address at the end of life. AIDS psychiatric care and palliative care need to be integrated and offered to persons throughout the course of illness. This concept serves as the introduction to the first section of this chapter and emphasizes the need for alleviating distress and suffering, finding meaning, maximizing life potential, and networking with families and loved ones to prevent suicide in persons with HIV and AIDS.

SUICIDE

Suicide is one of the most tragic of the psychiatric aspects of AIDS. Although suicide may or may not be associated with mental illness, it is frequently associated with psychiatric disorders in persons with medical illness. Persons with medical illnesses such as cancer, end-stage renal disease, Huntington's disease, and AIDS have been found to have a high prevalence of suicide,[1-11] and those who are suicidal have been found to have a high prevalence of psychiatric disorders such as mood disorders, substance use disorders, and psychotic disorders. In persons with AIDS, HIV-associated cognitive disorders, delirium, and dementia[12] further complicate the picture and increase suicide risk. Stigma and discrimination associated with HIV infection may play a dual role in the increased suicide risk in persons with HIV infection. Stigma leads to higher levels of distress and magnifies other psychiatric symptoms. Stigma and fear of discrimination result in alienation from friends and family. Although problems with disclosure were more prevalent in the first two decades of the HIV pandemic, some persons with HIV infection continue to hide their diagnoses from family and friends. This diminishes the network of psychosocial support so critical in suicide prevention.

The first half of this chapter addresses the magnitude of the problem of suicide in persons with AIDS, the sources of suicidality, the risk factors for suicide, the psychiatric and medical comorbidities, how to assess for suicide risk, and how to prevent the tragedy of suicide.

SCOPE

Suicide is the eleventh leading cause of death in the United States. Approximately 29,000 people commit suicide in the United States each year, with a rate of suicide of 10.8 per 100,000 in the general population. There are 10 to 25 suicide attempts for every completed suicide. The risk factors for suicide in general are all magnified in persons with severe medical illnesses such as AIDS. Most of the studies of the rate of suicide in persons with HIV infection and AIDS were done early in the epidemic. The rate of suicide in these studies ranges widely from 7.4 to 66 times greater than that in the general population,[8,9] or approximately 80 to 713 per 100,000 people.

PREVALENCE AND RISK

Suicide, medical illness, and psychiatric illness are inextricably linked in persons with HIV disease and AIDS. Suicide risk has been found to be higher in persons with chronic medical illness than in the general population.[1–4] Suicide is more prevalent in persons with end-stage renal disease, cancer, Huntington's disease, and AIDS.[5–11] In persons with AIDS, the wide range in suicide prevalence, from 7.4 to 66 times greater than the general population, reflects the multiplicity of disparate cohorts and times of studies.[8–11] Most studies indicate that persons with AIDS or HIV infection are at an increased risk for suicide. Marzuk et al.[9] studied the rate of suicide in New York City during 1985. He found that the suicide rate for men with AIDS from 20 to 59 years old was 36 times that of men from 20 to 59 years without a diagnosis of AIDS and 66 times that of men of all ages combined. Coté et al.[8] studied all death certificates indicating both AIDS and suicide in the United States from 1987 through 1989. He found a 7.4-fold higher rate of suicide in persons with AIDS. Drug overdose accounted for 39% of suicides, followed by firearms (25%) and suffocation (13%). Rajs and Fugelstad[13] reviewed 21 completed suicides in Stockholm over a period of 5 years. Medicinal drug overdose was also found to be the most prevalent suicide method. Older individuals[14] and women are particularly at a higher risk for suicide. In a sample of HIV-infected persons from Milwaukee, Wisconsin, and New York City, Kalichman et al.[14] found that 27% of respondents reported suicidal ideation within 1 week before the survey. In a more recent New York City autopsy study, Marzuk et al.[15] found HIV-positive men of African-American and Latino American ethnicity, aged 35 to 54 years, to be at the highest risk for suicide.

Erfurth et al.[16] in Munich documented that the two most common reasons for psychiatric consultation in patients with AIDS were for evaluation of suicidal behavior and treatment of depression. Suicidal behavior was present in 1 of 5 patients with HIV seropositivity or AIDS in a general hospital population.[10] Woller et al.[17] studied a cohort of HIV-infected gay men and found that suicidal behavior is related more to rejection by key persons or significant others than to disease stage or immune function.

MEDICAL COMORBIDITY

It is important to recognize that persons with HIV and AIDS have many other severe medical illnesses, some of which are associated with a high prevalence of suicide. Persons with AIDS are living longer, and some are living healthier lives. They are also subject to the same illnesses as the general population and also the aging population. Most persons with AIDS and access to care do not die of complications of AIDS, but die of other diseases, some related and some unrelated to AIDS or its risk behaviors. Persons with AIDS may develop cerebrovascular disease, cardiac disease, cancer, end-stage renal disease, end-stage liver disease, pulmonary hypertension, chronic obstructive pulmonary disease, diabetes mellitus, and thyroid disease. Many of these illnesses also carry a high prevalence of suicide by themselves, but when comorbid with HIV and AIDS they may heighten the risk of suicide.

In addition to comorbid medical illnesses, persons with AIDS also have HIV-related medical conditions that may predispose them to suicide. HIV nephropathy can lead to end-stage renal disease. HIV-induced cardiomyopathy can compromise cardiac function. Multiple neurologic conditions are also instrumental in contributing to considerable suffering. HIV-associated peripheral neuropathy is an extremely painful condition, and HIV myelopathy can lead to pareses and paralyses that are extremely debilitating. Additionally, opportunistic infections and cancers, although more rare with availability of highly active antiretroviral therapy (HAART), can cause severe illness in persons who lack access to care or who are nonadherent or unable to tolerate care. Severe wasting and protein energy undernutrition as well as intractable diarrhea from cryptosporidial infection can result in profound suffering and debilitation.

The complex illnesses associated with HIV infection and the comorbid medical conditions that develop in persons living longer with HIV disease can magnify and complicate suicide risk.

PSYCHIATRIC COMORBIDITY

In patients with HIV and AIDS, as in persons with other medical illnesses, suicide is related to psychiatric comorbidity. Mood disorders, especially major depressive disorder, substance use disorders, psychotic disorders, post-traumatic stress disorder, and cognitive disorders are all found to be associated with attempted and completed suicide in persons with AIDS. Persons with AIDS and psychiatric disorders are also vulnerable to the psychiatric side effects of medications, particularly those of the antiretroviral medications such as zidovudine-induced mania or efavirenz-induced depression or mania. It is important to recognize and address underlying psychiatric disorders in order to alleviate suffering and prevent suicide in this vulnerable population.

SOURCES OF SUICIDAL IDEATION, SUICIDE ATTEMPTS, AND SUICIDE

At the present time, routine screening for HIV infection in the United States is done only in the prenatal setting. Routine screening would measurably increase life expectancy and identify the 25% of HIV-infected individuals who are estimated to be unaware of their serostatus. The introduction of the concept of routine screening further complicates the issue of suicide, as did the introduction of home testing kits for HIV.

Some persons with HIV disease or AIDS may think of suicide in response to the exquisitely painful biopsychosocial challenges that they face. In individuals with HIV infection, suicidal ideation can occur at any time, from realization of being at risk to end-stage illness. From licensing of home HIV testing kits and routine screening for HIV infection to endstage AIDS, issues of suicide prevention are of major concern. Because persons may become suicidal before, during, and after HIV testing, routine screening and home HIV testing kits put individuals at risk for suicide. In an AIDS orientation course given by the author to third-year medical students from 1985 to 1995, one or two medical students each year stated that if they tested positive, they would commit suicide. The statements were entirely spontaneous and unsolicited. They were made during discussions of strong feelings aroused while caring for patients with AIDS.

Some persons with AIDS have risk behaviors such as drug use that have led to alienation from families or communities. They felt isolated, lonely, alienated, and expendable, even before the diagnosis of AIDS. A sense of expendability may be magnified by the stigma and discrimination related to HIV infection.

SUICIDE PREVENTION

The importance of taking a suicide history and evaluating for underlying psychiatric disorders cannot be overemphasized. Every patient with HIV infection should be screened for pain, distress, anxiety, depression, and substance use disorders. An integrated medical-psychiatric approach is most helpful in providing comprehensive care and addressing psychiatric problems. Some patients prefer to have the psychiatric care provided for them in the medical setting because they may view a psychiatric setting as yet another stigma. Furthermore, this integrated approach enables the members of a multidisciplinary team to work together to provide care, including physicians of multiple specialties, social workers, and nurses, as well as psychiatrists.

Suicide history-taking should include the following questions:

1. Have you ever tried to kill yourself?
2. What made you think of suicide?
3. Have you made any plans for suicide and, if so, what are they?
4. Have you ever thought of killing yourself before?
5. What would you accomplish by killing yourself?
6. Do you know anyone among your family members or friends who committed suicide?
7. Do you feel like you would be better off dead?
8. Do you feel like killing yourself now?

Far from harming the patient, talking about suicidal thoughts and feelings is highly relieving.

Persons with HIV infection may feel isolated and alienated. Thoughts of suicide, while on the one hand providing some measure of consolation and control, may be frightening and painful on the other. Sharing suicidal feelings with an empathic listener is not only relieving, but may enable the suicidal person to achieve a different perspective.

To prevent suicide in patients with HIV disease and AIDS, it is important to recognize dementia, delirium, depression, post-traumatic stress disorder, and psychosis. It is also important to understand the vulnerability to losses, stigma, and alienation. Persons with AIDS are also especially vulnerable to pain, pruritus, and multiple medical illnesses that increase the risk for suicide. Persons with HIV disease and AIDS respond extremely well to therapeutic modalities aimed at providing support and bolstering defenses and coping strategies. These include individual and group psychotherapy, crisis intervention, networking, treatment of psychiatric disorders, and use of relaxation techniques. The recognition and identification of stressors and precipitants are critical to prevention of suicide. Finally, to prevent suicide, it is most important to identify family members or friends who can be called on to stay with the patient and to provide a network of psychosocial support.

For the suicidal person with AIDS to resolve the suicide crisis, it is most important to establish a relationship, to restore hope, to restore or find meaning, and to develop goals. These require attention to the individual's philosophies of life and of death, to spirituality, and culture. It is important to recognize that every plan of care needs to be tailored to the needs, preferences, and background of the suicidal person.

The second half of this chapter addresses issues involved with the care of persons with AIDS at the end of life.

END-OF-LIFE CARE

The person with HIV infection needs to be able to have a way of preserving meaning and maintaining dignity and humanity from the day of diagnosis until the day of death. AIDS palliative care can be defined as comprehensive multidisciplinary care that focuses on maximizing life potentials independent of severity, stage, or prognosis. Although most clinicians emphasize the need for palliation at the end of life, palliative care can be more than end-of-life comfort care. Comfort takes on a greater role as curative care becomes less feasible and cure, care, and palliation are seen as part of a single smooth continuum.[18] The highest priority is to provide the utmost in comfort and security that care will be provided, that the patient need not fear abandonment by caregivers, and that all efforts to recognize and to alleviate symptoms will be made.

SYMPTOM MANAGEMENT

BIOLOGIC ASPECTS

With each symptom described, it is important to determine the specific cause of each symptom if at all possible. If the cause is reversible, efforts to do so need to be made, but even if the cause cannot be identified or alleviated, different avenues of relief may need to be pursued, depending on the basis for the symptom. In the interest of covering all of the biologic aspects of symptom management, this issue will be presumed to be part of the assessment of each of the following symptoms.

Pain

Pain is an incapacitating symptom in persons with any illness and is a devastating symptom in persons with AIDS. It is important to note that the risk of developing opioid dependence in the medically ill patient is extremely low, estimated to be 0.3%. Undertreated pain results in an increase in psychological distress and a reduction in the quality of life. Most pain related to severe illness can be adequately alleviated.

Pain is associated with increased risk of suicide in persons with HIV infection, as discussed in the first half of this chapter. Undertreatment of pain can also lead patients to request physician-assisted suicide. Pain is frequently undertreated in persons with AIDS, despite the needless suffering and the dangerous concomitant of suicide. Undertreatment of pain can result from inadequate assessment, unfamiliarity with management strategies, unconscious resistance and fears on the part of patients and caregivers, discrimination and stigma, and myths about analgesic use. Pain is best treated on an around-the-clock or standing order schedule rather than on an "as-needed" or "prn" basis, regardless of its etiology. As-needed orders for analgesia result in inadequate pain control when the length of time between doses is longer than the duration of the analgesic action of the medication ordered. The importance of standing orders for pain management has been described. It is stressful and depressing to be in pain, but it is even more upsetting to be in pain and to be faced with the humiliation of having to ask or beg for pain medication. As-needed orders should be reserved for rescue doses in the treatment of breakthrough pain in individuals who are on a standing analgesia regimen.

Long-acting narcotics such as long-acting morphine and fentanyl transdermal (Duragesic) system are most useful. Neuropathic pain responds to adjuvant or coanalgesic agents, including anticonvulsants and tricyclic antidepressants. Gabapentin (Neurontin) is extremely useful because it is not metabolized in the body and has no significant drug–drug interactions. Tricyclic antidepressants with low anticholinergic activity, such as nortriptyline, are effective and can provide relief from both pain and insomnia. Meperidine (Demerol) is contraindicated because its metabolite, normeperidine, is neurotoxic and can lead to confusion, tremors, myoclonus, and seizures.

It is important to recognize that persons with AIDS who are also drug dependent have more complex pain-related issues. Manipulative and sociopathic behaviors diminish when pain is adequately treated in persons with AIDS and drug dependence. Persons with HIV infection and opioid dependence have a higher tolerance for narcotics and need higher doses of potent analgesics to adequately treat their nociceptive pain. The prevalence of pain in persons with AIDS does not differ when populations of injection drug users (IDUs) are compared with non-IDUs. However, pain is greatly undermedicated in drug-dependent persons with AIDS. Pain control in persons with a history of drug dependence or who are active drug users can be adequately achieved by setting aside unnecessary concerns or hesitations. With previously addicted patients who are currently drug free, clinicians should follow the same guidelines for administration of analgesics that are recommended for persons who have never been addicted. For those patients who express concerns about use of opioids for pain relief, it is helpful to reassure them that adequate pain relief will not lead to relapse. Clinical research has shown that former drug users who have HIV infection do not have increased complaints of pain or greater need for opioids than those without addiction history.[19] IDUs with HIV infection and pain do not exaggerate their complaints and need dual treatment for addiction and pain. Agitation and behavioral dyscontrol result from both drug withdrawal states and severe pain. Agitation should be understood as an extreme manifestation of physiologic distress. IDUs and persons on methadone maintenance as agonist therapy for drug dependence have a high tolerance for opioids. For patients not on methadone maintenance but in heroin withdrawal, as is the case in many acute care settings in inner city hospitals, a methadone detoxification protocol is effective in treating heroin withdrawal.

When a person with AIDS and pain is maintained on a standing dose of methadone or treated with methadone for heroin withdrawal, the pain should be treated as a separate problem. Pain management needs to be carefully tailored to the needs of the individual, with an awareness of the psychological and social factors that may be contributing. Adequate pain management can provide comfort, relieve anxiety, alleviate suffering, and prevent suicide.

Itching

It is important to recognize and treat pruritus associated with AIDS and with its comorbid conditions, such as end-stage liver disease and end-stage kidney disease. Itching may be alleviated with doxepin cream for local use, doxepin systemically in low doses, or hydroxyzine.

Hiccups

Intractable hiccups are an extremely incapacitating symptom, especially at the end of life. Persistent hiccups can cause anorexia, weight loss, disabling insomnia, and depression. They can lead to overwhelming exhaustion and feelings of utter helplessness. Determining the cause may be helpful in directing specific treatment approaches. Antipsychotic medications, including chlorpromazine, haloperidol, and olanzapine, have been helpful in alleviation of symptoms. Hiccups may also be associated with nausea.

Nausea, Vomiting, and Diarrhea

Nausea, vomiting, and diarrhea are multifactorial and prevalent in end-stage AIDS. Almost any of the typical or atypical antipsychotic medications are effective as adjuncts or as treatments for nausea and vomiting. For intractable nausea and vomiting, ondansetron and granisetron along with low doses of olanzapine are extremely effective. For nausea and vomiting, as well as for diarrhea, it is important to identify and treat the cause. Often, in late-stage AIDS, it is difficult to resolve severe cryptosporidial diarrhea even with appropriate treatment. Exquisite humiliation and discomfort can result from uncontrollable watery diarrhea, and adults may need to wear absorbent undergarments. It is also crucial to alert caregivers to understandable feelings of discomfort or resentment attendant on having to repeatedly change and clean a patient after diarrheal accidents. Providing support for patient, family, and staff is crucial during this time. Providing symptomatic treatment and support are crucial and should be centered around relieving suffering and preserving dignity. Discussing feelings about loss of control can be relieving.

Dyspnea
Dyspnea is a frightening symptom at any time of life and adds to the distress at the end of life. Patients with dyspnea describe intense anxiety, panic, and fear of death by asphyxiation or drowning. It is reassuring to patients to know that at the end of life, if there is no hope for recovery, dying without intubation can be made more comfortable with the use of intravenous morphine. Morphine alleviates pain and dyspnea, along with the anxiety accompanying them. Olanzapine in low doses may also be helpful, along with a feeling of a breeze from a fan near the patient's bedside. Reassurance that the patient's wishes will be respected with regard to intubation and that the patient will not be abandoned but will be provided with comfort care and relief of distress and anxiety are essential.

PSYCHOLOGICAL ASPECTS

Distress
Persons with HIV disease and AIDS have high levels of distress from multiple sources, including symptoms, medical and psychiatric illness, discrimination and stigma, and social and financial stresses. Cohen et al.[20] found a 72% prevalence of distress, 70% prevalence of anxiety, and 55% prevalence of depression in a waiting room sample of patients at an HIV clinic. Distress at the end of life is considerably heightened by severe symptoms. It is important to identify and treat sources of distress.

Existential Anxiety
It is most important to be able to talk openly about death with persons with AIDS or any severe illness at the end of life. The patient may be reluctant to talk about death with family members for fear of overburdening them and may enter into a painful collusion of silence. Open dialog with patients about fears, philosophies, and spiritual beliefs can be extremely rewarding to both patients and the psychiatrist or caregiver who embarks on these discussions. Caring, compassionate, and empathic listening can be extremely supportive to patients and can also be a model for their beginning a dialog with family and loved ones.

Spiritual needs should be explored and addressed. These issues are covered in more depth in Chapter 34. It is important to involve chaplains if the patient is willing. Working with chaplaincy can provide an important level of consolation and care. It is important to explore whether patients have a belief in God and whether they have a specific religious affiliation. If patients feel they need to express angry feelings toward God, it may be important to do so in order to come to terms with the guilt this may have engendered. Some patients, on the other hand, may blame themselves for the illness and need to feel that they can be forgiven. It is especially important with HIV disease and AIDS that persons accept that it was a virus that caused them to be sick, not their behavior.

Psychiatric Disorders
Just as in suicide prevention, the recognition and treatment of psychiatric disorders is most important in order to alleviate suffering at the end of life. Delirium is highly prevalent in end-stage illness and often occurs in patients with end-stage AIDS. Persons with delirium respond well to olanzapine as a standing around-the-clock order. Efforts can be made to reverse the delirium, if this is possible and in keeping with the patient's wishes for care. In addition to delirium, patients may also have dementia, depression, anxiety, psychosis, and substance use disorders. Treatment with psychotherapy and medications may be indicated.

Social Factors

Alienation, isolation, and fear of dying alone have been addressed. It is important to address unresolved family conflicts and reunite patients with their families if possible. At times, patients are reluctant to disclose their diagnoses and isolate themselves to protect their families from awareness of AIDS. If it is not possible to resolve conflicts or to assist patients with disclosure, then a network of volunteers or even of caregivers can provide some modicum of support. One of the most valuable processes at the end of life is to help patients find meaning in their lives. This can be done as part of the therapeutic process, but also can be done through writing or dictating a life story. Being able to do a life review with a caring and compassionate listener is extremely therapeutic and provides a source of relief and comfort. Maintaining a sense that life has meaning and purpose is important throughout life and becomes more important at the end of life. The process helps patients maintain their dignity in the face existential anxiety and death. The psychotherapeutic process is also an extremely valuable part of care at the end of life. Patients are faced with profound separation anxiety and may be unable to express feelings to small children and teenagers whom they know that they will be leaving behind. The most significant countertransferential issues in psychotherapy at the end of life have to do with the profound sense of loss and sorrow that may reactivate unresolved mourning in the psychiatrist's life. It is important for the therapeutic process for the psychiatrist to be comfortable with strong feelings of sadness and even able to cry with a patient and hold hands at the end of life. However, it is also essential for psychiatrists to be sure that they are not over-identifying with the patient and that there is a colleague or team member with whom these feelings can be discussed and shared.

HOME VISITS

Psychosocial support at the end of life may entail visits to the home of the patient when the patient is confined primarily to bed as a result of weakness, loss of continence, and severe neurologic deficits and illness severity precludes outpatient visits. Home visits with a team comprising a nurse, social worker, psychiatrist, and member of the palliative care service can lead to a comfortable death with as much freedom from distress and fear as is possible. It is important to time such visits to include caregivers, especially family members, in the process. The psychotherapeutic process may consist more of holding hands and talking more briefly to the patient and accepting that the patient may need to sleep and may go in and out of delirium at times with end-stage illness. Here, acceptance, flexibility, and especially the psychiatrist's comfort with holding the patient's hand are of importance.

ADVANCE DIRECTIVES AND PRESERVATION OF SELF-DETERMINATION

Caregivers need to begin discussions early, while an HIV-seropositive person is healthy and can plan for the future. A healthy seropositive pregnant woman needs to be able to discuss her choice of a surrogate parent for her child, should she become ill, disabled, or die. All HIV-seropositive individuals should be encouraged to designate someone whom they trust to act on their behalf and to make medical decisions for them, should they no longer have the capacity to make these decisions for themselves. The advance directives can be documented in the form of a living will or medical durable power of attorney. The designation of someone trusted can be codified in a health care proxy, which is a document designating a health care agent. The process of making choices about advance directives should be part of a three-way discussion among the HIV-seropositive individual or person with AIDS, the person's primary physician, and the health care agent. The discussion may involve the patient's philosophy of life and death, belief systems, and resolution of conflicts about some of these difficult issues. The discussion should include all forms of decision-making,   luding medical care and end-of-life decisions such as do-not-resuscitate (DNR) orders and foregoing life-sustaining treatment.

ETHICAL ISSUES INVOLVED WITH FOREGOING LIFE-SUSTAINING TREATMENT

The evaluation of whether life-sustaining treatment should be initiated, maintained, foregone, withheld, or withdrawn depends on the values and preferences of the patient. Life-sustaining treatment is defined as mechanical ventilation, renal dialysis, chemotherapy, antibiotics, and artificial nutrition and hydration. Patients need to understand both the risks and benefits of artificial nutrition and hydration. They need to understand that tubes can be uncomfortable, that central lines can become infected, that intravenous lines can infiltrate. No distinction is made between withholding, withdrawing, or foregoing life-sustaining treatment. There are also some indications that when artificial hydration and nutrition are withheld, individuals need not be uncomfortable because of endogenous opioid secretion, as well as administration of analgesics for pain. Physicians have an obligation to relieve pain and suffering and promote the dignity and autonomy of dying patients in their care. This includes providing effective pain treatment even if it may foreseeably hasten death. Providing a model for comfort care and a nurturing, supportive environment includes changing many traditional health care practices and ensuring participatory decision-making styles.

ETHICAL ISSUES INVOLVED WITH DETERMINATION OF CAPACITY FOR DECISION-MAKING

Every individual should be presumed to have the capacity for decision-making and the right to self-determination. Every patient should be able to decide whether to stay in a health care facility, accept medical care, refuse procedures, or sign out against medical advice (AMA). When it appears to the physician that the patient is unable to understand or reason about his or her medical care, the physician can make a determination of decisional capacity. This determination is an assessment of a person's capabilities for understanding, communicating, and reasoning about specific issues. Mental illness per se, including dementia, schizophrenia, or depression, does not necessarily preclude decision-making. Any physician can determine decisional capacity. If an attending physician finds it difficult to make a determination, he or she can call upon a psychiatrist to assist. One of the most frequent concerns in the health care setting is whether or not an individual has the capacity to decide about DNR orders. The patient with HIV dementia may still be able to decide about a DNR order. To be able to give informed consent for DNR or no emergency cardiopulmonary resuscitation (CPR), an individual must be able to understand the following:

1. The general nature of the illness, its severity, and implications.
2. The meaning and implication of respiratory or cardiac arrest ("if my lungs or heart stop, I will die").
3. The distinction between CPR in an otherwise healthy person who has sudden trauma or arrhythmia and CPR in end-stage illness with severe compromise of health, immunity, organ function, and cognition.
4. The nature of CPR and the need for mechanical ventilation, intubation, and external cardiac massage.
5. The consequence of a DNR order.
6. The fact that an individual can change his or her mind about DNR.
7. A DNR order does not imply withholding or withdrawing care. Those are entirely separate issues.

Understanding issues of decisional capacity in individuals with HIV dementia can help preserve the delicate balance between safety and autonomy in the end-of-life care of persons with AIDS.

SUMMARY

Persons with AIDS are living longer, healthier lives because of good medical care, antiretroviral therapies, and prophylaxis for some of the previously fatal complications such as *Pneumocystis jiroveci* (formerly *carinii*) pneumonia (PCP). For persons living longer to live more comfortable lives, with preservation of independence and dignity, it is important to establish special integrated nurturing, supportive, and loving health care environments. Integrated medical and psychiatric care can alleviate distress and suffering, prevent suicide, and preserve dignity and autonomy in persons with AIDS from the time of diagnosis to the time of death.

REFERENCES

1. Barraclough B, Bunch J, Nelson B, et al. A hundred cases of suicide: clinical aspects. *Br J Psychiatry*. 1974;125:355–373.
2. Blumenthal SJ. Suicide: a guide to risk factors, assessment, and treatment of suicidal patients. *Med Clin North Am*. 1988;72:937–971.
3. Harris EC, Barraclough BM. Suicide as an outcome for medical disorders. *Medicine*. 1994;73:281–296.
4. McHugh PR. Suicide and medical afflictions. *Medicine*. 1994;73:297–298.
5. Abram HS, Moore GL, Westervelt FB. Suicidal behavior in chronic dialysis patients. *Am J Psychiatry*. 1971;127:119–124.
6. Breitbart W. Suicide in cancer patients. *Oncology*. 1987;4:49–54.
7. Schoenfeld M, Myers RH, Cupples LA, et al. Increased rate of suicide among patients with Huntington's disease. *J Neurol Neurosurg Psychiatry*. 1984;47:1283–1287.
8. Coté TR, Biggar RJ, Dannenberg AL. Risk of suicides among persons with AIDS: a national assessment. *JAMA*. 1992;268:2066–2068.
9. Marzuk PM, Tierney H, Tardiff K, et al. Increased risk of suicide in persons with AIDS. *JAMA*. 1988;259:1333–1337.
10. Alfonso CA, Cohen MA, Aladjem AD, et al. HIV seropositivity as a major risk factor for suicide in the general hospital. *Psychosomatic*. 1994;35:368–373.
11. Gala C, Pergami A, Catalan J, et al. Risk of deliberate self-harm and factors associated with suicidal behaviors among asymptomatic individuals with human immunodeficiency virus infection. *Acta Psychiatr*. 1992;86:70–75.
12. Alfonso CA, Cohen MAA. HIV-dementia and suicide. *Gen Hosp Psychiatry*. 1994;16:45–46.
13. Rajs J, Fugelstad A. Suicide related to human immunodeficiency virus infection in Stockholm. *Acta Psychiatr Scand*. 1992;85:234–239.
14. Kalichman SC, Heckman T, Kochman A, et al. Depression and thoughts of suicide among middle-aged and older persons living with HIV-AIDS. *Psychiatric Serv*. 2000;5:903–907.
15. Marzuk PM, Tardiff K, Leon AC, et al. Seroprevalence among suicide victims in New York City, 1991–1993. *Am J Psychiatry*. 1997;154:1720–1725.
16. Erfurth A, Naber D, Goebel FD. AIDS disease and psychopathology-observations by the psychiatric consultation service of an internal medicine clinic. *Fortschr Neurol Psychiatry*. 1989;57:469–473.
17. Woller W, Arendt G, Kruse J, et al. Prediction of suicidality in HIV-positive men [abstract]. *Int Conf AIDS*. 1993;9:896.
18. Cohen MAA, Alfonso CA. AIDS psychiatry: Psychiatric and palliative care and pain management. In: Wormser GP, ed. *AIDS and Other Manifestations of HIV Infection*. 4th ed. San Diego: Elsevier Academic Press; 2004:538–576.
19. Ferrando SJ. Substance abuse and HIV infection. *Psychiatric Ann*. 2001;31:57–62.
20. Cohen MA, Hoffman RG, Cromwell C, et al. The prevalence of distress in persons with human immunodeficiency virus infection. *Psychosomatics*. 2002;43:10–15.

SECTION VII

Policy Issues

CHAPTER 39

Prevention and Education Strategies

Michael D. Knox, Tiffany Chenneville

An estimated 5 million people are infected worldwide each year with the human immunodeficiency virus (HIV).[1] The United States has over 40,000 new acquired immunodeficiency syndrome (AIDS) cases[2] and about the same number of new HIV infections annually. These statistics are appalling because research has demonstrated that HIV infection and AIDS prevention programs work.[3] There are effective prevention models for all routes of HIV transmission and all populations at risk.[4–6] Successful disease prevention activities include education and access to information, counseling, HIV testing, and prevention supplies, including latex condoms and sterile injection equipment. The cost of preventing HIV infections varies, but it always represents a small fraction of the cost of providing the life-long pharmaceutical treatment required following a diagnosis of HIV infection.[7]

The traditional nomenclature of primary, secondary, and tertiary prevention can be applied to HIV disease and AIDS. The clinician has a role at all levels, which progresses along a continuum from that of educator at the primary prevention level to that of treatment provider at the tertiary prevention level. The role of the clinician at the primary prevention level is that of an educator who provides instruction to uninfected persons about behaviors that promote good health and reduce the likelihood of HIV transmission. This includes educational programs and messages for patients, at-risk populations, and the general community. Counseling and risk assessment are also important prevention strategies at this level. At the secondary prevention level, the role of the clinician includes not only HIV transmission reduction strategies, but also early intervention for those infected. The goal at this level is to control disease progression for HIV-infected individuals and to prevent further spread of the disease. Secondary prevention can include early testing and identification of those infected in order to prevent transmission by those who may be unaware of their infection. Partner notification and providing appropriate support to HIV-infected patients to assist them in developing and maintaining a repertoire of risk reduction behaviors are important as well.

Finally, at the tertiary prevention level, the role of the clinician broadens to include intensive treatment for infected individuals. This includes reducing viral load and treating the physical and mental health of the patient by providing the necessary foundation for maintaining safer behaviors and maximizing quality of life. Treatment is covered in depth elsewhere; this chapter focuses on the clinician's role in HIV disease and AIDS primary and secondary prevention. It is important to point out, however, that treatment options change rapidly and that keeping up to date is crucial. Continuing education is available through the federally funded AIDS Education and Training Centers that educate clinicians nationwide.

ASSESSMENT OF RISK

Behavioral risk assessment is a necessary and important component of HIV prevention.[6] Clinicians should incorporate screening for behavioral risk factors into the routine office visit with every new patient as part of an initial intake and on a regular basis with existing clients. The results can aid in clinical intervention, provide a focus for risk reduction strategies or referrals, and provide opportunities for education and counseling. For patients, a behavioral risk assessment provides an opportunity to ask questions and discuss concerns, which may increase positive changes in their behavior.

A thorough behavioral risk assessment includes a frank discussion about sexual and drug (including alcohol) use behaviors. This can only happen after good rapport between clinician and patient has been established. Given the sensitive nature of these topics, it is important to discuss the purpose of the assessment with the patient and to reassure him or her that information gathered will remain confidential. Table 39.1 includes risk assessment techniques recommended by the National Network of STD/HIV Prevention Training Centers.[6]

A thorough clinical risk assessment elicits symptoms of early HIV infection and other sexually transmitted infections (STIs). The clinician assesses for signs or symptoms consistent with chronic infection and problems associated with STIs (e.g., genital ulcers, warts, blisters, or other lesions) or HIV infection (e.g., headaches, diarrhea, fatigue, fever, chills, night sweats, skin lesions, rash, weight loss, oral thrush). When conducting a drug use risk assessment, the clinician must gather specific information about the types of drugs injected and whether clean needles were or are used.

When conducting a sexual risk assessment, the primary goal is to elicit accurate clinical and behavioral information, including the identification of specific risk behaviors. First, and

TABLE 39.1 Risk Assessment Techniques

Recommendations	Examples
Begin with nonthreatening questions	• Ask about history of STIs
Make no assumptions	• Avoid personally held stereotypes
	• Ask all patients about sexual history and practices
Be tactful and respectful	• Use appropriate nonverbal language
	• Communicate acceptance by head nodding and making eye contact
Be clear and ask direct questions about specific behaviors	• Avoid medical jargon
	• Clarify when necessary
Be nonjudgmental	• Recognize patient anxiety
	• Recognize your own biases
	• Avoid biased language, such as "You should . . ."
Use open-ended questions	• "Tell me about your current sexual practices." instead of "Are you sexually active?"
Avoid closed-ended (yes/no) questions	
Encourage the patient to talk when necessary	• "Say it in your own words"
"Normalize" behaviors so as to elicit honest responses from patients	• "Sometimes people have anal intercourse. Have you ever had anal intercourse?"

most important, the clinician must determine if the patient has been having sex. Although this seems obvious, the clinician must clarify definitions of sexual practice. For example, some patients may not report oral sex when responding to questions about whether or not they have been sexually active. Therefore it is important for the clinician to clarify what the patient means by "having sex." Once it has been established that the patient has been sexually active, it is important to determine the number and gender of sexual partners, both current and past. Avoid assumptions; it is not enough for clinicians to ask patients about their marital status or sexual identity. Marriage between heterosexuals does not preclude same-sex behavior among one or both partners. Furthermore, some who identify themselves as "heterosexual" may have same-sex partners and others who identify themselves as "homosexual" may have opposite-sex partners. Therefore the clinician must assess behaviors and avoid making inferences based on labels or self-descriptions.

Clinicians must inquire about the HIV status and history of STIs among sexual partners, keeping in mind that this information may be unknown. In completing the risk assessment, the clinician also may ascertain how the patient meets sexual partners (e.g., the Internet, bars, bathhouses, circuit parties, public venues, etc.). The clinician should then inquire about the various types of sexual activity in which the patient engages (i.e., oral, anal, vaginal) and the extent to which condoms or other barrier contraceptives are used, if at all. Further inquiry about condom use may involve questions such as the following[6]:

- What has your experience been with condom use?
- How frequently do you use condoms?
- Do you use condoms during certain sexual acts but not during others?
- Do you use condoms with certain partners but not with others?
- Are there factors or situations that interfere with your use of condoms?
- Do you feel confident about your ability to use condoms correctly?
- Did you use a condom the last time you had sex?

If conducting these assessments is too time-consuming for regular office visits, consider prescreening. The use of self-administered questionnaires or computer-, audio-, or video-assisted questionnaires are appropriate for the prescreening process. In addition, ancillary staff may conduct brief interviews with patients. The clinician can use the results of the pre-screening to more efficiently conduct a thorough risk assessment. Clinicians may consider using the HIV-risk screening instrument (HSI), which is a 10-item scale designed to discriminate between low- and high-risk behaviors associated with HIV infection.[8] Questions on the HSI elicit information about whether or not patients have engaged in specific risky behaviors, as opposed to the frequency with which patients engage in those behaviors, based on research that suggests participants are likely to respond more accurately when responses required are categorical in nature (i.e., yes, no, don't know). The specific risk factors assessed on the HSI include history of sexual intimacy with more than one sexual partner, history of anal sex and the extent to which condoms were used during anal sex, history (or sexual partner with history) of STIs, history of bartering for sex, history (or sexual partner with history) of injection drug use, and history of sexual intimacy with men who have had sex with men. Many questions on the HSI are phrased to elicit information about whether or not the behaviors listed have occurred within the past 10 years.

Besides time constraints, it is important to recognize certain barriers to effective risk assessment. Patients' perceptions that they are being stigmatized by a clinician certainly is one barrier. However, many patients may not only be comfortable discussing their sexual behavior, but may actually expect clinicians to gather such information. The discomfort associated with discussing sexual behavior often lies with the clinician. Clinicians not only report discomfort asking personal questions about sexual behavior, as well as discomfort responding to issues that arise in response to these questions.[9,10] Clinicians sometimes lack confidence in their ability to make the client comfortable, especially when discussing same-sex relationships. Finally, misconceptions held by the clinician regarding sexual behavior and level of risk act as barriers to effective risk assessment. These barriers can be addressed by developing specific policies and procedures for conducting risk assessments. This may include identifying specific questions to be asked during the assessment, developing a plan for responding to information that might surface, determining how information will be integrated into the patient's overall care, and training staff how to perform prescreenings or thorough risk assessments. Practice and experience will increase clinician comfort levels.

PATIENT EDUCATION

HIV infection prevention must become a high priority for all mental health professionals. Clinicians must educate teenagers and young adults who do not know how to properly use and remove a condom. We must educate pregnant women about mother-to-child transmission. We should teach our patients to take the necessary personal precautions to minimize the possibility of transmission of this deadly disease. This requires a frank and open discussion of sex and drug use with our patients and members of the community with whom we come in contact. A clinician might find it useful to use a model of a penis or an educational chart to provide patients with an explicit demonstration of the proper use of condoms. The correct procedure for removing the condom without spilling the contents should be emphasized. Clinicians should also be able to demonstrate the proper use of a female condom. It is important that clinicians gain proficiency in these demonstrations and overcome any barriers they have in terms of their comfort level with providing this type of experiential education. Clinicians should also keep in mind the sensitive nature of this educational material. Some patients, especially those suffering from certain mental illnesses, may become anxious or agitated in response to this type of explicit demonstration. Good clinical training and sound professional judgment will be imperative when confronting these issues. Furthermore, normalizing these behaviors is likely to help put patients at ease, which is why it is so important for clinicians to increase their proficiency and comfort levels.

Patient education should also emphasize behavior-focused prevention messages.[6] Education should extend beyond instructions on condom use to include discussions about abstinence, being faithful to one's sexual partner, personal and mutual masturbation, safe use of needles, and the need for screening of other STIs. Furthermore, clinicians must be prepared to respond to misconceptions about HIV infection. The identification of misconceptions requires a thorough assessment of a patient's knowledge and attitudes about HIV disease. Understanding what patients know about the transmission of HIV and what their concerns are will guide clinicians' attempts to correct misconceptions. Patients' misconceptions about their relative risk of infection or the interaction between STIs and HIV are common. For example, middle-aged, married patients may not consider themselves at risk for infection based on the misconception that HIV affects only homosexuals, the sexually promiscuous, or drug users. In addition, some patients may be unaware that STIs increase susceptibility to and transmissibility of HIV. These misconceptions should be assessed and addressed by the clinician on an individual basis. It is important to note that psychiatric patients may be particularly vulnerable to contracting STIs and, once an STI is contracted, diagnosis is likely to go undetected because of socioeconomic factors and limited access to medical care, thus increasing the risk of HIV infection among mentally ill populations. (Please refer to Chapter 18 for more detailed information on STIs.)

Once misconceptions have been corrected, tailored educational interventions that include behavioral goals to address high-risk behaviors (e.g., sexual and drug use behaviors) can be developed.[6] Interventions should be based on the results of an individual risk assessment that focuses on problem behaviors, attitudes, and individual circumstances, as well as information on the type and frequency of high-risk behaviors engaged in by the patient. More detailed information about behavioral risk assessment is discussed later in this chapter. With regard to patient attitudes, the clinician must determine patients' perspectives on their level of risk, their confidence or self-efficacy with regard to the ability to change high-risk behaviors, their intention or readiness for change, and any ambivalence they are experiencing about the perceived benefits and barriers to change. Individual circumstances to be considered include the relationship dynamics that exist between the patient and others with whom the patient engages in high-risk behavior (i.e., Who has the power?); environmental or situational triggers (i.e., Where and under what circumstances are problem behaviors most likely to occur?); and barriers to the development of replacement behaviors (i.e., What are the perceived negative effects of new behaviors?).

Readiness to change is important when developing behavioral goals and can be assessed along a continuum.[6] On one end are patients who do not recognize a need to change; in this case, it is the clinician's responsibility to present evidence to the contrary by providing information in a didactic format or through storytelling. Alternatively, some patients recognize the need to change, but are faced with certain barriers; it is the clinician's responsibility to discuss these barriers and to make suggestions accordingly. Finally, on the other end of the continuum are patients who exhibit a readiness to attempt specific behavioral changes. It is important to remember that change occurs over time and in incremental stages; this is especially important for patients who are not ready for extreme behavioral changes. In such cases, opportunities must be provided for change to occur in small steps.

Follow-up is a vital component of patient education.[6] Clinicians must establish a system for monitoring a patient's progress toward behavioral goals. When behavioral goals are met, the clinician must reinforce the patient's efforts and anticipate future problems or situational changes using a series of "What if . . . ?" questions (e.g., What if you find yourself in a situation with a new partner who is not accustomed to using condoms?). If, on follow-up, a clinician finds that the patient is not meeting behavior goals, further assessment of attitudes and individual circumstances, with the goal of redesigning the tailored intervention, is crucial.

Providing HIV disease education to patients may present unique challenges. Although there does not appear to be a significant difference in AIDS knowledge between mentally ill patients and the general population, certain conditions have been correlated with sexual risk behaviors.[11] For example, patients with schizophrenia, especially those with positive and excited symptoms, have been found to be more likely to engage in risky sexual behavior whereas patients presenting with symptoms of depression and anxiety have been found to be less likely to engage in such behavior. Research suggests that mental health patients mirror the general population in terms of the fallacies held about AIDS, including overestimating the risk of exposure from casual contact. Clinicians must rely heavily on their knowledge of psychiatric diagnoses and symptomatology when designing prevention efforts. Providing knowledge without a framework within which to use that knowledge will be futile, especially with certain patients. Consider a patient with schizophrenia whose knowledge about HIV disease is high, but whose psychotropic medication adherence is low. The latter must be addressed to control symptoms that might interfere with the ability of the patient to use his or her knowledge about HIV disease to avoid high-risk behavior.

COMMUNITY LEADERSHIP

The clinician, as a community leader, may be able to influence public opinion regarding HIV infection and AIDS education in the schools, condom distribution, and needle exchange programs and through the creation of "AIDS Awareness" campaigns in the community. Knowledge is the key to prevention, and clinicians can and should take advantage of opportunities to present information about AIDS at local community events. Clinicians can create informational displays about AIDS to be used in their own offices and in public venues throughout the community. Clinicians should know what community and web-based resources are available and should attend continuing education events to keep up to date on this rapidly changing epidemic so that they can disseminate accurate information to patients and members of the community.

HIV TESTING AND EARLY DETECTION

Effective prevention programs also include HIV testing and early detection. When persons who carry the virus have been identified, education and counseling must target the behaviors that place their partners and others at risk. Testing and counseling form a proven prevention strategy.[1] This combination helps people learn how HIV is transmitted and, depending on the results of the test, take steps to avoid becoming infected or infecting others.

Rapid HIV testing is highly recommended, given the high percentage of individuals who are tested for HIV but never return for their results. Individuals with HIV infection who are unaware of their diagnosis are at risk for unknowingly spreading the disease to others. Rapid HIV antibody tests produce results within minutes to hours, which helps ensure that patients are informed of their diagnosis, will receive the information they need to manage the disease, and can prevent its spread. Results from rapid HIV antibody tests are considered preliminary, and any positive results should be confirmed via other, more reliable tests (e.g., enzyme-linked immunosorbent assay [ELISA] followed by Western blot assay). Patients must understand that a negative HIV antibody test result does *not* guarantee that the person is not currently infected or will not become infected the next day. We should teach our patients to treat all people as if they are infected and to take the necessary personal precautions to minimize the possibility of transmission of this deadly virus.[7]

Pre- and post-HIV test counseling is imperative, and this type of counseling can present unique challenges in mental health settings.[12] Although informed consent is necessary for HIV testing and counseling in any setting, issues of capacity often arise when providing these services for the mentally ill. It is important to remember that capacity to consent is not defined by the presence of a mental disorder, but rather the patient's ability to comprehend the information presented and to draw reasonable conclusions based on that information. For example, a patient presenting with delusions may or may not be competent to consent depending on the content of the delusions. Clinicians also must assess the patient's capacity to cope with test results and be prepared to confront difficult situations that might arise. Certain qualities such as empathy, respect, warmth, and genuineness, while important in all therapeutic relationships, become especially important when providing pre- and post-HIV test counseling to patients with mental illness.

PERINATAL TRANSMISSION

An estimated 200 million women become pregnant each year, about 2.5 million of whom are known to be HIV-infected.[4] The education, testing, and counseling of these women, and the provision of medication necessary to reduce the risk of mother-to-child transmission, is one of the most important, successful, and easily implemented prevention strategies. Barriers that may prevent HIV testing during pregnancy include mental illness, language barriers, cultural differences, misperceptions regarding risk, time pressures, insurance reimbursement, and clinicians' fear of offending patients. Clinicians must be certain that mentally ill patients who are pregnant receive appropriate prenatal care, including HIV counseling and testing. Clinical consultation regarding mother-to-child transmission is available from the National Perinatal

HIV Consultation and Referral Service* (See Chapter 24 for more information on HIV in neonates.)

PREVENTION FOR MENTALLY ILL PERSONS WITH HIV INFECTION

Primary prevention efforts are aimed at helping individuals avoid acquiring HIV infection. Prevention for HIV-infected patients, on the other hand, is aimed at helping individuals avoid the spread of HIV. Even among couples in which both partners are infected, continued unprotected sexual activity is not recommended because different strains of the virus exist, some of which are more difficult to treat. Furthermore, other STIs can be transmitted that complicate the course of treatment for HIV-positive individuals. Prevention for HIV-infected patients is particularly important with mentally ill populations, given that research suggests that many people with mental illness engage in high-risk behaviors.[13] Clinicians who care for HIV-infected patients with mental illness, therefore, have a unique opportunity to help change risky sexual behaviors, thus limiting the spread of this disease.

Most people with HIV disease, including those with mental illness, remain sexually active, exemplifying the need for interventions designed to reduce unsafe sex practices among HIV-positive individuals.[14] HIV disease prevention messages must be reinforced during each patient encounter.[6] A patient's knowledge and understanding of HIV transmission should be assessed and documented frequently, as well as the patient's recent engagement in behaviors that increase the risk of HIV transmission. As described elsewhere, a patient's capacity to understand and draw reasonable conclusions based on information presented should be continually assessed in light of presenting symptoms of mental illness. Based on this assessment, the clinician should provide the patient with strategies for preventing transmission to others. Some research indicates that "loss-framed approaches," which focus on the negative consequence of unsafe sex for patients and their partners, are more effective than "gain-framed approaches," which focus on the positive consequences of safer sex.[14] Research suggests that intensive (6 to 15 hours), small group cognitive-behavioral HIV-risk reduction interventions are most effective with mentally ill populations.[13,15] Interventions should include knowledge, attitudes, motivation, behavior, and cognitive skills components. Modeling, role play, rehearsal, and other behavioral skills training methods are recommended in an effort to increase patients' perceived self-efficacy to change risky behaviors. Also extremely important for this population is that HIV risk reduction interventions be culturally tailored and implemented on an ongoing basis, given that behavior changes are likely to be relatively short term.

Clinicians must educate patients about the relationship between STIs and HIV and dispel myths held by patients regarding antiretroviral treatment, viral load, and the transmissibility of the virus.[6] Many patients incorrectly believe that treatment and/or a low viral load preclude transmission and, as a result, resume high-risk behaviors. A unique problem encountered by women with HIV infection is engaging in unprotected sex in an attempt to conceive. Clinicians should inform their female patients of the risk of transmission to others, including the unborn infant, and, if necessary, should provide these patients with referrals for preconception counseling and care. Finally, partner notification is considered a key component of HIV disease prevention for HIV-positive individuals. Although partner notification laws vary by state, the clinician's role, regardless of state law, should include counseling of patients who want to disclose their HIV status but need help in doing so and support for patients who have exposed someone to HIV and request that the individual be notified.

Barriers exist regarding prevention for positives. Clinicians have reported the following obstacles to discussing sexual and drug use behaviors with their HIV-positive patients: fear of offending the patient; time pressures; lack of confidence in skills to change risky behavior;

---

*National Perinatal HIV Consultation and Referral Service, telephone: 888-448-8765 confidentiality and the sometimes conflicting duty to protect unknown victims of harm; and general communication barriers, including difficulty initiating the conversation.[9] A willingness to overcome these barriers and familiarity with the issues associated with high-risk behavior are necessary precursors to effective prevention for HIV-positive persons. Some of the strategies discussed previously for conducting a risk assessment can be used when assessing patient risk and reinforcing prevention messages for HIV-infected individuals (see Table 39.1).

The National HIV/AIDS Clinicians' Consultation Center[†] recommends using a risk behavior checklist when providing prevention for HIV-positive individuals.[9] The first component includes education on less risky sexual behaviors, including information about abstinence, mutual masturbation and oral sex, and limiting the number of sex partners. The second component involves encouraging avoidance of risky situations, including people or places that increase the likelihood of risk-taking behavior. Limiting the use of alcohol and other drugs also is recommended, especially in situations that might lead to sexual behavior. The third component includes condom education, including a discussion about types of condoms used for vaginal and anal sex, the potential benefit of condoms or barriers for oral sex, and the need to always carry condoms. The fourth, and final, component includes disclosure of HIV status to sexual partners and discussions about safer sex with sexual partners.

OTHER PREVENTION STRATEGIES

Other crucial prevention strategies include postexposure prophylaxis and the treatment of other sexually transmitted diseases and substance abuse. Postexposure prophylaxis (PEP) involves prescribing antiretroviral medication to persons exposed to HIV. PEP is used after occupational exposure to blood products.[6] Health care workers' average risk of contracting HIV via exposure to HIV-infected blood is approximately 0.3%, although factors such as deep injury and visible blood on the device responsible increase risk for infection. Following exposure, PEP should be initiated as soon as possible, ideally within hours, although PEP has been started even if the interval since exposure has exceeded several days. When choosing which antiretroviral drugs to prescribe, factors to consider include whether or not the person exposed is pregnant and if the virus to which the person has been exposed is known or suspected to be resistant to certain antiretroviral drugs. The use of PEP for persons exposed to HIV via sexual or injection drug use activity is also appropriate.[‡]

The identification and treatment of STIs also is important. Annual screenings are recommended unless the patient is considered to be at high risk for HIV (e.g., multiple anonymous partners), in which case screening for STIs should occur at 3- to 6-month intervals.[9] Screening is used as a disease control measure, the goal of which is to identify asymptomatic individuals who may be at increased risk for disease, in hopes that patients identified via screening will comply with prescribed interventions.[6] Screening programs for STIs are a cost-effective and acceptable way to help control HIV. STIs to screen for include gonorrhea, chlamydia, syphilis, genital herpes, and trichomoniasis, among others.

The clinician's role in identifying and treating substance use is another important component of prevention. Injection and noninjection drug use substantially increases the risk for HIV infection. Although injection drug users have the highest prevalence rates for HIV, substantially elevated rates of HIV infection are also present among crack cocaine users and those with other substance use disorders, including alcohol abuse.

---

†*National HIV/AIDS Clinicians' Consultation Center, telephone: 800-933-3413.*
‡*For more information about PEP, please contact the National Clinicians' Post-Exposure Hotline (PEPLine), telephone: 888-448-4911.*

SUMMARY

HIV is usually spread by individual human behavior. We know which behaviors put people at risk and how to reduce or eliminate these risks.[7] There is still no cure for HIV infection, no vaccine, and no topical microbicide for vaginal and anal tissues. Disease prevention strategies must be aggressively implemented in all clinical practices to address this epidemic in an effective and efficient manner.

REFERENCES

1. UNAIDS/World Health Organization. *AIDS Epidemic Update*. Geneva: UNAIDS/World Health Organization; December 2004.
2. Centers for Disease Control and Prevention. HIV/AIDS surveillance report 2003. Available: http://www.cdc.gov/hiv/stats/hasrlink.htm. Accessed March 30, 2005.
3. Auerbach JD, Coates TJ. HIV prevention research: accomplishments and challenges for the third decade of AIDS. *Am J Public Health*. 2000;90:1029–1032.
4. UNAIDS. *Report on the Global HIV/AIDS Epidemic*. Geneva: UNAIDS; July 2002.
5. Valdiserri RO, Ogden LL, McCray E. Accomplishments in HIV prevention science: implications for stemming the epidemic. *Nat Med*. July 2003;9:881–886.
6. Centers for Disease Control and Prevention. Incorporating HIV prevention into the medical care of persons living with HIV: recommendations of CDC, the Health Resources and Services Administration, the National Institutes of Health, and the HIV Association of Infectious Diseases Society of America. *MMWR Morb Mortal Wkly Rep*. 2003;52(RR-12):1–24.
7. Knox M. AIDS prevention leadership. *J HIV/AIDS Soc Serv*. 2005;4(3):3–6.
8. Gerbert B, Bronstone A, McPhee S, et al. Development and testing of an HIV-risk screening instrument for use in health care settings. *Am J Prev Med*. 1998;15:103–113.
9. Graves D. HIV prevention: preventing transmission from HIV-positive to HIV-negative individuals. Available: http:/www.ucsf.edu/hivcntr/Consultation_Library/PWP.html. Accessed February 8, 2006.
10. Nolte S, Sohn MA, Koons B. Prevention of HIV infection in women. *J Obstet Gynecol Neonatal Nurs*. 1993;22:128–134.
11. McKinnon K, Cournos F, Sugden R, et al. The relative contributions of psychiatric symptoms and AIDS knowledge to HIV risk behaviors among people with severe mental illness. *J Clin Psychiatry*. 1996;57:506–513.
12. Oquendo M, Tricarico P. Pre- and post-HIV test counseling. In: Cournos F, Bakalar N, eds. *AIDS and People with Severe Mental Illness: A Handbook for Mental Health Providers*. New Haven, Conn: Yale University Press; 1996:97–112.
13. Kelly JA. HIV risk reduction interventions for persons with severe mental illness. *Clin Psychol Rev*. 1997;17:293–309.
14. Richardson JL, Milam J, McCutchan AL, et al. Effect of brief safer-sex counseling by medical providers to HIV-1 seropositive patients: a multi-clinic assessment. *AIDS*. 2004;18:1179–1186.
15. Otto-Salaj LL, Kelly JA, Stevenson LY, et al. Outcomes of a randomized small-group HIV prevention intervention trial for people with serious mental illness. *Community Ment Health J*. 2001;37:123–144.

CHAPTER 40

Physician Assisted Suicide and Voluntary Euthanasia

Marshall Forstein

Clinicians who care for people with human immunodeficiency virus (HIV) infection are inevitably asked about the late stages of illness and how they will treat the patient who is terrified of suffering from unbearable physical, emotional, or spiritual pain. Suicidal ideation and behavior have been clinical concerns from the beginning of the HIV epidemic. Risk factors that predict suicidal ideation and suicidal behavior in people infected with HIV have been well documented in the literature over the course of the epidemic, providing insights for clinicians and public health professionals to attend to those who are at greatest risk.[1-3]

More complicated for both researchers and clinicians is the issue of HIV-infected patients wanting to end their lives prematurely in the context of an inextricably deteriorating mental or physical illness. Co-temporally over the last several decades with the HIV epidemic is the greater public and professional interest in end-of-life issues, including the right to refuse treatment and the right to assist in ending suffering.

DEFINITION OF EUTHANASIA AND PHYSICIAN ASSISTED SUICIDE

Voluntary euthanasia is the administration of lethal medications to a patient by a physician with the expressed intention of ending the patient's life. For purposes of this chapter, instigation is by the patient of sound mind and is to be distinguished from unlawful "mercy killing." Physician assisted suicide is defined as a physician providing medications or advice to enable patients to end their own lives. Legal and ethical distinctions exist between voluntary euthanasia and physician assisted suicide, and there are important psychological and practical issues as well. Many terminally ill patients have access to medications that could be lethal and yet do not use them to end their own lives. Many physicians prescribe medications with the knowledge, if not the intent, to provide the means for patients to end their lives.

This chapter will focus specifically on the growing social, medical, and ethical issues of physician assisted suicide and voluntary euthanasia in the person with HIV or acquired immunodeficiency syndrome (AIDS). Are suicidal ideation and behavior and physician assisted suicide and voluntary euthanasia related? Are HIV-infected people who contemplate suicide during the course of illness at greater or lesser risk for deciding to act or request assistance at the end of life? Do requests for physician assisted suicide or voluntary euthanasia in the course of deteriorating illness arise out of the same underlying dynamic issues or social concerns at all points along the course of illness from the asymptomatic phase to end-of-life situations? Why do some act to end their own lives and some request the participation of others?

It is beyond the scope of this chapter to completely review the entire literature and debate on physician assisted suicide and voluntary euthanasia. Much has been written about requests for physician assisted suicide in general and in particular the experience in The Netherlands and Oregon, where voluntary euthanasia has been legalized.[4–6]

Although most jurisdictions in the United States do not have legislation supporting physician assisted suicide or voluntary euthanasia, and many have legislation prohibiting such action by physicians, it is clear from both research and clinical practice that physicians are not infrequently asked about their beliefs and practices of these. It is also clear, given the potential legal and professional issues, that requests for physician assisted suicide and voluntary euthanasia among patients with AIDS that are accommodated by physicians are under-reported. This chapter briefly reviews the history of suicide and HIV disease and the current state of knowledge about physician and patient attitudes and beliefs about physician assisted suicide and voluntary euthanasia. Finally, conceptual and current clinical issues are discussed.

HISTORICAL CONTEXT

Probably no pandemic in the history of the world has been complicated by the particular human behaviors that facilitate transmission. Unlike the hapless victims of the plague and the influenza epidemic of 1918, HIV disease is an epidemic that highlights the role of drugs and sex throughout the cultures and societies of the entire world. The stigma associated from the very beginning with behaviors that accrued social opprobrium has left an indelible mark on the people infected, affected, and at continued risk. Early on, HIV infection was known as Gay Related Immune Deficiency Syndrome (GRID), forever delineating the "guilty" from the "innocent" victims as HIV spread throughout the world. Although HIV infection is now a disease not contained in the initial populations, the stigma associated with contracting the disease is even greater, because the assumption continues that humans make all decisions based on rational estimations of risks and benefits. Early in the course of HIV spread, in the hopes of lessening the burden of blame, therapists and physicians discouraged making the route of transmission an issue of acceptance for treatment, applying the same approach to care to all. From a social policy standpoint, this made great sense to encourage testing and treatment. However, from a psychological perspective, although it presumably did not "matter" to the providers how someone got infected, it did to the individual; how people became infected was inextricably and intricately part of the coping defenses and capacity to manage the illness and subsequent behaviors that continued to put them and others at risk.

Since the beginning of the epidemic, the diagnosis of HIV infection has caused great physical, psychological, and spiritual suffering. Even with the advent of significant treatments that can prolong life, many people face an uncertain future, challenging even those with resilient coping mechanisms. In the third decade of the epidemic, HIV infection is increasingly a disease of vulnerable, stigmatized, and marginalized people who suffer from the comorbidity of psychiatric disorders, including substance abuse; other medical problems; and impaired psychosocial functioning as a precursor to or consequence of living with HIV disease.[7,8] Concerns about active efforts to end life in this context are suffused with issues affected by cultural beliefs and fears of being expendable and less valued, reminiscent of the Tuskegee syphilis experiment.

This author frames the years from 1981 (with the identification of the first cases in the medical literature) as having three phases for purposes of conceptualizing psychological and social issues that may bear on coping and perhaps suicidal ideation and requests for hastened death. These three phases can be designated as described in the following sections.

PHASE I: BEFORE HIGHLY ACTIVE ANTIRETROVIRAL TREATMENT

Phase I, before the advent of highly active antiretroviral therapy (HAART), corresponds to the initial experience of individuals who became infected before they could even be aware of the risk certain behaviors created. This also corresponds to the period in which stigma and isolation of highly marginalized social groups occurred and shame and blame were clearly evident. This period was marked by profound losses of entire social groupings and reported high rates of suicide that were never acknowledged except in certain settings. Infected individuals agonized about how they would die before their time, and the uninfected who had engaged in the same behavior as their friends who were sick and dying tried to understand the meaning behind why they were spared. Society became divided into those who were HIV-positive and those who were uninfected. Kaposi's sarcoma lesions and wasting syndrome were the scarlet As of the end of the twentieth century. Young people coming into their sexuality who witnessed the generation ahead of them dying off began to wonder when rather than if they would get infected.

PHASE II: THE ADVENT OF HIGHLY ACTIVE ANTIRETROVIRAL TREATMENT

The advent of HAART in 1996 brought the beginning of the concept that HIV infection might be considered a chronic but manageable disease. After so little success during the early years of AIDS, medical researchers jumped at the opportunity to find some hope that like other infectious diseases, HIV disease also would be conquered. When the HAART era began, amazing stories of physical rebounding from death's door were not uncommon. In addition, younger people began to have less personal experience with friends and peers dying of AIDS, leading many to diminish the importance of self-protection as HIV infection became considered a "manageable chronic disease."

PHASE III: THE PRESENT TIME

A decade after the beginning of HAART, some people with HIV infection have continued to be unable to benefit from treatment, for a variety of complex biologic, social, political, economic, and psychological reasons. Many began to put their lives back together, but treatment did not work equally well for all, and the world of those infected became divided into those for whom treatment was working and those for whom it failed. Individuals agonized over why they might be progressing when others on the same regimens were staying healthy. Some suffer from medication adherence fatigue, and others contend with so many difficult aspects of life that continued adherence to treatment becomes interrupted by psychiatric illnesses, substance use, and economic and social disruptions in their lives.

REVIEW OF THE LITERATURE ON SUICIDALITY AND HIV

Although clinicians have written about the psychological issues associated with suicidality in people with HIV disease,[9] research studies are variable in the conclusions about HIV infection being an independent risk factor for suicidal ideation, attempts, and completions. Research has not yet delineated the impact of these three phases on issues of suicidality or interest and requests for hastened death among people infected with HIV. Most of the data reported in the literature refer to the phase I and II periods, as described previously.

The first reports from 1988 to 1992 about suicidality in HIV disease were from AIDS register–based or postmortem studies. Initial reports in New York City, California, and Texas showed significantly elevated relative risk for suicide (relative to age-controlled expected rates) in patients who died of AIDS: 66, 17.2, and 16.3 times, respectively. The National Center for Health Statistics in 1992 showed a relative risk for suicide of 7.4, the expected rate for HIV-negative status. Several concerns need to be noted. First of all, these were retrospective studies of completed suicides. Second, there was no correlation of the suicides with psychiatric or neuropsychological impairment, such as HIV dementia, delirium, central nervous system (CNS) neoplasms, or metabolic dysfunction, that might affect mental status and hence impulsivity, executive dysfunction, and judgment. Additionally, it is not clear whether AZT monotherapy (which had been shown to reduce the incidence of HIV dementia) or any of the other prophylactic medications for opportunistic infections that were known to affect brain function might have influenced the risk for suicidal behavior in patients with AIDS. Steroids, antimicrobials, and antineoplastic agents have all been implicated in causing changes in mental state, from depressed mood to overt mania, further compromising the individual's ability to manage difficult affective states or process what being sick with AIDS means in the personal and social context. Furthermore, because the vast majority of subjects studied were men who had sex with men, there was no established epidemiologic information about base rates of suicide in that group compared to the general population. Rates of suicide in the general population do not necessarily correlate with class or racial oppression. A further caveat with all the studies was that the conclusions could not be generalized to the developing countries.

Of significance, many studies reported rates of suicidal ideation and behavior that were higher than base rates in patients with preexisting psychiatric illness.[2]

Bonnet et al.[10] reported on cause of death among HIV-infected patients in France from 1998 to 1999, after the beginning of the HAART era. Six percent of deaths were attributed to suicide or overdose.

Roy[11] examined 149 HIV-positive substance-dependent patients and found 44.3% had attempted suicide and 55.7% had not. Significantly more who attempted were female, and they scored higher on the Childhood Trauma Questionnaire (CTQ) for childhood emotional abuse, sexual abuse, physical abuse, and emotional and physical neglect.

Komiti et al.[12] reviewed 18 studies from 1989 to 2000. Different sample sizes, control groups, stage of HIV illness, time period (pre- or post-HAART), and methods of assessing psychiatric comorbidity do not permit a simple conclusion regarding the causative factors of suicidal ideation or behavior in the HIV-infected populations studied. The lack of consistency in methodologies, a variety of perspectives in what constitutes a real suicidal behavior, and the stigma associated with sexual orientation of the subject and knowledge about HIV status contribute to the confusion about what particular factors may explain the increased relative risk for suicide in HIV disease reported in many studies. Some studies report a direct link between HIV serostatus and suicidal ideation and behavior, whereas others suggest particular psychological pathways or psychosocial variables that preceded or derived from HIV infection that might contribute to increased suicidal risk rather than HIV itself: having a current or recent partner with AIDS, unemployment, bereavement, poor adaptive social functioning, depression, and hopelessness. Some reports suggest that there is greater risk for suicidal ideation (if not attempts) at different phases of HIV infection: new HIV diagnosis, change in acute medical status, length of illness. Some authors report no difference in risk according to stage of illness. Conflicting reports that advanced illness both increased and decreased suicidal ideation and behavior further confound the interpretation of the relationship between suicide and HIV status. Furthermore, what is not at all clear from the limited studies is the impact of HAART treatment on suicidal ideation and behavior. Several very important questions remain. What is the impact of successful HAART treatment on suicidal ideation and behavior? How do comorbidity of psychiatric illness, substance use, and hepatitis C infection affect outcomes? Does the risk for suicide increase when HAART fails for patients or patients fail to adhere to HAART and subsequently become more advanced in their illness? Given that more people in the United States are living longer on HAART, does advancing illness in the study subject in spite of treatment lead to increased hopelessness? What is the impact of bereavement on suicidal behavior? The question remains as to whether greater visibility of people living longer with HIV disease lessens the level of stigma associated with HIV, a factor often noted as contributing to social isolation and suicidality.

The literature on suicidal behavior in HIV-infected females is less extensive, although it appears that females may be less affected by HIV status alone and more affected by comorbid substance use or social factors such as employment, housing, lack of support, relationship issues, and finances. Limited information suggests that minority women may have fewer suicidal concerns than nonminority women. Suicidal behavior appears to be increased in HIV-positive women who have a psychiatric diagnosis at follow-up.[13,14]

Cooperman and Simoni[3] assessed prevalence, timing, and predictors of suicidal ideation and attempted suicide in 207 HIV-positive women in New York City. Of the 26% who reported attempting suicide since their HIV diagnosis, 42% acted within the first month after HIV diagnosis, and 27% acted within the first week. Contrary to expectations, having children and being employed were also positive predictors, whereas spirituality was negatively associated only with suicidal ideation, not attempts. Diagnosis of AIDS, physical or sexual abuse, and psychiatric symptoms were positive predictors of both ideation and behavior. As in previous studies, HIV-positive Black and Hispanic women had a lower prevalence of suicidality than HIV-positive White women. Larger studies of women are needed to interpret the findings thus far. Inequities in access to care, psychosocial expectations by gender role, and cultural beliefs appear to be important though not clear factors in understanding suicidal ideation and attempts in women with HIV infection.

Suicidal ideation and attempts among HIV-positive psychiatric patients are less well documented. One study of 190 HIV-positive patients (68% male) in an HIV mental health clinic reported 26% had suicidal ideation within 30 days of the admission to an inpatient psychiatric facility. Forty-nine percent reported a plan, and 48% continued intent during hospitalization.[15] Depression was diagnosed in 64%, drug dependence in 52%, and depressive personality in 50% of study participants. Greater risk for suicidal ideation and attempt or plan was associated with dual diagnosis, unstable personality disorder, and poor social function.

Bing et al.[8] reported that nearly half of the population being treated for HIV infection screen positive for depression: 36% for major depression and 26.5% for dysthymia. Depression is reported by many studies as a risk factor for suicidal behavior and self-harm. Depression is also often mentioned in the clinical arena as a potential motive for requests for physician assisted suicide and voluntary euthanasia, implying that with appropriate treatment such requests might diminish or cease. Certainly, regardless of the validity of such a presumed association, patients with HIV disease must be screened and treated for depression.

As the prevalence of HIV infection continues to rise in the psychiatric patient population, more studies will be needed to understand the particular contributions HIV and psychiatric illness make in conferring higher risk for suicidal ideation and behavior.

In comparing suicide in HIV disease and AIDS with suicide in other medically ill populations, risk for suicide appears to be elevated. Harris and Barraclough,[16] in a meta-analysis of studies between 1966 and 1992 investigating the prevalence of suicide in 63 different medical disorders including HIV disease and AIDS, reported that of the studies of HIV disease and AIDS that met criteria for inclusion in the meta-analysis, there was an increased risk representing almost a 7-fold increase compared with the expected rate. Although HIV disease and AIDS were not the highest risk for suicide of all studied medical diseases, they are higher than traditional diseases such as Huntington's chorea (3-fold risk), multiple sclerosis (2-fold risk), malignant neoplasms (1.4- to 2.5-fold risk), renal disease (14-fold risk), spinal cord injury (4-fold risk), and systemic lupus erythematosus (4-fold risk).

Some of the additional risk for HIV disease and AIDS was attributed to them being a relatively new disease, and the social stigmatization associated with the disease. Additionally, some researchers have found a strong association between mental illness, particularly depression, and suicidal patients with medical illness. Methodologic problems with finding cases of depression may account for some of the discrepancy in this association.

For clinicians working with patients with HIV disease and AIDS, this increased risk for suicidal ideation and behavior suggests the benefits of screening for depression throughout the course of illness.

PHYSICIAN ASSISTED SUICIDE AND VOLUNTARY EUTHANASIA

Observations about physician assisted suicide and voluntary euthanasia in patients with HIV infection must be viewed in the larger context of the growing support in the United States and many countries for the "right to die." Over 60% of the population now favors the legalization of voluntary euthanasia for patients with terminal illness.[17,18] Physicians have participated in this public debate, even to the publication of proposals for implementing voluntary euthanasia.[19] One of the most recent studies reported on attitudes by physicians and the general public regarding physician assisted suicide and voluntary euthanasia.[20] Asked to choose between the legalization of physician assisted suicide and an explicit ban, 56% of physicians and 66% of the public supported legalization, 37% of physicians and 26% of the public preferred a ban, and 8% of each group was uncertain. If physician assisted suicide was legal, 35% of physicians said they might participate if requested, 22% would participate in either physician assisted suicide or voluntary euthanasia, and 13% would participate only in assisted suicide. Not surprisingly, support for physician assisted suicide was lowest among strongly religious physicians, a tendency that has been reported in other studies of religious attitudes and physician assisted suicide.[21] In the Netherlands, where voluntary euthanasia has been legalized, 54% of physicians report having participated in at least one death.[22]

The HIV infection and AIDS epidemic has provoked considerable support and controversy around the "right to die."[23] Both patients with AIDS (90% in an Australian sample[24] and 55% in a New York City sample[25]) and providers support the desire for the legalization of physician assisted suicide and voluntary euthanasia. Physicians who had many patients with AIDS were more likely to support and more often willing to participate in assisted suicide. Slome et al.[26,27] reported on an increase from 28% of physicians in 1990 to 48% in 1995 who said they would likely or very likely grant a request by a patient with AIDS for assisted suicide.

Most research around physician assisted suicide and voluntary euthanasia focuses on the physician's reactions to hypothetical questions about willingness to participate in voluntary euthanasia or providing means for patients to take their lives. A few studies have examined the patient's point of view.

Bindels et al.[28] showed that in a nationwide study, 38% of deaths included medical decisions concerning the end of life (MDEL). Of all deaths, 2.1% were brought about by either euthanasia or physician assisted suicide. Of the 131 male homosexual participants diagnosed with AIDS between 1985 and 1992 taking part in a cohort study in Amsterdam, all had died before 1995, before the widespread availability of HAART. Of that cohort, 22% died by physician assisted suicide or voluntary euthanasia and in another 13% MDEL had been made—more than one third made decisions at the end of life. The authors remarked that the greatest difference between the groups (physician assisted suicide or voluntary euthanasia versus MDEL) was age at time of diagnosis, with 72% aged 40 or more in the assisted suicide or voluntary euthanasia group compared with 38% in the natural death group. Of note was the increased risk for physician assisted suicide with longer duration of survival after diagnosis with AIDS. Furthermore, it was noted that most of the patients would have died within 1 month even without assisted suicide or voluntary euthanasia based on physiologic parameters.

One hypothesis was that men who lived longer had more experience with seeing other men with AIDS suffer and die and had a greater opportunity to discuss their own wishes as the end of life approached. The authors concluded that because the decision for physician assisted suicide or voluntary euthanasia did little to shorten life, it could be viewed more as a type of extreme palliation applied at the terminal phase of a lethal disease.

Breitbart et al.[25] examined interest in physician assisted suicide among ambulatory HIV-infected patients. Of the 378 patients recruited, 90% met Centers for Disease Control and Prevention (CDC) criteria for AIDS. Self-report measures assessed pain, depression, physical symptoms, psychological distress, and social supports. Included in the questionnaire were attitudes and interest in physician assisted suicide. Sixty-three percent of the patients supported policies favoring it, and 55% considered it a personal option. The strongest predictors of interest correlated with psychological distress: depression, hopelessness, suicidal ideation. Contrary to many assumptions, interest in physician assisted suicide was not associated with pain intensity, pain-related functional impairment, extent of HIV disease, or symptoms.

In study in Europe, Andraghetti et al.[29] investigated the perspectives of over 1,300 HIV-infected persons from 11 European Union member states between 1996 and 1997. Of the respondents, 78% agreed with the legalization of euthanasia in case of severe physical suffering, 47% if there was severe psychological suffering, and 24% simply at the patient's request. For physical suffering with a clear patient request, respondents approved of alleviation of pain with double effect (81%), medical euthanasia (62%), and physician assisted suicide (45%). Of all respondents, 50% reported they would consider euthanasia for themselves if all treatment options were exhausted. Of interest, social indicators such as employment and educational level were significantly associated with attitudes rather than indicators of disease status.

Given the first wave of people infected with HIV, most of the literature reports on studies of gay men. Little evidence exists for the impact of important variables such as gender, race, ethnicity and cultural beliefs, drug use (addiction versus recreational), parenting status, or religious background on the rates of request for physician assisted suicide or voluntary euthanasia. Even among men, the data were gathered before the period in which profound changes in survival and functional capacity improved with HAART.

Studies are needed to distinguish the rates of physician assisted suicide and voluntary euthanasia from three different periods since the beginning of the epidemic: phase I—first wave with profound personal experience of loss in peer group and community, with little treatment for underlying HIV disease; phase II—era of HAART with profound changes for some in survival and recovery of function; phase 3—discovery of limitations of HAART, fatiguing adherence, and increasing prevalence of comorbid psychiatric and other significant medical disorders.

ORIGINS OF THE DESIRE FOR PHYSICIAN ASSISTED SUICIDE AND VOLUNTARY EUTHANASIA

Are people with HIV infection who request physician assisted suicide or voluntary euthanasia more or less similar to those who have explored suicidal ideation or had attempts? If there is some significant correlation between early interest in suicide (either preexisting to HIV infection or as a consequence) and physician assisted suicide, how does the looming end of life affect the meaning of such interest? And if in fact there is no association between the two, perhaps the very nomenclature *physician assisted suicide* is unfortunate in that it confuses the real meaning of the request and prevents a more considered discussion about end-of-life issues. For clinicians, and much of the public, especially those with strong religious and moral beliefs, the very word *suicide* conjures up an intolerable possibility that is always seen as destructive and necessarily requires active intervention to prevent at all costs. It is possible, however, to discern in an individual situation if the request for physician assisted suicide or voluntary euthanasia is fueled by the same internal experience as that which precipitates acute or chronic suicidality.

As in the case of suicide by people with AIDS, it has been assumed that the desire to end one's life was a result of wanting to end pain and suffering. Many factors, however, appear contributory to this wish to die prematurely: depression, hopelessness, psychological distress, isolation, and lack of social support. Before the advent of HAART, patients often deteriorated with painful loss of function, wasting, and disfigurement. In the Netherlands, where voluntary euthanasia is legal, 25% of patients with AIDS died by voluntary euthanasia before the availability of HAART. Unfortunately, there is a lack of evidence concerning the impact of a good response to HAART, or of a failure of HAART in the context of many people responding well, on the prevalence of completed suicides or requests for physician assisted suicide or voluntary euthanasia. After almost a decade of antiretroviral treatment, the emergence of resistant strains, significant side effects, treatment adherence fatigue, and a more marginalized, impoverished and multiply diagnosed patient population could affect the base rates of suicidal ideation, suicidal attempts, and requests for physician assisted suicide and voluntary euthanasia. Thus the current understanding about origins of the desire for physician assisted suicide and voluntary euthanasia from the research may lag behind what is already being seen in clinical practice. Evidence about the impact of HAART and the beginning failures of HAART in certain populations on suicidal ideation or requests for assisted suicide is currently lacking.

Clinically it is important to appreciate the subtle and meaningful differences between acute or chronic suicidality as a coping mechanism or symptom of impulsivity and the considered so-called "rational" decision to end one's life while still able to make a coherent decision. Although clinicians are taught that suicidal ideation, intent, and behavior are all part of a continuum, there is little empirical research examining the intrapsychic processes in a social context to clarify the meaning of suicidal ideation in managing anxiety, fear, and existential crises. The value of considering the ending of one's life is elaborated in the writing of existentialists such as Camus and Sartre. In fact, soon after the advent of the HIV epidemic, references to Sartre's *The Plague* were often used to provide a context for understanding the individual and social response to epidemics.

Lavery et al.[30] reported on a qualitative study intended to look at the meaning and intent of patients considering physician assisted suicide. The analysis yielded two factors that accounted for the desire for assisted suicide or voluntary euthanasia—disintegration and loss of community. As in other studies and clinical work, these factors contribute to a perception of loss of self.

Disintegration includes the impact of pain, loss of motor and cognitive function, wasting, and loss of bowel and bladder control, which leads to increasing dependency on others for basic body functions and requires a level of trust that caregivers will provide what is needed. Loss of personal dignity, autonomy, and self-control are all factors leading to the decision to end life before it happens naturally.

Loss of community included the progressive loss of participation in the world, the community, and close personal relationships. Fears of rejection by others and loss of mobility, leading to social isolation, contribute to the perception that there is nothing left for which life is worth living. Dementia and the accompanying loss of verbal capacity, thought generation, and processing of interpersonal experiences further contribute to this sense of losing the self. These factors combine to create a sense of loss of self—the perception that the fundamental essence of their being was irrevocably eroding. The desire for physician assisted suicide is seen as a way of limiting this loss of self.

It is important to recognize how rooted in the social experience is the development of the sense of losing the self. Factors that might help explain the increased rate of interest in physician assisted suicide in HIV disease and AIDS include the various ways in which social stigmatization occurs as a result of many different type of loss of community—disownment by families because of drug use or sexual orientation or history of physical or sexual abuse, both of which are more prevalent in more recently infected individuals. Much of the historical trauma encountered by people with HIV infection or AIDS may be reexperienced by becoming infected and at each stage along the illness.

For many gay men, earlier rejection and isolation from families of origin led to attempts with variable success to fashion "chosen families" for social and psychological support. Yet even men who were successful in creating such supports have been on the forefront of requesting the right to self-determination at the end of life. Questions remain as to the extent to which social supports and a sense of community can override individual concerns about control, autonomy, and dependency. Thus the dialectic between fears of disintegration and the capacity of the social support system to contain such fears must be examined and may fluctuate over time during the course of the illness.

Often, at a more deeply rooted psychological level are two competing beliefs—that one is not entitled to a self as evidenced by one's experience in the world and the abuse at the hand of others and the will to live and find the true self through the morass of developmental assaults, betrayals, and the rejection by others. Whereas acute suicidality may be predominantly a failure of coping mechanisms in a crisis, the request for physician assisted suicide or voluntary euthanasia may embody the realization and acceptance of the terminality of AIDS and the wish to bring closure to life sooner rather than later, foreclosing any further perceived abuse, disintegration, and abandonment.

Collectively, studies that show prevalence of suicidal ideation, attempts, and completion does not necessarily help in understanding the requests for physician assisted suicide or voluntary euthanasia. Although many people with HIV consider physician assisted suicide and voluntary euthanasia, there is little clear information about the real frequency of self-administration of medications to end one's life. Some studies suggest the incidence may be under-reported, given the legal and ethical issues involved.

Studies have not adequately explored more deeply psychodynamic meanings and implications of patients requesting physicians to provide the means for them to end their lives. Unlike suicidal patients who are infinitely resourceful at finding means of self-destruction, the quest for a painless, sure way to terminate one's life represents at some level the need to remain intact, both physically and emotionally. What does it mean to ask one's physician to provide the means or to act on one's behalf? How are these requests similar or different? What does it mean for an individual to want a physician to be the active agent in causing death (voluntary euthanasia), as opposed to requesting a more passive role in providing a prescription for that intended purpose at the patient's own hand? How does the interest in physician assisted suicide and voluntary euthanasia change over the course of illness for a particular person? How do individuals accommodate and manage the wish to avoid disintegration respond to engagement of providers and social supports as illness progresses? What can we learn about the personality differences between patients who need to have the power over the timing of their death and those who can tolerate the uncertainty and dependency on others to care for them until the very end of life.

It is important for all clinicians to assess the presence of acute suicidality in all HIV-infected patients regardless of symptoms and presence of psychiatric disorders and to actively engage terminally ill patients in a discussion of their wishes and intentions about their death. Physicians are often uncomfortable in discussing end-of-life issues. Patients can be afraid to provoke anger, detachment, or rejection from their physicians by raising such requests, but harbor fears about intolerable pain, loss of integrity, and ability to control their course. Many factors contribute to the request for a premature death. Attention to depression, cognitive impairment, and pain is essential, as well as to the existential concerns about the meaning of life and death and the sense of hope and despair in the process of final integration or dissolution of self.[31,32]

Psychiatrists are particularly poised to attend to the fears of loss and disintegration of self, formulating how earlier experiences, attachments, and trauma can resurface as precipitants to acute suicidality in the course of HIV illness or as a request for physician assisted suicide or voluntary euthanasia. Although studies begin to provide some insight into the factors that contribute to such requests, each individual's life course, personal philosophy, level of attachment to others, religious beliefs, and capacity to tolerate uncertainty, dependence, and loss of control must be considered in the clinical setting, bearing witness to the journey of the final stages of life.

SUMMARY

Physician assisted suicide provokes important issues for all of medicine. Although evidence shows more than half of patients and almost that many physicians favor legislation allowing for physician assisted suicide and voluntary euthanasia, only a relatively small percentage of people with terminal illness actually avail themselves of the practice even when permitted. Clearly, the need to have control over one's ultimate destiny does not mean the inevitable exercise of that control. Back[33] summarizes the impact of this issue as follows:

This small group of patients who describe an interest in assisted suicide can be seen as articulating a widespread public fear that the dying process represents a kind of destruction of humanness, a final indignity, and that medical care commonly falters in responding to these existential and spiritual concerns. Thus the issues raised by requests for physician assisted suicide resonate far beyond the small group of people determined to hasten their death in this way . . . Physician assisted suicide seems to be a window into a particular set of concerns that patients have about dying—relating to loss of self, loss of dignity, and the social context of dying. Understanding these concerns may shed light on what palliative medicine can do for all dying persons, whether they desire physician assisted suicide or not.

REFERENCES

1. McKegney F, O'Dowd M. Suicidality and HIV status. *Am J Psychiatry*. 1992;149:396–398.
2. Starace F. Epidemiology of suicide among persons with AIDS. *AIDS Care*. 1995;7(suppl 8):S123–S128.
3. Cooperman NA, Simoni JM. Suicidal ideation and attempted suicide among women living with HIV/AIDS. *J Behav Med*. 2005;28:149–156.
4. Block SD, Billings JA. Patient requests for euthanasia and assisted suicide in terminal illness. *Psychosomatics*. 1995;36:445–455.
5. Sullivan AD, Hedberg K, Fleming DW. Legalized physician-assisted suicide in Oregon: the second year, *N Engl J Med*. 2000;342:598–604.
6. van der Maas PJ, van der Wal G, Haverkate I et al. Euthanasia, physician-assisted suicide, and other medical practices involving the end of life in the Netherlands, 1990–1995. *N Engl J Med*. 1996;335:1699–1705.
7. Atkinson JH, Grant I, Kennedy CJ, et al. Prevalence of psychiatric disorders among men infected with immunodeficiency virus: a controlled study. *Arch Gen Psychiatry*. 1998;45:859–864.
8. Bing EG, Burnam MA, Longshore D, et al. Psychiatric disorders and drug use among human immunodeficiency virus-infected adults in the United States. *Arch Gen Psychiatry*. 2001;58:721–728.
9. Forstein M. Suicidality and HIV infection. In: Cadwell S, Burnham R, Forstein M, eds. *Therapists on The Front Line: Challenges in Psychotherapy with Gay Men in the Age of AIDS*. Washington, DC: American Psychiatric Press; 1994:111–146.
10. Bonnet F, Morlat P, Chene G, et al. Causes of death among HIV-infected patients in the era of highly active antiretroviral therapy, Bordeaux, France, 1998-1999. *HIV Med*. 2002;3:195–199.
11. Roy A. Characteristics of HIV patients who attempt suicide. *Acta Psychiatr Scand*. 2003;107:41–44.
12. Komiti A, Judd F, Grech P, et al. Suicidal behaviour in people with HIV/AIDS: a review. *Aust N Z J Psychiatry*. December 2001;35:747–757.
13. Brown G, Rundell J. A prospective study of psychiatric aspects of early HIV disease in women. *Gen Hosp Psychiatry*. 1993;15:139–147.
14. Simoni J, Nero D, Weinberg B. Suicide attempts among seropositive women in New York City. *Am J Psychiatry*. 1998;155:1626–1627.
15. Haller DL, Miles DR, Suicidal ideation among psychiatric patients with HIV: psychiatric morbidity and quality of life. *AIDS Behav*. 2003;7:101–108.

16. Harris E, Barraclough B. Suicide as an outcome for medical disorders. *Medicine*. 1994;73:281–296.
17. Blendon RJ, Szalay US, Knox RA. Should physicians aid their patients in dying? The public perspective. *JAMA*. 1992;267:2658–2662.
18. Genuis SJ, Genuis SK, Chang W-C. Public attitudes toward the right to die. *Can Med Assoc J*. 1994;150:701–708.
19. Quill TE, Meier DE, Block SD, et al. The debate over physician-assisted suicide: empirical data and convergent views. *Ann Intern Med*. 1998;128:552–558.
20. Bachman JG, Alcser KH, Doukas DJ, et al: Attitudes of Michigan physicians and the public toward legalizing physician assisted suicide and voluntary euthanasia. *N Engl J Med*. 1996;334:303–309.
21. Burdette AM, Hill TD, Moulton BE. Religion and attitude toward physician assisted suicide and terminal palliative care. *J Sci Study Religion*. 2005;44:79–93.
22. Chochinov HM, Wilson KG, Enns M, et al. Desire for death in the terminally ill, *Am J Psychiatry*. 1995;152:1185–1191.
23. Haghbin Z, Streltzer J, Danko GP. Assisted suicide and AIDS patients: a survey of physician's attitudes. *Psychosomatics*. 1998;39:18–23.
24. Tindall B, Forde S, Carr A, et al. Attitudes toward euthanasia and assisted suicide in a group of homosexual men with advanced HIV disease [letter]. *J Acquir Immune Defic Syndr*. 1993;6:1069–1070.
25. Breitbart W, Rosenfeld BD, Passik SD. Interest in physician assisted suicide among ambulatory HIV infected patients. *Am J Psychiatry*. 1996;153:238–242.
26. Slome L, Moulton J, Huffine C, et al. Physicians' attitudes toward assisted suicide in AIDS. *J Acquir Immune Defic Syndr*. 1992;5:712–718.
27. Slome LR, Mitchell TF, Charlebois E, et al. Physician-assisted suicide and patients with human immunodeficiency virus disease. *N Engl J Med*. 1997;336:417–421.
28. Bindels PJE, Krol A, vanAmeijden E, et al: Euthanasia and physician-assisted suicide in homosexual men with AIDS. *Lancet*. 1996;346:499–504.
29. Andraghetti R, Foran S, Colebunders R, et al. Euthanasia: from the perspective of HIV infected persons in Europe. *Br HIV Assoc HIV Med*. 2001;2:3–10.
30. Lavery JV, Boyle J, Dickens M, et al. Origins of the desire for euthanasia and assisted suicide in people with HIV-1 or AIDS: a qualitative study, *Lancet*. 2001;35:747–757.
31. Breitbart W, Rosenfeld B, Pessin H, et al. Depression, hopelessness, and desire for hastened death in terminally ill patients with cancer. *JAMA*. 2000;284:2907–2911.
32. Chochinov HM, Wilson KG, Enns M, et al. Depression, hopelessness, and suicidal ideation in the terminally ill. *Psychosomatics*. 1998;39:366–370.
33. Back A. Desire for physician-assisted suicide: requests for a better death? *Lancet*. 2001;358:344–345.

Index

A

AAN. *See* American Academy of Neurology
AAPI. *See* Asian American Pacific Islander Initiative
abacavir, 28, 30
abuse
    abusive relationships, 6, 281
    and psychological experience of infection, 104
    sexual, 281, 407
    See also substance abuse
acquired immunodeficiency syndrome. *See* AIDS
ACT-UP. *See* AIDS Coalition To Unleash Power
acupuncture, 367, 369
    effectiveness of, 372, 373
acyclovir, mental status changes and, 123
addiction, 183
    "pseudo-addiction", 183
adenotonsillar hypertrophy, 66
adherence
    to antiretroviral therapy, 31–32, 43–44
        adherence level needed (95 percent), 225, 229
    barriers to, 43–44
    medication holidays, 32
    personality and, 105
    psychotherapy and, 357
    substance use and psychiatric disorders and, 130
    surveys of potential for, 56
adjustment disorders, 72, 80–81
    cognitive behavioral stress management, 83
    Coping Effectiveness Training, 83
    pharmacologic interventions, 84
    psychotherapy and, 83
    stress vs. distress, 79
    treatment considerations, 83–84
    See also psychological reactions; stress
adolescents
    cultural expectations, 227–228
    family-based prevention programs, 331–332
    family influences, 328, 330
    HIV/AIDS in, 259–266
        depression and, 263
        prenatal care in pregnancy of, 251–252
        psychiatric aspects, 226–228
    in-utero infected cohort, 228
    mental health problems and self-harm behaviors, 304–305
    risks of sexually transmitted diseases, 192–193
    sexual victimization and, 228
    special populations
        African Americans, 226–228
        Asian and Pacific Islander Americans, 234
        gay, lesbian, bisexual (GLB), 304–305
        Hispanic Americans, 219, 220
        young men who have sex with men (YMSM), 290
    STI screening for, 192–193
    See also children
adrenal insufficiency, 204
advance directives, 88, 390–391
African Americans, 223–231
    African American HIV/AIDS Response Act (2005), 324
    down low lifestyle, 224, 228
    Gay Men of African Descent (GMAD), 295
    HIV/AIDS and, 223–231
        children and adolescents, 226–228
        mental illness and, 224–225
        poverty and, 7–8
        prevention of, 230
        statistics, 223
        transmission and risk factors, 4, 223–224
        treatment of, 229–230
    lithium contraindicated for, 229
    mental illness in, 225–226
aging, 268–269
    See also older adults
AI/ANs. *See* American Indians and Alaska Natives
AIDS, 18, 20–21
    clinical AIDS-defining conditions, 18, 20, 48
    definition of, 14
    See also HIV; HIV/AIDS
AIDS Awareness campaigns, 399
AIDS Coalition To Unleash Power (ACT-UP), 288
AIDS Education and Training Centers, 396
AIDS-related complex (ARC), 74–75
AI-SUPERPFP. *See* American Indian Service Utilization, Psychiatric Epidemiology, Risk and Protective Factors Project
Alaska Natives. *See* American Indians and Alaska Natives
alcohol use, 43
    cognitive dysfunction and, 129
    HCV infection and, 130
    HIV risk and, 127
    low alcohol metabolism rate in APIs, 237
    sleep disorder and, 141, 142
    withdrawal from, and psychotic symptoms, 119

alprazolam, 143
    drug interactions, 151, 153
alternative medicine, 347, 365
    alternative medical systems, 368–369
    defined, 366
    See also complementary and alternative medicine
Alzheimer's disease
    Clinical Dementia Rating, 57
    dementia, 50
    Global Deterioration Scale, 57–59
Ambien. See zolpidem
American Academy of Neurology (AAN), criteria for neurocognitive impairment, 48–50, 54
American Indians and Alaska Natives (AI/ANs), 241–249
    background and context, 242
    cultural perspectives on psychiatric conditions, 245–247
        depression, 246–247
        post-traumatic stress disorder, 245, 247
        substance use, 245–246
    HIV/AIDS trends and patterns, 242–244
        location, 244
        modes of transmission, 243–244
        risk factors, 243–244
    Indian Health Service (IHS), 244, 247
    languages and communication, 244
    mortality and morbidity levels, 242
    prevention strategies, 248
    psychiatric epidemiology, 244–245
    service provision, 247–248
    terminology, 241 (footnote)
    websites and resources, 248 (footnote), 249
American Indian Service Utilization, Psychiatric Epidemiology, Risk and Protective Factors Project (AI-SUPERPFP), 245
amitriptyline, 175
amphetamines, 119
    drug interactions, 158
    See also methamphetamine; methylenedeoxymethamphetamine
amphotericin, 27, 123
amprenavir, 282
anal sex, and HIV transmission, 17
angel dust (phencyclidine), 119
antibodies, 13, 23
    antibody status
        psychological reactions to disclosure of, 74–75
        psychological reactions to notification of, 72–73
        psychological reactions to testing, 73–74, 385
    autoantibodies, 16
    HIV antibody test, 13, 19, 23, 400
        limitations of, 34
anticonvulsants
    for mania, 273
    for pain, 174, 177–178
antidepressants, 77, 90
    African-Americans and, 229
    drug-drug interactions, 95, 153–157
    medical inpatients and, 205
    for mood disorders, 94–95
    for pain, 173–176
    St. John's wort and, 152, 160, 375
    for sleep disorders, 145
antifungal agents, mental status changes and, 123
antihistamines
    for pain, 174
    for sleep disorders, 145
anti-psychiatry movement, 343
antipsychotic medications, 123–125, 208, 229
    ADA guidelines on, 271
    atypical, 124–125, 229
        for delirium, 207
        for HIV-psychosis, 270
    drug interactions, 124–125
    first-generation (neuroleptics), 124, 229
        extrapyramidal reactions, 98, 133, 208, 229
    second-generation, 124, 229
    See also neuroleptics
antiretroviral therapy, 27–32
    adherence to, 31–32, 43–44
        adherence level needed (95 percent), 225, 229
    in children, 255, 261, 265
    combination antiretroviral therapy (CART), 14, 20
    complementary and alternative medicine and, 367
        risks and warnings, 374–376
    drug-drug interactions
        analgesics and, 178–179
        antidepressants and, 95
        anxiolytics and, 90
        psychotropic drugs and, 149–160
    herbal medicines and, 375
    highly active antiretroviral therapy (HAART), 14, 43–44, 149
        and "phases" of HIV infection/disease, 406
        psychological attributions to, 75–76
    historical context, 27, 406
    hormonal contraceptives and, 282
    initiation of, 14, 20, 27
    medications listed, 28–29
    in pregnancy, 251–254, 280
    principles of, 27–28
    psychological conditions and
        panic disorder, 89
        psychosis, 122–123
        sleep disorders, 140
        stress, 75–76, 88
    resistant strains, 20–21, 24, 31, 225, 280
    salvage regimens, 20
    side effects of, 72, 89, 122–123
    stress and, 75–76, 88
    toxicity of, 27, 94
    treatment regimens, 28–31
    See also adherence; postexposure prophylaxis; specific drugs
antisocial personality disorder (ASPD), 102, 105, 109
antiviral agents, mental status changes and, 123
anxiety disorders, 5, 45, 86–92
    behavioral treatments for, 81
    conditions that may mimic, 89–90

in HIV-positive patients, 89
    behavioral treatments for, 81
    pharmacotherapy of, 90–91
Hospital Anxiety and Depression Scale (HADS), 56
psychological stressors, 86–89
rates of, 86
screening for, 55–56
in special populations
    homeless, 310
    men who have sex with men (MSM), 293
    women, 281
    women who have sex with women (WSW), 303
substance abuse and, 132
anxiolytics, 77, 264–265
    metabolism and drug interactions, 153
APICHA. *See* Asian and Pacific Islander Coalition on HIV/AIDS
APIs. *See* Asian and Pacific Islander Americans
ARC. *See* AIDS-related complex
aripiprazole, 124, 125
Asian American Pacific Islander Initiative (AAPI), 239
Asian and Pacific Islander Americans (APIs), 232–240
    epidemiology, 232–233
    future research, 238
    geographic location, 233
    homophobia and, 234
    language barriers, 239
    low drug metabolism rate, 237
    as model minority group, 232
    Model Minority Myth, 236–237
    prevention and intervention programs, 238–239
    psychiatric issues, 236–238
        diagnoses, 236–237
        patient encounters, 236–237
        psychiatric disorders, 236
    psychosocial factors, 233–235
        cultural attitudes, beliefs, and values, 234
        help-seeking patterns/access to services, 235
        immigrant status, 234–235
        knowledge and perceptions about HIV/AIDS, 233
        social support, 235
        substance use, 235
    research and practice implications, 239
    risk factors, 232–233
    therapy considerations, 237
    translator use, 237
Asian and Pacific Islander Coalition on HIV/AIDS (APICHA), 295
ASPD. *See* antisocial personality disorder
assessment. *See* psychiatric assessment; risk assessment
asymptomatic stage, 18, 19–20
Atarax. *See* hydroxyzine
atazanavir, 29, 30
atomoxetine, 158
atovaquone (Mepron), 9, 21, 25
    drug interactions, 153
attention deficits, in infants and children, 115
autoantibodies, 16
autoimmune thyroiditis. *See* Graves' disease
autonomic nervous system, 380
Axis I diagnoses, 44–47
Ayurveda, 368
azidothymidine (AZT). *See* zidovudine
azithromycin (Zithromax), 21
    drug interactions, 153
AZT. *See* zidovudine

B

Bach flower remedies, 371
baclofen, for pain, 178
bacterial infections, 188–189
bactrim. *See* sulfamethoxazole/trimethoprim
BAEP. *See* brainstem auditory evoked potential
Bailey Scales of Development, 264
barbiturates, 143
    drug interactions, 152
Bartonella henselae, 122
Bartonella quintana, 310
BDI. *See* Beck Depression Inventory
Beck and Hamilton rating scales, 42, 226
Beck Depression Inventory (BDI), 55–56, 129, 226
    medical inpatients and, 205
behavioral therapy. *See* cognitive-behavioral therapy
Benadryl (diphenhydramine), 145
benzodiazepines
    for anxiety symptoms, 84, 90–91, 132
    for mania, 208
    metabolism and drug interactions, 153
    for pain, 175, 176
    for sleep disorders, 143–144
bereavement
    African-American children and, 227
    chronic state of, 290
    coping groups, 360
    as a stressor, 82
    support group interventions, 83–84
Biaxin. *See* clarithromycin
bioelectromagnetic-based therapies, 365, 370
biofeedback, 359, 370
biopsychosocial aspects, 7–8, 378–382
    implications for disease management and clinical practice, 380–381
    interaction of psychosocial aspects of HIV/AIDS and physiology, 378–380
        depression, 379
        disclosure, 378–379
        social support, 379–380
        stressful life events, 379
bipolar disorders, 45
    high risk behaviors and, 344
    in medical inpatients with HIV/AIDS, 201
    treatment of, 97–98, 208
Blacks. *See* African Americans
blood exposure, 32
blood transfusion, 18, 32
borderline personality disorder (BPD), 101, 102
    countertransference issues, 106
    diagnosing in the gay context, 103

borderline personality disorder (BPD) (*cont.*)
　psychoeducation for, 108–109
　screening for, 109
　and stigma of HIV, 104
　and treatment adherence, 105
　treatment approaches for, 107–108
boundaries, 363
BPD. *See* borderline personality disorder
brain
　abortive infection in, 15
　atrophy, 14–15
　autoantibodies, 16
　neuroimaging, 116–117
　regions with HIV-infection/virus load, 14–15
　white matter lesions, 15, 116, 131
　See also central nervous system
brain mapping. *See* electrophysiology and brain mapping
brainstem auditory evoked potential (BAEP), 65
breast feeding, and HIV transmission, 17, 250, 251, 256, 259, 280
Brief Symptom Inventory, 226
bupropion, 95
　drug interactions, 157, 178
buspirone, 132

C

CA. *See* capsid (CA) protein
California
　2005 legislative action, 324
　Proposition 96, 321, 325
　Sexual Abuse in Detention Elimination Act (2005), 324
CAM. *See* complementary and alternative medicine
Camus, literature of, 411
Canadian AIDS Treatment Information Exchange (CATIE), 375
candida dermatitis, 164
candidal esophagitis, 20, 321
cannabis, 119
capacity for decision-making, 391–392
Capgras' syndrome, 122
capsaicin, 178
capsid (CA) protein, 11
carbamazepine, 97, 132
　drug interactions, 152, 157–158
　for mania, 207, 273
　for pain, 177
CARE Act. *See* Comprehensive AIDS Resource Emergency (CARE) Act
caregivers
　for children with HIV/AIDS, 262
　education for, 256–257
　stress and, 80, 88–89
CARES program, 309, 310, 314
CART. *See* antiretroviral therapy; combination antiretroviral therapy
CATIE. *See* Canadian AIDS Treatment Information Exchange
rCBF. *See* regional cerebral blood flow

CBSM. *See* cognitive behavioral stress management
CBT. *See* cognitive-behavioral therapy
CCR5 (cysteine-cysteine chemokine receptor 5), 12, 13, 21
CD4 cell, 12
　bone marrow production of, 13
　coreceptors, 13
　receptors, 12, 13
CD4 cell count, 13–14, 23
　disease progression and, 18–21, 24
　initiation of antiretroviral therapy and, 14, 20, 27
　late symptomatic stage disease (AIDS) and, 18, 20
　mortality risk and, 14
　stress and, 380
CD8 cell, 14
CDC clinical disease stages. *See under* Disease stages
CDC-guidelines, on partner notification, 196
Center for Mental Health Services, 343
central nervous system (CNS), 14–16
　brain regions with HIV-infection/virus load, 14–15
　HIV/AIDS-related infections or neoplasms, 45, 48, 121–122, 203
　lymphoma, 94, 203
　opportunistic infections, diagnosis, 201–203
　pathophysiology of, 14–16
　See also brain; cognitive disorders; *specific CNS disorders*
cervical dysplasia, 20, 24
cervical ectopy, 278
cervical Papanicolaou smear, 24, 193
cervix, invasive squamous cell carcinoma of, 20
Cesarean section, 17, 253, 280
CHAMP Family Program, 331
character dimensions, 101, 102
chemokines, 16
chemotherapy, complications of, 48
chemotherapy drugs, mental status changes and, 123
Childhood Trauma Questionnaire (CTQ), 407
children, 259–266
　antiretroviral therapy in, 255, 261, 265
　attention deficits in, 115
　cognitive functioning/disorders, 115
　disclosure of child's HIV/AIDS status, 228, 262
　disclosure of parents' HIV/AIDS status to, 83, 227
　electroencephalograms for, 263
　family roles and, 80
　HIV/AIDS in, 259–266
　　epidemiology, risk factors, and consequences, 259–260
　　hyperactivity and, 264
　　intervention and psychological/psychiatric treatment, 263–265
　　learning disabilities and, 261
　　neurocognitive aspects of, 260–261
　　neuropsychological testing for, 264
　　pharmacologic treatment of, 264–265
　　psychiatric aspects, 226–228
　　psychological impact of, 262–263
　　retroviral medications and, 261
　　supportive and cognitive therapy for, 264

testing and, 264
    vaccination recommendations, 254
  HIV-negative, with HIV-positive parents, 227
  mental status assessment of, 263–264
  pain and, 164
  stress and, 80–81
  See also neonates and infants
Children's Memory Scale (CMS), 264
Chinese medicine
  acupuncture, 367, 369, 372, 373
  Chinese herbs, 317, 367, 373
  Traditional Chinese Medicine (TCM), 365, 368, 373
  treatment effectiveness studies, 373
chiropractic manipulations, 369
chlamydia, 188, 189, 195, 402
chloral hydrate, 145
chlorpromazine, 124
  and deinstitutionalization of mental patients, 342
  for delirium, 207
  for hiccups, 388
chronic illness, HIV as, 71, 76–77
cidofovir, 26
citalopram, 272
clarithromycin (Biaxin), 21, 26
  drug interactions, 153
clindamycin, 25
Clinical Dementia Rating, 57
clomipramine, for pain, 175
clonazepam, 90
  for mood disorders, 98
  for pain, 177
clonidine, for hyperactivity in children, 264–265
clozapine, 124, 125
  drug interactions, 158
  for psychosis, 208
club drugs, 43
CMS. *See* Children's Memory Scale
CMS Long Delay, 264
CMV. *See* cytomegalovirus
CNS. *See* central nervous system
cocaine, 119, 127
  anxiety and, 90
  drug interactions, 159
cognitive-behavioral HIV-risk reduction interventions, 401
cognitive behavioral stress management (CBSM), 83, 379
cognitive-behavioral therapy (CBT), 88, 359, 370
  effectiveness outcomes for, 372, 373
  for sleep disorder, 142, 359
cognitive disorders, 5–6, 15, 46–47, 111–118
  assessment and neuropsychological testing, 113–114
  characteristics of, 111–113
  cognitive complaints, 115
  course and progression of cognitive decline, 113
  diagnosis criteria, 111–113
  Global Deterioration Scale, 57–59
  HIV-associated dementia (HAD), 111, 112, 274–275
  minor cognitive motor disorder (MCMD), 14–15, 49–50, 111, 112, 131
  neuroimaging, 116–117
  neurologic assessment for, 84
  percentage of HIV-1-infected patients with, 48
  special populations, 115–116
    homeless people, 310
    infants and children, 115, 225–226, 260–261
    men who have sex with men (MSM), 293
    older adults, 116, 274–275
    substance users, 116
  substance abuse and, 129, 131
  test performance and functional abilities, 115
  See also HIV-associated dementia; psychological and neuropsychological testing
cognitive impairment assessment, 84
cognitive impairment criteria, 48–50, 54
combination antiretroviral therapy (CART), 14
  initiation of, 20
  See also antiretroviral therapy
community-based prevention programs, 332
comorbid medical conditions
  medically ill patients with HIV/AIDS, 198–211
  pain syndromes, 161–187
  psychotropic drug interactions with antiretroviral medication, 149–160
  sexually transmitted infections, 188–197
comorbid physical conditions, 43–44
comorbid psychiatric disorders, 3, 5–6, 44–47
  in medically ill patients with HIV/AIDS, 198–211
    changing scope of the HIV epidemic, 199
    depression, 205–206
    diagnostic evaluation, 204–205
    differential diagnosis, 201–204
    disorders and their treatment, 205–208
    epidemiology of, 199–201
    most frequently diagnosed disorders, 199–201
  personality characteristics and, 6–7
  See also special populations; specific disorders
compassionate continuity of care, 363
complementary and alternative medicine (CAM), 365–377
  alternative medical systems, 368–369
    Ayurveda, 368
    homeopathy, 368–369
    naturopathy, 369
    Traditional Chinese Medicine, 368
    treatment effectiveness outcomes, 373
  alternative medicine, defined, 366
  biologically based systems, 367–368
    treatment effectiveness outcomes, 371–372
  complementary medicine, defined, 366
  energy therapies, 369–370
    bioelectromagnetic techniques, 370
    Qigong, 368, 369
    Reiki, 369
    Therapeutic Touch, 369, 370
  integrative medicine, defined, 366
  manipulative and body-based techniques, 369
    treatment effectiveness outcomes, 372

complementary and alternative medicine (CAM) (*cont.*)
  mind-body interventions, 370
    treatment effectiveness outcomes, 372–373
  National Center for Complementary and Alternative Medicine (NCCAM), 347, 366
  prevalence of use in HIV/AIDS, 366–367
  reasons for use in HIV/AIDS, 367
  risks, warnings, and dangerous interactions, 374–376
  terminology, 366
  treatment effectiveness studies for CAM modalities, 370–371
    alternative medical systems, 373
    collaboration between conventional medicine and CAM practitioners, 371
    outcomes for biologically based methods, 371–372
    outcomes for manipulative/body-based interventions, 372
    outcomes for mind-body interventions, 372–373
    placebo effect, 370–371
    problems and dilemmas in CAM research, 374
Composition A, 367
compound Q, 366
Comprehensive AIDS Resource Emergency (CARE) Act, 248
compulsiveness, as temperament trait, 102
computed tomography (CT), 116, 264
condoms, 17
  condom distribution in prisons, 322, 325–326
  cultural factors affecting use, 218
  female condom, 398
  and HIV risk reduction, 43, 134, 195
  instruction on use of, 398
  question in sexual history-taking, 192
confidentiality
  of HIV testing results, 321–322, 325
  issues in family-oriented care, 333–334
  of medical records, 321–322, 325
Confusion Assessment Method, 90
consent, for HIV testing, 252, 321
contraceptives. *See* hormonal contraceptives
coping
  coping effectiveness training, 83, 359
  personality and, 104–105, 106
  skills training, 88
  with stress, 81
  styles, 6
    active vs. denial-based, 81
coreceptors, 13
core proteins, 12–13
Cornell Scale for Depression in Dementia, 272
corticosteroids
  mental status changes and, 123
  for pain, 175, 178
cortisol
  hypercortisolemia, 380
  in stress responses, 82, 380
cost
  of medical care, 7–8, 311
  medications, 310–311

countertransference, 106, 361, 362, 390
crack cocaine, 119, 127, 402
cranio-electrical stimulation, 370
criminalization of the mentally ill, 343, 344
Crixivan (indinavir), 145
cryptococcal meningitis, 27
  diagnosis, 202
  mood-disorder symptoms and, 94
  psychotic disorder and, 121
Cryptococcus neoformans, 26–27
Cryptosporidium, 164
crystals, 370
CT. *See* computed tomography
CTLs. *See* cytotoxic T lymphocytes
culturally sensitive services, 311, 314
culturally specific therapies, 361
CXCR4 (cysteine-X-cysteine receptor 4), 12, 13, 21
CYP3A4 inducers/inhibitors, 152
CYPP450 enzyme inhibition, 150–152
cysteine-cysteine chemokine receptor 5 (CCR5), 12, 13
cysteine-X-cysteine receptor 4 (CXCR4), 12, 13
cytokines, 13, 14
  CNS toxicity of, 15–16
  proinflammatory, 15, 16
  Th1 vs. Th2, 14
cytomegalovirus (CMV), 20, 25–26, 188, 189, 190
  diagnosis, 202
  mood-disorder symptoms and, 94
  testing for, 205
  valproic acid for treatment of, 207
cytotoxic T lymphocytes (CTLs), 14, 82

D

Dalmane (flurazepam), 143
dapsone, 21, 25, 123
Davis v. Hopper (1999), 323
DBT. *See* dialectical behavior therapy
decision-making capacity, determination of, 391–392
dehydroandrosterone (DHEA), mood disorders and, 96
deinstitutionalization of the mentally ill, 342–343
delavirdine (Rescriptor), 28, 30, 144, 145
  drug interactions, 152
delayed ejaculation, 7
Delirium Assessment Scale, 90
delirium, 46, 47
  end-stage illness and, 389
  etiology of, 206
  hypoactive and hyperactive variants, 206
  in medical inpatients with HIV/AIDS, 206–207
  mimicking anxiety disorder symptoms, 90
  superimposed (hepatic encephalopathy), 201
  treatment of, 206–207, 389
dementia, 5–6
  Alzheimer's type, 50, 57
  Clinical Dementia Rating, 57
  Cornell Scale for Depression in Dementia, 272
  HIV-associated dementia complex (HADC), 42, 46–47, 49, 56–57
  HIV Dementia Scale, 52

in HIV-infected homeless people, 310
in medical inpatients, 199–201
in older adults, 116
percentage of HIV-1-infected patients with, 48
risk factors for, 49–50
See also HIV-associated dementia (HAD)
Demerol. *See* meperidine
demographics, shifting, 199
denial, 355–356
Depakote, 229
Department of Health and Human Services, 312
Department of Housing and Urban Development (HUD), 310
depression, 5, 6, 72, 263, 379
antibody status notification and, 72–73
assessment/rating scales
Beck Depression Inventory, 55–56, 129, 205, 226
Brief Symptom Inventory, 226
Cornell Scale for Depression in Dementia, 272
Geriatric Depression Scale (GDS), 272
Hospital Anxiety and Depression Scale (HADS), 56
Patient Health Questionnaire depression scale (PHQ-9), 271–272
Symptom Checklist-90, 55–56
diagnosis and symptoms, 93–94
differential diagnosis, 271–272
electroconvulsive therapy, 272
HIV/AIDS disease progression and, 379
insomnia and, 140–141
in medical inpatients, 199–200, 205–206
in older adults, 270–272
risk factors, 94
screening for, 55–56
in special populations
African Americans, 225, 226, 229
American Indians and Alaska Natives, 246–247
children and adolescents with HIV/AIDS, 263
homeless people, 310
men who have sex with men (MSM), 293–294
older adults, 270–272
women, 281
women who have sex with women (WSW), 302, 303
spirituality and, 350
Stressor-Support-Coping Model for Psychosocial Intervention, 272
Symptom Checklist-90, 55–56
treatments, 77, 132, 229, 272
cognitive behavioral stress management intervention, 379
psychotherapy plus imipramine, 359
See also antidepressants; depressive disorders; mood disorders
depressive disorders, 44–45
major depressive disorder (MDD), 129
substance abuse and, 129, 130, 132
desipramine, 132
drug interactions, 178
for pain, 175

Desyrel. *See* trazodone
dextran sulfate, 366
dextroamphetamine, 95, 132, 206
for pain, 176
DHEA. *See* dehydroandrosterone
diabetes mellitus, risk from antipsychotic medications, 125, 270
diagnosis
Axis I diagnoses, 44–47
personality disorder and, 105
differential diagnostic considerations, 43
of HIV-associated minor cognitive motor disorder, 49–50
and initial medical evaluation, 23–24, 40–42
psychiatric diagnosis of medically hospitalized patients, 189–211
psychological testing and, 48–62
See also psychiatric assessment
dialectical behavior therapy (DBT), 107
diarrhea, 388–389
didanosine, 28, 30
dietary supplements, 367
diffusion tensor imaging (DTI), 116
Diflucan. *See* ketoconazole
dinitrochlorobenzene (DNCB), 366
diphenhydramine (Benadryl), 145
disabled individuals, 8, 9
disclosure of HIV/AIDS status, 378–379
to children, age-appropriateness of, 83
of children's status with HIV/AIDS, 228, 262
for men who have sex with men (MSM), 292–293
reluctance about, 8
disease progression, 18–21
and cognitive disorders, 111–113
and psychiatric morbidity, 6–7
psychological impact at different stages, 72–76
stress and immune parameters, 81–82
See also disease stages
disease stages, 18–21
acute HIV infection, 18, 19
asymptomatic stage (CDC clinical disease Stage A), 18, 19–20
disease phases (chronological), 406
early symptomatic stage (CDC clinical disease Stage B), 18, 20
late symptomatic stage (CDC immunologic Stage 3; AIDS), 18, 20–21
milestones in HIV care, 87–88
stresses associated with, 86–89
See also disease progression
distress
end-of-life care for, 389
"spiritual distress", 347–348
stress-distress spectrum, 79–85
divalproex sodium, 132
DNCB. *See* dinitrochlorobenzene
DNR. *See* do-not-resuscitate (DNR) orders
domestic violence, 281
dong quai, 375
do-not-resuscitate (DNR) orders, 391

Doral (quazepam), 143, 144
doxepin
  for itching, 388
  for pain, 175
drug abuse. *See* substance abuse
drug history, 150
drug interactions
  analgesics, 178–179
  antidepressants, 95
  antipsychotic medications, 124–125
  anxiolytics, 153
  differential diagnosis and, 204
  herb-drug interactions, 374–375
  psychotropic drug interactions with antiretroviral medications, 149–160, 270
    basic pharmacology, 149–150
    non-nucleotide reverse transcriptase inhibitors (NNTRIs), 152
    protease inhibitors, 150–152
    taking a drug history, 150
  substances of abuse, 159
  See also specific drugs
drug resistance, 26, 31
DTI. *See* diffusion tensor imaging
duloxetine
  for depression, 272
  metabolism and drug interactions, 157
  for pain, 175
dyspnea, 389
dysthymia, 5

E

echinacea, drug interactions, 160
Ecstasy (methylenedeoxymethamphetamine), 43, 129, 159
education. *See* prevention and education strategies
EEGs. *See* electroencephalograms
efavirenz, 29, 30
  drug interactions, 152, 272
  neuropsychiatric side effects, 30
  panic disorder and, 89
  psychosis and, 122–123
  sleep disturbances and, 66, 67, 140
  teratogenicity of, 282
electroconvulsive therapy, 96, 272
electroencephalograms (EEGs), 64, 263
electromagnetic therapy, 370
  effectiveness outcomes of, 373
electrophysiology and brain mapping, 63–68
  electroencephalograms (EEGs), 64
  electroencephalography, 63–65
  evoked and event-related potentials, 65–66
  quantitative electroencephalography (qEEG), 64–65
emtricitabine, 28, 30
encephalitis, 25
encephalopathy
  AZT for, 256
  HIV-associated progressive encephalopathy (HIV-PE), 261
  in HIV-positive children, 255–256

encephalopathy, in HIV-positive children, 255–256
endocrinologic conditions, 204
end-of-life care, 386–392
  advance directives and preservation of self-determination, 390–392
  do-not-resuscitate (DNR) orders, 391
  ethical issues of determination of capacity for decision-making, 391–392
  ethical issues of foregoing life-sustaining treatment, 391
  health care proxy, 390
  living will, 390
  medical durable power of attorney, 390
home visits, 390
medical decisions concerning the end of life (MDEL), 409
symptom management, 387–390
  biologic aspects, 387–389
  diarrhea, 388–389
  distress, 389
  dyspnea, 389
  existential anxiety, 389
  hiccups, 388
  itching, 388
  nausea, vomiting, and diarrhea, 388–389
  pain, 387–388
  psychiatric disorders, 389
  psychological aspects, 389–390
  social factors, 390
See also physician assisted suicide and voluntary euthanasia
energy therapies, 365
enfuviritide, 29, 30–31
envelope glycoprotein, 11, 12
env gene, 11
epidemiology, 3–11
  challenges of living with HIV, 7–8
  co-occurring psychiatric disorders, 5–6
  implications for mental health and substance abuse services, 8–9
  psychiatric, 5–6
  of psychiatric disorders in medical inpatients, 199–201
  psychiatric morbidity
    disease progression, and mortality, 6
    factors associated with, 6–7
  and risks, 3–5
  See also special populations
EPRs. *See* extrapyramidal reactions
Epstein-Barr virus testing, 205
erectile dysfunction, 159, 295
ERP. *See* event-related potential
escitalopram, 85, 95
estazolam (ProSom), 143
eszopiclone (Lunesta), 144
ethambutol, 26
ethical issues, 324–326
  end-of-life care, 383–392
    determination of capacity for decision-making, 391–392
    foregoing life-sustaining treatment, 391
    suicide and, 383–392

mental illness and prisons, 341–346
physician assisted suicide and voluntary euthanasia, 404–414
Principles of Medical Ethics, 324–325
ethnicity, and HIV transmission incidence, 4
euthanasia. *See* physician assisted suicide and voluntary euthanasia
event-related potential (ERP), 65–66
evoked and event-related potentials, 65–66
brainstem auditory evoked potential (BAEP), 65
event-related potential (ERP), 65–66
somatosensory evoked potentials (SEPs), 65
existential and spiritual therapies, 360
existential anxiety, 389
existential crisis, 348
extrapulmonary tuberculosis, 20
extrapyramidal reactions (EPRs), 98, 133, 208, 229, 270

F

FACIT. *See* Functional Assessment of Cancer Therapy
false positive results, 55
family. *See* patient's family
family and couples therapies, 360–361
family-centered approach to care, 329–330
fatigue
hormone therapy and, 96
sleep disturbance contributing to, 137
vs. sleep disturbance, 66–67
fearfulness, as temperament trait, 102, 103
felbamate, for pain, 177
fentanyl, for pain, 170, 387
flecainide, for pain, 178
fluconazole, 27, 270
flucytosine, 27
fluoxetine, 132
drug interactions, 157, 178
for pain, 175
serotonin syndrome and, 90, 157
fluphenazine, for pain, 176
flurazepam (Dalmane), 143
fluvoxamine, drug interactions, 152
fMRI. *See* functional magnetic resonance imaging
Folstein-McHugh Mini-Mental Status Examination, 42
forensic considerations, 341–346
fosamprenavir, 29, 30
foscarnet, 26
free radicals, 368
functional abilities testing, 115
Functional Assessment of Cancer Therapy (FACIT) Spiritual Well-being Scale, 350
functional magnetic resonance imaging (fMRI), 116
fusion inhibitors, 29, 30–31

G

GABA. *See* γ-aminobutyric acid
gabapentin (Neurontin), 98
drug interactions, 158
for pain, 177, 387
gag gene, 11
gag polyprotein, 11
galantamine, 275
γ-aminobutyric acid (GABA)
receptor agonists, 84
ganciclovir, 26
mental status changes and, 123
garlic supplements, drug interactions, 160
Gay and Lesbian Medical Association, 305
gay, lesbian, bisexual, or transgender (GLBT), 243, 289, 296, 348
See also homosexuality
gay, lesbian, or bisexual (GLB), 289, 304–305
Gay Men Health Crisis (GMHC), 288
Gay Men of African Descent (GMAD), 295
"Gay-Related Immune Disorder" (GRID), 288, 405
GDS. *See* Geriatric Depression Scale
General Health Questionnaire, 42, 129
genital herpes, 193, 402
genital ulcerative disease, 188, 278
genitourinary infections, 192
genogram, 332
Geriatric Depression Scale (GDS), 272
geriatric individuals. *See* older adults
GHMC. *See* Gay Men Health Crisis
gingko biloba
for dementia, 368
drug interactions, 160
ginseng, drug interactions, 160, 375
GLB. *See* gay, lesbian, or bisexual
GLBT. *See* gay, lesbian, bisexual, or transgender
Global Deterioration Scale, 57–59
glycoprotein coat (gp160), 11, 12
antibodies to, 13
GMAD. *See* Gay Men of African Descent
gonorrhea, 188–189, 195, 321, 402
gp41, 11, 12, 21
gp120, 11, 15, 21
gp160, 11, 12
granisetron, for nausea and vomiting, 388
Graves' disease, 204
GRID. *See* "Gay-Related Immunodeficiency Disorder"
grief
psychotherapy for, 356, 359
work, 83–84
See also bereavement
Grooved Pegboard psychomotor speed test, 54
group psychotherapy, 108, 360
growth hormone dysregulation, 67
guided imagery, 359

H

HAART. *See* antiretroviral therapy
HAD. *See* HIV-associated dementia
HADC. *See* HIV-associated dementia complex
HADS. *See* Hospital Anxiety and Depression Scale
Halcion. *See* triazolam
hallucinogens, 119
haloperidol, 123, 124
for delirium, 207
for hiccups, 388
for pain, 173, 176
for psychosis, 208

Halstead-Reitan Impairment Index, 54
harm avoidance, as temperament trait, 102, 103
hashish, 119
HAV. *See* Hepatitis A virus
hawthorn, 375
HBV. *See* Hepatitis B virus
HCV. *See* Hepatitis C virus
Health Resources and Services Administration (HRSA), 309, 312
heath care, HIV transmission during, 32–34
hepatic encephalopathy, 201
Hepatitis A virus (HAV), 194
   vaccination, 24, 194
Hepatitis B virus (HBV), 43, 188, 189, 190, 191, 194
   in HIV-infected homeless people, 310
   and HIV risk, 4
   prisons as reservoirs for, 321
   testing, 193
   vaccination, 24, 194
hepatitis C virus (HCV)
   comorbid, 43, 188, 189, 190–191
   education and counseling, 195
   in HIV-infected homeless people, 310
   neuropsychiatric complaints and, 201–204
   prisons as reservoirs for, 321
   substance abuse disorders and, 130
   testing, 193
herbal treatments, 159–160, 367
   as antimicrobial therapies, 368
   Chinese herbs, 367, 371, 373
   effectiveness studies, 371–372
   herbal supplements, 367
   herb-drug interactions, 374–375
   as immune therapies, 367
   risks, warnings, and dangerous interactions, 374–375
herpes, 24
   genital herpes, 193, 402
   herpes encephalitis, and psychotic disorder, 121
   herpes simplex virus 2 (HSV-2), 188, 189, 190
   herpes simplex virus, testing for, 205
   herpes zoster, 24
      recurrent multidermatomal, 20
heterosexism, 289, 295
heterosexual contact, and HIV incidence, 4, 9, 17, 32
hiccups, 388
highly active antiretroviral therapy (HAART). *See* antiretroviral therapy
high risk behaviors. *See* risks
High Sensitivity Cognitive Screen (HSCS), 52
Hispanic Americans, 215–222
   cultural factors and, 217–221
      culturally sanctioned sexual behaviors, 220
      homosexuality, 219
      la familia (familiarismo), 217–218
      language, 217
      machismo, 218–219
      marianismo (Virgin Mary in likeness), 219
      poverty, 219
      religion, 220–221
      sexually transmitted infections, 220
      substance use and abuse, 219–220
   HIV/AIDS
      epidemiology, 215–216, 218
      risk factors, 216–217, 221
      statistics, 216–218
   population growth rate, 215
   translator use and, 217
history, medical/psychological
   behavioral risk, 191–192
   drug, 150
   HIV cognitive, 51–52, 53–54
   medical/psychiatric, 24, 40–42
   psychological/neuropsychological, 50–52
   sexual, 41, 192, 314
   sexually transmitted infections, 191–192
   substance abuse, 40–41
   substance use, 192
   suicide, 386
HIV (human immunodeficiency virus), 11–14
   acute infection, 18, 19
   antibodies/antibody test, 13, 19, 34, 400
   challenges of living with, 7–8
   changing scope of HIV epidemic, 199
   diagnosis and initial medical evaluation, 23–24
   diagnostic criteria, 49
   disease progression/stages, 18–21
   genome, 11
   genotype, 24, 31
   HIV-1, 11
   HIV-2, 11
   infection and pathogenesis, 13–16
   latent state, 12
   medications other than antiretroviral, 153–160
   milestones in care, 87–88
   provirus, 12
   replication, 12–13
   resistant strains, 24, 31
   retrovirus, defined, 11
   structure, 11–13
   transmission, 16–18
      assessment of source of, 34
      categories, 3–5
      occupational, 32–34
      vertical, 250–251
      virus entry into host cell, 12
   treatment, 23–35
      barriers to, 43
      of medical complications of, 25–27
   triple diagnosis, 127–129
   See also antiretroviral therapy; HIV/AIDS
HIV-1 ribonucleic acid (RNA) test, 23
HIV/AIDS
   as a chronic medical illness, 71, 76–77
   biopsychosocial aspects, 378–382
   core principles of care, 312
   disease progression, 6–7, 18–21
   epidemiology overview, 3–11
   rates, 3–5
   risk factors, 4–5
   See also AIDS; HIV; *special populations*

HIV-associated dementia (HAD), 14, 15, 16, 111
  clinical staging system for, 56–57
  course and outcome, 275
  diagnosis of, 57–59, 112, 275
  mood disorders and, 94
  in older adults, 116, 274–275
  pathogenesis, 274
  risk factors, 274
  in substance users, 131
  subtypes, 275
  symptoms, 274
  treatment, 275
HIV-associated dementia complex (HADC), 42, 46–47, 49
  clinical staging system for, 56–57
HIV-associated progressive encephalopathy (HIV-PE), 261
HIV Dementia Scale, 52
HIV testing, 312, 400
  antibody test, 13, 19, 23, 400
    limitations of, 34
  California Proposition 96 and, 321
  compulsory, WHO position on, 321
  confidentiality of results, 321–322, 325
  enzyme-linked immunosorbent assay (ELISA), 400
  false positives, 23
  home HIV testing kits, 385
  informed consent and, 252, 321
  mandatory, 321–322
  negative results despite HIV presence, 19, 400
  pre- and post-test counseling, 356, 400
  in prenatal care, 251–253, 385, 400
    barriers to, 400
    "opt-out" approach, 252–253
  of prisoners, 321–322, 325
  RNA polymerase chain reaction testing, 19
  suicide and, 385
  Western blot, 23
HNRC HIV-Neurobehavioral Research Center neuropsychological battery, 54, 55
holistic medicine. *See* complementary and alternative medicine
holistic treatment, 347
homeless, HIV/AIDS among, 308–315
  culturally sensitive services, 311, 314
  mental illness and, 309–311, 313
    access to mental health care/medications, 310
    challenges, 309–311
    complicated medical problems, 310
    funding agency support for research and clinical services, 311
    identification and acceptance of illness, 309–310
    identification of culturally sensitive services, 311
    inadequate infrastructure, 311
    lack of skills development for independent living and employment, 311
    limited resources, rising health costs, and cutbacks in entitlements, 311
    nonadherence to treatment, 310–311
    risk reduction, 311
    stigma, 310
    substance use, abuse, and dependence, 311, 343
    unstable housing, 310
  poverty, HIV/AIDS and, 308–309
  recommended strategies for success, 314–315
  repeated homelessness, 313
  strategies for success, 312
    core principles of care, 312
    prevention, 312
    risk assessment, 312
    therapeutic alliance, 312
  successful planning and programs, 313–314
    CARES program, 309, 310, 314
    core issue of housing, 314
    Housing Opportunities for People with AIDS (HOPWA), 314
    integrated care, 313–314
    Tenderloin Collaborative Work Group (TCWG), 313–314
homeopathy, 368–369
homophobia, 234, 289, 295–296, 305
  internalized, 293
homosexuality
  African Americans, 224
  American Indians and Alaska Natives, 243, 244
  Asian and Pacific Islander Americans, 234, 236
  assumptions about sexual behavior and, 289
  coming out, 301–302
  community-based organizations, 288
    AIDS Coalition To Unleash Power (ACT-UP), 288
    Gay Men Health Crisis (GMHC), 288
  gay, lesbian, bisexual, or transgender (GLBT), 243, 289, 296, 348
  gay, lesbian, or bisexual (GLB), 289, 304–305
  Hispanic Americans, 219
  and HIV transmission, 4–5
  organized religions and, 349
  See also lesbians; men who have sex with men (MSM); women who have sex with women (WSW)
Hopkins Verbal Learning Test-Revised, 54
HOPWA. *See* Housing Opportunities for People with AIDS
hormonal contraceptives, 278, 280
  antiretrovirals and, 282
  herb-drug interactions and, 375
Hospital Anxiety and Depression Scale (HADS), 56
hospitalization. *See* medical hospitalization
Housing Opportunities for People with AIDS (HOPWA), 314
HPV. *See* human papillomavirus
HRSA. *See* Health Resources and Services Administration
HSCS. *See* High Sensitivity Cognitive Screen
HSI (HIV-risk screening instrument), 397
HSV-2 (herpes simplex virus 2), 188, 189, 190
HUD. *See* Department of Housing and Urban Development
human immunodeficiency virus. *See* HIV
human papillomavirus (HPV), 188, 189, 190, 194, 279
Huntington's disease, 383, 384

hydromorphone, for pain, 169
hydroxyzine (Atarax), 132, 145
hyperactivity, in children with HIV, 264
hypercortisolemia, 380
hypericin. *See* St. John's wort
hyperthermia, 366
hypnosis, 359
    effectiveness of, 373
hypnotics, 143–145
hypocretin neurons, 138
hypogonadism, 45, 204, 206
hypothalamic-pituitary-adrenal (HPA) axis, 380
hypothalamus, 138
hypothyroidism, 204

I

IADL. *See* instrumental activities of daily living
identity (self-concept) changes, 357
IDUs. *See* injection drug users
IFN-γ. *See* interferon-γ
IHS. *See* Indian Health Service
IL-1. *See* interleukin-1
IL-4. *See* interleukin-4
IL-6. *See* interleukin-6
Illinois
    2005 legislative action, 324
    African American HIV/AIDS Response Act (2005), 324
imipramine, 359
immune system
    function and aging, 269
    neuronal interaction with, 82
    stress and, 82, 380
    use of herbs and, 367
    use of massage and, 372
immunology, 14–16
    immune parameters, stress, and disease progression, 81–82
    inflammatory response to HIV-1, 15–16
    systemic immunopathogenesis, 14
impulsivity, as temperament trait, 102
IN. *See* integrase
Indian Health Service (IHS), 244, 247
Indians. *See* American Indians and Alaska Natives
indinavir (Crixivan), 29, 30, 145, 282
    drug interactions, 272
infants. *See* neonates and infants
inflammatory response to HIV-1, 15–16, 21
influenza vaccination, 24
informed consent, and HIV testing, 252, 321
injection drug users (IDUs)
    complicating conditions in, 130
    homelessness and, 309, 310
    reactivation of old infections, 130
    risks of HIV/AIDS, 4–5, 17, 127
    See also substance abuse; *special populations*
insomnia, 138–140
    See also sleep disorders
Institute of Medicine (IOM)
    Committee on Lesbian Health Research Priorities, 299
    Lesbian Health, 305–306

instrumental activities of daily living (IADL), 115
integrase (IN), 11
integrative medicine, 366, 367
interferon-γ (IFN-γ), 16
interferon alpha, 130, 201
interleukin-1 (IL-1), 13, 16
interleukin-4 (IL-4), 16
interleukin-6 (IL-6), 16
interpersonal therapy (IPT), 359
intravenous drug abuse. *See* injection drug users
intubation, 389
in utero infection, 228
    See also vertical transmission
invasive squamous cell carcinoma of the cervix, 20
Invirase. *See* saquinavir
IOM. *See* Institute of Medicine
IPT. *See* interpersonal therapy
isolation, social, 7, 356–357, 390, 412
itraconazole (Sporanox), drug interactions, 153

J

Jakob Creutzfeldt virus, testing for, 205

K

Kaiser, Jon, 370
Kaletra, 152
Kaposi's sarcoma, 18, 20, 24, 369
kava, drug interactions, 160
ketamine, 159
ketoconazole (Nizoral), drug interactions, 153
KFARY. *See* Kosovar Families Addressing Risk in Youth
Konefal, Dr., 370
Korean plants, 371
Kosovar Families Addressing Risk in Youth (KFARY), 331–332
Krieger, Delores, 370
Kunz, Dora, 370

L

Laing, R. D., 343
lamivudine, 28, 30
    for mania, 207–208
    panic disorder and, 89
lamotrigine, 98
    drug interactions, 158
    for mania, 273
    for pain, 177
latent stage. *See* asymptomatic stage
latent state, 12
legal issues
    advance directives, 390–392
    civil commitment law, 342
    concerning prisons/prisoners, 323–324, 342–343
    outpatient treatment statutes, 345
    regulations concerning HIV testing, 34
    suicide and end-of-life care, 383–392, 404–414
lemon balm, 368
lesbian, gay, bisexual (LGB). *See* gay, lesbian, or bisexual (GLB)
lesbian, gay, bisexual, or transgender (LGBT) *See* gay, lesbian, bisexual, or transgender

lesbians
    Gay and Lesbian Medical Association, 305
    health care access for, 305–306
    Institute of Medicine (IOM)
        Committee on Lesbian Health Research
            Priorities, 299
        Lesbian Health, 305–306
    lack of standard definition for, 299, 300
    Mautner Project for Lesbians with Cancer, 306
    National Lesbian Health Case Survey
        (NLHCS), 303
    See also homosexuality; women who have sex with
        women
leukopenia, 273
levorphanol, for pain, 169
LGB (lesbian, gay, bisexual). *See* gay, lesbian, or
    bisexual (GLB)
libido, 45
lidocaine, for pain, 178
lipodystrophy, 56, 88
listeriosis, 20
lithium, 97, 132, 229
    contraindicated for African-Americans, 229
    drug interactions, 158
    for mania, 207, 273
    toxicity, 158, 207, 229
liver function
    alcohol and substance abuse and, 43–44
    cirrhosis, 201
    hepatic encephalopathy, 201
living will, 390
local anesthetics, for pain, 174–175
long terminal repeat (LTR), 16
lopinavir, 29, 30
lorazepam, 90, 143, 207
    metabolism and drug interactions, 153
LTR. *See* long terminal repeat
lumbar puncture, 204–205
Lunesta (eszopiclone), 144
lymphoma, CNS, 94, 203

M

MA. *See* matrix (MA) protein
MacArthur Foundation National Survey of Midlife
    Development in the United States (MIDUS),
    303, 304
MAC infection. *See Mycobacterium avium* complex
    (MAC) infection
macrophage inflammatory protein (MIP)-1α, 16
macrophages
    chronic activated state, 13
    infection of, 13, 15
magnetic-based therapies, 365, 370
magnetic resonance imaging (MRI), 116
    for children, 264
    functional magnetic resonance imaging (fMRI), 116
    with gadolinium contrast, 204
magnetic resonance spectroscopy (MRS),
    116, 117
major depressive disorder (MDD), 129
malignancies. *See* neoplasms

mania
    accompanying psychotic episodes, 120, 121
    diagnosing, 97
    in HIV-infected homeless people, 310
    manic disorders, 45
    in medical inpatients with HIV/AIDS, 201,
        207–208
    in older adults, 272–273
    treatment of, 97–98, 132, 207–208, 273
maprotiline, for pain, 175
marijuana, 159, 368
massage therapy, 367, 369
    effectiveness studies, 372
matrix (MA) protein, 11
matrix metalloproteinases (MMPs), 16
Mautner Project for Lesbians with Cancer, 306
MBSR. *See* Mindfulness-Based Stress Reduction
    (MBSR) Program
MCMD. *See* minor cognitive motor disorder
MCP-1. *See* monocyte chemoattractant protein-1
MDD. *See* major depressive disorder
MDEL (medical decisions concerning the end of
    life), 409
MDMA. *See* methylenedeoxymethamphetamine
Medicaid, 309
medical comorbidity. *See* comorbid medical
    conditions; comorbid psychiatric disorders
medical durable power of attorney, 390
medical history. *See* history, medical/psychological
medical hospitalization
    and changing scope of HIV epidemic, 199
    psychiatric co-morbidities in HIV/AIDS inpatients,
        198–211
    psychiatric diagnosis and treatment, 198–211
    and relapse of primary psychiatric disorders, 201
medical treatment, 23–35, 198–211
    adherence to, 21–23
    barriers to, 43
    initial evaluation, 23–24
    of medical complications of HIV, 25–27
    medications other than antiretroviral, 153–160
    psychosis as a complication of, 122–123
    of substance users with HIV infection, 130–131
    treatment of medical complications of HIV,
        25–27
    treatment regimens, 28–31
    See also antiretroviral therapy; treatment
        considerations
medication holidays, 32
medications, adherence to. *See* adherence
meditation, 367, 370
    perceived effectiveness of, 372, 373
meningitis, 164
Mental Health: Culture, Race, and Ethnicity, 244
mental health services, epidemiologic implications,
    8–9
mental illness
    civil commitment laws, 342, 343
    criminalization of the mentally ill, 343, 344
    deinstitutionalization of the mentally ill, 342–343
    high risk behaviors and, 344

mental illness (*cont.*)
  HIV prevention/education for persons with, 401–402
  incarceration for nonviolent crimes, 343
  "mercy arrests", 343
  mistreatment of the mentally ill, 342–343
  outpatient treatment statutes, 345
  in prisons, 341–344
  recommendations, 344–345
  serious mental illness, defined, 341–342
  substance abuse and, 343
  See also psychiatric disorders; *specific disorders*
Mentalization-Based Therapy, 107–108
mental status changes, drugs associated with, 122–123
mental status examination, 41–42, 52, 263–264
men who have sex with men (MSM), 288–298
  HIV/AIDS among, 4, 288–298
    assumptions about sexual behavior and, 289
    discussing sex and risk behaviors with, 294
    diversity among, 288–289, 295–296
    HIV disclosure, 292–293
    HIV epidemiology among, 290–291
    HIV prevention for MSM, 291–292
    HIV testing and counseling, 292
    homelessness and, 308
    mental health treatment for, 293–294
    providing care to, 289–290
    racial/ethnic minority MSMs, 295–296
    risk assessment, 291–292
    treatment for sexual dysfunction, 295
  risks of HIV/AIDS, 4–5, 17
  sexually transmitted diseases and, 188
    screening for, 192–193
  in special populations
    African Americans, 224, 295
    American Indians and Alaska Natives, 243
    Asian and Pacific Islander Americans, 232–233, 234, 235, 236, 295
    Hispanic Americans, 218, 219, 221, 295
  suicide rates, 227
  young men who have sex with men (YMSM), 290
meperidine (Demerol), for pain, 170, 173
  contraindications, 387
Mepron. *See* atovaquone
metabolic syndrome, 125, 270, 271
methadone
  and efavirenz, 152, 159
  methadone maintenance treatment (MMT)
    drug interactions and, 158
    HIV-positive patients in, 128–129, 130
  for pain, 169, 388
methamphetamine, 119, 129
  anxiety and, 90
  drug interactions, 159
  unprotected sex and, 235
methotrexate, mental status changes and, 123
methotrimeprazine, for pain, 176
methylenedeoxymethamphetamine (MDMA, Ecstasy), 43, 129
  drug interactions, 159

methylphenidate, 95, 132, 206
  for hyperactivity in children, 264–265
  for pain, 176
mexiletine, for pain, 178
mianserin, for pain, 175
midazolam, 143
  drug interactions, 151, 153
Midlife Development in the United States (MIDUS), 303, 304
MIDUS. *See* MacArthur Foundation National Survey of Midlife Development in the United States
mind-body interventions, 365, 370
Mindfulness-Based Stress Reduction (MBSR) Program, 372
Mini-Mental State Examination (MMSE), 52
Mini-Mental Status Examination, Folstein-McHugh, 42
Minnesota Multiphasic Personality Inventory-2 (MMPI-2), 56
minor cognitive motor disorder (MCMD), 14–15, 20, 49, 111
  diagnosis of, 49–50, 112
  in substance users, 131
MIP-1α. *See* macrophage inflammatory protein (MIP)-1α
mirtazapine (Remeron), 95, 145
  metabolism and drug interactions, 157
MMPI-2. *See* Minnesota Multiphasic Personality Inventory-2
MMPs. *See* matrix metalloproteinases
MMSE. *See* Mini-Mental State Examination
MMT (methadone maintenance treatment), 128–129, 130, 158
modafinil, 158
  for depression, 206
  for pain, 176, 177
molindone, for psychosis, 208
monoamine oxidase (MAO) inhibitors, 375
monocyte chemoattractant protein-1 (MCP-1), 15, 16
monocytes, infection of, 13
mood disorders, 49, 89, 93–100
  diagnosis and symptoms, 93–94, 97, 271–272
  mania, 97–98
  misdiagnosed as schizophrenia, 226
  in older adults, 270–273
  risk factors, 94
  suicide among HIV/AIDS patients with, 98–99, 385
  treatment modalities, 94–96
    antidepressants, 94–95
    electroconvulsive therapy, 96
    electroconvulsive treatment, 96
    hormones, 96
    inpatient care, 96
    psychostimulants, 95–96
    psychotherapy, 96
  in women who have sex with women (WSW), 303
mood stabilizers, 157–158
morbidity. *See* psychiatric morbidity
morphine
  for dyspnea, 389
  for pain, 169, 387

MRI. *See* magnetic resonance imaging
MRS. *See* magnetic resonance spectroscopy
MSM. *See* men who have sex with men
muscle relaxation techniques, 359
Mycobacterium avium complex (MAC) infection, 20, 21, 26
Mycobacterium avium intracellulare (MAI), 164
Mycobacterium tuberculosis, 130
myopathy, 65

N

narcissistic personality disorders, 103, 104, 105
narcolepsy, 138
National Center for Complementary and Alternative Medicine (NCCAM), 347, 366
National Household Survey of Drug Abuse, 302
National Institute of Mental Health (NIMH)
    Consortium on Families and HIV/AIDS, 331
    Epidemiological Catchment Area Program, 343
    Office of AIDS, 331
National Institutes of Health (NIH), 309, 312
    National Center for Complementary and Alternative Medicine, 347, 366
National Lesbian Health Case Survey (NLHCS), 303
National Network of STD/HIV Prevention Training Centers, 396
National Perinatal HIV Consultation and Referral Service, 400–401
Native Americans. *See* American Indians and Alaska Natives
natural killer (NK) cells, 82
naturopathy, 369
nausea, 388–389
NC. *See* nucleocapsid (NC) protein
NCCAM. *See* National Center for Complementary and Alternative Medicine
needles
    cleaning of, 17, 192
    free needle programs, 17
    needle stick exposure, 18
    reuse of, 18
    sharing, and HIV, 4
    syringe exchange programs, 134, 322
nef (negative regulatory factor) gene, 11
nefazodone (Serzone), 145
    drug interactions, 151, 152, 157
nelfinavir, 29, 30
    in women, 282
neonates and infants, 250–258
    attention deficits in, 115
    cognitive functioning/disorders, 115
    developmental and neurobiologic issues, 255–256
    HIV/AIDS among, 250–258
        epidemiology, 250
    HIV-positive infant, 254–257
        antiretroviral medications, 255
        developmental and neurobiologic issues, 255–256
        diagnosis, 254
        initiation of treatment decisions, 255
        presentation of untreated children, 254–255
        psychiatry liaison and, 256–257
        treatment, 254
    preterm infants, 280
    vertical transmission, 250–251, 279–280
        implications for prenatal care, 251–252
        implications for treatment at labor and delivery, 252–254
        prevention of, 251
neoplasms, CNS, 45, 48
    diagnosis, 203
    and psychotic disorder, 121–122
neurobehavioral evaluation, 50–59
neuroimaging, 116–117
    for children, 263–264
neuroleptic malignant syndrome (NMS), 98, 124, 133
neuroleptics, 98, 124–125
    atypical, 124–125, 132
    drug interactions, 151–152, 158
    extrapyramidal reactions (EPRs), 98, 209
    for pain, 173, 176
neurolinguistic psychology, 370
neurologic assessment for cognitive impairment, 84
Neurontin. *See* gabapentin
neuropathic pain, 177
neuropathies in HIV/AIDS-infected patients, 164
neuropsychological testing. *See* psychological and neuropsychological testing
neurosyphilis
    in psychotic disorder, 121
    in substance users, 130
nevirapine (Viramune), 29, 30
    drug interactions, 152
    prenatal administration, 17, 253
    for sleep disorder, 144
New Republic, 343
NF6B. *See* nuclear factor NF kappa B
NIH. *See* National Institutes of Health
NIMH. *See* National Institute of Mental Health
NIMH Multisite HIV Prevention Trial, 284
NIMH neuropsychological battery, 53–54, 113, 114
Nizoral. *See* ketoconazole
NK. *See* natural killer (NK) cells
NLHCS. *See* National Lesbian Health Case Survey
NMS. *See* neuroleptic malignant syndrome
NNRTIs. *See* non-nucleoside reverse transcriptase inhibitors
non-nucleoside reverse transcriptase inhibitors (NNRTIs)
    drug interactions, 151, 152
    herbal treatments contraindicated with, 375
nonopiod analgesics, for pain, 167–168
non-rapid eye movement (NREM) sleep, 137–138
norepinephrine, in stress responses, 82
nortriptyline, for pain, 175
Norvir. *See* ritonavir
notification, partner, 196
novelty seeking, 102, 103, 105–106
NRME. *See* non-rapid eye movement (NREM) sleep
NRTIs. *See* nucleoside reverse transcriptase inhibitors
NSAIDS, for pain, 167–168
nuclear factor NF kappa B (NF6B), 12, 16
nucleocapsid (NC) protein, 11

nucleoside reverse transcriptase inhibitors (NRTIs), 28, 30
   drug interactions, 151, 152
nutritional supplements, 371
nutritionists, 367

O

obsessive compulsive disorder, AIDS-related, 89
occupational exposure, 32–34, 209, 402
   during mental health care, 32–33
   See also postexposure prophylaxis
olanzapine, 124, 125, 132
   for delirium, 207, 389
   for dyspnea, 389
   for hiccups, 388
   for mania, 132, 208
   for nausea and vomiting, 388
   for pain, 173, 176
   for psychosis, 133, 208
older adults, 267–276
   cognitive disorders, 116
   HIV-associated dementia (HAD), 274–275
     course and outcome, 275
     differential diagnosis, 275
     pathogenesis, 274
     risk factors, 274
     symptoms, 274
     treatment, 275
   mood disorders, 270–273
     depression treatment, 272
     depressive spectrum, 270–272
     differential diagnosis, 271–272
     mania, 272–273
     presenting symptoms, 271
   normal aging and HIV infection, 268–269
     immune system function and aging, 269
     pharmacokinetic changes and aging, 269
   psychiatric disorders, HIV, and aging, 269
   psychotic disorders, 269–270
     HIV-related psychosis, 270
     schizophrenia, 269–270
   risk, diagnosis, course, treatment, and aging, 267–268
     diagnosis, course, and aging, 268
     epidemiology, 267
     risk and aging, 267–268
     treatment, 268
   STI screening, 192–193
   substance use disorders, 273
ondansetron, for nausea and vomiting, 388
opioid agonists, 159
   See also methadone
opioid analgesics, for pain, 168–173
opioid side effects, 172, 173
opportunistic infections, 25–27, 201–203
oral candidiasis ("thrush"), 18, 20
oral contraceptives. See hormonal contraceptives
oral hairy leukoplakia, 18, 20
orexin (hypocretin) neurons, 138
otitis media, 164
oxazepam, metabolism and drug interactions, 153
oxcarbazepine, 158
oxycarbamazepine, 97
oxycodone, for pain, 169

P

p6 (core protein), 11, 12
p7 (core protein), 12
p17 (core protein), 12
p24 (core protein), 12–13
pain syndromes, 45, 161–187
   children and pain syndromes, 164
   drug interactions: analgesics and anti-HIV drug therapies, 178–179
   management, 165–167, 387–388
     assessment issues, 165
     barriers to, 180–181
     multimodal approach, 166–167
     pain measurement/assessment tools, 166
     and substance abuse, 179, 181–184
   neuropathies in HIV/AIDS-infected patients, 164
   nonpharmacologic interventions, 179
   pharmacotherapies for, 167–178
     adjuvant analgesics, 173, 174–175
     anticonvulsant drugs, 177–178
     antidepressants, 173–176
     corticosteroids, 178
     neuroleptics and benzodiazepines, 176
     nonopiod analgesics, 167–168
     opioid analgesics, 168–173
     opioid side effects, 173
     opioid side effects, medications to relieve, 172
     oral and topical anesthetics, 178
     psychostimulants, 176–177
   prevalence of, 161–162
   specific pain syndromes, 162–163
   treatment, 131, 387–388
   undertreatment of, 180, 387
   women and, 163–164
   World Health Organization (WHO) guidelines, 167
panic disorder, 5, 89
Pap smears, 24, 193
Parkinsonism, 16
   antipsychotic medications and, 124, 229
paroxetine, for pain, 175
Parran, Thomas, 196
partners
   medical evaluation and treatment, 196
   notification and referral, 196
   stresses for, 88–89
patient education. See prevention and education strategies
Patient Health Questionnaire depression scale (PHQ-9), 271–272
patient's family, 328–337
   couple or family assessment and intervention, 332–336
     action plan, 333
     confidentiality issues, 333–334
     family and couples therapies, 360–361
     genogram, 332
     systematic assessment, 332–333
     therapeutic relationship, 332, 334–336

family assessment, 330
family factors that adversely affect health, 330
family factors with salutatory effects on health, 331–332
  CHAMP Family Program, 331
  community-based prevention programs, 332
  family-based prevention programs, 331–332
  Kosovar Families Addressing Risk in Youth (KFARY), 331–332
  Project Care, 332
  WiLLOW program, 332
"family of choice" vs. "family or origin", 331
impact of HIV/AIDS on couples and familics, 329–330
special issues for gay couples, 332
PCP. *See* phencyclidine (PCP); *Pneumocystis jeroveci* pneumonia (PCP)
PD. *See* personality disorder
pediatric AIDS. *See* children
peer educators, 238
pelvic inflammatory disease (PID), 20, 194
pemoline
  for depression, 206
  for pain, 176, 177
penicillin, 194
pentamidine, 25
PEP. *See* postexposure prophylaxsis
perinatally-infected children, stress and, 80–81
perinatal transmission, 250, 253, 279–280, 400–401
  National Perinatal HIV Consultation and Referral Service, 400–401
peripheral neuropathy, 20
persistent lymphadenopathy (PGL), 19
personality, 101–105
  character dimensions, 101, 102
  characteristics, 6
  coping, and self-transcendence, 104–105
  high-risk behaviors and, 103–104
  models of, 101–102
  psychological experience of infection and, 104
  temperament traits, 101–102
  treatment adherence and, 105
personality disorder (PD), 46, 101–110
  antisocial personality disorder (ASPD), 102, 105
  and Axis I diagnoses, 105
  borderline personality disorder (BPD), 101, 102, 104, 105, 107–108
  character dimensions, 101, 102
  clusters A-C, 46, 102
  diagnosis of, in HIV-positive population, 102–103
  epidemiologic perspectives, 102
  future research directions, 109
  health care policy, 109
  models of personality, 101–102
  narcissistic personality disorders, 103, 104, 105
  personality, maladaptive behavior, and illness response, 103–105
    personality and high-risk behaviors, 103–104
    personality and psychological experience of infection, 104

personality and treatment adherence, 105
personality, coping, and self-transcendence, 104–105
substance abuse and, 129
temperament traits, 101–102
treatment considerations and implications, 105–109
  countertransference issues, 106
  group psychotherapy, 108
  individual psychotherapy, 106–108
  other interventions and considerations, 108–109
  psychopharmacology, 108
PET. *See* positron cmission tomography
PGL. *See* persistent lymphadenopathy; progressive generalized lymphadenopathy
pharmacology, of drug actions/interactions, 149–150
phases of disease. *See* disease stages
phencyclidine (PCP), 119, 159
phenobarbital, drug interactions, 152, 153
phenytoin, 177
  drug interactions, 152
phosphodiesterase inhibitors, 295
physical dependence, defined, 183
physician assisted suicide and voluntary euthanasia, 404–414
  definition of euthanasia and physician assisted suicide, 404–405
  historical context, 405–406
  legislation concerning, 405, 409
  literature review on suicidality and HIV, 406–409
  medical decisions concerning the end of life (MDEL), 409
  observations on, 409–410
  origins of the desire for, 410–413
  phases of HIV infection/disease, 406
    Phase I: before highly active antiretroviral treatment, 406
    Phase II: advent of active antiretroviral treatment, 406
    Phase III: present time, 406
  rates of, 409–410
  "right to die", 409
  terminology, impact of, 410
  vs. "mercy killing", 404
PID. *See* pelvic inflammatory disease
pill fatigue, 32
pimozide, for pain, 176
PIs. *See* protease inhibitors
The Plague (Sartre), 411
PML. *See* progressive multifocal leukoencephalopathy
Pneumocystis carinii. *See Pneumocystis jeroveci*
Pneumocystis jeroveci pneumonia (PCP), 18, 20, 25
  delirium and, 206
  gender non-specificity, 279
  massage in treatment of, 369
  in prisoners, 321
  in substance users, 130
pneumonia vaccination, 24
pol gene, 11
pol polyprotein, 11
polyneuropathy, 65
polysomnography, 66–67, 139–140

positron emission tomography (PET), 116–117
postexposure prophylaxsis (PEP), 18, 34, 209, 402
   for occupational exposure, 33, 34
   for sexual assault, 33
post-traumatic stress disorder (PTSD), 45, 379
   cognitive-behavioral group interventions and, 381
   comorbid with HIV/AIDS, 94
   delayed onset of, 304
   relapse with HIV treatment, 88
   risk for in HIV population, 89
   in special populations
      American Indians and Alaska Natives, 245, 247
      Asian and Pacific Islander Americans, 236
      men who have sex with men (MSM), 293
      women, 281
      women who have sex with women (WSW), 302, 303–304
   symptoms, 381
poverty and HIV/AIDs, 7–8, 219, 260, 278
   homelessness and, 308–309
   stress of HIV and, 74
power of attorney, medical, 390
PR. *See* protease
prayer, 350, 367, 370
   perceived effectiveness of, 373
pregabalin, for pain, 177–178
pregnancy
   antiretroviral therapy during, 251–252, 253–254, 280
   Cesarean section, 17, 253, 280
   contraception and, 279–280
   HIV testing/screening, 251–253, 385, 400
      "opt-out" approach, 251, 252–253
   and HIV treatment, 28
   prenatal care, 251–254
   prevention of vertical transmission, 251–254
   sexuality and, 279–280
   substance abuse in, 8
   treatment at labor and delivery, 252–254
   See also breast feeding; vertical transmission
prenatal care, 251–254
   See also pregnancy
prevention and education strategies, 395–403
   AIDS Education and Training Centers, 396
   assessment of risk, 396–398
      barriers to, 397–398
      behavioral risk screening, 396–398
      drug use risk assessment, 396
      HIV-risk screening instrument (HSI), 397
      prescreening, 397
      sexual risk assessment, 396–397
   barriers regarding prevention for positives, 401–402
   community leadership, 399–400
   HIV testing and early detection, 400
   for mentally ill persons with HIV infection, 401–402
   National Network of STD/HIV Prevention Training Centers, 396
   other prevention strategies, 402
   patient education, 398–399
   postexposure prophylaxis (PEP), 18, 33, 34, 209, 402
   primary, secondary, and tertiary prevention, 395–396
   risk behavior checklist, 402
   sexually transmitted disease identification and treatment, 402
   specific prevention programs, 312, 328
      African American and, 230
      Asian and Pacific Islander Americans (APIs) and, 238–239
      community-based, 332
      family-based, 331–332
      focus on individuals, 238
      for men who have sex with men (MSM), 291–292
      parent-oriented, 331
      peer educators, 238
      for prisoners, 319
      for women, 283–284
   substance abuse identification and treatment, 402
primaquine, 25
Principles of Medical Ethics, 324–325
prisoners, HIV/AIDS among, 5, 316–327, 341
   associated conditions, 321
   barriers to diagnosis and treatment, 317–318
   condom and syringe distribution, 322, 325–326
   confidentiality of medical records, 321–322, 325
   disease control, 318–319
   educational materials, 318
   ethical issues, 324–326
   HIV testing issues, 321–322, 325
      California Proposition 96, 321, 325
   legal issues, 323–324
      2005 California legislative action, 324
      2005 Illinois legislative action, 324
      2005 Texas class action lawsuit, 324
      The African American HIV/AIDS Response Act (2005), 324
      safety issues for inmates, 323
      segregation of HIV-positive inmates, 323
      Sexual Abuse in Detention Elimination Act (2005), 324
      U.S. Justice Department study, 323–324
   mental illness and, 5, 341–343
   prevalence, 316–317
   prevention programs, 319
   Stop Prison Rape, 323
   transmission and sexual behavior, 319–321
      consensual and nonconsensual sex, 319–320, 323–324
      sexual assaults, 319–320, 323–324
      substance abuse and, 320–321
   treatment of psychiatric illness in context of HIV/AIDS, 344
   See also prisons
prisons
   deinstitutionalization of the mentally ill, 342–343
   HIV and, 341
   mental health treatment in, 343–344
      in context of HIV/AIDS, 344
   mental illness in, 341–344
      serious mental illness, 341–342

recommendations, 344–345
situation in the correctional system, 342–343
civil commitment law, 342
deinstitutionalization, 342–343
mistreatment of mentally ill, 342–343
substance abuse and the mentally ill, 343
See also prisoners, HIV/AIDS among
procarbazine, mental status changes and, 123
progressive generalized lymphadenopathy (PGL), 59
progressive multifocal leukoencephalopathy (PML), 20
diagnosis, 203
mood-disorder symptoms and, 94
in prisoners, 321
and psychotic disorder, 121, 122
proinflammatory cytokines, 15, 16
Project Care, 332
Proposition 96, 321, 325
ProSom (estazolam), 143
protease (PR), 11
protease inhibitors (PIs), 29, 30
adverse metabolic effects, 125
and benzodiazepines, 143
drug interactions, 125, 150–152
herbal treatments contraindicated with, 375
protozoan infection (trichomoniasis), 188, 189, 191, 194
pruritus, 373, 388
psychiatric assessment, 39–47, 50–59
Axis I diagnoses, 44–47
anxiety disorders, 45
bipolar disorders, 45
cognitive disorders, 46–47
depressive disorders, 44–45
pain, 45
personality disorders, 46
psychotic disorders, 44
sexual dysfunction, 45
suicidal behaviors, 46
barriers to risk reduction, 43
barriers to treatment and adherence, 43–44
of children, 263–264
clinical approach to, 40–42
for cognitive impairment, 84
differential diagnostic considerations, 43
history, 40–41, 50–52
initial assessment, 23–24, 40
mental status examination, 41–42, 52
of neurocognitive impairment, 50–59
neuropsychological, 53–55
substance abuse, 43–44
symptom validity, 54–55
psychiatric comorbidity. See comorbid psychiatric disorders
psychiatric diagnosis and treatment of medically hospitalized patients, 198–211
medical hospitalization and changing scope of HIV epidemic, 199
psychiatric disorders
antedating HIV infection, 39, 201, 356
coupled with substance use and HIV disease, 127–129
psychiatric treatment of, 131–133

end-of-life care and, 389
HIV/AIDS and, 5–6, 9, 44, 224–225, 309
homelessness and, 309–311
treatment in correctional institutions, 344
in medically ill patients with HIV/AIDS, 198–211
diagnostic evaluation, 204–205
differential diagnosis, 201–204
disorders and their treatment, 205–208
epidemiology of, 199–201
mania, 207–208
provider issues, 209
psychosis, 208
system of care, 208–209
system of care issues, 208–209
older adults and, 269
in prisons/prisoners, 341–344
serious mental illness, defined, 341–342
triple diagnosis, 127–129
See also comorbid psychiatric disorders; mental illness; special populations; specific disorders
psychiatric epidemiology, 5–6
psychiatric morbidity, 6–7
See also comorbid psychiatric disorders
psychiatric support for medical care providers, 209
Psychodynamic Partial Hospitalization, 107–108
psychoeducation, 108–109
psychological and neuropsychological testing, 48–62
for children, 264
for cognitive disorders, 113–114
false positive results, 55
functional abilities testing, 115
functional indicators, 56–59
global deficit scores, 114
history, 50–52
HIV cognitive history, 53–54
HNRC neuropsychological battery, 54, 55
mental status examination, 41–42, 52
neuropsychological assessment, 53–55, 199
NIMH neuropsychological battery, 53–54, 113, 114
psychological functioning, 55–56
standard deviations, 50
symptom validity, 54–55
psychological functioning, 55–56
psychological reactions, 71–78
distinguishing between normal and pathologic psychological reactions, 76–77
HIV/AIDS as a chronic medical illness, 76–77
psychological impact at different stages of HIV/AIDS, 72–76
psychological attributions to highly active antiretroviral therapy, 75–76
reactions to antibody status notification, 72–73
reactions to antibody testing in women, 73–74
reaction to disclosure of antibody status, 74–75
seven existential "postures" of vulnerability/resistance, 76
treatment considerations, 77

psychomotor disorders, 6
psychopharmacology, 108
psychosexual dysfunction, 7
psychosis. *See* psychotic disorders
psychosocial aspects. *See* biopsychosocial aspects
psychosocial challenges, 7
psychosocial interventions, 380
psychostimulants, 95–96, 132
   drug interactions, 158
   medical inpatients and, 205
   for pain, 174, 176–177
psychotherapeutic strategies, 355–364
   boundaries, 363
   burnout, 363
   challenges amenable to psychotherapy, 355–358
      adjustment to medical illness, 356
      changes in developmental progression, 357–358
      changes in identity, 357
      grief, 356
      preexisting psychiatric disorders, 356
      response to initial infection, 355–356
      spirituality, 358
      stigmatization, 356–357
      treatment adherence, 357
   countertransference, 361, 362, 390
   peer support and supervision, 362
   specific techniques, 358–361
      cognitive-behavioral therapy (CBT), 359
      culturally specific therapies, 361
      existential and spiritual therapies, 360
      family and couples therapies, 360–361
      group therapies, 360
      interpersonal therapy (IPT), 359
      psychodynamic psychotherapy, 359–360
   transference, 361–362
   See also psychotherapy
psychotherapy
   for adjustment disorders, 83
   for anxiety disorders, 91
   for borderline personality disorder, 107–108
      Mentalization-Based Therapy, 107–108
      Psychodynamic Partial Hospitalization, 107–108
      Supportive Therapy for Borderline Patients, 107–108
      Transference-Focused Psychotherapy, 107–108
   burnout, 363
   countertransference, 106, 361, 362, 390
   family-centered approach, 329–330, 332–336
   individual, for anxiety disorders, 88
   for mood disorders, 96
   peer support and supervision for, 362
   for personality disorders, 106–108
      group psychotherapy, 108
      idealizing needs, 106, 107
      mirroring needs, 106, 107
      twinship or alter-ego needs, 106, 107
   for substance users with HIV infection, 131–132
   transference, 361–362
   See also psychotherapeutic strategies

psychotic disorders, 44, 119–126
   antipsychotic medications, 123–125
   associated with HIV-related medical conditions, 121–122
   differential diagnosis, 123
   in medical inpatients with HIV/AIDS, 208
   new-onset
      etiology and presentation of, 120–121
      in medical inpatients, 208
   preceding HIV infection, 119
   primary vs. secondary psychosis, 120
   psychosis as a complication of medical treatment, 122–123
   psychosis associated with substance abuse/dependence, 122, 132–133
   in special populations
      homeless people, 310
      men who have sex with men (MSM), 293
      older adults, 269–270
   treatment of HIV-associated psychosis, 123–125, 270
psychotropic drugs
   interactions with antiretrovirals, 149–160
   metabolism and interactions, 153–160
PTSD. *See* post-traumatic stress disorder
pyrimethamine, 25

Q

qEEG. *See* quantitative electroencephalography
Qigong, 365, 368, 369
QLI. *See* quality of life index
quality of life
   and anxiety disorders, 86
   impact of pain on, 161, 164–165
   self-transcendence level and, 105
"quality of life" crimes, 343
quality of life index (QLI), 105
quantitative electroencephalography (qEEG), 64–65
quazepam (Doral), 143, 144
quetiapine, 124, 125, 132
   for delirium, 207
   for mania, 208
quinolinic acid, 16

R

race, and HIV transmission incidence, 4
RANTES, 16
rapid eye movement (REM) sleep, 66, 137–138
rCBF. *See* regional cerebral blood flow
rectal intercourse, HIV transmission and, 17
recurrent multidermatomal herpes zoster, 20
regional cerebral blood flow (rCBF), 116
regulatory genes, 11
Reiki, 365, 369
religious and spiritual considerations, 347–354
   communication about spirituality, 352
   end-of-life care and, 389
   intrinsic vs. extrinsic religiosity, 350
   organized religion, 349–350
   psychotherapeutic strategies and, 358, 360

religion vs. spirituality: distinctions, 348–350
"Religious of Spiritual Problem" (*DSM-IV-TR*), 348
research on religion and spirituality and health/mental health, 350–352
  belief in a higher power, 351
  depression and, 350
  prayer/"distant healing", 350
  substance abusers and, 351–352
  "wellness-spirituality", 350
"spiritual distress", 347–348
therapeutic interventions, 352–353
REM. *See* rapid eye movement (REM) sleep
Remeron. *See* mirtazapine
Rescriptor. *See* delavirdine
resistance. *See* drug resistance
Restoril. *See* temazepam
retrovirus, defined, 11
rev (regulator of virion protein expression) gene, 11
reverse transcriptase (RT), 11
  See also non-nucleoside reverse transcriptase inhibitors; nucleoside reverse transcriptase inhibitors
Rey 15-Item Test, 54
ribavirin, 366
rifabutin, 26
risk assessment, 291–292, 312, 314, 396–398
  barriers to, 397–398
  drug use risk screening, 396
  HIV-risk screening instrument (HSI), 397
  National Network of STD/HIV Prevention Training Centers, 396
  prescreening, 397
  recommended techniques, 396
  screening for STDs, 193, 396–397
  sexual risk assessment, 396–397
  suicide risk assessment, 77
risks
  behavioral risk and sexually transmitted infections, 191–192
  discussing risk behaviors with HIV-positive MSM, 294
  high risk behaviors, 128, 291
    behavioral interventions to reduce, 291
    in Hispanic communities, 220
    mental disorders and judgement about, 225
    in mentally ill people, 344
    novelty seeking, 102, 103, 105–106
    in prisoners, 319–321, 344
    psychotic disorders and, 44
  of HIV/AIDS, 3–5, 16–18, 221, 308
    cognitive reserves and, 49
    in health care setting, 32–34
    psychiatric illness and, 44
  risk behavior checklist, 402
  risk environments, 4, 43
  risk reduction, barriers to, 43
  risk reduction interventions, 134–135
  Sexual Risk Behavior Assessment Schedule, 134–135

situations posing no risk, 16–17
of subsequent psychiatric disorders, 6
of suicidal behaviors, 46, 383–384
See also risk assessment; *special populations*
risperidone, 124, 125, 132
  for delirium, 207
  for HIV-associated psychosis, 133
  for mania, 208
  for psychosis, 208
ritonavir (Norvir), 29, 30
  drug interactions, 125, 150–152, 153, 157–159, 178, 270
  serotonin syndrome and, 90
  for sleep disorder, 144, 145
  in women, 282
role transitions, 359
RT. *See* reverse transcriptase
Ryan White Comprehensive AIDS Resource Emergency (CARE) Act, 248

S

St. John's wort, 366
  contradictions for use, 375
  for depression, 368
  drug interactions, 152, 160, 375
salvage regimens, 20
SAMHSA. *See* Substance Abuse and Mental Health Services Administration
saquinavir (Invirase), 29, 30
  drug interactions, 178, 272
Sartre, literature of, 411
schizoaffective disorders, 5, 208
schizophrenia, 208, 225
  high risk behaviors and, 344
  in older adults, 269–270
sedative hypnotics, 143–145
  metabolism and drug interactions, 153
seizures, 63–64, 95
selective serotonin reuptake inhibitors (SSRIs)
  for anxiety/depression, 84, 90, 95, 132, 229
  for children, 265
  drug interactions, 151, 272
  hyperserotonergic syndrome, 272
  obsessive compulsive disorder, 89
  for pain, 174, 175
self-directedness, 102
self-transcendence, 102, 104–105, 106
self-transcendence scale (STS), 105
SEPs. *See* somatosensory evoked potentials
seroconversion, 13
serotonin syndrome, 90, 157, 159
sertraline, 85, 95, 272
Serum Multiple Analysis-m6 (SMA 6), 46
Serzone. *See* nefazodone
SET. *See* Structural Ecosystems Therapy
set point, viral, 19, 20
sexual abuse, 281
  Childhood Trauma Questionnaire (CTQ), 407
sexual assault, postexposure prophylaxis for, 33
sexual avoidance, 71–72

sexual dysfunction, 7, 45
    delayed ejaculation, 7
    erectile dysfunction, 159, 295
    treatment decisions, 295
sexual history, 41, 192, 314
sexually transmitted infections (STIs), 188–197, 402
    assessment and screening for, 191
    asymptomatic in initial stages, 192
    bacterial infections, 188–189
    education and counseling, 194–195
    female-to-female transmission reported, 300
    history assessment, 191–192, 312
    and HIV, 4–5, 188, 401
    partner management, 195–196
        medical evaluation and treatment, 196
        notification and referral, 196
    partner notification, 194
    prevention and treatment of, 193–196
        behavioral management, 194–195
        Hepatitis B and Hepatitis A virus, 190, 194
        human papillomavirus (HPV), 190, 194
        medical management, 193–194
        National Network of STD/HIV Prevention Training Centers, 396
        partner management, 195–196
        pelvic inflammatory disease (PID), 194
        syphilis, 194
        trichomoniasis, 194
    prisons as reservoirs for, 321
    protozoan infection, 191
    risk assessment, 396–397
    risks of, 290
    screening and detection, 191, 192–193, 396
        sexual and substance use history, 192
    in special populations
        Asian and Pacific Islander Americans, 233
        Hispanic Americans, 220
        homeless, 309
        prisoners, 321
    viral infections, 190–191
        cytomegalovirus (CMV), 190
        Hepatitis viruses, 190, 194
        herpes simplex virus 2 (HSV-2), 188, 189, 190
        human papillomavirus (HPV), 190, 194
Sexual Risk Behavior Assessment Schedule, 134–135
sexual victimization, 228, 344
shingles, 164
sildenafil, 159, 295
single photon emission computed tomography (SPECT), 116, 117
sinusitis, 164
sleep, 66–67
    determinants of, 138
    hypothalamus and, 138
    non-rapid eye movement (NREM) sleep, 137–138
    normal sleep characteristics, 137–138
    NREM-REM cycle, 138, 140
    polysomnography, 66–67, 139–140
    rapid eye movement (REM) sleep, 66, 137–138

sleep apnea, 66
sleep disturbance, 66–67
slow-wave sleep (SWS), 66, 139–140
    See also sleep disorders
sleep disorders, 137–146
    alcohol and substance induced, 141
    antiretroviral therapy, 140
    assessment of, 139
    comorbid with HIV/AIDS, 94
    current treatment practices, 141–145
    determinants of sleep, 138
    insomnia, 138–140
        in HIV infection, polysomnographic changes, 139–140
        psychiatric disorders and, 140–141
        rebound insomnia, 143
    narcolepsy, 138
    normal sleep, characteristics of, 137–138
    NREM and REM sleep, 138, 140
    pharmacologic treatments, 142–145
        antidepressants, 145
        antihistamine, 145
        barbiturates, 143
        benzodiazepines, 143–144
        chloral hydrate, 145
        nonbenzodiazepine hypnotics, 144
        sedative hypnotics, 143–145
    psychiatric disorders and, 140–141
    stress and, 82
    See also sleep
slow-wave sleep (SWS), 66, 139–140
SMA 6. See Serum Multiple Analysis-m6
social-cognitive personality model, 102
social detachment, as temperament trait, 102
social isolation, 7, 356–357, 390, 412
social networks, 7, 390
    network of mutual commitment, 331
    See also patient's family
social stigma. See stigma
social support, 379–380
socioeconomic effects of HIV/AIDs, 7–8
somatosensory evoked potentials (SEPs), 65
Sonata (zaleplon), 144
special populations
    African Americans, 223–231
    American Indians and Alaska Natives (AI/ANs), 241–249
    Asian and Pacific Islander Americans (APIs), 232–240
    children and adolescents, 259–266
    Hispanic Americans, 215–222
    homeless, 308–315
    men who have sex with men (MSM), 288–298
    neonates and infants, 250–258
    older adults, 267–276
    patient's family, 328–337
    prisoners, 316–327
    statistics
        estimated AIDS cases compared, 218
        estimated HIV cases compared, 217
        survival rates compared, 217

women, 277–287
women who have sex with women (WSW), 299–307
SPECT. *See* single photon emission computed tomography
spirituality, 347–354
  caregivers and, 352–353
  communication about, 352
  defined, 348–349
  end-of-life care and, 389
  existential anxiety, 389
  existential crisis, 348
  expressions of, 348–349
  FICA Brief Spiritual Screening Instrument, 352
  four existential issues, 348
  Functional Assessment of Cancer Therapy (FACIT) Spiritual Well-being Scale, 350
  intrinsic life force, 348–349
  meditation, 367, 370
  psychotherapeutic strategies and, 358, 360
  in psychotherapy for personality disorder, 107
  religion vs. spirituality: distinctions, 348–350
  "Religious of Spiritual Problem" (*DSM-IV-TR*), 348
  research on religion and spirituality and health/mental health, 350–352
    belief in a higher power, 351
    depression and, 350
    prayer/"distant healing", 350
    substance abusers and, 351–352
    "wellness-spirituality", 350
  self-transcendence, 102
  spirit, meaning of, 348
  "spiritual distress", 347–348
  spiritual leaders, 348
  therapeutic interventions, 352–353
Sporanox. *See* itraconazole
SSRIs. *See* selective serotonin reuptake inhibitors
stages of HIV disease progression, 18–21
standard deviations, 50
stavudine, 28, 30
steroids, 25
  neurotoxic effects of, 94
  See also cortisol; testosterone
stigma, 72, 293
  health consequences of, 328
  HIV status disclosure and, 74–75
  psychotherapy for stigmatization, 356–357
  suicide risk and, 383
  women and, 74
stimulants. *See* psychostimulants
stimulus control, in sleep disorder treatment, 142
STIs. *See* sexually transmitted infections
Stop Prison Rape, 323
Streptococcus pneumoniae vaccination, 24
stress, 79–85, 379–381
  chronic, 379, 380
  cognitive behavioral stress management (CBSM), 83, 379
  coping with, 6, 81
  disease progression and, 81–82
  family stress, 329

  immune parameters and, 81–82, 380
  management techniques, 83, 372, 373, 379–381
  Mindfulness-Based Stress Reduction (MBSR) Program, 372
  psychological stressors, 86–89
  severe life stressors, 82
  stress-distress spectrum, 79–85
  stressful life events, 379
  treatment considerations, 83–84
  vs. distress, 79
  See also anxiety disorders; post-traumatic stress disorder
Stressor-Support-Coping Model for Psychosocial Intervention, 272
Structural Ecosystems Therapy (SET), 361
STS. *See* self-transcendence scale
substance abuse, 43–44
  addiction, 183
  criminalization of, 8
  defined, 183
  epidemiologic implications for services for, 8–9
  history of, 40–41
  identification and treatment, 402
  in the mentally ill, 343
  National Household Survey of Drug Abuse, 302
  noninjection drug use, 127
  pain management and, 179, 181–184, 387–388
  preexisting comorbid psychopathology, 201
  in pregnancy, 8
  "pseudo-addiction", 183
  psychiatric disorders and HIV, scope of the problem, 127–129
  psychosis and, 44, 122
  spirituality and, 351–352
  symptoms mimicing anxiety disorders, 89–90
  tolerance, physical dependence, vs. addiction/abuse, 183
  See also injection drug users; substance use; *special populations*
Substance Abuse and Mental Health Services Administration (SAMHSA), 309, 312
substances of abuse, drug interactions, 159
substance use
  cognitive disorders and, 116
  coupled with psychiatric disorders and HIV disease, 127–129
    psychiatric treatment of, 131–133
  directions for future research, 135
  history, 192
  HIV risk reduction interventions, 134–135
  psychotic disorders and, 119
  risk assessment, 396
  self-help groups, 131–132
  sleep disorder and, 141
  in special populations
    African Americans, 225
    American Indians and Alaska Natives (AI/ANs), 243–244, 245–246
    Asian and Pacific Islander Americans, 233, 235
    Hispanic Americans, 219–220
    homeless people, 311, 343

substance use (*cont.*)
   older adults, 273
   prisoners, 320–321, 343
   women who have sex with women (WSW), 302, 303
  syringe exchange programs, 134
  treatment in HIV-infected patients, 133–134
  See also substance abuse; substance use disorders
substance use disorders, 127–136
  coupled with psychiatric disorders and HIV disease, 127–129
   HIV risk behaviors, 128
   HIV seroprevalence in treatment settings, 128
   psychopathology and substance abuse in clinical samples of patients with HIV, 128–129
   psychopathology and substance abuse in research cohorts, 129
   scope of the problem, 127–129
  medical aspects of HIV infection in substance users, 129–131
   common HIV-associated and other medical problems, 129–130
   medical treatment of substance users with HIV, 130–131
  in medical inpatients, 199–201
  in older adults, 273
  treatment in HIV-infected patients, 133–134
  treatment in older adults, 273
  triple diagnosis, 127–129
suicide, 383–386
  as coping mechanism vs. "rational" decision, 411–412
  history-taking, 386
  literature review on suicidality and HIV, 406–409
  medical comorbidity, 384–385
  methods used, 384
  prevalence and risk, 384
  prevention, 386
  psychiatric disorders and, 98–99, 383–384, 385
  risk assessment, 77
  scope of, 384
  sources of suicidal ideation, suicide attempts, and suicide, 395
  in special populations
   African-Americans, 227
   Asian and Pacific Islander Americans, 236
   women, 282
  suicidal behaviors, 9, 46, 263, 384
   inpatient care for, 96
  suicidal ideation, 5, 46, 384
   sources of, 395, 410–413
  See also physician assisted suicide and voluntary euthanasia
sulfadiazine, mental status changes and, 123
sulfamethoxazole, 25
sulfamethoxazole/trimethoprim (SMX/TMP; Bactrim), 153
Supportive Therapy for Borderline Patients, 107–108
survivor guilt, 76, 290
SWS. *See* slow-wave sleep

syphilis, 188, 189, 194, 195
  neurosyphilis, 121, 130
  in prisoners, 321
  syphilis screening, 193, 402
  Treponema pallidum, 196
syringe exchange programs, 134, 322
  See also needles
systemic immunopathogenesis, 14
systemic viral pathogenesis, 13
Szasz, Thomas, 343

T

tadalafil, 159, 295
tardive dyskinesia, 124, 229, 270
tat gene, 11
Tat protein, 11, 15
TB. *See* tuberculosis
TCM. *See* Traditional Chinese Medicine
TCWG. *See* Tenderloin Collaborative Work Group
temazepam (Restoril), 143
  metabolism and drug interactions, 153
Tenderloin Collaborative Work Group (TCWG), 313–314
tenofovir, 28, 30
testing. *See* HIV testing; psychological and neuropsychological testing
testosterone
  deficiency, 204, 206
  mood disorders and, 96
Texas, 2005 class action lawsuit, 324
Therapeutic Touch, 365, 369, 370
thioridazine, for psychosis, 208
thrombocytopenia, 177, 273
"thrush". *See* oral candidiasis
thyroid deficiency, 204
Titicut Follies, 343
TNF-α. *See* tumor necrosis factor-alpha
tocainide, for pain, 178
tolerance, defined, 183
topiramate, 98
  drug interactions, 158
touch therapies, 369
Toxoplasma gondii, 25
toxoplasmosis, CNS, 20
  diagnosis, 202
  mood-disorder symptoms and, 94
  in prisoners, 321
  psychotic disorders and, 120, 121
Traditional Chinese Medicine (TCM), 365, 368
  treatment effectiveness studies, 373
Trail Making Test, 54
trait-dispositional personality model, 102
transference, 361–362
Transference-Focused Psychotherapy, 107–108
transmission, 16–18
  blood transfusion/exposure and, 18, 32
  female-to-female, case reports of, 299–300
  high-risk sexual behaviors, 17
  injection substance abuse and, 17
  occupational, 32–34, 209, 402
  situations posing no risk, 16–17

through medical care, 18, 32
transmission categories, 3–5
vertical transmission, 17–18, 115, 250–260, 400–401
virus entry into host cell, 12
trazodone
    for anxiety/insomnia in substance users, 132
    drug interactions, 157, 178
    for insomnia/sleep disorders, 84, 145
    for pain, 175
    toxicity, 157
treatment adherence. *See* adherence
treatment considerations, 77
    personality disorder, 105–109
    psychological reactions, 71–78
    stress/adjustment disorders, 83–84
    suicide risk assessment, 77
    See also medical treatment; *specific disorders*
treatment, medical. *See* medical treatment
Treponema pallidum, 196, 204
triazolam (Halcion), 143
    drug interactions, 151, 153
trichomoniasis, 188, 189, 191, 194
tricyclic antidepressants, 90, 95, 132
    for children, 265
    for pain, 174, 387
trimethoprim, 21, 25
    sulfamethoxazole/trimethoprim, 153
trimetrexate, 25
triple diagnosis, 127–129
    psychiatric treatment and, 131–133
tuberculosis
    extrapulmonary, 20
    in HIV-infected homeless people, 310
    Mycobacterium tuberculosis, 130
    prisons as reservoirs for, 321
    pulmonary, 24
tuberculous meningitis, and psychotic disorder, 121
tumor necrosis factor-alpha (TNF-α), 13, 15–16, 67
tumor necrosis factor-delta (TNF-δ), 67

U
unemployed individuals, 9

V
vaccinations
    for children with HIV, 254
    HAV and HBV, 24, 194
    for HIV prophylaxis, 24
valganciclovir, 26
valproate, 158
    for mania, 273
    for pain, 177
valproic acid, 97
    for mania, 207, 273
    side effects of, 273
vardenafil, 159, 295
venlafaxine
    for depression, 272
    metabolism and drug interactions, 157
ventricular enlargement, 14
ventrolateral preoptic nucleus (VLPO), 138
vertical transmission, 17–18, 115, 250–251, 260
    implications for prenatal care, 251
    implications for treatment at labor and delivery, 252–254
    National Perinatal HIV Consultation and Referral Service, 400–401
    prevention of, 251, 253–254
    risk of, 250
    types of, 250, 260
        perinatal, 250, 253, 279–280, 400–401
        postnatal (breast feeding), 250, 251, 256, 259, 280
        in utero, 250, 279
vif (virion infectivity factor) gene, 11
Vif protein, 11
vincristine, mental status changes and, 123
Vineland scale, 264
viral infections, 190–191
viral load, 13, 19
viral pathogenesis, systemic, 13
viral resistance, 20–21, 24, 31, 225, 280
viral set point, 19, 20
Viramune. *See* nevirapine
virology, 11–16
    See also HIV (human immunodeficiency virus)
visualization, 370, 373
vitamin C, 366, 368
    risks/warnings about, 375
vitamin supplements, 366, 368
    effectiveness studies, 371
VLPO. *See* ventrolateral preoptic nucleus
vomiting, 388–389
vpr (viral protein R) gene, 11

W
WAVE (Women, AIDS, and Violence Epidemic), 5
Wescler Intellectual Scales for Children, 264
white matter lesions, 15
WHO. *See* World Health Organization
WiLLOW program, 332
Wiseman, Frederick, 343
women
    abusive relationships and, 6, 281
    HIV/AIDS among, 7–8, 277–287, 282
        anxiety and, 281
        common manifestations, 279
        depression and, 5, 282
        epidemiology, 277–278
        HIV illness, 278–279
        injection drug-related transmission, 127
        pregnancy and contraception, 279–280
        prevention, 283–284
        proportion of AIDS cases, 4
        provider access, 283
        psychiatric complications, 281–282
        psychosocial factors, 282
        risk factors, 278
        sexuality and pregnancy, 279–280
        stigma and, 282
        suicide and, 282

women (*cont.*)
- transmission categories/rates, 4, 103–104, 233
- treatment, 282–283
- pain and, 163–164
- psychological reactions to antibody testing, 73–74
- sexually transmitted diseases and, 188–197
- stress and, 81
- WAVE (Women, AIDS, and Violence Epidemic), 5
- *See also* women who have sex with women; *special populations*

women who have sex with women (WSW), 299–307
- access to health care, 305–306
- coming out, 301–302
- incidence and risk factors for HIV/AIDS, 299–310
- myth of "lesbian immunity", 301
- psychiatric aspects of HIV in, 302–305
- sexual practices, 300
- *See also* homosexuality; lesbians; women

World Health Organization (WHO)
- guidelines on pain, 167
- position on compulsory HIV testing, 321

WSW. *See* women who have sex with women

Y

YMSM. *See* young men who have sex with men
yoga, 370
young men who have sex with men (YMSM), 290

Z

zalcitabine, 28, 30
zaleplon (Sonata), 144
Zamora, Pedro, 290
zidovudine (AZT), 28, 30
- drug interactions, 152
- for encephalopathy, 256
- for HAD, 275
- prenatal administration, 17–18, 28, 251, 253
- with valproic acid, 97

ziprasidone, 124, 125, 207
- drug interactions, 158

Zithromax. *See* azithromycin
zolpidem (Ambien), 144
- metabolism and drug interactions, 153

Zubrod Performance Scale, 56–57